Small Animal Emergency and Critical Care for Veterinary Technicians

Third edition

Andrea M. Battaglia, LVT

Section Supervisor, ICU/INC/ER
Cornell University Hospital for Animals
Cornell University
Ithaca, New York

Andrea M. Steele, MSc, RVT, VTS (ECC)

ICU Technician
Intensive Care Unit, Health Sciences Centre
Ontario Veterinary College
Guelph, Ontario, Canada

ELSEVIER

ELSEVIER

3251 Riverport Lane
St. Louis, Missouri 63043

SMALL ANIMAL EMERGENCY AND CRITICAL CARE FOR
VETERINARY TECHNICIANS, ED 3   ISBN: 978-0-323-22774-2

Previous editions copyrighted 2007, 2001

Library of Congress Cataloging-in-Publication Data
Small animal emergency and critical care for veterinary technicians /
[edited by] Andrea M. Battaglia, Andrea M. Steele. -- Third edition.
     p. ; cm.
  Preceded by Small animal emergency and critical care for veterinary
technicians / Andrea M. Battaglia. 2nd ed. c2007.
  Includes bibliographical references and index.
  ISBN 978-0-323-22774-2 (alk. paper)
  I. Battaglia, Andrea M., editor. II. Steele, Andrea M., editor. III.
Battaglia, Andrea M. Small animal emergency and critical care for veterinary
technicians. Preceded by (work):
  [DNLM: 1. Emergencies--veterinary--Handbooks. 2. Animal
Technicians--Handbooks. 3. Critical Care--Handbooks. SF 778]
  SF778
  636.089'6025--dc23   2015012799

Content Strategist: Shelly Stringer
Content Development Manager: Ellen Wurm-Cutter
Senior Content Development Specialist: Maria Broeker
Associate Content Developmental Specialist: Katie Gutierrez
Publishing Services Manager: Jeff Patterson
Project Manager: Jeanne Genz
Designer: Julia Dummit

Printed in U.S.A.

Last digit is the print number: 9   8   7   6   5   4   3   2

 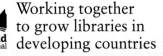

To the veterinary technicians who have dedicated their careers providing the best patient care possible to the emergent, critically ill or injured small animal patient. Saving lives is your specialty.

Contributors

Amy Breton, CVT, VTS (ECC)
Emergency Head Technician
Veterinary Emergency & Specialty Center
Waltham, Massachusetts

Daniel Chan, DVM, DACVECC, DECVECC, DACVN
Senior Lecturer in Emergency and Critical Care
Clinical Nutritionist
Department of Clinical Science and Services
The Royal Veterinary College
North Mymms, Hertfordshire, Great Britain

Jim Clark, DVM, MBA
Professor
U.C. Davis School of Veterinary Medicine
Davis, California
Founder and Co-Owner
Pet Emergency & Specialty Center
San Rafael, California

Jennifer Collins, RVT
Neurology Technician
Clinical Studies
University of Guelph
Guelph, Ontario, Canada

Harold Davis, BA, RVT, VTS (ECC) (Anesthesiology)
Manager
Small Animal Emergency & Critical Care Service
William R. Pritchard Veterinary Medical Teaching
   Hospital
University of California, Davis
Davis, California

Jessica Davis, BA, RVT, VTS (ECC)
MedVet Medical and Cancer Centers for Pets
Cincinnati, Ohio

Jennifer Devey, DVM, DACVECC
Emergency and Critical Care Consultant
Saanichton, British Columbia, Canada

Pam Dickens, CVT
Animal Care Center
New Port Richey, Florida

Charlotte Donohoe, BA, RVT, VTS (ECC)
Emergency Veterinary Referral Coordinator/Triage
Ontario Veterinary College
University of Guelph
Guelph, Ontario, Canada

Julie Hirsch-Fitzpatrick, AS, CVT, VTS (ECC)
Public Relations and Referral Specialist
Saint Francis Veterinary Center of South Jersey
Woolwich Township, NJ

Fiona James, DVM, MSc, DVSc, DACVIM (Neurology)
Assistant Professor
Department of Clinical Studies
Ontario Veterinary College
University of Guelph
Guelph, Ontario, Canada

Deborah Kingston, ACA, AHT, RVT
Specialty Technician
Department of Cardiology
Ontario Veterinary College
University of Guelph
Guelph, Ontario, Canada

Jody Nugent-Deal, RVT, VTS (Anesthesia) and (CP-Exotics)
Supervisor
Department of Small Animal Anesthesia
University of California Davis, Veterinary Medical
   Teaching Hospital
Davis, California

Louise O'Dwyer, MBA, BSc (Hons), VTS (Anesthesia, ECC), DipAVN (Medical & Surgical), RVN
Clinical Director
PetMedics Veterinary Hospital
Manchester, Greater Manchester, Great Britain

Angela Randels-Thorp, CVT, VTS (ECC, SAIM)
Veterinary Technician Manager
1st Pet Veterinary Centers
Chandler, Arizona

DeeDee Schumacher, CVT, VTS (ECC), MEd
Professor
Veterinary Technology
Des Moines Area Community College
Ankeny, Iowa

Nancy Shaffran, CVT, VTS (ECC)
Private Lecturer/Consultant
International Veterinary Academy of Pain
    Management: 2015-2017 President
Erwinna, Pennsylvania

Kenichiro Yagi, BS, RVT, VTS (ECC, SAIM)
Manager
Intensive Care Unit/Blood Bank
Adobe Animal Hospital
Los Altos, California

Preface

The *Small Animal Emergency and Critical Care for Veterinary Technicians* has evolved into this full color edition with other new features to assist the reader in caring for the critically ill or injured small animal patient.

Other new features of this edition include:

- Medical math challenges and scenario-based training exercises throughout the book and the accompanying Evolve website, to encourage the reader to practice what they are learning from the text.
- Technician notes highlighting important points and information that the author thinks crucial for best patient care practices.
- A chapter dedicated on how to achieve better communication. Excellent communication is essential in creating a cohesive team or positive client experience.
- New contributors with a variety of experience from private specialty practices, emergency clinics, and academia to provide updated information.

Small Animal Emergency and Critical Care for Veterinary Technicians provides a valuable resource for veterinary technicians and students interested in this specialized area. Oftentimes it is the veterinary technician who begins the life-saving procedures before the veterinarian on duty has a chance to join the team, making knowledge of these procedures paramount.

The book is divided into three sections. The first section focuses on the critically ill patient and therapies used to support these dynamic patients.

Chapters dedicated to emergency receiving, shock, cardiopulmonary resuscitation, and trauma introduce the second section. Each chapter details specific situations encountered in the emergency room. The type of emergency is defined and many life-saving procedures described.

The technician involved in emergency and critical care medicine is often required to work a variety of shifts and expected to handle client communications during very difficult times. The final section includes chapters focusing on how to be a healthy shift worker and how to improve communication skills.

We think you will find this resource useful in providing the best possible care for the critically ill or injured small animal. Emergency and critical care medicine is very dynamic, and veterinary technicians should continue their education on a daily basis through publications, continuing education seminars, and practical experience.

Thank you for your continued dedication and desire to provide the best possible care for your small animal patients.

Acknowledgments

I never imagined in 1997 when I signed the contract for the first edition, I would be involved with a third edition 17 years later.

First, I want to recognize all of you who have approached me over the years with kind words of appreciation for this work. You have been the catalyst for the third edition.

Shelly, Maria, Jeanne, and the many others on the Elsevier team who have been involved with making the third edition the best, thank you for all of your support and commitment to creating our visions into a reality.

It has been a great pleasure working with you, Andrea Steele; your contributions go far beyond the words on these pages.

To the many veterinary technicians I have worked with over the years; your dedication and commitment to making sure all the patients receive the best care possible is admirable. Countless numbers of time I have watched you work through your back pain, bite wounds, hunger, and sometimes tears to take care of just one more…and return the following day (or night) with a renewed sense of energy and passion. My respect for all of you is immeasurable.

And finally, to my greatest teachers and fans…Audrey, Hannah, Rhiana, Dave, Mom and Dad…your love, friendship, and support are never ending and I could not have done this without all of you.

Andrea M. Battaglia, LVT

I have been fortunate throughout my career as a Registered Veterinary Technician to meet the "right people at the right time." Starting way back in 1995, Dr. Kathy Hrinivich, a new graduate at the time, was very wise in pointing me in the right direction to help me choose veterinary technology as my career path. I will be forever grateful for her prompting! After graduation, Dr. Karol Mathews became my mentor in the ICU at the Ontario Veterinary College. Her influence on both my career as an ICU Technician and my work as a Technician Educator has been immense, and for that I want to thank her from the bottom of my heart. Both Harold Davis, BA, RVT, VTS (ECC, Anesthesiology), and Nancy Shaffran, CVT, VTS (ECC), have shaped my career as a Technician Educator in immeasurable ways, and have become my close friends over the years. They may not realize it, but they are my idols, and I want to be like them when I grow up. Finally, I want to thank Andrea Battaglia, LVT, who through a chance meeting at the International Veterinary Emergency and Critical Care Symposium just a few years ago, allowed me to become a co-editor of the next edition of her famous book. Andrea, thank you for taking a chance on me! For all my work colleagues at the Ontario Veterinary College, thank you for putting up with me…I know that this can be a challenge. ☺

Finally, my husband Mark and children Madi and Ethan have supported and encouraged me in everything I have done, and for that I will always be grateful. Taking risks has never been my strength, but they have encouraged me to step outside of my comfort zone.

Andrea M. Steele, MSc, RVT, VTS (ECC)

Contents

SECTION I: CRITICALLY ILL SMALL ANIMALS

1 Critical Thinking—Skill of Observation and Interpretation, 2
Andrea M. Battaglia
Defining Critical Thinking, 3
Discovering How Critical Thinking Impacts Decision-Making, 3
Developing Critical Thinking Skills, 4
Delivering Information Received, 5
Sustaining the Development and Use of Critical Thinking, 6

2 Monitoring of the Critically Ill or Injured Patient, 9
DeeDee Shumacher
Physical Examination, 13
Clinical Pathologic Monitoring, 14
Packed Cell Volume and Total Plasma Protein Measurements, 16
General Guidelines for Interpretation of Packed Cell Volume and Total Plasma Protein Measurements, 17
Hematologic Analysis, 17
Electrolyte and Chemistry Analyzers, 19
Urine Volume and Specific Gravity, 21
Blood Gas Analysis, 22
Colloid Osmotic Pressure, 25
Lactate Concentration, 27
Coagulation Tests, 28
Device-Based Monitoring, 30
Pulse Oximetry, 30
Blood Pressure, 32
Electrocardiogram Monitoring, 35
End-Tidal Carbon Dioxide Monitoring, 37
Central Venous Pressure, 39
Multiparameter Monitoring Equipment, 40

3 Patient's Lifeline: Intravenous Catheter, 43
Andrea M. Battaglia and Julie Hirsch-Fitzpatrick
Types of Intravenous Catheters, 44
The Anatomy of the Multi-Lumen Catheter Kit, 44
Choosing the Right Catheter, 45
Vascular Access Points, 46
Placement, 46
Prevention and Management of Complications During Placement, 53
Stabilization, 54
Intraosseous Catheterization, 56
Challenges, 57
Maintenance, 58

4 Fluid Therapy, 61
Charlotte Donohoe
Body Water, 62
Patient Assessment, 63
In-Hospital Monitoring of Fluid Therapy Patients, 66
Fluid Types, 69
Delivery Systems, 73
Complications of Fluid Therapy, 74

5 Transfusion Medicine, 78
Kenichiro Yagi
Whole Blood and Components, 79
Blood Sources, 83
Blood Collection, 90
Blood Administration, 96
Transfusion Reactions, 100
Alternate Transfusion Products and Methods, 102

6 Nutritional Support for the Critically Ill Patient, 106
Daniel L. Chan
Nutritional Assessment, 107
Goals of Nutritional Support, 107
Summary, 120
Products Listed, 120

7 Oxygen Therapy Techniques, 123
Andrea M. Steele
Definitions/Acronyms, 124
How to Assess the Need for Oxygen, 124
How to Assess Oxygen Levels, 124
How to Deliver Oxygen, 126
Oxygen Toxicity, 132
Conclusion, 132

8 Mechanical Ventilation, 135
Andrea M. Steele
Important Terms, 136
Indications for Mechanical Ventilation, 137
Mechanical Ventilation Strategies According to Disease Type, 138
Placing the Patient on the Ventilator, 138
Nursing Considerations for Long-Term Ventilator Patients, 140
Troubleshooting, 142
Weaning from the Ventilator, 143
Summary, 143

9 Pain Assessment and Treatment, 146
Nancy Shaffran
Physiology of Pain, 148
Assessment and Recognition, 148
Pain Relief, 149
Pure (Full) Agonists, 153
Mixed Agonist and Antagonist Opioids, 153
Antagonists, 154
Topical Analgesia, 154
Local Infiltration, 155
Alpha$_2$ Agonists, 155
Alpha$_2$ Antagonist Reversal, 156
Constant Rate Infusion (CRI), 156
Epidural Anesthesia and Analgesia, 160
Monitoring Drug Effects, 160
Pain Management Checklist, 160

10 Anesthesia in the Critically Ill or Injured Patient, 165
Jennifer J. Devey
Introduction, 166
Goals for Success, 166
Preanesthetic Stabilization, 168
Preanesthetic Preparedness, 169
Setting Up for Major Surgery, 170
Drugs, 170
Analgesics, Local Anesthetics, and Preanesthetic Agents, 171
Neuromuscular Blocking Agents, 176
Intubation, 177
Maintaining a Patient Under General Anesthesia, 178
Controlled Ventilation, 179
Monitoring, 179
Electrocardiography, 181
Pulse Oximetry, 181
Supportive Measures Needed During Anesthesia, 183
Anesthetic Emergencies and Complications, 184
Recovering the Patient, 188

11 Isolation Techniques in Clinical Practice, 191
Louise O'Dwyer
Infection Risks in Veterinary Clinics, 192
Infection Control Programs, 192
Isolation Protocols, 201
Isolation Facilities, 202

SECTION II: EMERGENCY CARE FOR SMALL ANIMALS

12 Emergency Receiving, 208
Andrea M. Battaglia
Preparation—The Readiness Assessment, 209
Facility, 210
Assessment of the Emergent Patient, 212

13 Management of Patients in Shock, 223
Harold Davis
Types of Shock, 224
Oxygen Delivery, 224
Pathophysiology of Shock, 224
Initial Assessment and Recognition, 226
Therapy, 228
Monitoring, 231
Summary, 232

14 Cardiopulmonary Resuscitation Current Practice, 234
Harold Davis
Preparation, 235
Recognition, 236
Phase One: Basic Life Support, 237
Phase Three: Post–Cardiac Arrest Care, 244
Summary, 245

15 Traumatic Emergencies, 247
Jennifer J. Devey
Introduction, 248
Readiness, 248
Patient Assessment, 253
Trauma Triad of Death, 256
Resuscitation, 256
Analgesia, 259
Wounds, Bandages, and Splints, 259
Surgical Resuscitation, 260

Basic Monitoring, 260
Advanced Monitoring, 261
Postresuscitation Care: The First 24 Hours, 262
Nutrition, 262
Communication, 263
Assessment and Management of Specific
   Injuries, 263
Conclusion, 267

16 Hematologic Emergencies, 269
Kenichiro Yagi
Hemostasis, 269
Clinical Assessment, 276
Anemia, 280

17 Cardiovascular Emergencies, 292
Deborah Ann Kingston
Diagnosis of Heart Disease, 293
Overview of Cardiac Physiology and
   Pathophysiology, 302
Heart Failure, 303
Identifying Patients Who May Have Heart
   Failure, 304
Monitoring Therapy for Heart Failure, 307
Cardiac Arrhythmias, 308
Heartworm Disease, 312
Cardiac Tamponade and Pericardial Effusion,
   314
Feline Aortic Thromboembolism, 315

18 Respiratory Emergencies, 319
Andrea M. Steele
Patient Presentation, 319
Be Prepared, 321
Obtaining Vascular Access, 322
Rapid Intubation Sequence, 322
Primary Survey and Minimum Database, 323
Secondary Survey, 323
Continued Management, 325
Common Respiratory Emergencies, 325
Traumatic Conditions, 325
Airway Disorders, 328
Pulmonary Edema, 329
Pneumonia, 329

19 Gastrointestinal Emergencies, 332
Jennifer J. Devey
Vomiting, 333
Diarrhea, 333
First Aid Measures, 333
Physical Examination, 334

Resuscitation of the Critical Patient, 335
Diagnosis, 336
Medical Treatment, 337
Monitoring, 340
Record Keeping, 340
Anesthesia and Surgery, 340
Postoperative Care, 341
Specific Gastrointestinal Emergencies, 342
Conclusion, 348

20 Metabolic and Endocrine Emergencies, 351
Angela Randels
Diabetic Ketoacidosis, 352
Hypoadrenocorticism (Acute Addisonian
   Crisis), 356
Case Study, 361
Hypercalcemia, 362
Hypocalcemia, 365
Hypoglycemia, 368

21 Urologic Emergencies, 373
Andrea M. Battaglia and Andrea M. Steele
Urinary Obstruction, 374
Kidney Disease, 383
Treatment of Acute Kidney Injury, 385
Treatment of Chronic Kidney Failure, 387
Conclusion, 389

22 Reproductive Emergencies, 391
Amy Breton
Four Phases of Ovarian Cycle, 391
Reproductive Emergencies in Females, 392
Reproductive Emergencies in Males, 400

23 Ocular Emergencies, 404
Pam Dickens
Globe, 407
Eyelid, 409
Cornea, 410
Anterior Chamber, 411
Lens, 411
Conclusion, 412

24 Neurologic Emergencies, 414
Fiona James and Jennifer Collins
Seizures, 415
Vestibular Disorders, 420
Spinal Cord Injury, 422
Peripheral Nervous System Emergencies, 426
Head Trauma, 427
Rabies, 429
Conclusion, 429

25 Toxicologic Emergencies, 431

Jessica D. Davis

Fundamentals of Treatment, 433

Decontamination: Prevention of Further
   Absorption, 433

Activated Charcoal, 436

Lipids, 436

Supportive Care, 437

Specific Types of Toxicities, 437

Environmental Toxins, 446

Pharmaceuticals, 447

Metals, 448

Toxicology in the Veterinary Hospital, 450

Conclusion, 450

26 Avian and Exotic Emergencies, 452

Jody Nugent-Deal

Hospital Preparedness, 453

Preparing for CPR for the Avian, Reptilian, and
   Small Animal Exotic Patient, 453

Avian Emergencies, 454

Exotic Small Mammal Emergencies, 465

Common Emergencies in Rabbits, 474

Common Emergencies in Rodents, 476

Reptile Emergencies, 476

27 Disaster Medicine, 488

Amy N. Breton

Legal Issues, 490

Types of Disasters, 490

Triaging, 492

Owner in the Disaster, 493

Self-Protection, 493

Common Emergencies, 494

Search and Rescue Canines, 495

Surgery, 498

Record Keeping, 498

Rechecking Appointments, 499

Helping the Local Veterinary Infrastructure, 499

Personal Recovery after the Disaster, 499

Structure of a Disaster, 500

Becoming Involved, 501

Joining a Team, 501

Disaster Training, 503

Conclusion, 504

SECTION III: PRACTICE MANAGEMENT

28 The Art of Scheduling, 508

Andrea M. Battaglia

Sleep Deprivation, 510

Creating the Optimal Shift for Employees, 510

Helpful Hints for Day Sleeping, 512

Working the Night Shift, 513

Conclusion, 513

29 Client Communication in an Emergency, 515

Jim Clark

Why Communication Matters, 515

Fielding Telephone Calls, 516

Initial Greeting of Clients, 517

Expressing Empathy, 517

Communicating Effectively with Emergency
   Clients, 517

Presenting Critical Care Estimates, 518

Exam Room Communication, 519

Presenting Estimates, 520

Discussing Euthanasia, 520

Communicating with Challenging Clients, 521

Communicating with Referral Practices, 521

Critically Ill Small Animals

This section introduces many technical skills needed to care for the critically ill small animal. Commonly used supportive therapies and procedures for maintaining the critically ill patient through anesthesia are included.

1 Critical Thinking—Skill of Observation and Interpretation

Andrea M. Battaglia

KEY TERMS

Communication
Compassion fatigue
Critical thinking
Moral distress
Shared mental model

CHAPTER OUTLINE

Defining Critical Thinking
Discovering How Critical Thinking
  Impacts Decision-Making
Developing Critical Thinking Skills

Delivering Information Received
Sustaining the Development and Use
  of Critical Thinking

LEARNING OBJECTIVES

After studying this chapter, you will be able to:
- Define critical thinking.
- Learn how to develop and use critical thinking skills.
- Maintain passion for learning and prevent burn out.

> *"No problem can withstand the assault of sustained thinking."*
>
> *Voltaire*

Veterinary emergency and critical care medicine continues to evolve, providing higher levels of care. Many 24-hour emergency and critical care facilities have been established throughout the country and many more are in various stages of planning and development. One must be able to interpret their observations correctly in order to provide immediate and appropriate care for the critically ill or injured patient. This is a skill set needed to be successful in this specialized area. (Figures 1-1 to 1-4). For example, a decreased response during a neurologic evaluation might indicate a need for change in the treatment plan to improve the patient's prognosis; a change in posture might indicate a need to implement a pain management program. Many options in the form of monitoring and diagnostic equipment are available to provide optimal patient care; however, these tools cannot replace a veterinary technician. In this technologic age, it must not be forgotten that the "hands on" skills of observing, interpreting, and monitoring are essential for providing excellent complete patient care.

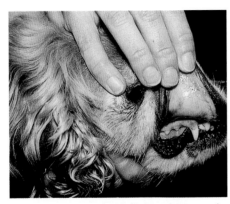

FIGURE 1-1 Icterus mucous membrane color in a cocker spaniel with liver disease.

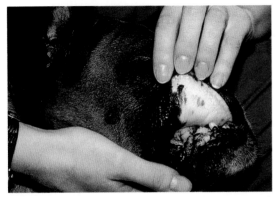

FIGURE 1-2 Pale mucous membrane color in a boxer with a packed cell volume of 13%.

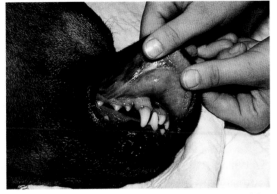

FIGURE 1-3 Brick red mucous membranes in a mixed breed with septic shock.

DEFINING CRITICAL THINKING

Critical thinking is a term commonly used to describe a skill necessary to be successful in the human nursing field and has been considered essential for more than 50 years. Many definitions have been created in attempts to capture the meaning of critical thinking.

Critical thinking refers to the ability to rationally make a decision regarding the patient on the basis of thorough consideration of data discovered through investigation, analysis, and evaluation. The American Philosophical Association (APA) defined critical thinking as purposeful, self-regulatory judgment that uses cognitive tools such as interpretation, analysis, evaluation, inference, and explanation of the evidential, conceptual, methodologic, criteriologic, or contextual considerations on which judgment is based. Applying critical thinking to everyday practice is imperative in order to provide excellent patient care (Figure 1-4).

DISCOVERING HOW CRITICAL THINKING IMPACTS DECISION-MAKING

The following eight elements of thought have been listed as the essential parts of critical thinking: information gathering, focusing, remembering, organizing, analyzing, generating, integrating, and evaluating. Knowledge, experience, problem-solving, and decision-making abilities are qualities one must have to be able to incorporate critical thinking independently and successfully.

Nursing care is an action that will lead to results. It is never a thoughtless, insignificant act and the veterinary technician must apply a multidimensional approach in order to proceed with the right decision to provide the best patient care possible and prevent medical errors.

Treatment sheets are plans for patient care needs during the course of a day that should be shared with the medical care team. It is important to always think outside of the written orders and to always remember to treat the patient, not just complete a sheet or request. Patient care needs can develop over the course of hospitalization. For example, the large, recumbent patient too weak to move may develop decubital sores if not assisted to move or provided adequate padding. A slight change in a respiratory pattern may indicate the need for oxygen therapy.

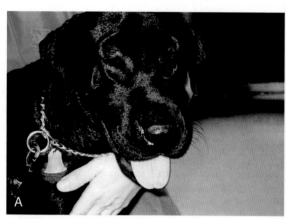
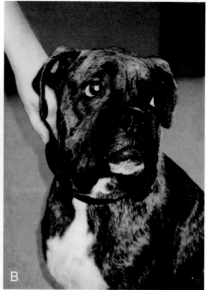

FIGURE 1-4 The Labrador puppy **(A)** and boxer **(B)** are experiencing an anaphylactic reaction. Both had severe facial swelling and showed signs of respiratory difficulty as the condition progressed. Because of breed conformation, assessment was more difficult in the boxer than in the Labrador puppy; however, because of the history of recent vaccinations and observations of hives on other areas of the body, a diagnosis could be made and treatment initiated.

DEVELOPING CRITICAL THINKING SKILLS

The hospital environment needs to foster critical thinking by respecting all members of the team as an integral part of the patient's healthcare. A **shared mental model** must be part of the hospital culture to be successful. This is accomplished through effective **communication,** collaboration, appropriate staffing and delegation, recognition, and leadership. A culture of safety is also important—a culture in which team members can perform their duties knowing errors will be addressed respectfully and placing blame is not the focus. Providing patient safety and creating better systems to prevent errors is the primary goal.

The veterinary technician new to the profession can continue to develop his or her critical thinking skills by practicing how to gather information through investigation when a patient's status changes or is admitted into the hospital. Being involved with implementation of a treatment plan, after the medical team has decided the best approach, assists in developing an understanding of the systematic approach needed.

Appropriate staff is essential to be able to provide excellent nursing care. Time is needed to be able to transfer and receive information about individual patients.

Ask the following questions when introduced to a patient:

1. What is the reason for the patient being hospitalized?
2. What is the current status of the patient?
3. Are other chronic conditions (e.g., seizures, diabetes mellitus) present?
4. Should additional procedures or diagnostic tests be scheduled?
5. What is the plan of treatment, including types of medication prescribed and reasons the specific medication has been selected? *(Investigate if there are any questions about the medication being administered, including mode of action, dose, and route of administration.)*
6. What is the patient's response to treatment?
7. What pain management techniques should be prescribed and why are these techniques selected?
8. Are successful handling techniques being used? *(If techniques are aggressive, ensure appropriate actions have been taken to limit harm to staff and patient.)*
9. What is the patient's response when receiving treatment?
10. Have the patient's nutritional requirements been achieved?

Evaluate the following observations:

1. Consideration of any breed predispositions (e.g., von Willebrand's disease for a Doberman or airway disease in a brachiocephalic breed)
2. The current position of the patient (e.g., Is the patient comfortable?)
3. Respiratory pattern and/or rate
4. Response of the patient when approached
5. Proper functioning of indwelling tubes, including intravenous (IV) catheters, urinary catheters, feeding tubes, abdominal or chest drains; and evaluation of site(s) of insertion
6. The presence of a specific unidentified nursing care that should be implemented
7. The unique nursing contribution that could provide additional benefit to this patient

Concept mapping has been another tool used to help develop critical thinking skills. It involves using key concepts and determining how they relate to one another. This exercises the right side of the brain, also known to be the creative hemisphere. It is important for the productive and analytic phases of creative thinking.

Tanner's clinical judgment model is a rubric based on four concepts: noticing, interpretation, responding, and reflection.

- *Noticing* is the first step in beginning the process. This involves recognizing an observation or information that deviates from what is considered normal.
- *Interpretation* is successful when there is an understanding of what is normal and expected. Once interpretation of the observation occurs and the appropriate response is defined, prioritization of the data received and development of a plan are initiated.
- *Responding* appropriately involves many soft skills including the ability to display confidence and leadership and to communicate clearly and efficiently. The patient's needs and response to treatment are considered and the responder must have excellent technical skills.
- *Reflection* is a transparent process. An evaluation of the decisions made, the institution of the plan, and the general technical performance occur. Reviewing patient response is included. The goal is to always consider methods that improve nursing care (Figure 1-5).

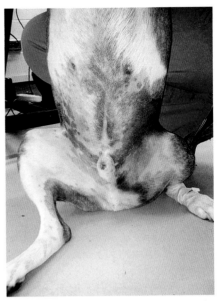

FIGURE 1-5 A 2-year-old hound mix presented with vomiting, lethargy, and anorexia. Based on the owner's history including ingestion of a child's toy and garbage by the dog, a foreign body was assumed the primary concern. Further evaluation of the patient included observations of bruising on the ventral abdomen. It was determined further diagnostics were necessary to correctly diagnose and treat the patient.

DELIVERING INFORMATION RECEIVED

Communicating the information received through observation, verbal requests, or written instructions is also an important part of nursing care. The Joint Commission (TJC) analysis of sentinel events revealed failure in communication was the most frequent problem cited in most of the events. Another study in the *Journal of the American Medical Association (JAMA) of Internal Medicine* disclosed that 200 errors were made in the wrong diagnosis and treatment of a patient attributable to communication failures between the patient and doctor. TeamSTEPPS® is an open source program developed by the Department of Defense's Patient Safety Program in collaboration with the Agency of Healthcare Research & Quality (AHRQ) program. The goal is to provide **S**trategies and **T**ools to **E**nhance **P**erformance and **P**atient **S**afety. Part of the program involves the implementation of systems to avoid communication breakdowns that result in errors. Acronyms have been created to be introduced to all members of the healthcare team so that all healthcare members have a clear understanding of how information should be delivered.

BOX 1-1 | Example of an SBAR

Scenario
Dr. Smith is at the scrub sink preparing for surgery. One of the in-house patients is displaying concerning behavior and the veterinary technician responsible for patient care needs to update the veterinarian.
   Critical care technician (CCT) presenting an SBAR

Situation (S)
"Dr. Smith, *Jerry Klein*, the coonhound in cage 9 who had surgery for a gastric dilation volvulus last night, is increasingly anxious and is beginning to vocalize and chew the bars on the cage."

Background (B)
We have taken him for a walk and the owner stated he has separation anxiety.

Assessment (A)
He does not appear painful (lying down comfortably and temperature, pulse, respirations [TPRs] within normal limits) and has responded well to the fentanyl continuous rate infusion (CRI).

Recommendation (R)
I would like to give him trazodone for his anxiety.

BOX 1-2 | Example of the I-PASS

Scenario
The day shift technician is introducing the first patient to the evening shift technician.
I—Felix is a 5-year-old male castrated cat who presented with a urinary blockage at 9 AM.
P—Bladder was large and firm and all blood work was normal. Urinary catheter was passed with a small amount of resistance. No history of urinary blockage. No complications under anesthesia.
A—We will continue IV fluid therapy and monitor urine output, antibiotics, and pain management through the night.
S—Use caution when handling. Felix became fractious after recovery. Owner had warned us that he can be challenging when feeling well. We will be removing urinary catheter in the morning and observing if Felix urinates during the day. Hope to send home tomorrow evening.
S—Night tech: I understand we will be monitoring urine output through the night and maintain the IV fluid therapy, pain management, and antibiotics. Use caution when handling; goal is to send home tomorrow evening. When will we begin to feed Felix?

The SBAR (**S**, situation; **B**, background; **A**, assessment; **R**, recommendation) is a quick and concise method that can be adopted by the hospital for consistency in how to provide information about a patient (Box 1-1).

Once the critically ill or injured patient is hospitalized, the assessments of the patient's condition will continue to occur throughout the day. The transfer of the patient between shifts is important and a common source of error if communication is not clear on the patient treatment orders, updates, and status.

I-PASS (**I**ntroduction, **P**atient summary, **A**ction list, **S**ituation awareness/contingency planning, **S**ynthesis by receiver) is a method that has been proven to be successful in improving the way in which information is delivered and received (Box 1-2).

The acronyms implemented by the hospital can also be shared with the clients. This will help develop a shared mental model throughout the entire healthcare team, which should include the owner of the pet.

The veterinary technicians will need to communicate patient care needs, results of diagnostics, and many other details throughout their shifts. It is important to also follow through with written communication that will serve as part of the legal medical record. Highlighting important changes that may have occurred, clinician's requests, observations, and procedures that have been performed are details that are included within the treatment sheet. This also assists in ensuring information is received accurately.

SUSTAINING THE DEVELOPMENT AND USE OF CRITICAL THINKING

Compassion fatigue and **moral distress** are common terms describing conditions that ultimately can lead to poor performance and burn out. This occurs in many healthcare professions and has been noted as the cost for caring.

Compassion fatigue has been defined as deep physical, emotional, and spiritual exhaustion; it develops from the repeated exposure, for extended periods of time, to suffering and death and also from the continuous support of people who are experiencing intense emotions.

Moral distress occurs when one is aware of the appropriate ethical action to take but is unable or forced to take action contrary to personal and professional values.

As members of the veterinary healthcare team caring for animals that are critically ill or injured, we will face situations that could lead to feelings of helplessness and frustration. It is important to establish an environment where all members of the team are encouraged to take regular breaks and incorporate care for the caregivers.

Warning signs of compassion fatigue include the following:

- Avoidance behaviors
- Emotional numbness
- Anxiety/stress
- Loss of sense of humor
- Sleep disturbance
- Eating disorders
- Irritability
- Over-reactive behavior
- Poor attendance
- Loss of confidence in abilities
- Self-medication with drugs or alcohol

> *TECHNICIAN NOTE* It is important to note the signs and begin the healing.

The first step is awareness; then incorporating the following will help:

- Accept that you can be negatively impacted by the trauma of caring for others.
- Find allies.
- Prioritize self-care and practice relaxation techniques.

The veterinary technicians involved with caring for our critically ill and injured patients need to make caring for themselves a priority. Wellness is one of the components to being successful. Without a state of well-being it will be very difficult to incorporate critical thinking daily. When we are exhausted and feeling frustrated, we tend to use our limited energy to complete the minimal requirements. Following an order as it is written without thinking about why we are to use the specific approach and if we can improve upon the care begins to occur. This will result in a lack of job satisfaction and ultimately burn out.

As stated by Jack Kornfield, a Buddhist monk, "If your compassion does not include yourself, it is incomplete."

Veterinary technicians can help to create an optimal emergency and critical care center by always having the desire to improve how they observe, evaluate, and deliver patient care. To accomplish this goal, they must educate themselves, learn new skills, and share new information they have obtained through continuing education and experience with the entire staff. Maintaining good communication skills (verbal and written) is essential for establishing a solid foundation to accomplish the main goal—providing the best nursing and medical care for the critically ill or injured small animal patient.

SUGGESTED READINGS

Alfaro-LeFevre R: *Critical thinking, clinical reasoning and clinical judgment: a practical approach*, ed 5, St Louis, 2013, Elsevier.

Benner P, Hughes RG, Sutphen M: Clinical reasoning, decision making and action: thinking critically and clinically. In Hughes RG, editor: *Patient safety and quality. An evidence based handbook for nurses, Healthcare Res Qual*, April 2008, pp 87–109.

Brown MN, Keeley SM: *Asking the right questions: a guide to critical thinking*, ed 10, Saddle River, NJ, 2012, Pearson Education.

Condon BB: Thinking unleashed, *Nurs Sci Quart* 25(3):225–230, June 2012.

Critical Thinking Website: *Learning the art of critical thinking*. Available at www.critcal thinking.org/pages/becoming-a-critic-of-your-thinking/html.

Figley CR, Roop RG: *Compassion fatigue in the animal care community*, Washington, DC, 2006, Humane Society Press.

Gerdman JL, Lux K, Jacko J: Using concept mapping to build clinical judgment skills, *Nurs Educ Pract* 13:11–17, May 2013.

Moorman DW: Communication, teams and medical mistakes, *Ann Surg* 245(2):173–175, Feb 2007.

Scheffer BK, Rubenfeld MG: A consensus statement on critical thinking in nursing, *J Nurs Educ* 39(8):352–359, Nov 2000.

TeamSTEPPS program. Available at www.teamstepps.ahrq.gov.

The 4As to rise above moral distress: *American Association of Critical Care Nurses*: Aug 2008. Available at www.aacn.org.

SCENARIO

Purpose: To provide the veterinary technician an opportunity to determine the most efficient way to communicate concerns.

Stage: Level III emergency and critical care facility. Overnight shift.

Scenario

Patient 1: It is 11:00 PM and one of the patients is exhibiting behavior that is concerning. It is a 7-year-old German shepherd that arrived in critical condition with a hemoabdomen around 9:00 PM. Initial diagnostics including radiographs revealed a splenic mass. It appeared on the chest radiographs as no metastasis and the owners decided to proceed with treatment. Removal of the splenic mass was performed by the surgeon on call. The surgery went well and the mass was removed without incident. The recovery was uneventful. A transfusion was given and the dog is currently on fluid therapy, pain management, and antibiotics. The dog is now exhibiting signs of discomfort including restlessness and an inability to relax. Heart rate is 156 beats/minute and pulses fair. Temperature 100° F and respiratory rate pant. Mucous membranes pale pink. The veterinarian in house is admitting other patients and unable to address concerns. They asked for you to contact the surgeon on call.

Questions

- Would you consider obtaining other information before contacting the surgeon on call?
- Are there any other observations needed before determining the appropriate response?
- How would you choose to present the information?

Patient 2: It is 1:00 AM. An 18-week-old Rottweiler puppy arrives because owners stated the puppy was lethargic and vomited. The puppy had been sent home 12 hours earlier from the referring veterinarian because fluid therapy and antiemetics had improved condition. It was assumed the puppy had ingested something and had a mild gastritis. Nothing abnormal was revealed on the initial blood work, radiographs, or ultrasound performed at the referral hospital. The owners provided a complete vaccination history on the initial exam.

You note after taking the temperature that there is a small amount of dark stool on the thermometer. The temperature is 102.5° F, heart rate 130 beats/minute, respiratory rate 30 breaths/minute. Mucous membrane pink and tacky. Puppy is responsive but quiet.

Discussion

- Would you consider obtaining any more information from the owners?
- What other diagnostics would you need to prepare a plan?
- How would you present information to the attending veterinarian?

Discussion

Patient 1

- Would you consider obtaining other information before contacting surgeon on call?
- Yes. Quick assessment tests including PCV, TS, BG, AZO.
- Are there any other observations needed before determining appropriate response?
- Yes. Review the treatment sheet and note if the patient had urinated postoperatively. In this case, the patient had not, and when walked urinated large amounts. Post walk, the patient rested comfortable through the rest of the night.
- How would you choose to present information?
- If walk had not resolved anxiety and discomfort, the SBAR would have been used to present to veterinarian over the phone.

Patient 2

- Would you consider obtaining any more information from the owners?
- Yes. Review of vaccination history and travel history. When asked for specifics it was discovered the vaccines had been given by breeder and last one received at 14 weeks of age. Puppy had been to obedience and agility classes.
- What other diagnostics would you need to prepare a plan?
- Yes. Would consider suggesting a test for the parvo virus.
- How would you present information to the attending veterinarian?
- Would present the findings in a SBAR format and include in the response reasons for wanting to perform a parvo test before moving puppy out of exam room.

2 Monitoring of the Critically Ill or Injured Patient

DeeDee Shumacher

CHAPTER OUTLINE

Physical Examination
Clinical Pathologic Monitoring
Packed Cell Volume and Total
  Plasma Protein Measurements
General Guidelines for Interpretation
  of Packed Cell Volume and Total
  Plasma Protein Measurements
Hematologic Analysis
Electrolyte and Chemistry Analyzers
Urine Volume and Specific Gravity
Blood Gas Analysis

Colloid Osmotic Pressure
Lactate Concentration
Coagulation Tests
Device-Based Monitoring
Pulse Oximetry
Blood Pressure
Electrocardiogram Monitoring
End-Tidal Carbon Dioxide Monitoring
Central Venous Pressure
Multiparameter Monitoring
  Equipment

KEY TERMS

Auscultation
Azotemia
Capnography
Central venous pressure
Chemosis
Coagulation
Colloid osmotic pressure
Ecchymosis
Electrocardiogram
End-tidal volume
Hemolysis
Iatrogenic
Icterus
Lactate
Lipemia
Oscillometric
Palpation
Petechia
Polyuria
Postrenal oliguria
Prerenal oliguria
Primary hemostasis
Pulse oximetry
Renal oliguria
Secondary hemostasis
Third-space losses

LEARNING OBJECTIVES

After studying this chapter, you will be able to:

- Describe the three main types of monitoring utilized in an emergency and critical care setting.
- Explain the importance of complete and accurate record keeping.
- Understand the importance of a complete physical examination and its correct interpretation.
- Understand the importance of proper sample collection.
- Describe, perform, and interpret common clinical pathologic tests.
- Understand the merits and limitations of device-based monitoring.
- Interpret the results of device-based monitoring.
- Integrate monitoring devices with other monitoring techniques to improve patient care.

Accurate and continuous monitoring is essential for the care of critically ill and injured animals. There are three main categories of monitoring, including physical hands-on examination, clinical pathologic monitoring, and device-based monitoring. Each piece of information obtained through the utilization of all types of monitoring will provide the necessary information to determine how the patient is responding to therapy. Documentation of all diagnostic results and exam findings is also an essential part of complete patient care. Without standardized record keeping, monitoring is not useful for patient care and can lead to erroneous conclusions. Records for critical patients can be in the form of a table, flow sheet, or dot plot form (Figure 2-1).

IVRC
IOWA VETERINARY
REFERRAL CENTER

24-HOUR ORDERS

M T W TH F ST SN

Date_____ Day #_____

Service_____ am DVM_____ pm DVM_____

PROBLEMS

	Today	lb		1st Shift		2nd and 3rd shift	
B		kg					
W	Yesterday	lb		Tech services		Tech services	
		kg		1 2 3		1 2 3	

Discharged by: Tech_____Time_____Page #_____

#	MEDICATIONS	FREQ	6	7	8	9	10	11	N	1	2	3	4	5	6	7	8	9	10	11	M	1	2	3	4	5
M1																										
M2																										
M3																										
M4																										
M5																										
M6																										
M7																										
M8																										
M9																										
M10																										
M11																										
M12																										
M13																										
M14																										
#	EXERCISE/FOOD/WATER	FREQ	6	7	8	9	10	11	N	1	2	3	4	5	6	7	8	9	10	11	M	1	2	3	4	5
E1	Outside Walk/Sling/Carry																									
E2	Water																									
E3	Food/type: Amt:																									
E4	Food comsumption																									
E5	Special instuctions																									
E6																										
#	LAB/RADIOLOGY	FREQ	6	7	8	9	10	11	N	1	2	3	4	5	6	7	8	9	10	11	M	1	2	3	4	5
L1																										
L2																										
L3																										
L4																										
L5																										
#	FLUIDS AND ADDITIVES	FREQ	6	7	8	9	10	11	N	1	2	3	4	5	6	7	8	9	10	11	M	1	2	3	4	5
F1																										
F2																										
F3																										
F4																										
F5																										
F6																										
F7																										
F8																										

FIGURE 2-1 A record for a critical patient. (Courtesy of Iowa Veterinary Referral Center.)

#	LAB/RADIOLOGY	FREQ	6	7	8	9	10	11	N	1	2	3	4	5	6	7	8	9	10	11	M	1	2	3	4	5
L1																										
L2																										
L3																										
L4																										
L5																										
#	VITALS AND MEDICAL ORDERS	FREQ	6	7	8	9	10	11	N	1	2	3	4	5	6	7	8	9	10	11	M	1	2	3	4	5
V1	Temp/Pulse/Respiratory rate																									
V2	MM/CRT/LOC																									
V3	Pulse strength (0 to 3)																									
V4	Blood pressure																									
V5	Pain score (0 to 5)																									
V6	Note V/D/U																									
V7	Weight																									
V8																										
V9																										
V10																										
V11																										
V12																										
V13																										
V14																										
V15																										
V16																										
V17																										
V18																										
V19																										
V20																										
V21																										
V22																										
V23																										
V24																										
V25																										
V26																										
V27																										
V28																										
V29																										
V30																										
V31																										
V32																										
V33																										
V34																										
V35																										
V36																										
V37																										
V38																										
V39																										
V40																										

FIGURE 2-1 cont'd A record for a critical patient.

Continued

Catheter/Tube	Site	Date placed	Day #

DEFAULT ORDERS: q2h; Record fluids q6h; mm CRT, Pulses, LOC, Note V-D-U-BM-food-water, flush catherters q12h; TPR, q24h, Weigh
Alarm; RR<18 or >40, HR <72 or >150 (D), 180 (C), BP<80 or >150, I<99 or >104 Pulse strength; 0 = absent, 1 = weak, 2 = normal, 3 = strong

FLUIDS FLOW CHART

Fluids:

Time	Amt	Total	Amt	Total	Amt	Total	Amt	Total	Amt	Total	Amt	Total	Amt	Total
24-hr Total														

VITAL SIGNS FLOW CHART

Time	T	P	R	mm	CRT	LOC	Ur/Fec	V/D	Pulse	Pain	PCV	TS	BP	Glu	Lac

Technicians and Assistants	Shift	Technicians and Assistants	Shift

Time	Treatments and Observations

FIGURE 2-1 cont'd A record for a critical patient.

The following should be included on the form: a space to record the time when the monitoring was completed, the monitoring values, and the name or initials of the person who completed the monitoring. The ideal form should also include an area where tech notes can be documented. These notes include anything performed by the team or caused by the patient to allow for consistency in communication during patient hand-offs. Only professional medical terminology is used when writing on the form because this is considered a legal document and part of the medical record.

> **TECHNICIAN NOTE** Consistency between shifts can also be maintained by completing rounds and discussing each patient with the oncoming shift. It is also important to remember that individual results obtained while monitoring a patient are important, but equally important is the ability for trends to be noticed at a glance.

PHYSICAL EXAMINATION

The importance of a thorough physical examination cannot be overstated. Technicians are an integral part of the patient's complete healthcare team. A technician's observations and serial physical exam findings are crucial for successful outcomes. Hands-on monitoring provides essential information about a patient and cannot be replaced by high-tech equipment. The physical examination includes patient observations, palpation, auscultation, and temperature.

Important observations include, but are not limited to, a patient's respiratory rate, depth, effort, and pattern; a patient's perceived level of pain; a patient's mental status; a patient's ins (intake, such as fluid therapy or oral intake) and outs (output, such as production of stool, urine, vomit, saliva); mucous membrane color; capillary refill time; level of mobility; and the patient's overall condition (Figures 2-2 through 2-4).

> **TECHNICIAN NOTE** Acute pain scales have been developed and are widely available on-line to make assessing a patient's level of pain much less subjective and aid in consistency of pain control between shifts. See Chapter 9: Pain Assessment and Treatment.

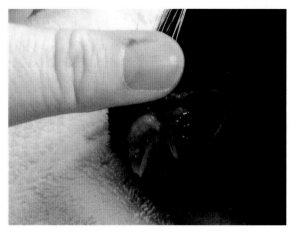

FIGURE 2-2 Pale mucous membranes.

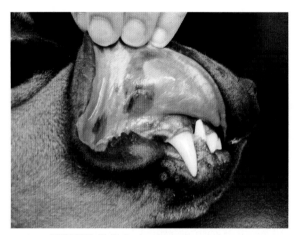

FIGURE 2-3 Brick red mucous membranes.

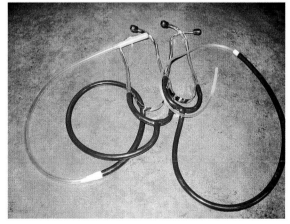

FIGURE 2-4 Esophageal stethoscopes.

Palpation is the process of using one's hands to assess a patient. The abdomen is an area that should be palpated on most patients. It is important to remember that too light a palpation can lead to missed findings and too aggressive a palpation can be uncomfortable or even harmful to the patient. Learning to correctly palpate each area of the patient is achieved by experience. Learning what feels normal on palpation will allow recognition of an abnormal finding when it is encountered.

Auscultation is the process of using a stethoscope to listen to the organs of the body. Most stethoscopes have a bell and a diaphragm.

> *TECHNICIAN NOTE* The bell of the stethoscope is used with light contact and allows low-frequency sounds to be heard and the diaphragm is used with firm contact and makes hearing higher frequency sounds easier.

Auscultation should always include multiple areas on both sides of the patient's body. The respiratory system and the gastrointestinal system are areas of the body that should be auscultated on most patients. It is important for the technician to become familiar with the stethoscope and listen to as many patients as possible to recognize the sounds of normal findings. This will make recognizing abnormal sounds much easier. Abnormal breathing patterns, abnormal sounds heard without a stethoscope, and coughing are indications for auscultation of the larynx and trachea, in addition to the lungs and heart. If gastrointestinal function is abnormal, a lack of gut sounds indicates the possibility of ileus. An esophageal stethoscope is a useful tool in the anesthetized patient or a patient that is on long-term ventilator use (Figure 2-5). It allows clear auscultation of the lungs and heart and may allow early detection of abnormalities such as pulmonary crackles or heart murmurs.

An elevated temperature may indicate infection, hyperthermia, or inflammation. A low temperature may indicate environmental hypothermia, poor perfusion, or a decreased metabolic rate secondary to medications (e.g., opioids) or disease (e.g., hypoglycemia, hypothyroidism). Metabolic rates are associated with temperature; therefore it is important to closely monitor a patient's temperature. This can be especially important in shock states or in anesthetized patients in whom vital organ systems such as cardiac function and coagulation can be adversely affected by hypothermia.

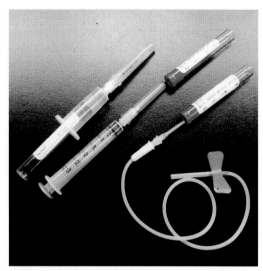

FIGURE 2-5 Blood collection systems. *(Top)* Vacutainer, *(middle)* syringe and needle; *(bottom)* butterfly catheter with needle adapter.

Continuous temperature monitoring, using esophageal or rectal probes, should be performed on anesthetized patients. Serial temperatures can also be taken using aural, axillary, or rectal thermometers. Ear infections, long ear canals, and environmental temperature can reduce the accuracy of aural thermometer readings. Rectal temperature may not reflect core temperature in poorly perfusing animals or those with stool in their colon. Axillary temperatures should be used with caution, especially with the newer 10-second thermometers available. Often the thermometer must be allowed to cycle until the temperature stabilizes.

> *TECHNICIAN NOTE* It should always be noted on the monitoring form how the patient's temperature was taken so the patient can continue to be monitored with the same method to obtain accurate trends.

CLINICAL PATHOLOGIC MONITORING

Reliable test results are only possible if samples are collected properly. Before a sample is collected a laboratory reference should be consulted to ensure proper container and sample handling techniques are utilized. Critical care patients frequently need serial blood samples drawn. It is important (especially in small, neonate, or anemic patients) to draw no more than 10% of the patient's total blood volume per week (Casal et al, 2014).

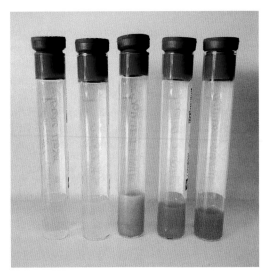

FIGURE 2-6 Varying degrees of hemolysis and lipemia in serum. *(Left)* Normal serum to *(right)* severely hemolyzed and lipemic serum.

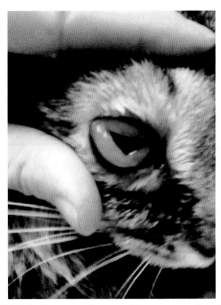

FIGURE 2-7 Severe chemosis. (Photo courtesy Kelsy Brue.)

> **TECHNICIAN NOTE** A chart kept with the patient that lists the amount of each blood sample collected can make it easier to monitor the total volume collected per week.

Long, large-bore catheters placed in central veins (e.g., jugular, medial or lateral saphenous) can provide the technician with a reliable sampling port. These central lines can be maintained for many days or indefinitely, depending on the type of catheter. Obtaining blood samples from a central line is often less stressful and more comfortable for the patient and also avoids the possible complications associated with multiple venipunctures. Use of the largest needle possible and proper aspiration of the syringe will help to minimize hemolysis. Use of Vacutainer needles and Vacutainer butterfly collection systems also helps to minimize hemolysis and premature activation of blood clotting (Figure 2-6). Sampling from a central line involves a three-syringe technique (two syringes containing saline flush and one sample syringe). Ensure that the amount of flush used, especially in the small patient, is not excessive, and always monitor blood volumes as mentioned previously.

Specific tests have exact requirements for sample handling and collection tubes and these protocols must be followed. For example, if collection tubes are not properly filled using their vacuum suction and too little blood mixes with the anticoagulant, then the sample will be diluted and the lab tests will provide erroneous results. Likewise, if too much blood is added to a sample tube with anticoagulant, the ratio will be incorrect and the blood may clot. Once a sample is placed in a tube it should be gently inverted 10 times to mix with the anticoagulant.

When a sample is being centrifuged, always balance the centrifuge to prevent uneven wear on the motor. The correct centrifuge speed should be used depending on the sample being processed. Serum and plasma must be removed from red blood cells immediately after centrifugation. If the serum or plasma is left to sit on the red blood cells, many lab results can be adversely affected. For example, if plasma remains in contact with red blood cells the cells continue to metabolize glucose at a rate of approximately 5% to 10% per hour, which will result in an erroneous glucose level measurement (Stockham et al, 2004). Blood samples should be run in a timely manner to avoid postcollection changes in values that will cause confusion when the results are being interpreted.

Serum or plasma color and clarity should always be evaluated and the results recorded in the patient record. This information can give important clues about the patient's disease process. Normal serum is clear and colorless (Figure 2-7). Common changes in serum color and clarity include the following:

- **Lipemia** (white, turbid)—Lipemic serum indicates high levels of fat in the blood and can occur if the animal has eaten recently. It can also be associated with various diseases such as acute pancreatitis, diabetes mellitus, hypothyroidism, and primary lipid disorders. The technician may need to repeat the test after withholding food for 12 hours (if appropriate).

> TECHNICIAN NOTE   Lipemic samples can also be refrigerated and recentrifuged at high speeds. This usually causes a fat layer to form at the top of the sample. The sample can then be aspirated from the tube and used. NOTE: Slight hemolysis often is noted in lipemic samples even if proper sample collection techniques are utilized.

- **Icterus** (yellow)—Icteric serum occurs most commonly in patients with liver disease or hemolytic anemia.
- **Hemolysis** (red)—Hemolyzed serum occurs usually as a result of poor sampling technique and handling; however, it can also indicate intravascular hemolysis associated with hemolytic anemia.

PACKED CELL VOLUME AND TOTAL PLASMA PROTEIN MEASUREMENTS

The packed cell volume (PCV) or hematocrit (HCT) and the total plasma protein (TP) measurements are important tools in the emergency and critical care patient. They are quick and simple to perform and provide a lot of information. The two tests should always be run together for more accurate interpretation of the patient's status.

INDICATIONS
Any hospitalized patient, especially those animals that may have the following:
- Dehydration
- Anemia
- Trauma
- Shock

EQUIPMENT
- Micro-HCT centrifuge
- Capillary tubes with or without anticoagulant, depending on the sample type
- Clay trays to seal the capillary tubes
- Card or slider tray tube reader to measure the PCV
- Refractometer to measure the TP

TECHNIQUE
Whole blood, either placed directly into anticoagulant-containing capillary tubes or removed from a properly filled EDTA (ethylenediaminetetraacetic acid) tube, or a heparinized syringe placed in a plain capillary tube may be used. Capillary tubes must be sealed with clay after the sample is inserted and before they are placed in the centrifuge. The clay end should face outward. At least two to three capillary tubes should be filled in case of breakage within the centrifuge.

After the sample has spun, three layers will be evident. The red cell column or PCV is closest to the clay. The buffy coat is a white or turbid layer just above the PCV and is composed of white cells and platelets. The third layer is the plasma protein layer.

Once the plasma is evaluated, the PCV is read using a micro-HCT tube reader—a slide rule used to estimate the PCV volume by measuring the percentage of total blood volume. The simplest type is a card with markings on it that are lined up with the red cell column to determine the PCV. In addition, wheeled micro-HCT readers are available in which the capillary tube is inserted in a groove and marked wheels are rotated under the sample to provide the PCV value. Both types have instructions on them. The buffy coat percentage also should be read and recorded.

A refractometer is a device used to determine the TP. The capillary tube is split above the buffy coat, and the plasma protein is blown onto the surface of the refractometer. The technician reads the refractometer by looking into the instrument at the column on the grid labeled *g/dl* (grams per deciliter). The line where the shaded area meets the light area is the TP. The refractometer should be calibrated regularly using distilled water, which has a specific gravity of 1.0.

Spun capillary tubes from each reading may be kept taped to a white piece of paper and labeled with patient information along with the date and time of collection. This provides a visual record of changes in the plasma protein color and clarity over time, which may provide valuable information on the patient's clinical course.

TROUBLESHOOTING
Erroneous readings can be made if the blood is clotted. Lipemia and hemolysis will falsely increase the TP measurement. Administration of Oxyglobin (OPK Biotech) hemoglobin (Hb) solution within 3 to 4 days will cause changes in the PCV that make it inaccurate.

The machine-calculated hematocrit (from a hematology analyzer) may be 1 to 3 points higher than a measured PCV from a spun micro-HCT tube as a result of trapping of plasma in the red cell column. Using proper centrifuge speeds and spinning the tube for at least 3 minutes will help minimize this artifact.

INTERPRETATION

Normal adult canine PCV is 37% to 55%, with lower values in puppies and higher values in sighthound breeds such as greyhounds. Normal adult feline PCV is 30% to 45%, also with lower values in young kittens. TP normal ranges are 5.4 to 7.5 g/dl in dogs and 5.7 to 7.6 g/dl in cats. These values also vary with age (Anthony et al, 2007).

Anemia is defined as a PCV measurement below the reference range. The PCV should always be interpreted along with the TP, because dehydration and splenic contraction (especially in dogs) affect the PCV. The TP can give important clues about whether dehydration or splenic contraction is affecting the PCV measurement. Dehydration will cause rises in the PCV because it is measured as a percentage of the blood volume. With dehydration, less water is found in the blood and the relative percentage of the PCV will increase without an actual increase in the red cell number. The TP value will also rise in this situation because relatively more proteins and less water are found in the plasma. Conversely, the PCV and TP values are good tools to gauge the effects of intravenous (IV) fluids and rehydration because they are expected to drop when diluted with IV fluids.

In dogs and cats, the spleen acts as a reservoir for red blood cells (RBCs) and can expand and contract. It will contract in response to exercise or blood loss and expand under the influence of sedation and anesthesia. This causes increases and decreases in the PCV, respectively, but does not change the TP measurement.

GENERAL GUIDELINES FOR INTERPRETATION OF PACKED CELL VOLUME AND TOTAL PLASMA PROTEIN MEASUREMENTS

- High PCV with the following:
  - Normal TP implies splenic contraction or breed-related high normal.

- Low TP implies protein loss or decreased RBC production with splenic contraction and dehydration (commonly seen in hemorrhagic gastroenteritis).
  - High TP implies dehydration.
- Low PCV with the following:
  - Normal TP implies anemia from erythrocyte destruction or decreased production.
  - Low TP implies blood loss or dilution from IV fluids (see Figure 2-7).
  - High TP implies protein overproduction with anemia as in bone marrow diseases or other chronic illnesses such as feline infectious peritonitis.
- Normal PCV with the following:
  - Low TP implies decreased protein production or increased loss from the gastrointestinal or urinary tract.
  - High TP implies dehydration with anemia or increased globulin production as in feline infectious peritonitis or other infectious diseases.

(NOTE: These guidelines only mention the most basic and common interpretations.)

> *TECHNICIAN NOTE* If abdominal or thoracic bleeding is suspected in a patient, a PCV measurement from a peripheral blood sample can be compared to the PCV measurement of blood from a thoracocentesis or abdominocentesis. If the PCV value of the centesis sample is comparable to that of the peripheral blood sample, an active bleed is indicated. If the peripheral blood sample value is considerably higher than that of the centesis sample, a previous bleeding episode is indicated.

HEMATOLOGIC ANALYSIS

Hematology analyzers provide complete blood counts, which typically include at least RBC, white blood cell (WBC), and platelet counts along with WBC differential counts and RBC indices (which are indicators of variations in size and color of RBCs that relate to RBC regeneration). A variety of automated veterinary specific hematology cell counters are available.

> *TECHNICIAN NOTE* It is important to remember that no machine can replace a manual blood smear examination. A blood smear is a very useful, inexpensive, and quick way to gain large amounts of information about a critical patient.

INDICATIONS

Most critical patients are likely to have problems that may cause complete blood count abnormalities. The following types of patients are particularly vulnerable:

- Patients with possible blood loss or anemia
- Patients with infectious or inflammatory conditions, such as fever and sepsis
- Patients with **petechiae** or **ecchymoses** suggesting platelet abnormalities (Figure 2-8)

EQUIPMENT

Point of care (POC) testing for hematology is available from multiple companies and is sometimes combined with chemistry analyzer functions. Most analyzers provide numeric results in addition to graphic results.

The equipment should be well researched before purchase, because each machine offers something different. Veterinary hematology analyzers are recommended over human analyzers because the variation in cell sizes can alter machine results significantly if they are not calibrated for that species.

The only equipment needed for a blood smear examination is a drop of fresh whole blood, microscope slides, standard Diff-Quik stains, immersion oil, and a microscope.

BLOOD SMEAR TECHNIQUE

Blood smear evaluation begins with a low-power scan of the smear to assess for platelet and RBC clumps and to determine whether WBCs are disproportionately clustered at the feathered edge (Figure 2-9). If agglutination is present, then a slide agglutination test using fresh whole blood or blood from an EDTA tube diluted 1:10 with saline on a slide should be performed. This will help the technician to distinguish between rouleaux formation and autoagglutination, which indicates an antibody attached to RBC membranes (characteristic of immune-mediated hemolytic anemia) (Figures 2-10 and 2-11).

At ×40 magnification, the smear should be examined at the monolayer where the cells are not touching

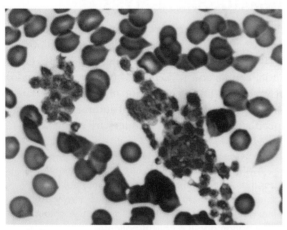

FIGURE 2-8 Petechia and ecchymosis on a dog's ventral abdomen. (Photo courtesy David Liss.)

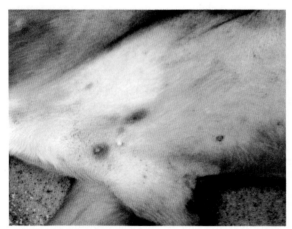

FIGURE 2-9 Severely clumped platelets on a blood smear.

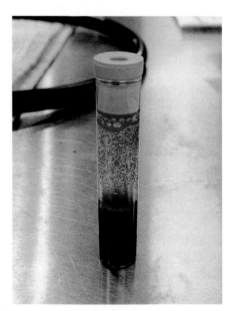

FIGURE 2-10 Autoagglutination in a purple top tube. (Photo courtesy Jamie Holms.)

each other. The technician should estimate the WBC count by multiplying the number of cells in one field by 1600. He or she should count several fields to ensure a representative sample. If the white cells are clustered at the feathered edge, then this estimate will be falsely lowered.

At ×100 magnification, the platelet count can be estimated by multiplying the number of platelets in a field by 15,000 (Cornell). RBC and WBC morphologic presentations should be evaluated at this field. Spherocytosis and inclusion bodies are some of the features that are important to notice.

For automated hematology analyzers, the technician should refer to specific instructions for specimen collection, handling, and processing. Most analyzers use blood collected into an EDTA (lavender top) tube that has been completely filled to ensure appropriate dilution of the blood in the anticoagulant.

TROUBLESHOOTING

Inappropriate smearing and staining can affect estimations of cell counts and morphologic abnormalities in blood smears. The blood must be evenly smeared in a monolayer, allowed to dry entirely, and stained within 2 hours of being smeared.

> *TECHNICIAN NOTE* When making a blood smear with anemic blood, the angle of the pusher slide should be increased. When making a blood smear with a very viscous sample, the angle of the pusher slide should be decreased.

Stains are affected by dilution from water, contamination, and exposure to formalin vapors. Stains should be discarded and changed regularly, as recommended by the manufacturer or a reference lab. Additionally, clumping of cells and counting from thick areas of the smear will cause errors in cell counts. If EDTA anticoagulated whole blood is used, then partially filled tubes will dilute the blood and cause erroneous cell counts.

> *TECHNICIAN NOTE* EDTA is the preferred anticoagulant for morphologic evaluation of cells. Heparinized samples can alter cell morphology and are not recommended.

INTERPRETATION

The technician should refer to a hematology atlas for pictures of cell morphologic changes that are significant in critical patients (e.g., spherocytes).

- Normal WBC counts in adult dogs are approximately 6000 to 17,000 cells per microliter of blood.
- Normal WBC counts in adult cats are approximately 5500 to 19,000 cells per microliter of blood.
- Normal platelet counts in adult dogs are approximately 160,000 to 430,000 cells per microliter of blood.
- Normal platelet counts in adult cats are approximately 300,000 to 800,000 cells per microliter of blood (Anthony et al, 2007).

The technician should refer to the reference lab used by the hospital or manufacturer of an automated hematology analyzer for specific reference ranges.

ELECTROLYTE AND CHEMISTRY ANALYZERS

Electrolyte and chemistry analyzers are now available as POC instruments that allow almost immediate results in a critical care setting. Rapid assessment of electrolyte levels and blood chemistries provides vital information that guides immediate therapy. The reference values for the individual machine should be used, because machines vary significantly and reference values for each machine are established separately. Reference values are readily accessible on most manufacturers' websites.

INDICATIONS

Many critical patients will benefit from POC testing of electrolytes and blood chemistry analysis.

Common emergencies that would cause electrolyte derangements include the following:

- Vomiting, diarrhea, or both
- Diabetes mellitus
- Urinary tract disease

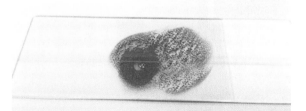

FIGURE 2-11 Positive slide agglutination test. (Photo courtesy Kenichiro Yagi.)

- Toxin ingestion
- Eclampsia

Patients with any potentially serious illness or trauma could benefit from blood chemistry testing to assess organ function.

EQUIPMENT

POC testing has become more affordable and common in veterinary practices. A variety of either portable or smaller bench-top instruments have been developed for veterinary practices. Many instruments that analyze electrolytes and some blood chemistry analyzers also can be used to perform blood gas analysis. Many analyzers allow the user to choose between performing individual tests and running complete panels. Performing complete panels is useful in making an initial diagnosis whereas running individual tests is very useful for rechecking values to determine how a patient is responding to therapy.

The main function of any critical care laboratory's electrolyte and chemistry analyzer is to provide rapid and accurate results at a reasonable cost. The buyer must take all of this into account before making a purchase. It is important to research not only the unit itself but also its associated costs such as reagents, standards, electrodes, annual maintenance, cleaning solutions, and conditioning solutions. Certain types of analyzers require more labor-intensive maintenance and may be more prone to technical difficulties. Consulting with current users of the same equipment may be helpful in the decision-making process. Internet message boards on sites such as the Veterinary Information Network have discussions on various pieces of POC equipment (Figure 2-12).

After the final decision is made regarding what type of analyzer to use, a technical manual should be acquired and read thoroughly. A maintenance protocol and cleaning schedule should be established. The staff should keep a technical support number close to the unit in plain view for unfamiliar users. All the unit's maintenance records must be kept, as well as detailed notes of technical support remedies to problems that arise, so that the next time the problem occurs it can be addressed more rapidly. When purchasing an analyzer, one should consider buying a yearly maintenance contract to ensure the analyzer can be repaired quickly if a major malfunction occurs. This purchase will increase the initial costs but will provide insurance for the times when the machine experiences problems and is unable to be repaired by the staff. Having a second, less

expensive, bedside analyzer for backup should also be a consideration.

Additional factors that influence the choice of analyzer include anticipated number of panels, the need for individual chemistries or full panels, reagent shelf life, and overall costs.

TECHNIQUE

The sample needed for most analyzers varies between individual machines; however, whole blood, serum, or plasma samples are common. Some analyzers allow testing of body fluids other than blood, which is useful in emergency or critical care settings. Good sample handling techniques are essential to avoid artifacts or damage to the analyzer.

TROUBLESHOOTING

As with all analyzers, it is optimal for the entire technical staff to be trained in the equipment's use. One or two well-trained technicians should be responsible for the day-to-day and general maintenance of the machine. Quality control (QC) for POC testing equipment (or any laboratory equipment) makes the difference between obtaining accurate or dangerously misleading, erroneous results. QCs should be run either according to a schedule or prior to a sample to ensure accuracy. Unexpected results, results that differ significantly from past data, or artifactual problems should prompt critical analysis of potential changes in the patient's condition. Each piece of equipment has its own list of sample factors that can interfere with the accuracy of results, and all staff members must be familiar with

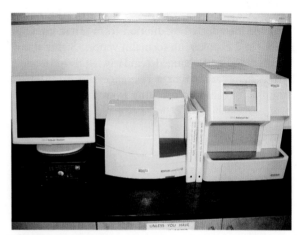

FIGURE 2-12 Idexx Laboratories in-house hematology and blood chemistry analyzers.

this list. For example, some analyzers will produce erroneous results if the sample is extremely lipemic.

INTERPRETATION

The goals of these blood tests are to provide a focal point for the organ system(s) that may be affected by the patient's disease process or injury and to monitor a patient's response to therapy. A general chemistry profile gives an indication of liver and kidney function, acid-base status, and plasma protein levels. Electrolyte values are run in conjunction with chemistry profiles and provide a more complete picture of a patient's condition. The technician should be familiar with life-threatening electrolyte abnormalities that require immediate attention. These include the following:

- Hyperkalemia, often seen with urethral obstruction, acute renal failure, or hypoadrenocorticism (Addison's disease)
- Hypocalcemia, often seen with eclampsia or hypoadrenocorticism
- Severe hypernatremia, often seen with nonketotic hyperosmolar diabetic crisis

The blood chemistry can also reveal life-threatening abnormalities that the technician should recognize. These include the following:

- Hypoglycemia, commonly seen in neonatal animals, toy breed puppies, and animals with sepsis or diabetic crisis
- Severe **azotemia** (elevations in blood urea nitrogen and creatinine values, indicating kidney failure)

Just as one panel will show one snapshot in time, a series of panels will show the effect of the clinician's treatment plan.

> **TECHNICIAN NOTE** As with all critical care monitoring, serial monitoring is most informative. The progress of the patient will dictate the frequency of electrolyte and chemistry analysis. Many computer-based patient charting systems allow for automatic graphing of serial results to give a very visual assessment of changes in patient values.

URINE VOLUME AND SPECIFIC GRAVITY

Measurements of urine volume and specific gravity are important tools for monitoring the emergency and

critical care patient. These tests provide information about renal perfusion (renal functionality) and are a means of assessing fluid resuscitation in critical patients. Whenever possible, these tests should be performed together to provide a more accurate interpretation of the patient's status.

INDICATIONS

Any hospitalized patient, especially those animals that may have the following:

- Dehydration
- Anemia
- Trauma
- Shock
- Suspected renal disease
- Electrolyte imbalances
- Hormonal imbalances
- Osmotic conditions (such as diabetes mellitus)

EQUIPMENT

Scale (to weigh patient and/or bedding)
Refractometer (to measure specific gravity)
Urine collection system (may be open or closed) (Figure 2-13)

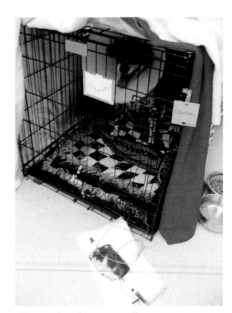

FIGURE 2-13 Closed urinary collection system. Note the severely hemorrhagic urine. (Photo courtesy Iowa Veterinary Referral Center.)

TECHNIQUE

A closed collection system is ideal for measuring urine volume. Other means of measuring urine volume include obtaining a free-catch specimen or measuring urine in the bottom of a cage. Towels or other absorbent materials can be weighed before being placed in a patient's cage. When soiled with urine these can be reweighed and an estimate of volume can be made.

> *TECHNICIAN NOTE* One milliliter (ml) of urine is equivalent to approximately 1 gram (g) of urine. Weighing hospitalized patients daily or even multiple times per day can also help estimate fluid gains and losses. It can be estimated that a 1-kilogram (kg) gain or loss is equivalent to 1 liter (L) of fluids gained or lost by the patient. It is important to remember that if a patient has third-space losses the patient will not have a decrease in body weight. **Third-space losses** occur when large volumes of fluids accumulate in body cavities such as pleural, peritoneal, or interstitial spaces as a result of certain disease processes. Technicians should monitor for signs of third-space losses as a result of pulmonary edema, ascites, protein loss, heart failure, renal insufficiency, or fluid overload.

INTERPRETATION

Ideally, urine production for dogs and cats should be 1 to 2 ml/kg/hour (depending on the ability of the kidneys to concentrate urine) (Mathews, 2006). Specific gravity values for dogs and cats should be approximately 1.030 and 1.035, respectively (Wamsley et al, 2004). If urine output is decreased (**oliguria**), possible causes include prerenal, renal, or postrenal causes or inadequate fluid resuscitation. In these cases it would be expected that the specific gravity of the urine would be increased. If this is not the case, renal insufficiency should be suspected. Possible causes of polyuria include fluid overload, hormonal imbalances, electrolyte abnormalities, osmotic conditions, or administration of glucocorticoids (dogs) or diuretic agents. The urine specific gravity of patients with **polyuria** is expected to be decreased. This, however, does not rule out renal insufficiency. As previously mentioned, other monitoring parameters should be assessed along with urine production and specific gravity to gain a more complete picture of a patient's status.

BLOOD GAS ANALYSIS

Blood gas analysis provides information about the acid-base status as well as the oxygenation and ventilation status (Figures 2-14 and 2-15). Acid-base and oxygenation disturbances are frequent occurrences in critical patients. The blood (and whole body) is normally maintained within a narrow pH range. Most cellular systems are dependent on this homeostasis and do not function normally when out of the normal pH range. It is also important to note that many of our pharmaceuticals work more efficiently within this pH range, and alterations in pH can result in changes to how the body reacts to various drugs.

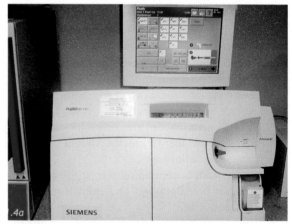

FIGURE 2-14 Siemens RAPIDlab blood gas analyzer. (Photo courtesy David Liss.)

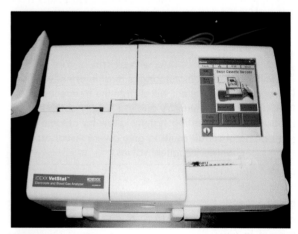

FIGURE 2-15 Idexx Laboratories VetStat blood gas and electrolyte analyzer.

Venous or arterial blood can be used for blood gas analysis, but only arterial samples give information about oxygenation. In the normal lung, arterial blood passes through the lungs and is saturated with oxygen. If a problem exists with gas exchange in the lung, then this will be reflected in the amount of oxygen that binds with the RBCs. The partial pressure of oxygen in arterial blood (PaO_2) will reflect the patient's oxygenation status. Venous samples can be used to give information about acid-base status and ventilation.

Blood gas analyzers can be "bedside" or bench-top devices. Most commonly available blood gas analyzers will also measure electrolyte levels and may also provide some other serum chemistry information, such as blood glucose or creatinine values. This information is very useful in the immediate assessment of an unstable patient.

INDICATIONS

Any critical patient may benefit from blood gas analysis. A blood gas analysis is particularly helpful in patients with the following:
- Respiratory emergencies including the following:
  - Pulmonary thromboembolism
  - Pneumonia
  - Congestive heart failure
- Metabolic emergencies including the following:
  - Urethral obstruction
  - Diabetic ketoacidosis or nonketotic hyperosmolar crisis
  - Eclampsia
  - Hypoadrenocorticism (Addison's disease)
  - Ethylene glycol toxicity
  - Any form of shock

EQUIPMENT

When considering blood gas equipment, reliability and ease of use are the first priorities. Different machines may analyze only blood gases; or they may analyze blood gases and electrolytes; or they may measure blood gases, electrolytes, and chemistries on a single blood sample. Consider if special sampling equipment is needed, such as arterial blood gas syringes, or if blood can be collected without anticoagulant. Many machines are cartridge based, whereas others have separate reagents within the machine. Depending on the volume of blood gases performed in your clinic, one type may prove more economical than the other.

All users should be instructed in the sampling and sample input procedures for the machine. Cartridge-based systems have the advantage of being small, and they do not require additional reagents; however, if a cartridge is overfilled or underfilled, the waste of a cartridge can become expensive. The large bench-top units are fast and very easy to use; however, the initial cost and maintenance can be significant since there are regular reagent and membrane replacements that need to be performed. Most QC and calibrations on this type of machine are scheduled. If a larger machine is in place, one person should be assigned to be in charge of blood gas equipment maintenance. Reading the technical manual and developing a close relationship with the machine's technical support branch will aid the technician in learning the maintenance duties. Most companies will offer a comprehensive training course with the purchase, to ensure "super users" are familiar with all aspects of the unit. All maintenance instructions should be followed precisely; if calibrations are needed, these must be done daily.

TECHNIQUE

Blood for blood gas analysis should be collected according to the manufacturer's instructions. Most machines use lithium heparin or sodium heparin as their preferred anticoagulant. Commercially available blood gas syringes and arterial samplers have minimum sample requirements to ensure the correct ratio of blood to anticoagulant. The machine may only require 0.125 to 0.3 ml of blood even though more may need to be drawn for the specific container. If using a heparinized syringe, the sample must be gently rolled in the hands to ensure mixing of the heparin with the blood. Using sodium heparin will result in inaccurate sodium measurements when obtaining electrolyte measurements.

Venous samples may be drawn from any peripheral or central vein. The status of the tissues in the area from which the blood was sampled can affect results. For example, a sample taken from a vein in a traumatized limb will yield different results than a sample taken from a vein that has more normal blood flow. Similarly, blood results taken from the hind limb of a cat with an aortic thromboembolism will differ markedly from those of a jugular sample taken from the same patient.

Arterial sampling should be done via an arterial puncture or arterial catheter using a 25- or 26-gauge needle. Arterial samples are most often collected from the femoral artery and the dorsal pedal artery. To puncture an artery, the technician should first palpate for a good pulse. Positioning for the sample is with either one or two fingers on the pulse. If using the one-finger method, then the technician should feel for the pulse, visualize the artery under his or her finger, and aim the needle at a 45-degree angle toward the pulse. The needle should enter the artery, and blood will travel into the self-filling syringe or into the capillary tubes. If using the two-fingered method, then the technician should assess for the pulse with two fingers spaced about 1 inch apart. The needle should be positioned at a 90-degree angle, halfway between the two fingers. On entering the artery, the blood should pulse up the syringe barrel. After the sample is drawn, any air bubbles should be expelled, the syringe should be capped tightly, and then the syringe should be rotated. If using an arterial capillary sampler, the blood should be allowed to fill the capillary tubes inside the sampler completely; then the needle should be removed and capped tightly. Ideally, samples should be analyzed immediately or within 15 minutes if stored at room temperature. If a sample cannot be analyzed immediately, then the technician should place the tightly capped syringe into an ice bath and analyze its contents within 1 hour. Most analyzers will require additional information, including the patient's identification number, the patient's temperature, and the percent of inspired oxygen the animal is breathing at the time of sampling (FiO_2). The percentage of oxygen in room air at sea level is 21%. For optimal results, a core temperature should be taken no more than 5 minutes before the blood is drawn. All of this information should be acquired and recorded before the sample is drawn.

An arterial catheter can be placed in a dorsal pedal artery using aseptic technique. A Luer-Lock injection cap may be placed on the end, through which a needle may be used to obtain a sample. If the catheter is also being used for direct arterial blood pressure measurements, a stopcock attached to the catheter and pressure tubing will allow for easy sampling access and flushing through the second port, which should be capped at all times. These catheters should be labeled as an arterial line and must be monitored frequently. An arterial line must also be flushed with heparinized saline (1 unit/ml heparin in 0.9% sodium chloride) and optimally heparin-locked (10 units/ml heparinized saline).

TROUBLESHOOTING

Acquiring a blood gas sample is fairly straightforward. Obtaining a venous blood gas sample uses the same technique as drawing a venous blood sample for other blood tests. Obtaining an arterial blood gas sample requires more skill, but the pulsatile flow of the blood in a syringe or capillary tube helps indicate the accuracy of the arterial puncture. Anatomically, a vein lies in close proximity to an artery, and a great chance exists that the vein may be punctured instead. Looking at the values and the clinical picture of the patient is the best way to gauge which sample has been drawn. If the patient appears to be clinically stable and the technician is confident in the accession, then he or she can assess the partial pressure of oxygen (PO_2) and the partial pressure of carbon dioxide (PCO_2) to help make the decision. If the patient is in respiratory distress and the PO_2 and PCO_2 numbers are within venous ranges, then a great possibility exists that the blood sample accession was executed properly. However, if the patient appears clinically stable and the blood work indicates more of a venous sample, then taking a known venous sample may be beneficial to compare measurements. If the PO_2 and PCO_2 values of both samples are comparable, then it is highly likely a vein was punctured in both accessions.

An arterial catheter is the optimal way to be consistent in accessions, although the risk of a significant bleed exists if the catheter apparatus is dislodged. The placement of arterial catheters requires more skill than that for a venous catheter, but technicians can become proficient with practice.

> *TECHNICIAN NOTE*   After multiple attempts to access the artery without success, the artery can begin to spasm and be rendered temporarily useless.

INTERPRETATION

This discussion focuses on the components of a blood gas analysis that examines the patient's acid-base and respiratory status (Table 2-1). Electrolytes are addressed in detail in their own section of this chapter.

Definitions
The following definitions should be noted:

- PaO_2 is the partial pressure of oxygen in the arterial blood. This value indicates how well the blood is

TABLE 2-1	Normal Blood Gas Values*			
SAMPLE	pH	PCO₂ (mm hg)	HCO₃⁻ (mm hg)	PO₂ (mm hg)
Dog venous	7.35-7.45	40-50	20-24	30-42
Dog arterial	7.35-7.45	35-45	20-24	90-100
Cat venous	7.3-7.38	41.8-50.8	19.4-23.4	38.6-49.6
Cat arterial	7.34-7.44	33.6-40.6	17.5-20.5	102.9-117.9

From Waddell LS: Blood gas analysis management tree, *NAVC Clin Brief* 10(1):18-19, 2012.
*In-house normal values should be established if the machine does not come with a published reference range.

being oxygenated. This value also indicates how well the lungs and pulmonary circulation are functioning.
- pH is a measure of the acidity or alkalinity of the blood. In general, pH measures the amount of hydrogen ions in the blood. The pH value has a narrow window of normalcy. If the value strays beyond normal, the buffering system is triggered to help compensate for the abnormal value. This value is affected by both metabolic and respiratory factors.
- PaCO₂ is the partial pressure of carbon dioxide (CO_2) in the circulating arterial blood and is an indicator of ventilation. Because CO_2 acts as an acid, excess CO_2 may cause acidosis or the body may hypoventilate to raise CO_2 levels to compensate for alkalosis. PaCO₂ is considered the *respiratory component* of a blood gas.
- HCO₃⁻ (or bicarbonate ion) is the major buffer in the body. The level of bicarbonate ion determines the "metabolic component" of a blood gas.
- BE is the base excess (the amount of base above or below the normal buffer level). A base *deficit* is how far away from zero a patient is to the *negative* and describes how many units of base are needed to return the patient to neutral. A base *excess* describes how far from zero a patient is to the *positive*. A base excess or deficit indicates a *metabolic* disturbance or compensation in the patient's blood chemistry.

Simple Blood Gas Analysis

The following information should be noted:
- A simple acid-base disturbance is one with a primary disorder and the appropriate compensation.

- A mixed acid-base disturbance has at least two separate, simultaneous disturbances.
- The technician should begin by determining whether an acid-base disturbance is present by comparing the pH to the normal range. If the pH is normal, usually an acid-base disturbance is not present. In certain circumstances, the pH may be normal, but the HCO₃, PaCO₂, or base excess (or a combination of these factors) values may be abnormal, indicating a compensated acid-base disturbance. If the pH is less than normal, the blood is acidemic. If the pH is greater than the normal range, the blood is alkalemic.
- Next the technician should examine the base excess and the bicarbonate ion level. If they are above normal, then either primary or compensatory metabolic alkalosis is present. Metabolic acidosis is a common disturbance and can be caused by conditions such as diabetic ketoacidosis or kidney failure. If the base excess and the bicarbonate ion levels are low, then either primary or compensatory metabolic alkalosis exists. Metabolic alkalosis is less common in small animal species but can be seen with vomiting.
- The technician should then compare the PaCO₂ measurement with the normal range. If it is high, then either a primary or a compensatory respiratory acidosis exists. If it is low, then either a primary or a compensatory respiratory alkalosis exists. A high PaCO₂ value is the definition of hypoventilation and commonly occurs in patients with respiratory depression for any reason, including anesthesia. Respiratory alkalosis can occur with hyperventilation, occasionally from pulmonary disease, or more commonly as a compensation for metabolic acidosis.
- The PaO₂ value should be between 90 and 100 mm Hg with normal lungs while the patient is breathing room air (FiO₂). The expected PaO₂ values for patients breathing different FiO₂ measurements should be approximately 5 × FiO₂. For example, an anesthetized patient breathing 100% oxygen should have a PaO₂ of about 500 mm Hg. Values less than these are indicative of hypoxemia, and oxygen therapy is generally indicated below 60 to 80 mm Hg (mild to severe hypoxemia).

COLLOID OSMOTIC PRESSURE

The definition of **colloid osmotic pressure** (COP) is the pressure exerted by colloid particles dissolved in a solution on a semipermeable membrane. To understand this concept, one should picture a bucket of fluid that is separated in the middle by a semipermeable membrane. This membrane will let smaller particles and water pass through to either side easily, but larger particles are forced to stay in their original compartments. Crystalloids are the smaller particles; colloids are the larger particles. If more colloid particles are found on one side compared with the other, the fluid and crystalloid particles will move from the side with the lower number of colloids (i.e., lower concentration) to the side with the higher number of colloids (i.e., higher concentration) to balance the pressure on the membrane. COP is the measurement of the pressure exerted on the capillary membrane by the colloid particles.

> **TECHNICIAN NOTE**   Importantly, it is the number of particles (not the size of the particles) that determines the COP. However, the size of the particle is what determines how long it is retained within the intravascular space.

Natural colloids are the proteins found in plasma. They consist of albumin, globulin, and fibrinogen. Synthetic colloids are water-based solutions that contain particles of several different sizes. Some examples are Dextran 70°, Hetastarch°, Pentastarch°, Voluven°, and Hb solutions (Hb-based oxygen carriers).

INDICATIONS

Blood COP is important to help determine whether the vasculature is allowing plasma proteins to leak into the interstitium or the compartment outside the vessel. If fluid is allowed to leak outside of the vasculature, edema or swelling will appear. Vasculitis and systemic inflammatory response syndrome are disease processes that will cause leaky vessels and low protein levels. In cases where hypovolemia is present, such as blood loss and shock, a low COP may indicate the need to rapidly expand the intravascular space. Colloid administration will draw water and electrolytes into the vasculature to help expand the circulatory system.

COP helps determine the concentration of plasma proteins in the blood. A lack of plasma proteins is an indication for the clinician to administer some kind of colloid, whether in plasma or in a synthetic colloid, to help restore fluid pressure balance. The large colloid particles will help draw fluid back into the vessels. Keeping the blood proteins at a consistent level helps maintain

the proper fluid balance to allow the body to function properly. On the other hand, if the COP is normal, indicating adequate plasma protein, but other clinical factors such as a high total protein reading arise, then this would indicate to the clinician that he or she may need to administer crystalloids to restore fluid balance.

EQUIPMENT

A colloid osmometer measures the COP of blood, plasma, or serum (Figure 2-16). The machine uses a semipermeable membrane that separates the plasma entry port from a protein-free solution. It is recommended to use heparinized whole blood samples for clinical ease, although plasma may be used as well. The machine must be well maintained to ensure accurate results. It must be calibrated every day with solutions of a known COP, and it must be flushed with saline daily and zeroed with saline before and after each use.

TECHNIQUE

The technician should draw a sample of whole blood into a heparinized syringe or Vacutainer tube treated with lithium heparin. He or she should check for clots by carefully rolling the tube between the hands and then expel a small amount of blood from the syringe (or insert a thin wooden stick into the blood in the tube and drag along the side). If there is no evidence of clotting, the technician should proceed with sampling.

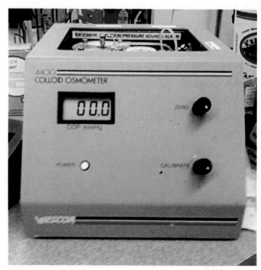

FIGURE 2-16 Wescore Inc. colloid osmometer. (Photo courtesy David Liss.)

TROUBLESHOOTING

Once synthetic colloids are administered, one cannot correlate the total solid measurement to the COP. The reading of the solids may not take into account the amount of particles added from the synthetic colloids; therefore the COP reading is the more appropriate number from which to extrapolate information.

INTERPRETATION

Normal values of whole blood range from 15.3 to 26.3 (mean 19.95) mm Hg in dogs and from 17.6 to 33.1 (mean 24.7) mm Hg in cats (Waddell, 2009).

LACTATE CONCENTRATION

Lactate is a byproduct of the breakdown of glucose in anaerobic conditions (when tissue oxygen delivery is inadequate). It is normal to have some lactate circulating in the bloodstream. The liver is responsible for clearing lactate from the body by converting it back to glucose or by oxidizing the molecule to CO_2 and water. Elevated lactate concentrations can serve as a marker for a diverse group of serious underlying conditions.

INDICATIONS

> **TECHNICIAN NOTE** Lactate concentrations are usually considered to be accurate indicators of inadequate tissue perfusion. Therefore any patient at risk of poor perfusion should have lactate levels monitored. This includes patients with the following:
> - Animals in shock or any patient suspected of being in shock
> - Animals with circulatory disturbances as in heart failure, thrombosis, or gastric dilation volvulus
> - Animals with trauma, especially crush injuries

EQUIPMENT

Both hand-held and bench-top machines are available to measure lactate levels. As lactate monitoring has become more common in veterinary medicine the number of machines on the market has increased and the price has improved dramatically. Each machine uses specific sample types; therefore checking with the manufacturer for the particular machine is important. Ideally, a literature search should be performed to ensure the machine has been validated for use in veterinary patients. Many lactate meters are marketed for athletes to monitor anaerobic metabolism, not for sick, hospitalized veterinary patients.

TECHNIQUE

Lactate level can be measured using venous or arterial blood samples. The samples must be analyzed within 30 minutes. The method of analysis varies by machine type.

TROUBLESHOOTING

As with any equipment, a certain amount of maintenance is to be expected. The smaller, hand-held machines are simpler. The technician must handle the calibrations and codes, but otherwise the machines are easy to set up and use. As mentioned earlier, the larger bench-top machines require much more maintenance and should be monitored and maintained by one or two individuals.

When preparing any blood for sampling, the blood should be tested for clots before insertion into the machine. The sample should also be mixed before sampling in order to ensure uniformity.

INTERPRETATION OF RESULTS

- Normal lactate levels: <2.5 mmol/L (dog), <1.5 mmol/L (cat)
- Mild increase: 3 to 5 mmol/L
- Moderate increase: 5 to 10 mmol/L
- Severe increase: >10 mmol/L (Mathews, 2006)

Increased lactate levels fall into one of two types of lactic acidosis: types A and B. Type A lactic acidosis is the result of tissue hypoxia, poor tissue perfusion, and shock. Gastric dilation volvulus and septic abdomens caused by intestinal perforation are two examples where lactic acid concentrations will be elevated.

Type B lactic acidosis can be categorized into one of four groups:

1. Systemic illness (diastolic murmur, rheumatic fever, infection, leukemia)
2. Drugs and toxins (ethanol, salicylates, methanol)
3. Heredity and congenital errors in metabolism (glucose 6-phosphatase deficiency)
4. Miscellaneous

The most important aspect of lactate analysis to consider is that one sample is only a snapshot of the patient's condition. Serial lactate levels provide a more accurate picture of a disease process. To correct the abnormality, the underlying cause of the lactic acidosis must be treated. For example, poor tissue perfusion and shock require boluses of fluids, either crystalloids or colloids, or both. Oxygen support may be necessary to reverse hypoxia. The inability to reduce plasma lactate concentrations may be a poor prognosticator of survival.

Treating lactic acidosis quickly and effectively will increase the patient's chances for survival. In general, tissue perfusion and oxygenation should be improved by aggressive fluid therapy with or without oxygen support, provided spontaneous ventilation is adequate.

COAGULATION TESTS

Coagulation abnormalities are common in patients who are critically ill. Coagulopathies can be associated with trauma and sepsis, as well as autoimmune, congenital, or idiopathic disease conditions.

> *TECHNICIAN NOTE* Determining the coagulation status of patients is imperative to assess the risk associated with diagnostic procedures and surgeries. For patients at substantial risk of bleeding, coagulation status should be determined before routine procedures such as cystocentesis are performed.

Tests of the patient's coagulation status that can be performed on site in the veterinary hospital include one-stage prothrombin time (PT), activated partial thromboplastin time (aPTT), activated clotting time (ACT), buccal mucosal bleeding time (BMBT), and platelet counts. Samples must be taken correctly for accurate coagulation tests. These tests determine whether deficiencies exist in different parts of the coagulation cascade. By identifying the part of the coagulation system that is abnormal, specific treatment including blood component therapy can be tailored to the exact problem.

INDICATIONS

Many patients in the critical care setting should have clotting function assessed either at presentation or during their treatment. Patients with any of the following diagnoses or differentials are at particular risk of coagulopathies:

- Rodenticide toxicity
- Thrombocytopenia
- Immune-mediated hemolytic anemia
- Sepsis
- Disseminated intravascular coagulopathy
- Protein-losing nephropathies
- Liver disease

- Immune suppression as a result of drug therapy
- Large-volume blood transfusion

EQUIPMENT

POC testing for coagulation function is available for veterinary patients. These analyzers use fresh whole blood or citrated blood and are most often used to analyze the PT and aPTT; however, they can also measure active clotting time (ACT).

The ACT test can also be run using special Vacutainer tubes filled with diatomaceous earth and/or ground glass particles. The only other equipment needed is a heating block, or the technician's axilla, and a timer. Special machines also exist to accurately time ACT.

Measurement of the buccal mucosal bleeding time (BMBT) requires a spring-loaded device that cuts two uniform incisions. Gauze squares or filter paper and a timer are also required to perform the test.

Manual platelet counts can be done from a blood smear, or automated counts can be performed using an automated hematology analyzer calibrated for veterinary species.

TECHNIQUE

In patients with possible coagulopathy, blood samples should be collected from peripheral veins rather than central veins to reduce the risk of excessive bleeding as a result of venipuncture.

Blood for PT/aPTT testing is collected in a sodium citrate (blue) tube, via a straight Vacutainer collection system or a Vacutainer tube holder with a Vacutainer butterfly line. Ideally, a "dummy tube" or other sample will be withdrawn first to remove any clotting factors activated during the venipuncture. The sodium citrate tube is then filled with the correct amount of blood (noted on the tube) to avoid dilution. The tube is checked for clots by inserting a wooden dowel and drawing it up the side of the tube. If no clot is present, then the sample is ready for analysis. The technician should follow directions for the particular POC analyzer to complete the process. If fresh whole blood is to be used, then the blood must be placed immediately into the warmed cartridge after venipuncture.

A manual ACT uses 0.5 to 2 ml of fresh whole blood, depending on the tubes being used. The venipuncture must be clean and blood must flow readily into the syringe. A venipuncture is performed using a needle and syringe, or Vacutainer collection system, into a pre-warmed ACT tube. A "dummy sample" may be collected first; however, if the technician is concerned about **iatrogenic** blood loss, this can be avoided. The tube is rotated five times to ensure that the sample is well mixed. The tube is then placed in a heating block at 37° C, or onto the technician's own axilla, and the time to formation of a clot is noted. The first reading is taken at 60 seconds. The technician does this by rotating the tube and doing a visual check for clot formation. If a clot is not present, then the tube is replaced in the heating block and checked every 5 to 15 seconds until a clot is noted.

The BMBT is performed with a spring-loaded device used to cut two uniform incisions, to standardize the size of the incision. The site used is the labial mucosa, which is exposed by folding the dorsal lip upward. A piece of gauze tied lightly around the muzzle can hold the lip back and increase venous hydrostatic pressure. The device is placed over the site with gentle pressure, and the trigger is released. Timing of the test begins at this time. Filter paper or gauze is held close to the incision site to absorb the blood. The actual incision site should not be touched because this will interfere with the test results. Timing is stopped once the flow has stopped and a clot is present. This value, reported in seconds, is the BMBT.

The technician calculates manual platelet estimates by counting the mean number of platelets in 5 to 10 microscope fields under ×100 oil magnification and multiplying this number by 15,000 (French, 1997). This estimates the number of platelets per microliter of blood. The smear should be examined for clumping and examined in a thin, uniform layer.

(The reader should refer to the section titled Hematologic Analysis for information regarding analyzers for automated platelet counts.)

TROUBLESHOOTING

The patient's disease process needs to be taken into consideration any time a blood sample is drawn. The patient with anemia can only afford to give enough blood that avoids dilution within the Vacutainer tubes to prevent iatrogenic blood loss. The area of venous access should be clipped and swabbed with a cotton ball soaked in alcohol, reducing sample artifact.

The most consistently accurate samples are those taken in one venipuncture. This will help prevent excess bleeding, hematoma, and clot formation, and it provides the sample most representative of the circulating blood.

Pressure bandages should be applied over the venipuncture site for no less than 5 minutes to minimize bleeding. If a patient has a known coagulopathy, then a pressure bandage may need to stay on the site for a longer period of time. The site and surrounding tissue need to be monitored closely for extraneous swelling.

Platelet clumping may occur if a sample is not collected using a Vacutainer tube or if the sample is not analyzed soon after collection. If this happens, the platelet count may be falsely read as low. The blood sample should always be mixed gently and well in the EDTA tube for best results.

INTERPRETATION

The PT and aPTT tests evaluate the extrinsic (external) and intrinsic (internal) and common portions of the clotting cascade. The coagulation cascade consists of many clotting factors that work in conjunction with each other and with vitamin K to maintain the body's ability to clot. Normal ranges for PT and PTT values will vary between analyzers. Normal values need to be established for individual machines. Prolonged results indicate a disruption in the coagulation cascade. If either the PT or the PTT reading is normal, and the other is prolonged, several clotting factors can be ruled out. This is important when a question exists as to which of the plasma products available needs to be administered.

> *TECHNICIAN NOTE* Both the BMBT test and the platelet count are two diagnostic tests to determine bleeding disorders caused by a **primary hemostasis**. Primary hemostasis problems are related to platelet or vessel disorders. These disorders include von Willebrand's disease, thrombocytopenia, thrombocytopathy, and vasculopathies. The BMBT is a good test to perform for possible vasculitis or thrombocytopenia (low platelets). A platelet count is directly related to clot formation function. If an animal has low platelets, it will have a diminished ability to form a clot. The platelets start the clotting process. If the platelets are not present, or do not work properly, a clot cannot form. If the clot cannot form, continual bleeding will occur unless pressure is applied to this area. This animal is now predisposed to bleeding even with minimal amounts of trauma.

ACT is a simple screening test for severe abnormalities in the intrinsic and common pathways of the coagulation cascade. It measures the time for the fibrin clot to form after activation by the glass particles, kaolin, or diatomaceous earth in the tubes. PT, PTT, and ACT are some of the diagnostics for determining whether a **secondary hemostasis** exists, or the ability to form a secondary clot is present. Bleeding disorders associated with secondary hemostasis are related to problems with the coagulation cascade. These are circumstances such as rodenticide ingestion, drug toxicity, and liver disease.

- Normal ACT time is 60 to 110 seconds for dogs and 50 to 75 seconds for cats.
- Normal BMBT range is 1.7 to 4.2 minutes for dogs and 1.4 to 2.4 minutes for cats.
- Normal platelet count is 150 to 500 $\times 10^3$ cells/μL for dogs and 200 to 600 $\times 10^3$ cells/μL for cats (Hackner, 1999).

DEVICE-BASED MONITORING

Over the past few years, more advanced, device-based monitors have become more affordable and thus more commonly used in veterinary medicine. This final category of monitoring helps technicians develop a clearer picture of how a patient is responding to treatment. It is important to keep in mind that although the equipment in this third category is more complex, it is no more important than the physical examination or clinical pathologic monitoring.

Either new or used monitoring equipment can be obtained. Because of the expense involved and the extent medical care depends on the results of monitoring, warranties and service contracts should be carefully scrutinized. Easily accessible, 24-hour technical service should be provided either by the companies supplying the machines or by the service contract provider.

One or two people should be appointed to maintain these machines; however, all staff members should have the manuals available to them in case of equipment failure. Because each piece of equipment is different, staff training should include instructions of how to work and maintain all monitoring equipment. Training can often be incorporated into the purchase agreement and be delivered by the technical staff of the equipment distributer.

Nothing can replace the veterinary technician in patient monitoring. Tools and machines may provide information that a physical examination or laboratory parameter cannot, but it is the person who assesses the information, determines its validity, and develops a diagnostic or treatment plan based on the findings.

Machines are not infallible and errors of false readings can occur. All unexpected abnormalities should be confirmed before treatment is adjusted. Confirming results may be as simple as getting another reading, but confirmation may also involve performing a second test. For instance, if the pulse oximeter is reading 75% but the patient has pink mucous membranes and is breathing normally, then the probe position should be checked before the patient can be assessed as being severely hypoxic.

PULSE OXIMETRY

Pulse oximetry noninvasively calculates the oxygen saturation of hemoglobin (Hb) using spectrophotometry. This gives information about arterial oxygen content and, consequently, tissue oxygen delivery. The saturation of Hb in the arterial blood is usually referred to as SaO_2; however, when measured by pulse oximetry rather than by an arterial blood gas, Hb saturation is referred to as SpO_2 and expressed as a percentage. Adult Hb molecules can exist in four forms: (1) oxyhemoglobin (oxygen bound to Hb), (2) deoxyhemoglobin, (3) carboxyhemoglobin (carbon monoxide bound to Hb), and (4) methemoglobin (an irreversible change in the shape of Hb that does not allow it to carry oxygen molecules). The pulse oximeter measures the amount of deoxyhemoglobin and oxyhemoglobin and calculates the relative percent of Hb that is saturated with oxygen.

The basic principle behind this technology is that deoxyhemoglobin absorbs red light but not infrared wavelengths, whereas oxyhemoglobin absorbs infrared wavelengths but not red light. A probe is applied to skin or mucous membrane, across an arterial bed, which emits light at both red and infrared wavelengths. The relative amounts of each wavelength detected by the probe, after the blood absorbs some of each wavelength, allow the saturated proportion to be calculated. The probe will only read pulsatile flow so that the SpO_2 is based on arterial blood levels.

Pulse oximeters display the strength of the pulsatile signal either in a waveform as a bar graph or in a color light–emitting diode (LED). This signal must remain strong because the accuracy of the oximeter decreases when pulsatile flow is not detected or is poorly detected. Most oximeters give a continuous display of the pulse rate. This should correspond to the palpable pulse rate and to the auscultated heart rate to ensure accuracy.

INDICATIONS

- Animals at risk for hypoxemia:
  - Patients with tachypnea or dyspnea
  - Patients that are anesthetized
  - Patients that are critically ill
  - Patients in rapidly deteriorating conditions
- Animals being monitored because they are receiving oxygen therapy or mechanical ventilation

EQUIPMENT

Pulse oximeters are available as hand-held portable monitors or as table-top monitors (Figure 2-17). They are often a component of parameter monitors. Table-top monitors display a waveform and a digital readout to help confirm an arterial signal and accurate reading.

The probe can be either a transmittance type (the probe has two pieces; one side of a clip contains a light-emitting diode [LED] that shines across tissue to a second piece that acts as a photodetector) or a reflectance type (both the LED and the photodetector are contained in a one-piece probe; the light is reflected off hard tissues back to the probe) (Figure 2-18). Both types of probes are used, but clip type transmittance probes are most common in veterinary practice.

TECHNIQUE

The probe is placed on skin and must remain in place for 20 to 30 seconds to obtain an accurate reading.

Probe placement options include the following:
- Tongue
- Lip
- Pinna of ear
- Prepuce and vulva
- Toe and toe web
- Metacarpus
- Ventral surface of the tail
- Axillary or inguinal skin fold
- Gastrocnemius tendon

Pigmented areas may not produce accurate readings. Haired areas may need to be clipped and cleaned to allow readings. Mucous membranes that are dry may not read accurately, and dampening with water will assist readings.

TROUBLESHOOTING

Potential sources of difficulty in obtaining pulse oximetry readings or accuracy include the following:
- Patient motion
  - Shivering or tremors
  - Seizure activity
- Poor perfusion states
  - Hypothermia
  - Hypovolemia
  - Vasoconstriction for other reasons
- Severe anemia
- Environmental light interference

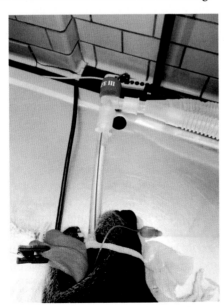

FIGURE 2-17 Pulse oximeter probe on a dog's tongue.

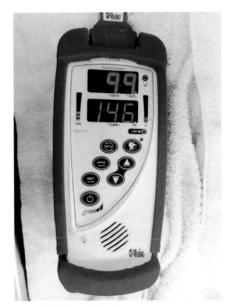

FIGURE 2-18 Masimo pulse oximeter.

- Pigmentation in skin, both natural and acquired, as in the following:
  - IV dyes used for diagnostic procedures (NOTE: Oxyglobin administration does not interfere with pulse oximetry; icterus may or may not interfere with it.)
- Abnormal Hb level
  - Methemoglobinemia
  - Carboxyhemoglobin or carbon monoxide toxicity

To help obtain an accurate reading, the area may need to be clipped and cleaned (if appropriate) or warmed. If ambient light is providing interference, then the probe can be covered. If the probe has been in position for more than 30 seconds and a strong signal is not obtained, then it can be repositioned.

If the probe is on the tongue of an anesthetized or unconscious patient, it should be repositioned every 5 to 10 minutes because the clips can occlude flow to the area. Moistening the tongue with water can also aid in obtaining an accurate pulse oximetry reading. Whenever low readings are obtained but the reading does not match the patient's clinical status, an arterial blood gas should be evaluated.

INTERPRETATION

A patient with normal lung function breathing room air (or 100% oxygen) should have an SpO_2 reading greater than 95%. Pulse oximetry cannot replace direct measurement of PaO_2 using arterial blood gases because SpO_2 does not correlate with PaO_2 in a linear relationship. At approximately 92%, the SpO_2 correlates to a PaO_2 of 60 mm Hg. Below this SpO_2 value, the PaO_2 rapidly declines to life-threatening levels. Patients with SpO_2 levels below 94% should be given supplemental oxygen.

Once the SpO_2 value is in the normal range, pulse oximetry cannot detect changes in arterial oxygenation until a significant change has occurred. This can be a serious limitation when the patient is being supplemented with high levels of oxygen. For instance, during general anesthesia when a patient is breathing 100% oxygen, the PaO_2 should be approximately 450 to 500 mm Hg. The oximetry reading will not drop until the PaO_2 has decreased below approximately 100 mm Hg, which is a very significant decline. Therefore pulse oximetry should not be the only method of monitoring respiratory function during general anesthesia or mechanical ventilation. Despite these limitations, it is considered a minimum standard of monitoring human patients under anesthesia and is a very useful noninvasive technique.

BLOOD PRESSURE

Measurement of arterial blood pressure (BP) provides important information about tissue perfusion and overall cardiovascular function. Arterial BP consists of three values: (1) systolic, (2) diastolic, and (3) mean arterial pressures. Systolic pressure is the pressure against the arteries generated by ventricular contraction, and diastolic pressure is the minimum pressure maintained between contractions. Mean arterial pressure is the average pressure during the cardiac cycle. The pulse pressure equals the systolic minus the diastolic pressure and is palpated at the femoral, dorsal pedal, lingual, or other arteries. BP measurements and pulse quality are important monitoring tools in an intensive care unit (ICU) because organ function declines and cell death can occur at BPs above and below critical values. Therefore changes in BP dictate many therapeutic interventions in patients.

INDICATIONS

- Patients with possible cardiovascular abnormalities of any cause including the following:
  - Shock
  - Heart disease
  - Systemic inflammatory response syndrome or multiple organ dysfunction syndrome
- Patients with a rapidly changing clinical status
- Patients that have received anesthesia
- Patients being mechanically ventilated
- Patients with primary diseases that are associated with hypertension including the following:
  - Chronic renal failure
  - Hyperthyroidism
  - Hyperadrenocorticism (Cushing's syndrome)

EQUIPMENT

BP can be monitored using direct or indirect techniques. The technician makes direct BP measurements via an arterial catheter, most commonly by an electronic pressure transducer. This is the same equipment that can be used for central venous pressure (CVP) measurement; however, the system may use special tubing for arterial systems and may be connected to the patient through a fluid-primed pressure dome. Additionally, the system may be kept patent using a unidirectional flushing device that continuously infuses pressurized saline. Manufacturers of electronic pressure transducers provide detailed information about this specialized equipment. The display will give values for systolic, diastolic, and mean pressure and preferably generates a continuous pressure wave.

Indirect or noninvasive BP can be measured in veterinary patients by automated oscillometric or ultrasonic (Doppler) techniques that work by occluding arterial pressure under a cuff. In oscillometric equipment, the machine inflates the cuff to pressures greater than systolic levels; then the cuff pressure is automatically gradually decreased and the microprocessor detects oscillations that change at systolic, mean, and systolic BP. Those values are reported on a display screen. The entire process is automated. Models are manufactured specifically for veterinary use.

In ultrasonic techniques, a manually inflated cuff is attached to an aneroid sphygmomanometer so that readings may be obtained. A small ultrasound probe placed directly over the artery transmits an audible signal of the pulse when the cuff pressure decreases enough to allow flow to return to the artery. Depending on the model, the cuff may either be separate from the ultrasound crystal or be attached to it. If separate cuffs are used, then human pediatric BP cuffs of varying sizes are usually used, although there are also veterinary specific, one-limbed cuffs currently available. Human pediatric cuffs must be modified for use with a Doppler system by tying a knot in one of the two limbs of tubing on the cuff (the other is connected to the sphygmomanometer). The probe is connected to a receiver-amplifier-speaker unit that is powered by a rechargeable battery. If background noise is significant or the noise of the probe disturbs the patient, then earphones may be connected to the receiver. The piezoelectric crystal in the probe is delicate and can be easily damaged. It should be wiped clean and covered with a manufacturer-supplied cover or a piece of gauze or foam (taped on the unit) when not in use. Alcohol will cause deterioration of the crystal and should never be applied directly to the probe. The cable that attaches the crystal to the receiver may also become worn with heavy use, leading to noise interference or poor performance. To help extend their lives, the wire cables should not be bent or kinked. Manufacturers recommend that the probes remain plugged into the unit, because the connectors can also be a source of wear and tear.

TECHNIQUE

Direct Arterial Pressure Monitoring

Direct arterial pressure monitoring is the gold standard for BP measurement. It is underused because of perceived technical difficulties in placing and maintaining arterial catheters, as well as lack of equipment. Arterial catheterization can become routine with practice. The availability of used monitoring equipment and transducers has substantially reduced costs and makes it affordable for any hospital dealing with critically ill or injured patients.

An arterial catheter can be placed in any artery; however, the most commonly used are the dorsal pedal and the femoral arteries. Femoral artery catheters may be harder to maintain because of the difficulties involved in wrapping and stabilizing that location. If a risk of bleeding exists, then it will be easier to maintain hemostasis if a more peripheral artery is catheterized.

Special arterial catheters are available, but commonly available IV catheters may be used (especially for short-term use). The area should be anesthetized with a topical anesthetic such as lidocaine/prilocaine, or 4% liposomal lidocaine, 15 to 30 minutes before the procedure. If being placed emergently, a lidocaine bleb may be used. Percutaneous methods or cut-down methods can be used to place the catheters. Short (1 to 1½ inches) over-the-needle catheters tend to be difficult to maintain for longer periods of time because they tend to kink. Longer catheters (arterial, through-the-needle, or those placed by Seldinger technique) may last longer. Once the catheters are placed, they must be secured well to prevent inadvertent dislodging and kinking. Aseptic technique should be observed during placement and maintenance of arterial catheters.

Arterial catheters are prone to thrombosis. Flushing can be accomplished manually by flushing with heparinized saline every 1 to 2 hours. Alternatively, the catheters can be connected to a low constant rate infusion of heparinized saline delivered by an infusion pump or a pressurized bag. Electronic pressure transducer systems work with disposable pressurized unidirectional flushing devices that are connected directly to the system. If a transducer system is not available, then BP can be measured directly using the same manometer method as for measuring CVP.

Indirect Blood Pressure Monitoring

BP is measured indirectly using either an oscillometric device or a Doppler ultrasound flow detector. Indirect techniques are less accurate but are noninvasive and require less skill than direct BP monitoring. There are advantages and disadvantages to both indirect blood pressure monitoring techniques.

Both methods entail placing a pressure cuff over an artery on the limbs or tail. Appropriate cuff size is important for accuracy of readings. The cuff width should be approximately 40% of the circumference of the limb or tail. Many cuffs have markings on them to indicate whether the fit is appropriate as the cuff is being placed. Some cuffs have markings on them indicating where the artery must come in contact with the cuff. A cuff that is too large can lead to artificially low readings, and a cuff that is too small can lead to artificially elevated readings. A piece of tape may be loosely applied to the cuff to prevent it from becoming disconnected when inflated, but must not inhibit full inflation.

> **TECHNICIAN NOTE** Always record the location on the animal that the blood pressure was taken and the size of the cuff that was used. This will allow subsequent readings to be taken using identical techniques and equipment so changes and trends in readings will be meaningful.

Oscillometric Devices

The technician should place an appropriately sized cuff distal to the elbow, around the midmetatarsal, or around the base of the tail. A lateral or sternal position gives more accurate readings, because the cuff should be near the level of the heart. The machine can be programmed to provide a single reading or repeated measurements over set time intervals. Most accurate readings in a conscious patient will be obtained with minimal restraint and minimal movement. Five readings should be obtained and averaged, discarding obviously different numbers. Weak pulse signals from poor flow, small arteries, shaking, and movement will interfere with the accuracy of the **oscillometric** device. Because of these limitations, it may be difficult to obtain readings using this method in very small dogs or cats, conscious animals, or animals in shock. It is very useful in anesthetized patients. Most oscillometric BP devices only measure mean arterial pressure (MAP) and then use proprietary algorithms to calculate systolic and diastolic blood pressure readings from the MAP. Because the MAP is the only measured value, it can be considered the most accurate of the three readings. In addition to BP

oscillometric devices, also measure pulse rate. A manual heart rate or pulse rate should be taken to confirm the accuracy of the blood pressure reading. If the manual rate matches the rate from the device, it can be assumed that the blood pressure reading is accurate as well.

There is a new type of oscillometric blood pressure monitor that is now available in veterinary medicine. Instead of only measuring MAP and calculating systolic and diastolic BP this new device measures all three readings. This new technology, called high-definition oscillometry (HDO), has shown promising results thus far. HDO is said to be more sensitive and able to take more accurate readings even in the face of arrhythmias. More studies using approved validation criteria need to be completed before this technology is embraced by veterinary medicine.

Doppler Ultrasound Flow Detectors

Doppler ultrasound flow detectors use an ultrasonic probe placed over an artery and an occluding cuff placed proximal to the probe (Figure 2-19). The area over the artery is clipped (usually just proximal to the palmar metacarpal pad, to the plantar metatarsal pad, or to the ventral surface of the tail base). The probe is covered with ultrasound coupling gel (or the skin over the artery is covered), and it is placed over the vessels and adjusted until a pulse is audible. The probe can then be secured in place with tape. If the patient has a very deep groove in the location of the arch, then the probe can be secured better by placing a gauze square or cotton ball over the top of the probe before taping it in place. If the tape is placed too loosely, then the signal may be weak. In small

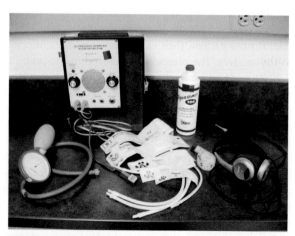

FIGURE 2-19 Parks Medical ultrasonic Doppler blood pressure monitor and accessories.

patients the lack of a signal may indicate that the tape has been placed too tightly.

A BP cuff is placed just proximal to the ultrasonic probe and inflated using a sphygmomanometer. The cuff should be held at the approximate level of the heart; then the cuff is allowed to deflate slowly. The measurement at which the sound of the blood flow first is audible is the systolic pressure. The level at which the sound changes is the diastolic pressure. The diastolic pressure is not always heard using this method.

Lack of perfusion or very poor pulses, hypothermia, severe vasoconstriction, and poor probe contact can lead to an absent or very weak signal. During anesthesia the concurrent use of other electrical equipment, especially electrosurgical equipment, can interfere with the flow signal. The Doppler method of BP requires more skill than the oscillometric method.

One of the significant advantages of the Doppler ultrasound flow detector over an oscillometric device is that the flow through an artery is transmitted by an audible signal. This allows use of the Doppler ultrasound probe for applications other than BP measurement. The quality and intensity of the audible pulse can be used to monitor blood flow. This can be done continuously in anesthetized or unconscious patients, allowing subjective but immediate detection of changes in cardiac output or heart rhythm. Doppler flow detectors can be used to determine the presence of flow in distal limbs whenever the technician is concerned about circulatory disturbances. This may be the case in patients with severe trauma to a limb or possible thromboembolic disease blocking blood flow. For example, cats with possible saddle thrombi can have lack of blood flow confirmed by placing the Doppler probe over each femoral artery. This is a more sensitive indicator of flow than digital palpation.

The Doppler flow probe can be placed on the surface of the cornea (after placing ultrasonic gel) to monitor for the presence of blood flow to the head. This technique can also be used to monitor the success of resuscitative efforts during cardiopulmonary resuscitation.

INTERPRETATION

Hypotension is defined as BP readings less than 80 mm Hg (systolic) or 60 mm Hg (mean) and always warrants treatment of underlying cause and continued monitoring. Below this level, shock (inadequate tissue perfusion and oxygen delivery leading to cellular death and organ damage) is expected. Controversy continues over the level of hypertension that should prompt treatment, and often the decision to treat will be based on concurrent clinical signs of hypertension. In general, patients with systolic BP readings equal to or greater than 180 mm Hg are at risk for end-organ damage (Brown et al, 2007).

In anesthetized and critically ill patients, BP trends are often more important for assessment of patient status than individual readings. Knowledge of a patient's BP trends, like other methods of monitoring discussed in this chapter, is an integral part of critical care treatment decisions.

TROUBLESHOOTING

The reader should review the individual method techniques for the specifics of troubleshooting. For indirect methods, localized poor flow, patient motion, inappropriate cuff size, and lack of consistent technique between readings will all lead to inaccurate or unobtainable readings. For Doppler ultrasound and direct arterial monitoring, operator skill will significantly affect the success of the method chosen, but both methods can be readily learned with practice.

ELECTROCARDIOGRAM MONITORING

The **electrocardiogram** (ECG) is a record of the electrical activity of the heart muscle used to monitor heart rhythm. Changes in the size or structure of the heart are also reflected in the ECG because those changes affect the direction and speed at which electrical impulses travel through the heart.

INDICATIONS

ECGs are used as diagnostic and monitoring tools. Many patients arriving at the emergency department or being treated in an ICU should have ECG tracings recorded at some point during the assessment or treatment, because heart function can be affected by many conditions other than primary cardiac disease. An ECG is often used to confirm arrhythmias suspected while listening with a stethoscope. Many arrhythmias are too subtle to be heard on auscultation or are intermittent, so normal auscultation does not negate the importance of ECG monitoring. In critically ill animals, continuous or serial intermittent ECG monitoring provides important information about trends in cardiovascular function.

Specific indications for ECG monitoring are the following:

- Trauma (especially with significant hemorrhage or possible thoracic cavity trauma)
- Shock (cardiogenic, hypovolemic, and distributive)
- Possible systemic inflammatory response syndrome or multiple organ dysfunction syndrome
- Syncope or collapse
- Anesthetized patients
- Poisoning or intoxication
- During cardiopulmonary cerebral resuscitation
- Cardiac or pulmonary disease
- Any auscultated arrhythmia
- During the IV bolus administration of drugs (i.e., calcium gluconate, sodium bicarbonate) that can produce arrhythmias

EQUIPMENT

ECG machines can provide results using a continuous display screen, a printout, or both. Because the technician can only gather accurate measurements by measuring waveforms and distances, printing capability is necessary for full assessment. A continuous display is important for monitoring of critical patients because their heart rhythms are expected to change over time.

ECG monitors also vary in the way they are connected to the patient. Traditionally, lead wires were connected to both the patient and the machine, limiting the mobility of the patient. Telemetry units have leads attached to the patient along with a battery pack, usually slung around the patient's neck or taped to the body, which wirelessly transmits an ECG signal to monitors placed in convenient locations. Many technicians have sewn custom vests of varying sizes that can hold the telemetry module in place on an active patient. Handheld monitors and smartphone cases and apps, without leads, are available. These small devices are held against the patient's chest and a tracing is obtained. Most models have some memory capabilities to store tracings and some have printout capabilities. Although the quality of these tracings often is not equal to that obtained with standard ECG leads, the quality of the equipment is improving; the major advantage is that a quick rhythm strip can be obtained in the examination room or at the patient's cage. Esophageal ECG devices are available for use in anesthetized patients. These devices tend not to be affected by other electronic monitoring equipment,

as with external devices. They should not be used in combination with electrocautery units.

TECHNIQUE

The technician should place the patient in the right lateral recumbent position, on the floor or on a table covered with paper or a nonconducting material (metal tables should be avoided). Dyspneic or fractious animals can have ECGs recorded in any position. These tracings cannot be compared with standardized measurements but may still be useful to provide rhythm information.

The electrodes may be attached to the skin by alligator clips, wire, or adhesive patches. The alligator clips may be less traumatic if the teeth are filed, the spring is loosened, or a gauze or paper towel patch protects the skin inside a clip. If clips or wires are placed, then the technician should saturate the area with alcohol or ECG paste to provide good contact. For long-term attachment of traumatic alligator clips, wire suture may be preplaced and the clips attached to the wire. To do this, a 20- or 22-gauge hypodermic needle is passed through the skin in the desired location and the wire is threaded through the needle. The needle is removed, leaving the wire in place. The ends of the wire are twisted together to prevent inadvertent removal. It is advisable to place tape around the ends of the wire for safety and as a visual reminder that wires have been placed. The ECG clips then are attached to the wires.

Alcohol should not be used if the leads are being attached during cardiopulmonary resuscitation (CPR) and, potentially, defibrillation because doing so is a fire hazard.

Alternatively, ECG patches can be applied to the skin or foot pads. To improve adhesion, the skin should be well shaved, cleaned with alcohol, and dried before patch placement. In recumbent patients the patches can be placed on the metacarpal and metatarsal pads and held in place using tape if necessary.

The standard lead II or six-lead ECG is recorded using three or four electrodes that are attached to the patient. Three- or five-lead ECG cables are available and electrodes are color-coded and labeled on the basis of the human anatomy: right foreleg (RA), white lead; left foreleg (LA), black lead; right hind leg (RL), green lead; left hind leg (LL), red lead; and the V lead (C), which is an exploring lead and is brown. A three-lead ECG cable does not have a brown or green (RL) electrode. In most emergency situations, the three-lead ECG is preferable since it can be rapidly attached, but if using a five-lead ECG, the four limb leads are attached and the V (brown) lead is not.

The ECG should be monitored on lead II for at least 1 minute, noting any abnormalities. Printing a 10-second strip, or multiple strips, ideally at both 50 and 25 mm/ second speeds, will allow for direct measurements and further interpretation. It is important to try and capture any intermittent abnormalities on the paper strip. The strip should be labeled with patient information and the date and time of the tracing, if the machine does not automatically perform this function.

More specialized and detailed ECGs are used in most cardiology practices, and are called nine-lead ECGs. A nine-lead provides the standard limb leads, I, II, and III, in addition to the aV_L, aV_R, and aV_F augmented limb leads, and the V_1, V_2, and V_3 chest leads. These types of ECGs are not typically used during emergency treatment, but, rather, are used as part of the diagnostic process.

TROUBLESHOOTING

> **TECHNICIAN NOTE** Electrical interference, movement of the patient, and respiratory motion are common factors that can create problems with obtaining a clear ECG tracing.

Check the electrodes to make sure good contact is achieved with the skin by both proper placement and sufficient application of alcohol or paste. Respiratory motion is usually seen as a regular undulation of the baseline as the chest rises and falls. As long as this is regular, it will not unduly interfere with interpreting a rhythm strip. Conversely, shivering, or 60-Hz cycle interference from other electrical equipment attached to the patient or nearby, can cause unreadable ECG tracings. This type of tracing will look like a rough or fuzzy baseline, or the whole tracing will irregularly move up and down on the paper. If this happens, then the technician should remove or move other electrical equipment, try moving the electrodes to more peripheral locations on the body, or do both to reduce the interference.

INTERPRETATION

A normal tracing shows a P wave, QRS complex, and T wave, which correspond to atrial depolarization (P wave), ventricular depolarization (QRS complex), and ventricular repolarization (T wave). When reading an ECG rhythm strip, the fundamental principles are to calculate the heart rate, look for overall regularity of rhythm, make sure a P wave is present for every QRS complex, and assess for abnormally shaped complexes such as ventricular premature contractions.

In an emergency or arrest situation, it is important to confirm that electrical activity (i.e., an ECG waveform) has an associated heartbeat and pulse. Electrical activity does not necessarily mean that the heart is beating. Additionally, electrical complexes and auscultated heartbeats may not produce enough heart function to generate a pulse pressure. This is called a *pulse deficit* and is commonly found in emergencies such as ventricular tachycardia. A pulse deficit represents a serious condition that must be addressed.

Each wave has a normal duration (milliseconds) and height (millivolts), as well as a normal interval between waves. These measurements are useful in determining the health of the electrical conduction system. Abnormalities are associated with conduction disturbances and can be associated with changes in the heart muscle or pericardial space.

END-TIDAL CARBON DIOXIDE MONITORING

Capnometry is the measurement of CO_2 level in a gas using spectrophotometry. Using this technology to record the concentration of CO_2 in a single end-exhaled (end-tidal) breath is called *capnography*. Capnography provides a noninvasive means of assessing CO_2 levels in the body. CO_2 is the major byproduct of tissue metabolism, and assessment of body levels gives important information about perfusion, metabolism, and ventilation. **End-tidal carbon dioxide** ($EtCO_2$) monitoring is a reasonable alternative to measuring the $PaCO_2$ using arterial blood gas analysis. All general anesthetic agents and many analgesics such as narcotics cause respiratory depression. This leads to a buildup of CO_2, or a respiratory acidosis, and because of this, $EtCO_2$ monitoring is always indicated in an anesthetized patient or when respiratory depression or hypoventilation is a concern.

INDICATIONS

- Monitoring of ventilation in spontaneously breathing anesthetized, or comatose, intubated patients
- Confirmation of endotracheal and feeding tube placement

- Monitoring of cardiopulmonary cerebral resuscitation
- Monitoring of patients undergoing mechanical ventilation

EQUIPMENT AND TECHNIQUE

Capnographs are either hand-held monitors or larger table-top monitors, often incorporated in a multiparameter monitor. A sensor or sampling tube is attached between the breathing circuit and the endotracheal tube or on the open end of the endotracheal tube if it is not attached to a circuit. $EtCO_2$ level can be measured with the sensor placed on the end of a tightly fitting face mask, although this technique is less accurate than when performed in an intubated patient. Special nasal cannulas can also be purchased that offer oxygen supplementation through one prong, and sample $EtCO_2$ on the other prong.

In sidestream-type monitors, a sample of gas is guided down a small-bore tube that exits near the end of the endotracheal tube (Figure 2-20). The sample is measured away from the end of the tube. In mainstream-type monitors, the measurement takes place exactly at the end of the tube. (The reader should refer to the following Troubleshooting section for more information on the difference between the two types.)

Both types of monitors display a numeric value, and most monitors also display a waveform. The waveform, or capnogram, is a graphic display of the changes in $EtCO_2$ over time. The shape of the capnogram provides

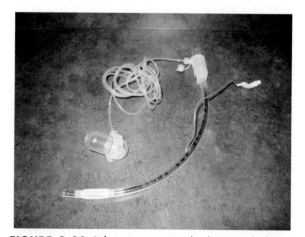

FIGURE 2-20 Sidestream capnograph tubing attached to an endotracheal tube. Note the tubing coming from the side of the adapter attached to the endotracheal (ET) tube and the long tube that takes the sample to the machine to be analyzed.

important information about respiratory patterns, technical problems such as endotracheal tube occlusion or excessive rebreathing, and patient perfusion. Most hand-held monitors do not provide capnograms, and some monitors will provide printouts of capnograms. Most multiparameter monitors can be equipped with capnography. (The reader should refer to the end of this chapter for more information about multiparameter monitors.)

TROUBLESHOOTING

Both sidestream and mainstream monitors have problems that may interfere with their accuracy and ease of use. With sidestream sampling, the small size of the sampling tube can lead to occlusion with secretions. Sidestream capnographs draw off a portion of the gas flow and may require increased oxygen flow rates (especially in small patients on low-flow closed circuit systems). Mainstream capnographs have heated sensors to prevent condensation of moisture from the exhaled gases. With long-term use, the inhaled gases can be heated enough to pose a risk of burns to the respiratory mucosa. Additionally, the larger device attached to the breathing circuit in a mainstream sampler adds significant dead space and weight to the tubing. Leakage of any portion in the breathing circuit (from the sidestream sampling tube) or at the level of a mainstream sensor can falsely lower readings. Mainstream monitors also require longer warm-up time and more frequent calibration that may make them unsuitable for use in an emergency or arrest situation.

Moisture can interfere with readings in both types of monitors. For this reason, the sensor should be positioned above the level of the patient so that moisture in the endotracheal tube does not accumulate in the sensor or tubing. Sampling tubing and sensor devices should be checked regularly for accumulations of respiratory tract secretions or condensation, especially if readings do not correlate with the status of the patient based on other monitoring values. If the patient is stable enough to permit disconnection of the device, then exhaling into the sensor will easily rule out mechanical failure of a capnograph.

INTERPRETATION

Normal arterial CO_2 concentration values for an anesthetized patient with normal perfusion and pulmonary function are about 35 to 45 mm Hg. The $EtCO_2$ is ≈ 5 mm Hg less than the arterial value (Sorrell-Raschi, 2009).

The waveform or capnogram produced by exhaled CO_2 has a unique shape.

> *TECHNICIAN NOTE* Changes in the shape of the waveform give information about respiration and anesthesia technical problems.

Basic analysis of the capnogram should include the following:
- Presence or absence of a waveform:
  - Absence of a waveform may indicate cardiac or respiratory arrest, apnea, disconnection of the breathing circuit, esophageal intubation or extubation, complete obstruction of the endotracheal tube, or malfunction of the monitor.
- Noting the actual $EtCO_2$ value and comparing it with normal reference ranges:
  - Elevated CO_2 levels can result from either increased CO_2 production (usually from increased metabolism, as in fever or seizure activity) or decreased elimination (i.e., hypoventilation).
  - Low CO_2 levels may indicate either decreased metabolism (as in hypothermia) or increased elimination (as with hyperventilation).
- Examination of the shape of the waveform:
  - If the baseline is above zero, then it usually indicates rebreathing of exhaled gases from exhausted soda lime or low fresh gas flow.
  - Gradual rise in the $EtCO_2$ reading without a normal plateau may indicate airway obstruction or a kinked endotracheal tube.
  - A sharply peaked wave may be caused by tachypnea or a leak in the circuit.
  - A sudden drop in the wave to very low or zero can indicate disconnection or a large leak, airway obstruction, extubation, or arrest.

CENTRAL VENOUS PRESSURE

Central venous pressure (CVP) measurement estimates the blood pressure (BP) within the right atrium by measuring pressure in the cranial or caudal vena cava. While CVP has been used for many years as an indicator of fluid status of the veterinary patient, recently the value of CVP has been questioned. While currently controversial, many clinicians still consider CVP a valuable tool and, therefore, we will focus on it here.

> *TECHNICIAN NOTE* Right atrial pressure is a good indicator of vascular volume, so CVP is useful for monitoring fluid therapy in hypovolemic patients or in patients at risk for volume overload.

INDICATIONS

Indications for CVP measurement include monitoring fluid therapy in patients that may be hypovolemic, such as in the following cases:
- Patients that have experienced trauma
- Patients with gastric dilation volvulus
- Patients with hemoabdomen

CVP measurement may also be indicated for monitoring patients at risk of volume overload such as in the following cases:
- Patients with preexisting heart disease that require IV fluid therapy
- Patients with right ventricular congestive heart failure
- Patients requiring high-volume IV fluid diuresis

EQUIPMENT

To measure CVP a central venous catheter must be placed in either the jugular, the femoral, or the saphenous vein. When placing a jugular catheter, the tip must be positioned at the entrance to the right atrium. For femoral or saphenous catheters, the tip must be positioned within the intrathoracic caudal vena cava, as close to the heart as possible. If the catheter tip is proximal to either of these locations, then the measurements do not accurately reflect pressures in the right atrium.

CVP measurements can be obtained using either a water manometer or an electronic pressure transducer. Water manometers are sold as disposable kits and usually consist of a clear plastic column that is marked in centimeters. Alternatively, a piece of plastic tubing can be taped to the wall of the cage with a metric ruler next to it for a "homemade" water manometer. The manometer is connected to the central venous catheter by extension tubing and a three-way stopcock. The setup is filled with heparinized saline from a syringe or fluid bag attached to the three-way stopcock. Vitamin B complex can be added to the fluids for better visualization of the fluid column. Single measurements are taken with a water manometer. Electronic pressure transducers are usually part of multiparameter monitors but may be standalone monitors as well. These monitors are attached to the patient's catheter using special extension tubing and the transducer. A display screen shows a pressure waveform and gives a continuous readout of the CVP.

TECHNIQUE

For all techniques, a freely flowing catheter without occlusions is essential. The patient must be in the same position for each reading to allow the technician to compare readings and record patient position at each measurement. Lateral recumbency is preferred because the zero point will never change, but sternal recumbency can also be used. A reference or zero point must be established by one of two methods. In the most widely used method, the three-way stopcock and bottom of the manometer are positioned at the level of the right atrium to establish a zero point. This level is at the height of the manubrium in a lateral patient or at the scapulohumeral joint with the patient in sternal recumbency. The manometer may be taped in place on the wall of the cage so that the reference point is kept constant. Alternatively, the manometer and stopcock may be held on a stable surface next to the down shoulder in a lateral patient or the elbows in a sternal patient (Figure 2-21). An imaginary line from the level of the right atrium to the manometer is drawn, and the value in centimeters to which this corresponds is set as the zero point and recorded for use in subsequent measurements. This value is subtracted from the final measurement to give an absolute CVP measurement.

To obtain a measurement using a water manometer, the stopcock is turned off to the patient and the manometer is filled with saline. The stopcock is then turned off

to the fluid bag or syringe, and the fluid level is allowed to equilibrate with the patient. The level of the meniscus is the CVP. This level will fluctuate with respiration because this changes intrathoracic pressure.

When using an electronic pressure transducer, a reference point is also established by placing the transducer in a set location. This may vary depending on the system used. Once the setup is in place, it can be left connected to the patient for continuous readout. The system and catheter should be flushed with heparinized saline every 4 to 6 hours or as directed by the manufacturer.

TROUBLESHOOTING

Inaccurate readings will be obtained if the following occur:

- Kinking or thrombi occlude the catheter.
- The tip of the catheter is not appropriately placed.
- The catheter is moved in or out of the vessel during readings.
- The reference point is not kept constant during readings.
- Patient positioning changes during readings.

INTERPRETATION

Normal CVP ranges from 0 to 10 cm of water (Farry, 2012). Values less than this suggest hypovolemia, and values greater than 10 cm of water suggest volume overload. Serial measurements are more useful to gauge response to therapy and trends in intravascular volume than are single numbers. Frequency of measurements depends on the stability of the patient and the potential for rapid deterioration. For example, a patient that has oliguric renal failure and is being given IV fluids may need CVP readings hourly to detect early signs of volume overload. Serial CVP measurements are often useful to guide treatment decisions in unstable patients. For example, the administration of IV fluid volumes can be tailored to responses in the CVP in a patient with traumatic hypovolemic shock.

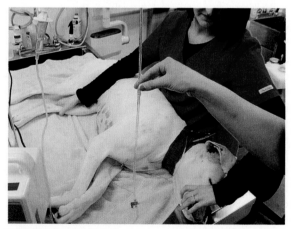

FIGURE 2-21 Central venous pressure measurement with dog in lateral recumbency.

MULTIPARAMETER MONITORING EQUIPMENT

Monitors are available that combine most of the functions discussed previously. These multiparameter monitors either are created for human medical applications and adapted for veterinary use or are designed specifically for the veterinary market.

The monitors can be purchased either in basic configurations (usually ECG, SpO_2, and noninvasive blood pressure [NIBP]) or as fully optioned monitors including the preceding measurements plus two IBP ports, temperature, capnography, and gas inhalant concentration. These monitors are often intended as anesthesia monitors but are useful for emergency and critical patients in other settings (Figure 2-22).

Combination monitors provide at-a-glance information about many body systems all on one screen, occupy less shelf or storage space than separate monitors, and often add features that may not be available when separate monitors are used (e.g., continuous core temperature readings). Disadvantages include cost, and certain features may not be as well adapted to veterinary species as others. For example, the pulse oximetry sensors included on some monitors may not be sized appropriately for veterinary patients. Additionally, combination monitors that provide noninvasive BP monitoring use oscillometric technology that may not function appropriately for very small patients.

When considering purchase of a combination monitor, it is important to decide which features will be useful for the practice and investigate the technology of each feature. Consider units that have been validated for veterinary patients, rather than humans. Warranty and service contracts are also important variables. Besides the equipment issues previously mentioned, warm-up time and calibration needs may affect a monitor's usefulness in an emergency situation and make it more suitable to the relatively controlled situation of an anesthetized patient.

The combination monitors can be mounted on a pole for portability or placed on a shelf for ease of monitoring.

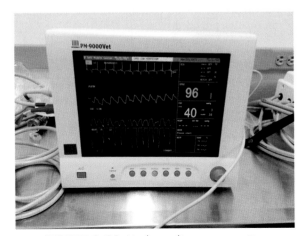

FIGURE 2-22 Mindray multiparameter monitor.

The technique of use and troubleshooting is similar to that mentioned in each monitoring section of this chapter.

MANUFACTURERS OF EQUIPMENT LISTED IN THE TEXT

Blood Gas, Chemistry, Hematology POC Analyzers
Vet Lab Station, Vet Stat, Catalyst, Lasercyte, Idexx Laboratories, Westbrook, ME

Lactate POC Analyzer
Lactate Scout, EFK Diagnostics, San Antonio, TX
Lacate Pro, faCT Canada Consulting, Quesnel, Canada

Osmometer
Wescor 4400 Colloid Osmometer, Wescor Inc., Logan, UT

Coagulation Testing Equipment
Coag Dx, Idexx Laboratories, Westbrook, ME
Surgicutt, International Technidyne Corp., Edison, NJ

Blood Pressure Monitoring Equipment
Dinamap Veterinary Blood Pressure Monitor, Critikon Incorp., Tampa, FL
Doppler Ultrasound, Parks Medical Electronics, Aloha, OR

Multifunction Monitors
Midray Medical, Mahwah, NJ
Cardell Monitors, Sharn Veterinary Incorp., Tampa, FL
Advisor Vital Signs Mutiparameter Monitor, Surgivet, Waukesha, WI

REFERENCES

Anthony E, Sirois M: Hematology and hemostasis. In Hendrix CM, Sirois M, editors: *Laboratory procedures for veterinary technicians*, ed 5. St Louis, 2007, Elsevier Mosby, p 35.

Brown S, Atkins C, Bagley R, et al.: Guidelines for identification, evaluation, and management of systemic hypertension in dogs and cats, *J Vet Intern Med* 21:542–558, June 2007.

Casal ML, Bentz AI: Neonatal care of the puppy, kitten and foal. In Bassert JM, Thomas JA, editors: *McCurnin's clinical textbook for veterinary technicians*, ed 8, St Louis, 2014, Elsevier, p 791.

Cornell College of Veterinary Medicine, Hematology Atlas. Available at https://www.eclinpath.com/hemostasis/tests/platelet-number/. Accessed Jan 2014.

Farry T: Monitoring the critical patient. In Norkus CL, editor: *Veterinary technician's manual for small animal emergency and critical care*. Ames, Iowa, 2012, Wiley-Blackwell, p 74.

Hackner S: Hematological emergencies. In King L, Hammond R, editors: *Manual of canine and feline emergency and critical care*, Shurdington, 1999, British Small Animal Veterinary Association, p 155.

Jack CM, Watson PM, Donovan MS, editors: *Veterinary technician's daily reference guide: Canine and feline*, ed 2, Ames, Iowa, Blackwell Publishing, pp 105–107.

Mathews KA: *Veterinary emergency and critical care manual*, ed 2, vol. 745. Guelph, Ontario, 2006, LifeLearn. 400–402.

OPK Biotech: Oxyglobin general interference with clinical chemistry laboratory analysis. Available at www.oxyglobin.com/laboratory_interference.php. Accessed Nov 2013.

Sorrell-Raschi L: Blood gas and oximetry monitoring. In Silverstein DC, Hopper K, editors: *Small animal critical care medicine*, St Louis, 2009, Elsevier Mosby, pp 878–882.

Stockham SL, Dolce KS: Glucose. In Cowell RL, editor: *Veterinary clinical pathology secrets*, St Louis, 2004, Elsevier Mosby, p 191.

Waddell LS: Colloid osmotic pressure and osmolality. In Silverstein DC, Hopper K, editors: *Small animal critical care medicine*, St Louis, 2009, Elsevier Mosby, pp 868–871.

Wamsley HL, Alleman AR: Physical and chemical aspects of urinalysis. In Cowell RL, editor: *Veterinary clinical pathology secrets*. St Louis, 2004, Elsevier Mosby, p 148.

ADDITIONAL READINGS

e-Clin Path On-line textbook: Cornell College of Veterinary Medicine. Available at https://www.eclinpath.com/. Accessed Dec 2014.

Ford RB, Mazzaferro EM: *Kirk and Bistner's handbook of veterinary procedures and emergency treatment*, ed 9, St Louis, 2012, Elsevier.

Mathers KA: *Veterinary emergency and critical care manual*, ed 2, Guelph, Ontario, 2006, LifeLearn.

Norkus CL: *Veterinary technician's manual for small animal emergency and critical care*, Ames, Iowa, 2012, Wiley.

Silverstein DC, Hopper K: *Small animal critical care medicine*, St Louis, 2009, Elsevier.

Wingfield WE, Raffe MR: *The veterinary ICU book*, Jackson, Wyo, 2002, Teton NewMedia.

SCENARIO

Purpose: To provide the veterinary technician the opportunity to build or strengthen his/her understanding of how the patient's monitoring parameters demonstrate the patient's response to treatment.

Stage: Busy emergency and referral clinic staffed with one emergency clinician, two veterinary technicians, one veterinary assistant, and one receptionist.

Scenario

Tuesday evening 6:30 PM.

Patient: 6-year-old, SF Doberman Pinscher HBC presents to clinic. The owner walks the dog into the clinic on a leash. Initial assessment indicates the dog has bright pink mucous membranes, CRT <1 sec; she is slightly tachycardic and has road rash on her abdomen. The owner is concerned about money and only consents to doing what is absolutely necessary to saving the dog's life. A PCV/TP is drawn and is 45% and 6.8 g/dl, respectively. A cephalic IV catheter is placed and the dog is started on IV LRS at twice the maintenance rate and is hospitalized for observation and pain control as needed. One hour later the dog's mucous membrane color is pale pink, CRT >2 sec; and her cranial abdomen appears distended and is painful.

Delivery

Write your initial concerns about this patient and how you would monitor this patient. Include monitoring parameters, frequency, and trends that you expect to develop if the patient is responding appropriately to treatment.

Write additional monitoring parameters that should be checked at 1-hour postpresentation and explain why it is important to determining how this dog is responding to treatment.

Discussion

- Compare and discuss your answers with your partner. If there are differences, present your reasoning to your partner and develop a monitoring plan that you both find appropriate.
- Additional monitoring details may be provided to the participants so they can evaluate how the patient is responding to treatment based on how the scenario continues to evolve.
- The discussion should continue with the additional information provided.

Key Teaching Points

- This exercise provides the veterinary technician the opportunity to consider an emergency case in a nonthreatening and nonemergency situation.
- The veterinary technician can evaluate his/her ability to assess how a patient is responding to therapy and make additional recommendations based on his/her findings.

MEDICAL MATH EXERCISES

You have a patient that weighs 32 lb. How much urine would you expect him to produce over the next 24 hr? (Your answer should be a range.)

Patient's Lifeline: Intravenous Catheter

Andrea M. Battaglia and Julie Hirsch-Fitzpatrick

CHAPTER OUTLINE

Types of Intravenous Catheters
The Anatomy of the Multi-Lumen Catheter Kit
Choosing the Right Catheter
  Material
  Size
Vascular Access Points
Placement
Prevention and Management of Complications During Placement
Stabilization

Peripheral Catheters
Jugular Catheter
Intraosseous Catheterization
Challenges
  Specific Breeds
  Neonates
  Fractious Feline And Cantankerous Canine
  Collapsed Vascular System and Other Challenges
Maintenance

KEY TERMS

Central line
Intraosseous
Jugular
Multi-lumen catheter
Venous access

LEARNING OBJECTIVES

After studying this chapter, you will be able to:

- Introduce many types of IV catheters.
- Discuss different placement techniques used in veterinary medicine.
- Understand the limitations and all access points for venous access.
- Prevent infection of intravenous catheters.

In the critically ill or injured small animal patient, an IV catheter must be properly placed and secured to function properly. It can be used to introduce drug and fluid therapies, blood products, and nutrition. The IV catheter can also be used to obtain multiple blood samples from a patient. This reduces the stress for the animal by avoiding frequent venipuncture and saves the technician time by providing a readily available port for blood sampling without the need for assistance.

Small animal patients in an emergency or critical care unit have diverse needs. Accessible vessels, size, species, and clinical presentation vary. The veterinary technician must become familiar with the various types and sizes of IV catheters available, the common **venous access** points on the animal, and the various procedures for placing IV catheters.

TYPES OF INTRAVENOUS CATHETERS

Many types of IV catheters are available. Through-the-needle catheter units and over-the-needle catheters are most commonly used in veterinary practice. Animals requiring long-term fluid therapy, drug therapy, or both will benefit from peripherally inserted central catheters (PICCs) or **multi-lumen catheters**.

Through-the-needle catheters usually are placed in the jugular vessels but also can be placed in the medial saphenous vein on cats and in the medial and lateral saphenous veins on dogs (Figure 3-1). This type of catheter is most commonly available in 8- and 12-inch lengths and is 18 or 20 gauge.

The over-the-needle catheters usually are placed in peripheral vessels but can also be used in the **jugular** vessels of smaller patients, including neonates. They are available in multiple gauges and lengths, ranging from 10 to 24 gauge in diameter and ¾ to 5½ inches in length.

THE ANATOMY OF THE MULTI-LUMEN CATHETER KIT

Multi-lumen catheters are available for delivering multiple fluid or drug therapies. Incompatible solutions can be administered simultaneously through this type of catheter. The lumens have separate entrance and exit ports to prevent any mixing of compounds. It is still important to understand the pharmacokinetics of the drugs being used to determine which drug is infused through the distal port. Some drugs will change the pH of the environment, which can inactivate or change other drug's action within the body.

Multi-lumen catheters are available in double, triple, or quadruple varieties, with a large selection of lengths and sizes. These catheters are placed using a guide-wire or an introducer that peels or detaches. Arrow International® manufactures the Twin catheter. It is a double-lumen catheter with an over-the-needle introduction design; these work very well in the peripheral vessels.

Antimicrobial impregnated central venous catheters are used most commonly in humans. These catheters are coated with minocycline and rifampin or chlorhexidine and silver sulfadiazine. They significantly reduce the microbial colonization and blood-stream infection that can occur with long-term indwelling catheter use in humans. The cost effectiveness of the catheters must be considered and used in a minority of human patients. Antimicrobial-impregnated central venous catheters are available as single-lumen or multi-lumen catheters in a variety of lengths and gauges. A guide-wire or sheath that detaches is used for introduction.

The multi-lumen catheter has two to four ports within one line and is available in various lengths to accommodate the need for central venous access. The cross section diagram illustrates how the lumens are designed to provide the option to deliver incompatible fluid therapies (Figure 3-2). The lumens will be different gauges and depend on how many lumens are chosen within the chosen catheter. Many companies design the catheters and it is important to determine what will meet your patient's

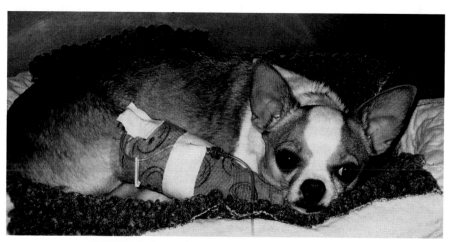

FIGURE 3-1 Long line in lateral saphenous vessel of a dog.

needs. It is recommended to have an assortment of sizes to provide the correct size for the patient.

Each lumen will have a specific priming volume and should be noted on the package insert. It is important to note the priming volume to avoid boluses of concentrated drugs that can be administered through the ports. The estimated volume for some extensions on the catheter is 0.02 ml of fluid/cm of catheter.

The ports on the multi-lumen catheters are color-coded to indicate the position of the ports on the distal end of the catheter. It is also helpful to the user to use the color code to determine the fluids or drugs that are attached to each port. The catheters are also marked with a black line or point to indicate the number of centimeters being advanced into the patient.

The guide-wire's primary purpose is to provide a pathway into the vascular system that allows the advancement of other catheters. Most wires have an anti-friction coating and are marked with a black line to assist in determining the number of centimeters advanced. There is a straight soft tip on one end and the J-tip on the other. The J-tip assists the correct central venous catheterization towards the right atrium during right subclavian catheterization in humans. It may be necessary to use the straight end of the wire in small or hypovolemic patients. It can be difficult to feed the catheter over the J-tip, but do not cut the wire. It is a braided wire and will unravel.

The tissue dilator is usually made out of rigid Teflon. This dilator is used to open the vessel for ease of passage of the catheter. The dilator can also be advanced to the hub, with the wire removed if the patient requires an immediate fluid or drug bolus. Once the patient is re-stabilized, the wire is passed to transfer the long-term, multi-lumen catheter.

Vascular access ports were introduced in the 1980s and were used most commonly in research animals and in people receiving chemotherapy. Universities and veterinary referral centers have found them to be very beneficial for patients on long-term cancer chemotherapy and for patients with chronic renal failure who need long-term fluid therapy.

The port is surgically placed subcutaneously. The catheter is surgically placed into the jugular vessel inserted into the port. The catheters are most commonly polyurethane or silicone; the ports are made of metal or plastic. The port has an inner diameter (septum) where injections are performed. This port can be located easily by palpating the septum and is accessed by puncture with a noncoring needle after the area is aseptically prepped. To avoid damaging the port, the technician should use only the needles recommended by the manufacturer.

Vascular ports are available in a variety of sizes, and single- and dual-chamber ports are available (Figure 3-3).

CHOOSING THE RIGHT CATHETER

MATERIAL

Critically ill small animals commonly need an IV catheter long term. It is necessary to be aware of the animal's treatment plan to choose the most appropriate catheter type.

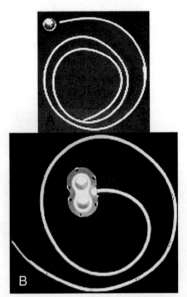

FIGURE 3-3 Vascular access ports. **A,** Single-chambered vascular access port. **B,** Dual-chambered vascular access port.

Cross Section of the Multi-Lumen Catheter

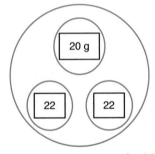

FIGURE 3-2 Cross-sectional diagram of multi-lumen catheter.

A variety of compounds are used to make indwelling catheters. Polyvinyl chloride, polyethylene, polypropylene, polyurethane, silicone elastomer (Silastic), tetrafluoroethylene (TFE, Teflon), fluoroethylenepropylene (FEP, Teflon), elastomeric hydrogel, and blends of these materials (e.g., Vialon, a polyurethane blend) are the most common. Some compounds are more reactive than others (depending on the type and rigidity of the compound). Researchers believe that leaching of plasticizers and stabilizing agents may contribute to the adverse reactions some animals have to catheters.

Catheters manufactured from silicone and polyurethane are less thrombogenic than those consisting of other materials. Catheters made of polyvinyl chloride, polypropylene, and polyethylene are the most reactive.

SIZE

The preferred gauge and length of catheter used in a patient depend on the purpose of the IV catheter and the size of the patient. Critically ill patients often need large volumes of fluids. Therefore the technician would use the largest-gauge catheter that can be placed.

Catheter length is very important in animals needing central venous pressure monitoring, a procedure used to monitor fluid therapy. Selecting the correct length can be estimated by performing measurements first. The points to include are the initial point of insertion of the catheter (mid-jugular vein) to the second rib space. The distal end of the catheter is placed cranial to the right atrium (Figure 3-4). In the cat or small dog, the technician can access the caudal vena cava by placing a catheter in the medial saphenous vessel. Radiographs should be taken

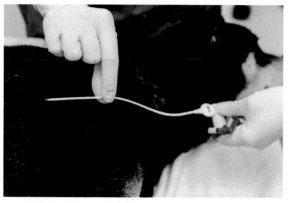

FIGURE 3-4 Measuring for correct length of catheter.

to confirm proper placement when using the catheter for central venous pressure monitoring purposes.

VASCULAR ACCESS POINTS

The best vascular access point to use on the small animal patient depends on many factors. The treatment plan, accessibility, and underlying disease process are the primary concerns.

For example, an animal with severe coagulopathies should not have a catheter placed in the jugular vein if avoidable because of the potential for uncontrolled hemorrhage around the insertion site. Traumatized limbs attributable to fractures, open wounds, or surgical wounds are painful and routinely require bandage changes. These locations should be avoided.

Cats with thromboembolism should not have catheters placed in either of their pelvic limbs.

It is also important to consider how the location of catheter placement will be maintained. Patients that are vomiting should ideally have their catheters placed in the lateral or medial saphenous vessels or jugular, and patients that have diarrhea or urinary incontinence should be placed in cephalic vessels or jugular.

The most common access points are the cephalic, lateral saphenous, medial saphenous, and jugular veins.

The jugular vessels are the best site if a patient needs prolonged fluid therapy or if multiple blood samples must be drawn. In a patient that may require an esophagostomy tube placement in the future, consider using the right jugular when possible, because an E-tube is normally placed on the left side.

Peripherally inserted central catheters (PICCs) are available for those situations when a **central line** is necessary but the jugular vessel is not an option for access. Long lines should be avoided in the animals that may be hypercoagulable because of the risk of intravascular clotting.

PLACEMENT

Correct placement of IV catheter units entails an understanding of catheter mechanics. All materials, including the catheter unit, heparinized saline, sterile bandage to cover the insertion site, and the materials needed to stabilize the unit, are readily available. *There are some studies suggesting heparinized saline is not necessary to maintain short catheters placed in peripheral vessels and*

in some cases is contraindicated. It is important that it is decided what the standard will be in the individual hospital.

Commercially available topical anesthetics such as lidocaine/prilocaine, 4% liposomal lidocaine cream, and amethocaine gel have been shown to provide some pain relief during catheter placement. This is not an option for emergent situations because it requires up to 1 hour for full affect and up to 15 minutes for partial relief once the topical anesthetic is applied. The cream is placed on the shaved skin and the area is covered with a bio-occlusive dressing before placement is attempted. Subcutaneous lidocaine blocks can be used as well and are most commonly used when the guide-wire technique is performed.

It is recommended the hospital initiates a "2 strikes you are out" rule to avoid having one person attempt venipuncture multiple times. It allows a fresh approach to a difficult placement.

A complete sterile prep is performed with complete removal of hair and scrub using a chlorhexidine-based solution. Some patients may have sensitivity to a scrub and it is important to research ingredients to confirm they are inert and safe for all species (Figure 3-5).

Placing over-the-needle catheters involves a four-step process after the site is shaved and surgically scrubbed. If the catheter is being placed in a limb, then

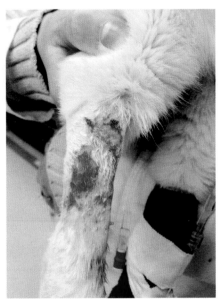

FIGURE 3-5 Reaction to scrub on leg of feline.

it is important to create a sterile field in which to work. This is accomplished by wrapping a sterile bandage around the distal portion of the catheter site. It is best to attempt placement as distal as possible, always keeping in mind the patient's conformation. The unit is placed into the vessel. Once a flashback is observed, the entire unit is advanced into the vein slightly to ensure that the stylet is placed in the vessel properly. The catheter is then advanced off the stylet into the vein. The stylet must be stabilized and not allowed to advance with the catheter. If this is not done the stylet can shear the end of the catheter. The stylet is then removed and the catheter is capped and flushed with heparinized saline (unless IV fluid therapy is started immediately through this catheter).

> **TECHICIAN NOTE** Once the stylet is removed from the catheter, it cannot be reinserted. This is a very risky maneuver and can cause shearing of the catheter.

Placing a catheter into the jugular vessel is a team effort. The person restraining and positioning the animal must work with the person placing the catheter. The animal usually is placed in lateral recumbence for this procedure, with the neck extended. A rolled towel placed under the neck can assist in visualizing the vessel. It may be necessary to try different angles of the head and extensions of the neck before the vessel can be visualized or palpated. A cat's vessels can be palpated and visualized easily when the neck is extended and the head rotated outward.

Placing obese animals or breeds with thick necks in a sitting position, with the head slightly elevated and turned away from the venipuncture site, facilitates access to the jugular vessel.

Box 3-1 illustrates a six-step process that involves the use of a peel-away sheath needle.

Box 3-2 illustrates a six-step process called the guide-wire technique (also called the Seldinger technique). An introducer (hypodermic needle), stylet, dilator, and catheter are used.

Box 3-3 illustrates a six-step process that involves the use of a catheter placement unit (through-the-needle catheter) that is contained in a sterile covering.

Box 3-4 describes a technique that uses a feeding tube and an over-the-needle catheter.

BOX 3-1 | Technical Tip: Peel-Away Sheath Technique

Items needed:

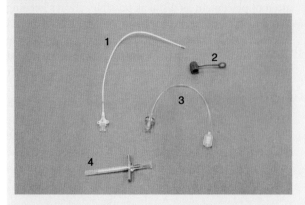

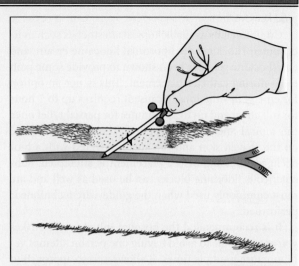

- Items for prepping, drape, and sterile surgical gloves
- #11 surgical blade
- Peel-away sheath introducer with catheter
- Heparinized saline
- Injection cap with extension line
- Materials needed for stabilization

1. Shave and surgically prep the site. Drape around the site. Sterile surgical gloves must be worn. Perform a small skin nick incision using surgical blade.
2. Insert the over-the-needle sheath through the small nick in the skin into the vessel.

3. Advance the needle sheath slightly to ensure that the sheath and the needle are seated in the vessel.
4. Stabilize the needle and advance the sheath (slightly rotating it back and forth) into the vessel.

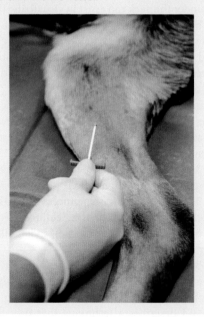

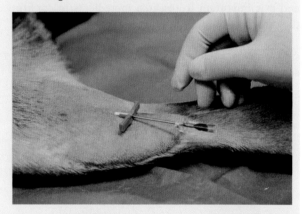

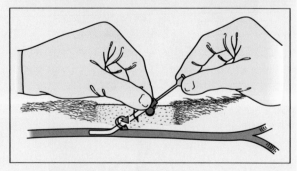

BOX 3-1 | Technical Tip: Peel-Away Sheath Technique—cont'd

5. Remove the needle and place a finger over the opening to prevent excessive hemorrhage or air embolus.

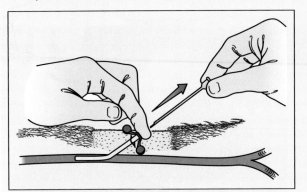

6. Insert the catheter through sheath.

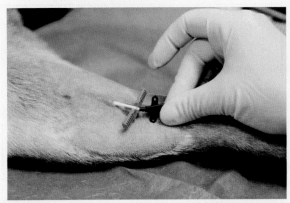

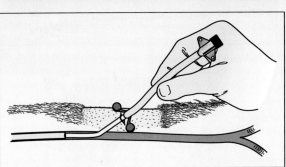

7. Cap and aspirate to remove air and until blood fills port.

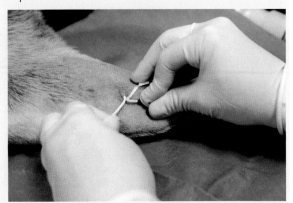

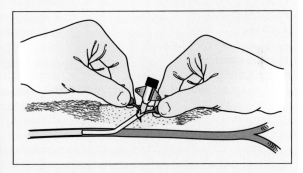

8. Flush the catheter with heparinized saline. Pull up and out on the tabs of the sheath. Slight hemorrhaging will occur around the site.

Gloves and surgical drapes were omitted from illustrations so that positioning of hands and catheter could be shown. Gloves must be worn and a sterile field provided.

BOX 3-2 | Technical Tip: Guide-Wire (Seldinger) Technique

Items needed:

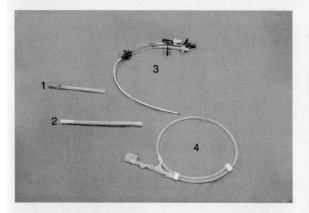

- Items for prepping, drape, and sterile surgical gloves
- #11 surgical blade
- Guide-wire
- Dilator
- Polyurethane IV catheter
- Heparinized saline
- Injection cap with extension line
- Materials for stabilization including sterile gauze

Shave and surgically prep the site. Drape around the site. Self-adhering disposable drapes are available or surgical drapes can be used. Sterile surgical gloves must be worn and surgical mask and gown suggested. Long hair is secure with a hair tie or surgical cap is worn. Maintain sterility throughout the procedure.

1. Perform a small nick incision using the surgical blade.
2. Insert the IV catheter into the vessel.

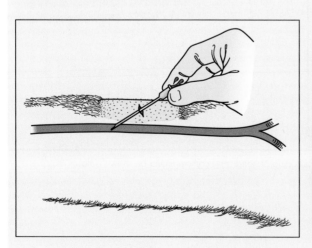

3. Place guide wire into vessel through the catheter (or needle if used as the introducer). For smaller animals, cats, and dehydrated patients, insert the straight end first.

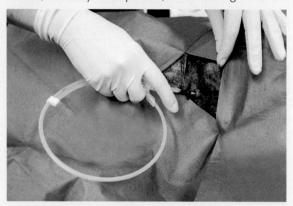

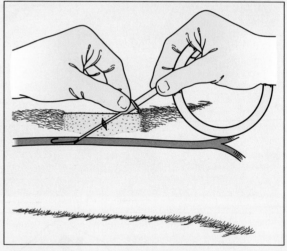

4. Remove the catheter from the vessel and off the wire.

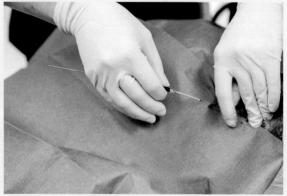

BOX 3-2 | Technical Tip: Guide-Wire (Seldinger) Technique—cont'd

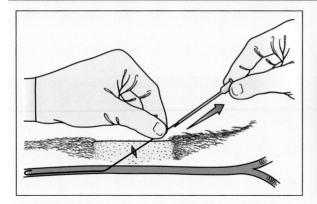

5. Place a dilator over the wire and into the initial insertion point. Rotate back and forth to facilitate insertion. Insert about 50% of the dilator, and then remove it. If the patient's status deteriorates suddenly, then this dilator can be inserted all the way, the wire can be removed, and fluid therapy can begin. After stabilization occurs, the wire can be reinserted, the dilator removed, and a long-term catheter placed.

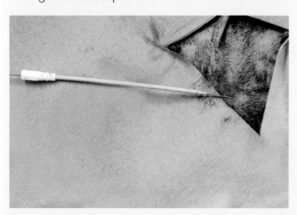

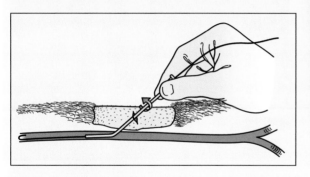

6. Place the IV catheter over the wire and into the vessel.

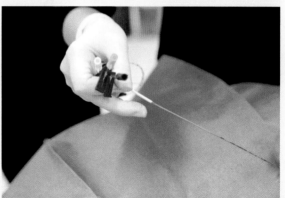

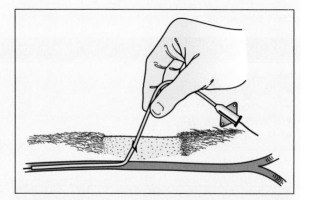

7. Remove the wire, clamping the extension before the wire is completely removed to prevent air embolus and cap the catheter. The air is withdrawn using a sterile needle and syringe. Once air is removed and blood has filled the port, flush it with heparinized saline.

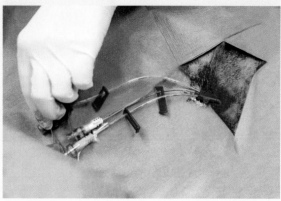

Continued

| **BOX 3-2** | Technical Tip: Guide-Wire (Seldinger) Technique—cont'd |

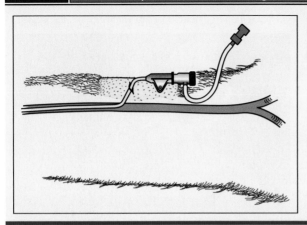

Gloves and surgical drapes were omitted from illustrations so that positioning of hands and catheter could be shown. Gloves must be worn and a sterile field provided.

| **BOX 3-3** | Technical Tip: Through-the-Needle Catheter Unit |

Items needed:
- Through-the-needle catheter unit
- Injection cap with extension line
- Heparinized saline
- Materials for stabilization

1. Insert needle through the skin and into the vessel.

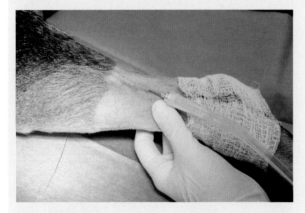

2. Advance the catheter into the vessel and lock it into the needle hub.

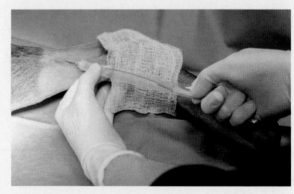

3. Remove the needle from the site.

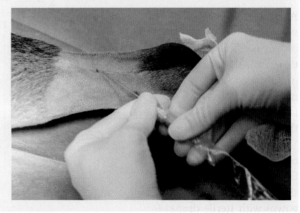

BOX 3-3	Technical Tip: Through-the-Needle Catheter Unit—cont'd

4. Place the needle guard over the needle.

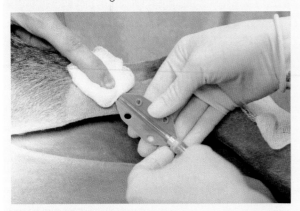

5. Apply pressure to the insertion site and remove the stylet.

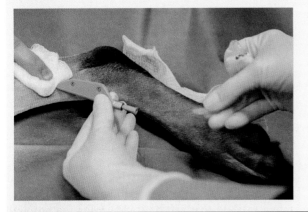

6. Aspirate to remove air from the catheter until blood is aspirated.
7. Cap and flush the catheter.

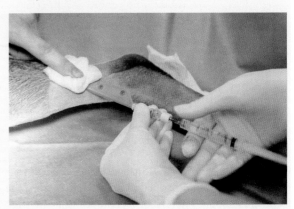

PREVENTION AND MANAGEMENT OF COMPLICATIONS DURING PLACEMENT

A complete sterile prep of the site is necessary to prevent catheter-related infections. A generous amount of hair is clipped away from the site. It is important to use clean, sharp, clipper blades to avoid clipper burns or cuts. Long-haired breeds will have their feathers removed from their limbs to prevent contamination. It is important to mention this to owners so they understand the reasons behind the removal of hair.

Maximal sterile barrier precautions are also highly recommended as deemed appropriate at your hospital. Consistent protocols should be followed. Studies have shown that the use of sterile gloves, masks, caps, and gowns with sterile drapes for the guide-wire technique has greatly reduced the rate of catheter infections in humans (Figure 3-6).

Air embolism has been reported to occur in humans during placement of central venous catheters using the guide-wire technique or peel-away sheaths as an introducer. This can occur when there is a negative central venous pressure and access to the central circulation through an open, unsealed catheter. It has been recommended while completing step 7 (see Box 3-2) when the guide-wire is removed, the extension tubing, once the wire passes a few centimeters out of port, should be clamped before the entire wire is withdrawn. The port is capped immediately once the wire is removed, the clamp is released, and air is withdrawn by aspirating using a needle attached to a syringe until blood fills the port. The syringe filled with air is removed and the port

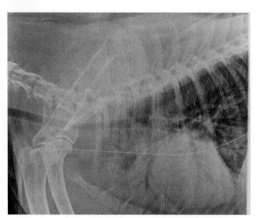

FIGURE 3-6 Guide-wire released accidently.

flushed with heparinized saline. Although this complication has not been described in veterinary patients, the technician should implement techniques to avoid possible air embolism.

If a peel-away sheath is being used as an introducer, it is very important that the person performing the technique places his/her finger immediately over the open sheath until he/she is able to feed the catheter into the vessel. This will prevent the sheath from being left open to air and will decrease blood loss.

When performing the guide-wire technique the proximal end of the wire is always held by the person performing this technique until the distal tip is completely out of the vessel. This will prevent the risk of having the wire pulled into the vascular system. If this complication happens, use of interventional radiology techniques is the preferred method for retrieval and removal.

If uncontrolled hemorrhage occurs during the placement of a catheter into the jugular vessel, surgically ligating the vessel may be necessary.

STABILIZATION

Once the catheter is in place, it must be stabilized properly. The wrap should provide additional catheter stabilization, increase patient comfort, and protect the insertion site. Multilayered wraps should be avoided in patients receiving cancer chemotherapy intravenously. The area above the insertion site should remain uncovered so that it can be checked frequently throughout the treatment period.

The other disadvantage of multilayer wraps is that they can retain moisture. Transparent, semipermeable

---

BOX 3-4	Technical Tip: Using an Over-the-Needle Catheter Unit and Feeding Tube for Jugular Catheter Placement

Items needed:
- 14-gauge over-the-needle catheter with a 5-French feeding tube or 16-gauge over-the-needle catheter with a 3.5-French feeding tube*
- Injection cap with heparinized saline
- Materials for stabilization

Before performing this technique, confirm that the materials are compatible. Some catheters are tapered differently on the distal end, and feeding tubes cannot pass through them.
1. Shave and surgically prep the site.
2. Insert a 14-gauge over-the-needle catheter through the skin, into the vessel.
3. Advance the catheter off the stylet into the vessel.
4. Introduce a 5-French feeding tube through the catheter, into the vessel. A drop of 50% dextrose at the catheter hub may facilitate feeding tube introduction.
5. Cap and flush the catheter with heparinized saline. Remove the over-the-needle catheter from the vessel up to the initial insertion point. Loop the line and stabilize it to the patient.

*For smaller patients, a 16-gauge over-the-needle catheter with a 3.5-French feeding tube can be used.

dressings are ideal but many times are not sufficient support for our small animal patients.

The following methods have been successfully used by the authors; however, it is important to incorporate a method that can be standard for the hospital. Following an established guideline can help minimize complications.

PERIPHERAL CATHETERS

Two ½-inch-wide pieces of tape, long enough to encircle the leg, are used for initial stabilization. The first is placed at the base of the hub. Tabs should be created on either side of the hub and the tape should be wrapped firmly around the leg. The second piece is placed, adhesive up, under the catheter, with equal lengths of tape on either side. It is crisscrossed around the catheter and wrapped around the leg. Tissue glue can be used to further stabilize the catheter. A small drop on either side of the hub is sufficient. Some animals may have a severe tissue reaction to the ingredients in tissue glue and, therefore, it should be used sparingly. This technique is very useful for active patients (especially fractious cats) or when quick stabilization is necessary.

A sterile gauze pad or a sterile adhesive bandage is placed over the catheter insertion site. Cast padding is placed underneath the proximal portion of the hub to create padding between the leg and the catheter. It is wrapped around the leg to provide additional support.

Rolled gauze is used for additional support and for securing extended injection ports. Adhesive wrap (Vetwrap® or Elastikon® works well) can then be used to cover the entire bandage. Injection ports should always remain uncovered for quick venous access. Occasionally, it is necessary to extend the wrap to the toes to assist circulation. Cats usually need this extended wrap.

JUGULAR CATHETER

For a through-the-needle type of jugular catheter, three pieces of tape long enough to encircle the patient's neck are needed for initial stabilization. The first piece is split 2 inches down the middle and placed so that the small strips are positioned along either side of the catheter. It is wrapped around the neck, incorporating the small strips for the final connection. The other pieces are placed on either side of the catheter and wrapped around the neck. (For additional stabilization, a piece of tape with tabs placed at the base of the catheter or needle guard and a drop of tissue glue [or sutures] is put on each tab of the butterfly so that it adheres to the neck. This is done before the tape is placed.) Cast padding is placed over the tape to provide additional support. Rolled gauze is placed over the cast padding. Adhesive wrap is applied to secure the entire bandage to the patient's neck. It is very important to check the tightness of the bandage around the neck after each layer is placed. If the patient shows any signs of discomfort or difficulty breathing, then the bandage should be removed immediately and rewrapped more loosely, using less material. Leashes should be placed around the shoulder, or a harness can be used (Figures 3-7 and 3-8).

Multi-lumen catheters have a hub with holes for suture material. Once the catheter hub is sutured in place, the insertion site should be covered with a sterile dressing such as a clear bio-occlusive dressing (such as Tegaderm™), or sterile adhesive bandage, before a light wrap is applied following the same layering procedure as mentioned previously.

Through-the-needle catheters that are placed in the lateral saphenous veins of dogs can be secured using the following technique. The catheter is withdrawn ½ inch

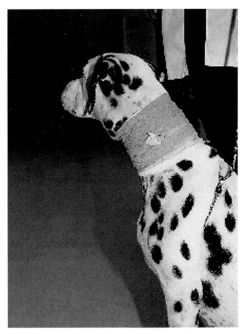

FIGURE 3-7 Leash should be placed around shoulder to prevent additional stress to jugular catheter site.

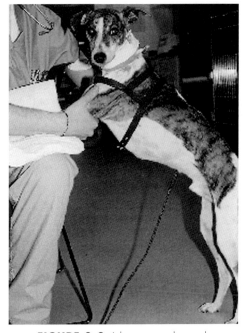

FIGURE 3-8 A harness can be used.

and the needle guard is placed pointing upward. A small piece of tape is placed on the catheter loop, with tabs on either side. The tabs are secured to the leg with tissue glue. This prevents the catheter from dislodging. Tape is used to secure the needle guard to the leg. A piece of cast padding is placed between the needle guard and the leg to provide a cushion. A sterile adhesive bandage or bio-occlusive dressing is again placed over the insertion site; then the entire needle guard and catheter site can then be wrapped. Rolled gauze is used for more stabilization. Then adhesive wrap is placed over the entire bandage.

Through-the-needle catheters placed in the medial saphenous veins of cats or small dogs can be secured using the following method (the patient remains in lateral recumbence for this step). The catheter is pulled out far enough to loop around the stifle. Two inches usually is sufficient. (When the catheter is looped out, bleeding should be expected.) A piece of tape is placed around the catheter (with tabs on either side), and tissue glue is used for further stabilization. A sterile gauze pad is placed at the insertion site, with tape to keep it in place, or sterile adhesive bandage or bio-occlusive dressing may be used. The patient is turned over carefully. The needle guard is placed along the lateral aspect of the patient's thigh and secured with tape. The catheter is secured using the same method and materials as previously mentioned.

Catheters placed in the medial aspect of the leg can also be wrapped without looping the catheter and leaving the needle guard on the medial side of the leg. The advantages of this method are less manipulation of the patient and a decreased risk of dislodging the catheter. The disadvantage (especially in cats) is the discomfort of the wrap. It extends to the toes, and a splint is needed, making it difficult for the patient to ambulate. It also must be changed frequently during the day because it is soiled easily.

INTRAOSSEOUS CATHETERIZATION

Intraosseous catheters have historically been used in veterinary medicine in neonates. They can also be placed in adult animals; however, adult bone density is significantly higher, and it may require more specialized equipment. In neonates, 20- or 22-gauge needles can often be used, whereas in adults a bone marrow needle is usually required. Catheters are typically placed in the proximal femur or humerus and used for drug, fluid, or blood administration when IV catheterization has failed.

More recently, a product originally created for advanced emergency response in humans has filtered to the veterinary market. This is the EZ-IO™ Intraosseous Infusion System, by Vidacare, and is comprised of a drill and specialized stainless steel cutting catheters. With this system, intraosseous access can be obtained in only a few seconds, allowing for rapid administration of drugs, fluids, or blood until intravenous access can be obtained. This system has indications for use during acute cardiovascular collapse and other critical emergencies, as well as during cardiopulmonary resuscitation (CPR).

There are a number of sites that can be used for the EZ-IO, including the tibial tuberosity, greater tubercle of the humerus, trochanteric fossa, and the wing of the ileum, although the tibial tuberosity and greater tubercle of the humerus are most recommended in veterinary patients.

The chosen site is palpated, shaved, and aseptically prepared. If time permits, infusion of 2% lidocaine will make things more comfortable for the patient, and a stab incision will facilitate passage through the skin. These two steps are skipped during critical emergencies, such as CPR. The catheter is seated firmly against the periosteum of the bone, before the trigger on the drill is depressed. The skin and bone should be held firmly by the restrainer, and the person performing the procedure will push hard against the bone to prevent the catheter from sliding. The drill trigger is depressed, while continuing to push against the bone. Once the medulla is reached, the catheter will stop its forward movement and the drill trigger is released (only a second or two). Remove and save the stylet, and aspirate the catheter. In most cases, bone marrow will be aspirated to confirm placement. Regardless of the presence of marrow, the catheter should be flushed with saline. It should flush readily, if placement is correct. Fluids or blood are attached by a luer-lock adapter to the catheter. Drugs are administered at the same dosage as with intravenous administration. Once shock is corrected, intravenous access should be attempted again for long-term fluid therapy.

The EZ-IO catheters are expensive, and the distributor recommends that they can be resterilized and reused up to 10 times, or until there is damage to the tip. The manufacturer cautions that the catheter and stylet are cut after being mated as a pair, however, so the pair must remain together; a stylet from another catheter will not match, and will therefore not drill through the bone smoothly.

CHALLENGES

SPECIFIC BREEDS

Placing catheters in basset hounds and dachshunds is very challenging because their limb structure and loose skin make it difficult to place and stabilize IV catheters. Other breeds with loose skin can also be a challenge.

Auricular veins may be used but it is important to use caution when securing the catheter to the pinna. Tape that is placed too tight can restrict blood flow to the distal end of the pinna. Sloughing can occur.

Visualizing and palpating the vessel are easier for the person placing the catheter when the skin is stretched and rotated upward by the handler. The technician should be very cautious about the degree of rotation. When the skin folds are released, the catheter port should be easy to access.

A small nick incision facilitates a smoother introduction of the catheter unit into the vessel. The catheter should be made of a rigid material such as Teflon, because it is less likely to kink while being advanced and will not migrate out of the vessel if stabilized properly.

Elation® works well in stabilizing catheters in animals with loose skin folds. It is strong enough to hold the layers of skin back in most cases.

NEONATES

Restraint is very important in facilitating a successful venipuncture in these animals. The jugular vessel is the most accessible vein.

The neonate should be cradled in the palms of the hands, using its arms as a support for the body. The animal should then be placed on its back, head toward the technician's fingers. For larger puppies, having the restrainer sit in a chair and use the thighs as a trough may help to facilitate positioning for a catheter. Forelimbs must be held firmly to the chest. (Wrapping the patient in a towel sometimes is effective but can limit the technician's ability to monitor the animal during this procedure.) The person placing the catheter extends the head back and rotates it slightly until the vessel can be visualized. Using the other hand, the over-the-needle catheter is introduced into the jugular vessel. The animal should be held in an upright position when securing the catheter (Figures 3-9 and 3-10).

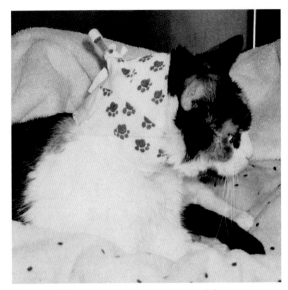

FIGURE 3-9 Jugular catheter in a diabetic cat.

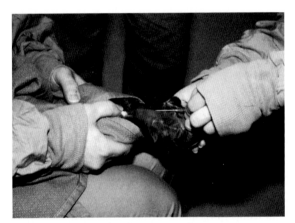

FIGURE 3-10 Restraining the neonate.

FRACTIOUS FELINE AND CANTANKEROUS CANINE

The restraining tools and the handler are the keys to successful IV catheter placement in aggressive animals. Risks should not be taken with animals that show any signs of aggression, and the supplies available for protection should always be used. Restraining tools include muzzles, cat bags, towels, and sedation. Consider asking for sedation orders for very stressed and aggressive patients. Taking these precautionary measures prevents injury to the animal and staff.

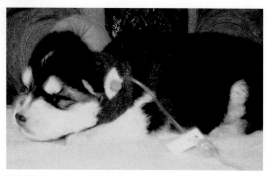

FIGURE 3-11 Jugular catheter in a neonate with a low-flow extension set attached.

The use of a catheter that acts as a multipurpose unit and has a long indwelling time is important. The following setup works well in the fractious animal: An 18-gauge, 12-inch through-the-needle catheter or a long, polyurethane catheter is placed in the lateral saphenous vein in the dog and the medial saphenous vein in the cat. A low-volume extension set is connected to the catheter. This setup allows access to a vessel at a distance. (Medex Inc., Hilliard, Ohio, makes a low-volume extension set with a 60-inch 1-ml line.) The technician is then free to draw blood or administer drug and fluid therapies through the extension set (Figure 3-11).

Putting an Elizabethan collar on the animal blocks its vision and makes it more difficult for the animal to bite. A leash is left around the animal's neck and the end placed outside the cage.

COLLAPSED VASCULAR SYSTEM AND OTHER CHALLENGES

A mini cut-down should be performed if an IV catheter cannot be placed quickly in an emergency situation. A hypodermic needle is used instead of a blade. The technician should hold a 20-gauge hypodermic needle like a pencil and, using the cutting edge of the bevel, make an incision through the skin, horizontally across the leg, to expose the vessel (the incision should begin distally). If the catheter placement is not successful, then incisions can be made parallel to the vessel, up the leg, until placement is successful.

Intraosseous cannulization also can be performed in an emergency. Intraosseous needles are available for this procedure. The most common sites include the medullary canal of the femur or humerus. Once the area is prepped with a local anesthetic, the needle is inserted into the greater tubercle of the humerus or the greater trochanteric fossa of the femur. Aspiration of bone marrow confirms the proper placement, or a radiograph can be taken.

Peripheral edema in the critically ill patient is not an uncommon condition. Wrapping the entire limb for 10 minutes may help displace the edema and allow for venous access. This may occur in patients with severe allergies, spider bites and bee stings, cardiac disorders, kidney injury, hypoalbuminemia, autoimmune disorders, or trauma.

MAINTENANCE

Proper placement technique, catheter choice, and site maintenance all play an important role in determining the indwelling time of an IV catheter. The guidelines for the placement and maintenance of the intravenous catheter can be included in the hospital's infectious disease prevention protocols. The IV catheter site should be assessed during treatment times and every 2 hours if the animal is receiving fluid therapy. Visual checks and palpation of the area above the catheter are performed throughout the day. Bandages should be changed every 24 hours or if they become wet or soiled. IV catheters must be flushed with heparinized saline every 6 to 8 hours if a continuous IV drip is not being administered. Disinfecting ports with an alcohol swab before injecting is also a very important part of preventing infection.

Once the bandage is removed, the site is evaluated for signs of redness or swelling. Infection can be categorized as local or systemic. Local infections are noted when the catheter site appears inflamed or there is purulent discharge. The animal may show signs of discomfort when the catheter is flushed or palpated. The site may be hot and swollen and patient may have an increased temperature. This is commonly called phlebitis, or inflammation of the vessel.

Systemic, or bacteremic, catheter-related infections are defined when there is a positive blood culture that strongly implicates the catheter as a source of infection. The catheter tip is cultured and the same bacteria are found in both the catheter tip and the blood culture. Clinically, the patient may have a fever, leukocytosis, and other signs associated with sepsis.

It is important the catheter is removed if infection is suspected. The catheter must be removed and the leg warm-packed every 4 hours until the swelling subsides. Culturing the catheter tips will assist in determining the cause and type of infection.

The catheter should be flushed to check for any leakage around the site, and the limb above the catheter should be palpated for evidence of subcutaneous fluid. If it is observed that fluid has been delivered subcutaneously, it is important to note the fluid and drugs being administered, and if they may be damaging to surrounding tissues. Infusion of other drugs or fluid may be necessary to prevent tissue necrosis.

The Centers for Disease Control and Prevention (CDC) do not recommend routine application of antimicrobial ointment to venous catheter insertion sites because of the potential to promote fungal infections and antimicrobial resistance. Chlorhexidine patches are used as an alternative. The patch slowly releases chlorhexidine, which is the only solution known to maintain its bactericidal effects in the presence of bodily fluids over a 7-day period in human studies.

If the catheter must be replaced, then the old one should be left in place (if still functional) until a new line has been established. It is important to maintain venous access at all times in the critically ill small animal. All fluid administration sets and fluid bags are changed when the IV catheter is changed.

The IV catheter is the patient's lifeline in many situations. The veterinary team must work together to place and maintain IV catheters properly. Written information about placement including date, location, type, and size of catheter used; appearance of the site before placement; and the person who placed the catheter is important to document on the medical record.

The entire staff must understand IV catheter placement, stabilization, and maintenance protocols to provide optimal patient care.

SUGGESTED READINGS

Frasca D, Dahyot-Fizelier C, Mimoz O: Prevention of central-venous catheter related infection in the intensive care unit, *Crit Care* 14:212, 2010.

Gabriel J: Infusion therapy part two: prevention and management of complications, *Nurs Standard* 22(32):41–48, 2008.

Guidelines for the prevention of intravascular catheter-related infections. Available at www.cdc.gov/hicpac/bsi/bsi-guidelines-2011.html. Accessed Nov 17, 2013.

Hanson B: Technical aspects of fluid therapy. In *DiBartola SP: Fluid therapy in the small animal practice*, Philadelphia, 1992, Saunders.

Mathews K, Brooks M, Valliant A: A prospective study of intravenous catheter contamination, *J Vet Emerg Crit Care* 6(1):33, 1996.

Publication of the Infusion Nurses Society: Infusion Nursing Standards of Practice, *J Infusion Nurs* 34(1S), 2011. Chapter 16: Prevention of intravascular catheter-associated infections. Available at www.ahrq.gov/legacy/clinci/ptsafety/chap16a.html. Accessed Oct 31, 2013.

Ueda Y, Odunayo A, Mann FA: Comparison of heparinized saline and .9% sodium chloride for maintaining peripheral intravenous catheter patency in dog, *J Vet Emerg Crit Care* 23:517–522, 2013.

Wysoki MG, Covey A, Pollak J, et al.: Evaluation of various maneuvers for prevention of air embolism during central venous catheter placement, *J Vasc Interv Radiol* 12:764–766, 2001.

SCENARIO

Purpose: To provide the veterinary technician with the opportunity to decide how to proceed with common situations that would require an IV catheter placement in a small animal patient.

Stage: Level I emergency critical care facility. Busy Wednesday late morning.

Scenario

A 40-kg, 2-year-old intact male Labrador retriever arrives after being hit by a car. He is alert and responsive. His heart rate is 140 bpm, CRT is 1-2 seconds, MMs are pink, and he is panting. Physical examination reveals an open radius-ulnar fracture of the right front limb with a mild amount of hemorrhage, a closed humeral fracture of the left front limb, and the presence of a few lacerations and abrasions on the ventral chest consistent with road rash. The patient is admitted and will require a CRI for appropriate pain management and crystalloid and colloid administration. Regular monitoring of lab values will require multiple blood draws throughout hospitalization.

Questions

- Identify ideal location to place the IV catheter.
- What type of IV catheter would be ideal for the location?
- What size would be selected? Include gauge and length.

Continued

SCENARIO—cont'd

- What type of pain control, if any, would be used?
- What type of catheter placement would you avoid?
- What type of catheter, if any, would you avoid using?

Key Teaching Points

- Provides opportunity for veterinary technician to recognize need for different approach to different situations.
- Encourages investigating other types of IV catheters available.
- Provides veterinary technician with opportunity to consider different venous access points.

Discussion

- Location: Jugular or medial/lateral saphenous.
- Reason: Cephalic vessels must be avoided because of fractures.

- Type/Size: **Option 1**—Peripheral over-the-needle catheter (18 gauge) + sampling long line (*PICC or through-the-needle 16-18 gauge*).
- Reason: Large-bore catheters ideal for optimal fluid delivery. Long line will allow for obtaining blood samples for multiple tests.
- Type/Size: **Option 2**—Multi-lumen catheter (7F, 20-30 cm).
- Reason: Multiple ports available for multiple fluid and drug therapies; also length will be dependent on location. If jugular is selected, length will be determined by noting landmarks, then confirmed by radiograph after placement. If medial or lateral saphenous selected, 30 cm will be adequate.
- Pain management: General pain management for emergent patients with fractures is always considered. More sedation may be required if multi-lumen catheter is placed.

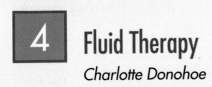

4 Fluid Therapy

Charlotte Donohoe

CHAPTER OUTLINE

Body Water
Patient Assessment
  History and Physical Exam
  Fluid Administration
  Emergency Admission
In-Hospital Monitoring of Fluid
  Therapy Patients
  Urine Production
  Blood Pressure
  Body Weight
  Central Venous Pressure

  Mentation and Physical Exam
   Findings
  Osmolality
Fluid Types
  Crystalloids
  Colloids
Delivery Systems
Complications of Fluid Therapy
  Volume Overload

KEY TERMS

Colloid
Crystalloid
Dehydration
Hypertonic
Hypotonic
Hypovolemia
Isotonic
Osmolality
Volume overload

LEARNING OBJECTIVES

After studying this chapter, you will be able to:

- Differentiate between body water compartments and understand the distribution of body water.
- Understand differences between isotonic/hypotonic/hypertonic crystalloids and know when it is appropriate to use them.
- Understand the concept of osmolality and describe how it affects body water compartments.
- Know the clinical signs associated with complications of fluid therapy and understand the importance of early detection.
- Know the appropriate vital signs and tools used to monitor fluid therapy patients and be familiar with what changes in these measurements indicate.

Intravenous fluid therapy plays a vital role in the supportive care and treatment that is available to veterinary patients in the emergency and critical care hospital setting. The vast majority of our patients require fluids to replenish losses they have experienced during surgical procedures, severe illness, or traumatic events. Fluid therapy is an important component in patient care and treatment for our critically ill or injured hospitalized patients.

Intravenous (IV) fluids may be used for many different reasons during treatment. Fluids are administered with the following goals: replacing volume deficits, maintaining appropriate hydration, providing nutrition, and facilitating administration of intravenous medications. The technician's knowledge, experience, and skill set are paramount in the safe delivery of intravenous fluid therapy. It is important that knowledge remains current and includes an understanding of the principles and practices associated with fluid delivery.

BODY WATER

Approximately 60% of an animal's body weight is contributed by body water. Water exists throughout the body and is maintained in various compartments in strictly regulated proportions. The intracellular space is the largest compartment of body water and represents approximately 40% of body weight. The extracellular compartment, holding a slightly smaller share of total body water, constitutes 20% of body weight. The extracellular space is comprised of the interstitial space and the intravascular space, which account for 15% and 5% of body weight, respectively. Transcellular fluid, found in the synovial joints, pleural space, aqueous humor, and cerebral spinal fluid (CSF), is also considered part of the extracellular compartment. Figure 4-1 illustrates the proportions of the various body water compartments.

Body water estimations for juvenile or senior patients must account for differences in body composition. Body water content is closer to 70% to 80% in pediatric patients and closer to 55% to 60% in geriatric patients.

Healthy animals maintain body water through drinking and digestion of food. Body water is lost through respiration, urination, and excretion under normal circumstances. A healthy animal loses approximately 50 ml/kg of fluid per day. In times of illness, water may not be ingested in appropriate amounts and excess body fluids may be lost through vomiting, diarrhea, or increased urination. Fluid therapy is used to restore and/or maintain body water in animals that are unable to keep up with their daily losses through eating and drinking. Fluids may be delivered via several different routes. Deciding on a route that is suitable for an individual patient requires consideration of the patient's individual needs:

Nursing considerations for fluid therapy include the following:

- What are the patient's history and clinical signs?
- What is the patient's cardiovascular status?
- How quickly does the patient require the fluids?
- What volume of fluids is needed?
- Will the patient be hospitalized due to its illness?

By considering these factors, an appropriate route for fluid delivery can be selected for the patient. Slower fluid delivery may be achieved per os (by mouth) or via subcutaneous administration. Oral delivery may require a feeding tube to facilitate delivery. Placement of esophagostomy or gastrostomy tubes allows the client to deliver predetermined volumes of fluid while caring for their pet at home. Subcutaneous fluids are typically delivered by the veterinary care team in the hospital setting and can be administered during a short office visit. Absorption of fluids delivered by either of these routes is relatively slow and would not be the recommended route of administration for patients that are not hemodynamically stable. See Table 4-1 for advantages, disadvantages, and contraindications regarding routes of administration.

Intravascular fluid delivery is achieved via peripheral catheter or central line. Intraosseous cannulas can be an

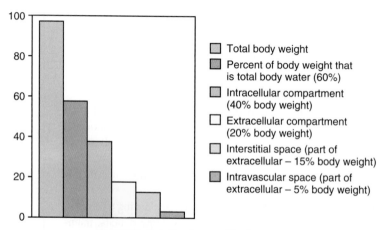

FIGURE 4-1 Distribution of body water.

alternative when intravenous access is difficult. Fluids may be delivered in relatively large volumes at high fluid rates by either of these routes, but rate is dependent on the size of the catheter's lumen and the length of the catheter. These routes are appropriate for moderately to severely compromised patients and require hospitalization and diligent monitoring throughout the duration of therapy (Table 4-1).

PATIENT ASSESSMENT

Once the route of fluid administration has been determined, the technician can assist the clinician in determining how much fluid the patient will require. Evaluation of the patient's vital signs, physical exam findings, and preliminary blood work help determine fluid volume deficit and/or degree of dehydration.

Dehydration involves a loss of body water from the extravascular compartment. **Hypovolemia** refers to a loss

of circulating volume from the intravascular compartment. Left untreated, severe dehydration leads to hypovolemia. Hypovolemia can exist in an adequately hydrated patient, such as one who experiences trauma. Trauma that involves hemorrhage can cause a volume loss from the intravascular compartment. The other compartments have not lost a significant volume of water so the patient would be considered adequately hydrated.

HISTORY AND PHYSICAL EXAM

A thorough physical exam yields information that allows the healthcare team to estimate the patient's hydration status. Obtaining a detailed history complements the physical exam findings by providing information including length of illness and frequency of fluid losses (for example, from vomiting, diarrhea, urination, or inappetence).

Evaluation of eye position, skin turgor, and mucous membrane (MM) moisture contributes information that

TABLE 4-1	Routes of Administration			
ROUTE	**INDICATIONS**	**CONTRAINDICATIONS**	**EQUIPMENT REQUIRED**	**TECHNICIAN NOTES**
Oral	Mild dehydration Short-term illness Small patients Animals with feeding tubes	Hypovolemia Shock Vomiting or nauseous animals Mentally inappropriate patients Decreased to absent gag/swallow reflex	Nasal/esophageal/percutaneous gastrostomy tube Syringes Baby bottles (neonates)	Confirm tube placement in appropriate location before administration of fluids Aspirate tubes before fluid administration/check residual volume
Subcutaneous	Mild dehydration Nonhospitalized animals	Hypovolemia Shock Hypothermia Dermal infection Skin wounds	Bag of sterile IV fluid for injection Administration set Needle (18-20 gauge) Isotonic crystalloid solution	Administer up to 10 ml/kg at each site Do not administer fluids under pressure because it can damage tissues and cause pain New sterile needle for each patient
Intravenous	Dehydration Hypovolemia Anorexia/vomiting/diarrhea of several days duration Surgical procedures IV drug administration	Patients medically managed at home are not ideal candidates for IV fluid therapy	Sterile fluids for injection Administration set IV catheter and supplies Dial volume set/burette or fluid infusion pump Technical staff	Consider the patient's clinical signs when choosing site for IV catheter When possible avoid areas likely to be contaminated
Intraosseous	Cardiovascular collapse Lack of IV access Neonatal patients Avian patients Short-term use until IV access is obtained	Skin lesions at site of insertion Fractures Osteomyelitis	Hypodermic needle (neonates) Spinal needle IO catheter (various types) Administration set Technical staff	Familiarity with landmarks is essential Fluids safe for IV administration are safe for IO administration

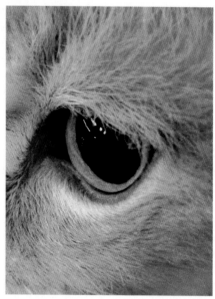

FIGURE 4-2 Evaluating the animal's eye position can provide clues to hydration status.

can be used to estimate the patient's *degree of dehydration* (Figure 4-2).

Eye Position

- Eyes become sunken in orbits in animals with moderate to marked dehydration

Skin Tent/Skin Turgor

- A fold of skin gently pinched should promptly return to normal position. Slow return to normal or standing independently suggests loss of elasticity and dehydration.
- Geriatric patients will have a slow skin tent.

Mucous Membrane Moisture

- Membranes should be moist and shiny.
- Dehydrated animals develop tacky to dry mucous membranes.
- Membranes may develop a dull appearance with loss of moisture.
- Panting animals may have dry mucous membranes from breathing with their mouths open.
- Nauseous patients may salivate excessively and may appear to have moist mucous membranes as a result. Measurements of the animal's vital signs are included in the physical exam. Evaluating the following parameters allows the technician to assess the animal's *intravascular volume status.*

Pulse Rate and Quality

- Heart rate typically increases in response to decreased intravascular volume.
- Femoral pulse quality may change as intravascular volume decreases.
  - Pulses become weak or thready.
- Dorsal pedal pulses may disappear.
  - Typically, pedal pulses disappear when blood pressure decreases and mean arterial pressure (MAP) is ≤60 mm Hg.
- In late (decompensatory) stage of hypovolemic shock, heart rate decreases.

Mucous Membrane Color and Capillary Refill Time

- MMs may remain pink in the face of hypovolemia; usually become dusky.
  - If volume loss is due to hemorrhage, MMs become pale pink to grey.
- MMs may develop dark color attributable to diminished perfusion.
- Capillary refill time (CRT) is prolonged in hypovolemic patient (3+ seconds).

Temperature

- Body temperature may be increased or decreased in the hypovolemic patient depending on the underlying condition.
  - Severe dehydration, poor perfusion, and marked hypovolemia typically lead to decreased body temperature.

FLUID ADMINISTRATION

A fluid therapy plan may be calculated once an estimate of the patient's perceived percentage of dehydration has been made (Table 4-2). The following equation can be used to determine the volume of fluid required to replace hydration deficit:

$$\text{Volume to deliver (ml)} = \%\text{ dehydration (decimal)} \times \text{body weight (kg)} \times 1000$$

or

$$\text{Volume to deliver (ml)} = \%\text{ dehydration (decimal)} \times \text{body weight (lb)} \times 500$$

For example:

A 25-kg dog presents to the hospital with a history of 2 days of vomiting and lethargy. He has dry mucous

TABLE 4-2	Estimating Percentage of Dehydration
Less than 5%	Subclinical—unable to appreciate hydration-related changes on physical exam History of illness involving fluid loss, not prolonged Normal mucous membranes, vital signs not appreciably changed
5%	Mucous membranes tacky or dry History of fluid loss
7%	Dry mucous membranes Prolonged skin tent Increased heart rate Pulse pressure/quality and blood pressure normal History of illness involving fluid loss, somewhat prolonged
10%	History of illness involving fluid loss, somewhat prolonged Dry mucous membranes Prolonged skin tent Increased heart rate Weak to thready pulse pressure Hypotension
12%	History of marked fluid loss Dry mucous membranes Prolonged skin tent Increased or decreased (decompensatory shock) heart rate Hypotension Pulses weak to absent Decreased body temperature ± cool extremities Diminished/abnormal mentation Sunken eye position

membranes and a prolonged skin tent and is tachycardic. He is estimated to be 7% dehydrated.

$$\text{Volume to deliver (ml)} = 25 \times 0.07 \times 1000$$
$$= 1750 \text{ ml of fluid to replace hydration deficit}$$

This volume is usually replaced over the first 24 hours of the patient's fluid therapy plan. In some situations, it may be desired that the dehydration deficit is replaced over a shorter period of time (≈12 to 18 hours). Extra caution with respect to monitoring is recommended to ensure that the patient can tolerate this fluid load. Expediting replacement of dehydration deficit is not recommended in respiratory or heart failure patients.

Ongoing daily losses must be addressed in addition to the hydration deficit. Maintenance fluid requirements are estimated between 40 and 60 ml/kg/day and are add-

ed to the hydration deficit to determine a fluid rate for each patient. Maintenance fluid requirements compensate for sensible losses (measurable losses such as urine) and insensible losses (immeasurable losses such as fecal matter and respiration).

For the 25-kg dog in the previous example, maintenance fluid volume would be:

- = 25 kg × 50 ml/kg/day
- = 1250 ml/day

To calculate the dog's fluid rate:

- 1750 ml to replace hydration deficit over 24 hours = 73 ml/hr
- 1250 ml to compensate for ongoing losses over 24 hours = 52 ml/hr
- The two volumes are added together since dehydration deficit is being replaced in conjunction with the maintenance fluids being delivered.

Ideally, this patient would receive 125 ml/hr for the first 24 hours of fluid therapy assuming that the animal is cardiovascularly stable. The patient should be evaluated frequently for any sign that he/she is not tolerating the rate of fluid administration. Extra consideration is warranted for patients whose perceived ongoing losses exceed what is normally expected. For example, an animal with profuse vomiting and/or diarrhea is going to require more than just the average maintenance fluids to keep up with ongoing losses.

EMERGENCY ADMISSION

Baseline data are collected through the use of minimally invasive procedures to further assess the hydration and volume status of the emergency patient. Blood collection at time of IV catheter placement is ideal since it evaluates the patient before the initiation of fluid therapy. In addition, by withdrawing blood from the newly placed catheter (before heparin/saline flush), the technician can avoid an additional needle stick for the patient. Several tests may be run on this sample without delay in most emergency-equipped hospitals. As a minimum database, packed cell volume (PCV), total solids (TS), stick blood urea nitrogen (BUN), and urine specific gravity (USG) should be evaluated (Figure 4-3).

PCV
- Dehydration can cause an increase in both PCV and TS measurements.
- Volume lost from hemorrhage may be accompanied by decreased PCV/TS values.

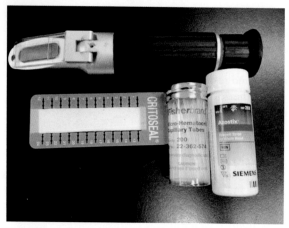

FIGURE 4-3 PCV/TS, BUN stick, and USG measurements should be obtained at time of admission and will help assess the animal's hydration and volume status.

- Dehydration may cause the PCV value to appear falsely elevated in the anemic patient.
- Decreases in PCV/TS values attributable to hemorrhage may not be immediately apparent.

Stick BUN

- Loss of body water causes the concentration of urea in the circulating blood to increase in dehydrated patients with normal renal function. BUN reading may be elevated at time of admission.

Urine specific gravity

- USG may be increased in the dehydrated patient with normal renal function.
  - The body conserves water and excretes waste in a smaller volume of water, thus increasing the USG.

IN-HOSPITAL MONITORING OF FLUID THERAPY PATIENTS

Once fluid therapy has been initiated, diligent patient monitoring is essential. The technician must record and trend any changes in body weight, urine production, blood pressure, central venous pressure, mentation, and physical exam findings.

URINE PRODUCTION

- In addition to USG, urine volume should be monitored in patients receiving fluid therapy.
- Patients with normal renal function should produce a minimum of 1 to 2 ml/kg/hr of urine while receiving fluids.

- Indwelling urinary catheters with a closed collection system facilitate measurement of urine production and USG.
  - This is particularly important in recumbent patients or animals with acute or chronic renal disease.
- Measurement of urine volume should occur every 2 to 4 hours.
  - More frequent (hourly) measurement is required in acute kidney injury patients or those thought to be in anuric renal failure.

BLOOD PRESSURE

Hypovolemic patients are often hypotensive on presentation. One of the goals of fluid therapy is to restore circulating volume and improve perfusion. Fluid therapy aims to restore circulating volume and eventually return blood pressure to near normal parameters.

- Blood pressure measurement must be used in conjunction with other vital parameter evaluation to estimate the patient's volume status and perfusion (Figure 4-4).
- Serial measurements are important during the resuscitation phase of fluid therapy.

BODY WEIGHT

Because such a large percentage of body weight is contributed by body water, it is helpful to monitor a patient's body weight as we strive to replace water losses through fluid therapy.

- Measured a minimum of once daily for fluid therapy patients.
- Weight gain or loss over short periods of time indicates fluid gain or loss.
- 1 kg of body weight corresponds to 1 L of fluid gained or lost (1 lb = 500 ml).
- As a patient's fluid deficit is corrected, weight gain is expected.

TECHNICIAN'S NOTE In addition to serial measurement of body weight, patients should be evaluated for third-space losses. This type of loss occurs when fluid shifts out of the vascular space and into a body cavity such as the pleural space, peritoneal space, or interstitial space. This intravascular fluid loss is not highlighted by a change in body weight since the fluid is still within the animal's body. However, the fluid *is* lost from the vascular space and the effects of this may be associated with a decrease in blood pressure and poor peripheral perfusion.

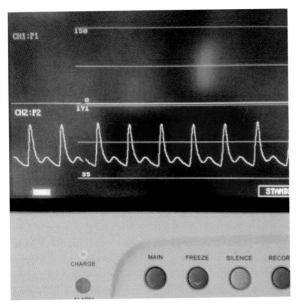

FIGURE 4-4 Direct arterial blood pressure measurement is a useful tool for advanced monitoring of the fluid therapy patient.

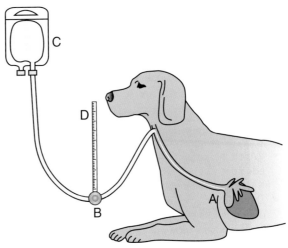

FIGURE 4-5 Central venous pressure (CVP) measurement. With the patient in sternal recumbency, a jugular venous catheter is advanced to the level of the right atrium (A) and connected to the stopcock (B). The stopcock is connected to an IV delivery system (C) and a manometer (D). (Redrawn from Allen DG: Ancillary aids to cardiopulmonary medicine. In Allen DG, Kruth SA, editors: *Small animal cardiopulmonary medicine*, Philadelphia, 1988, BC Decker, p 142.)

CENTRAL VENOUS PRESSURE

Central venous pressure (CVP) is an advanced monitoring tool that is useful in determining whether fluid volume has been adequately restored and for determining that the heart is able to cope with fluids administered. A central venous catheter is placed with the goal of having its tip in the cranial (or caudal) intrathoracic vena cava. Placement at this location allows estimation of right atrial pressure or preload. The catheter is attached to a fluid line that communicates either with a manometer or with an electronic transducer and monitoring equipment. The transducer and zero point of the manometer are placed at the level of the right atrium. Fluctuations in vascular volume are conveyed through the fluid line and interpreted through changes on the manometer or transducer and computer.

In the volume-depleted patient CVP is lower than in the euvolemic animal (Figure 4-5). Increases in CVP are expected as volume is restored, but also may indicate that forward flow through the heart is compromised. Careful assessment of the entire patient in conjunction with CVP measurement is needed to fully understand the success of fluid therapy. For example, if physical exam findings and vital signs are indicative of improved intravascular volume and perfusion and CVP is approaching normal, it is likely that fluid therapy has achieved its goal. In contrast, if the patient's evaluation is suggestive of continued hypovolemia and poor perfusion but CVP is normal or increased, it is likely that forward flow is not sufficient and the increase in right atrial pressure is a reflection of this rather than an indication that volume is restored.

- CVP varies slightly from patient to patient.
- Normal CVP is generally accepted as 0 to 10 cm H_2O or 0 to 7.5 mm Hg.
- Trending CVP is of more value than a single measurement.
- Patient position at time of measurement should be recorded on flow sheet since CVP can fluctuate slightly depending on position.
- Transducer or zero point on the manometer must be at the level of the right atrium.
  - In sternal recumbency use the scapulohumeral joint as a landmark.
  - In lateral recumbency use the manubrium as a landmark.
- Significant increases in CVP (more than 2 to 4 cm H_2O) or CVP >10 cm H_2O may indicate volume overload.

MENTATION AND PHYSICAL EXAM FINDINGS

The technician must be aware of status changes in patients who are receiving fluid therapy. As fluid volume deficit is replaced, the patient's mentation is likely to improve.

The technician should include thoracic and cardiac auscultation in his/her routine evaluation of the patient. Palpation of the patient's limbs and evaluation of the catheter limb/site are recommended at regular intervals.

TECHNICIAN'S NOTE

- Watch the patient's hocks for any loss of detail or edema.
  - Is often associated with volume overload.
- Thoracic auscultation may reveal moist lung sounds during fluid therapy.
  - The patient may not be tolerating fluid load.
- Cardiac auscultation may reveal irregular rhythms such as a gallop rhythm.
  - Patient is not tolerating fluid load.

OSMOLALITY

A *mole* is a unit of measurement used in science when enormous quantities of very small particles are quantified. An *osmole* is also a unit of measurement, but one that is used more frequently when discussing fluid therapy. An osmole represents the number of moles of a substance that contribute to osmotic pressure, that is, the pressure required to stop a solvent from passing through a membrane into a solution via osmosis.

Osmolality is a measurement of how many osmoles exist in a kilogram of solvent. Osmolarity is a similar measurement, but considers the number of osmoles in a liter of solution. When discussing blood plasma or fluid therapy, these terms can be used interchangeably because the difference between them is small enough that it is insignificant. Osmolality is an important concept in the discussion of fluid therapy because it is intricately involved in the movement of body water. It is impractical for most veterinary practices to maintain the equipment to measure plasma osmolality, an osmometer. It is generally accepted that cats have a measured serum osmolality of 310 mOsm/kg and dogs 300 mOsm/kg. The *measured* osmolality accounts for particles in the solution that are osmotically effective (they contribute osmotic pressure and do not cross a membrane) as well as particles that are not osmotically active (they pass freely through a membrane and exert negligible osmotic pressure). In contrast, *calculated* osmolality accounts only for particles that contribute

significantly to the osmolality of a solution. Different formulas can be used to calculate serum osmolality based on the concentrations of certain solutes in the blood. Generally speaking, the higher the concentration of the solute, the more it contributes to serum osmolality (because of the higher number of particles present) and the more likely it is included in the calculated osmolality equation. One of the most osmotically active solutes in the body is sodium. It dominates the extracellular fluid compartment and does not freely flow through all membranes. Sodium is regularly included in the calculation of osmolality, as is glucose. Potassium and urea exert less impact than sodium because they move freely across the cell membrane. They do not contribute significantly to osmolality and are considered ineffective osmoles. Nevertheless, they are included in the osmolality calculation; particularly if/when their concentrations are greater than normal. The following equation can be used to determine calculated osmolality:

$$\text{ECF osmolality} = 2\,(\text{Na} + \text{K}) + (\text{glucose}/18) + (\text{BUN}/2.8)$$

NOTE: This equation assumes that glucose and BUN are measured in milligrams per deciliter. If they are measured in millimoles per liter, the division by 18 and 2.8, respectively, can be omitted.

$$\text{osmolality} = 2\,(\text{Na} + \text{K}) + \text{glucose}\,(\text{mmol/L}) + \text{BUN}\,(\text{mmol/L})$$

Osmolality increases when an animal becomes dehydrated because the loss of water creates an increase in sodium concentration. It follows that in a volume-overloaded patient, osmolality decreases. When serum osmolality increases, osmoreceptors signal a release of antidiuretic hormone (ADH), which causes water conservation. Conversely, a decreased serum osmolality suppresses ADH release, decreases water reabsorption, and leads to an increase in sodium concentration.

Measurement and/or calculation of osmolality can help guide fluid therapy in the critical care setting. Rapid changes in osmolality place the patient at risk for cerebral edema. As fluid administration decreases osmolality in the dehydrated patient, changes can be monitored to ensure it is not changing too rapidly. Hyperglycemic hyperosmolar diabetic patients benefit from osmolality trending as well because their osmolality is dramatically affected by the glucose concentration in their serum.

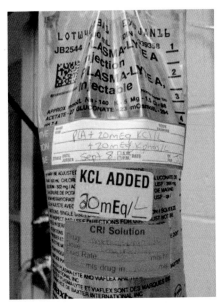

FIGURE 4-6 A bag of crystalloids may contain numerous medications for continuous infusion. Bags should be well-labeled at all times.

FLUID TYPES

CRYSTALLOIDS

Fluid therapy in veterinary medicine relies almost exclusively on crystalloid solutions for replacement and maintenance of body water. Crystalloids are a mixture of water, sugar, and salt and flow freely between body water compartments. When delivered to the intravascular space, crystalloids quickly travel to the interstitial space so that only approximately ¼ of the volume administered remains in the intravascular space.

Several different crystalloids are used in veterinary patients (Figure 4-6). They vary slightly in their electrolyte content, pH, sugar content, presence or absence of a buffer, and buffer type. Replacement solutions are **isotonic,** meaning they have a sodium and chloride content similar to those of the extracellular fluid. The osmotic pressure created by isotonic solutions is the same as the fluid to which they are being compared. Intravenous administration of an isotonic crystalloid does not change the osmotic pressure within the vasculature significantly and does not cause dramatic fluid shifts between compartments. Replacement solutions are chosen to initiate

volume resuscitation in the dehydrated or hypovolemic patient (Table 4-3).

Maintenance crystalloids are **hypotonic** solutions that are not suitable for initial volume resuscitation. Their sodium and chloride content is lower than that of the intravascular space. These solutions also leave the intravascular space rapidly and are more effective at replenishing the extravascular space, more specifically, the intracellular space. As a result of their tendency to rapidly leave the IV space, hypotonic crystalloids are not suitable for treatment of hypovolemia in the critical care patient (Table 4-4).

Hypertonic crystalloid solutions are most often reserved for use in conjunction with isotonic solutions in the treatment of marked hypovolemia. Hypertonic solutions have a higher solute content than that to which they are being compared. With respect to a hypertonic crystalloid, the fluid has a sodium content that is greater than that found in the blood plasma in the intravascular space. The high sodium content increases the osmotic pressure in the compartment and causes fluid to shift into the IV space, thus increasing intravascular volume (Table 4-5).

> **TECHNICIAN'S NOTE** Hypertonic saline (HTS) is a potent volume expander but must be used with caution.

Because the increased osmotic pressure causes fluid to shift from the interstitial and intracellular compartments, HTS should be avoided in dehydrated patients. Side effects associated with the use of HTS include hypernatremia, hyperchloremia, hyperosmolality, and metabolic acidosis. Patients with previously diagnosed cardiac compromise or those with hypernatremia are poor candidates for HTS. Rapid infusion has been associated with bronchoconstriction and may cause rapid, shallow respirations.

HTS is a potent intravascular volume expander but is also useful in head trauma patients. Its effects include a decrease in intracranial pressure, which is beneficial when treating brain injury (Tables 4-6 and 4-7).

COLLOIDS

Colloid solutions are another important fluid used frequently in the emergency and critical care setting. These solutions contain large, high molecular weight particles that cannot travel freely between body water compart-

TABLE 4-3 | Isotonic Replacement Fluids

SOLUTION	OSMOLALITY (mOsm/L)	SODIUM (mEq/L)	POTASSIUM (mEq/L)	CHLORIDE (mEq/L)	CALCIUM (mEq/L)	BUFFER	TONICITY	INDICATIONS
Lactated Ringer's	273	130	4	109	3	Lactate	Isotonic	Dehydration Hypovolemic shock Vomiting Diarrhea Acute kidney injury Metabolic acidosis
Plasma-Lyte A	294	140	5	98	0	Acetate gluconate	Isotonic	Dehydration Hypovolemic shock Vomiting Diarrhea Acute kidney injury Metabolic acidosis
0.9% NaCl	310	154		154			Isotonic	Dehydration Hypovolemic shock Vomiting Diarrhea Hyperkalemia Metabolic alkalosis
Normosol-R	296	140	5	98			Isotonic	Dehydration Hypovolemic shock Vomiting Diarrhea Hyperkalemia Metabolic alkalosis

TABLE 4-4 | Hypotonic Crystalloid Solutions

SOLUTION	OSMOLALITY (mOsm/L)	SODIUM (mEq/L)	POTASSIUM (mEq/L)	CHLORIDE (mEq/L)	CALCIUM (mEq/L)	BUFFER	TONICITY	INDICATIONS
Plasma-Lyte M	363	40	13	40			Hypotonic	Replacement/maintenance of extravascular volume
0.45% NaCl	155	77		77			Hypotonic	Maintenance of extravascular volume
5% dextrose in H$_2$O (D$_5$W)	253						Hypotonic	Extravascular volume replacement Congestive heart failure Hypernatremia

ments. The molecules are too large to pass through a healthy capillary membrane and when delivered intravenously they remain within the intravascular compartment. The presence of these large particles increases the oncotic pressure within this space and results in the movement of body water into the vasculature. The fluid shift into the intravascular space increases the vascular volume and leads to improved blood pressure and perfusion.

Colloids are very effective volume expanders. For this reason, smaller volumes of colloids achieve similar results to larger volumes of **crystalloids.** This is an added benefit in patients that are unable to tolerate large volumes of fluid. Furthermore, in the hypovolemic large breed dog, administration of a colloid in conjunction with a crystalloid can significantly decrease the crystalloid volume needed to replenish intravascular volume.

TABLE 4-5 | Hypertonic Crystalloid Solutions

SOLUTION	OSMOLALITY (mOsm/L)	SODIUM (mEq/L)	POTASSIUM (mEq/L)	CHLORIDE (mEq/L)	CALCIUM (mEq/L)	BUFFER	TONICITY	INDICATIONS
3% NaCl	1026	513		513			Hypertonic	Hypovolemic shock Intravascular volume expansion
7.5% NaCl	2464	1232		1232			Hypertonic	Hypovolemic shock Intravascular volume expansion
Normosol-M + 5% dextrose	363					Acetate	Hypertonic	Intravascular volume expansion

TABLE 4-6 | Summary of Dosage Guidelines for Intravenous Fluid Administration*

SOLUTION	INDICATIONS	CONTRAINDICATIONS	RATE (GUIDELINE ONLY)
Isotonic crystalloids	Hypovolemic shock	Volume overload Congestive heart failure	10-20 ml/kg bolus over 15-20 min; reassess and repeat if necessary
Hypertonic crystalloids	Hypovolemic shock Head trauma	Hypernatremia Severe dehydration	4 ml/kg
Synthetic colloids	Hypovolemic shock Trauma	Coagulopathy Renal disease	10-20 ml/kg/day (canine) 10-15 ml/kg/day (feline)
Isotonic crystalloids	Ongoing illness Maintenance	Congestive heart failure Volume overload	50-60 ml/kg/day

*It is important to recall that each patient must be evaluated as an individual. The following fluid rates are guidelines only and may not be appropriate for some patients.

As colloids are delivered, fluid moves out of other body water compartments and shifts into the IV space. In times of illness, it is possible that these other compartments are already experiencing some degree of volume loss. The concurrent administration of crystalloid fluids with colloids decreases the amount of fluid borrowed from the extravascular compartment. It avoids further disruption of volume status in the interstitial and intracellular spaces. Crystalloids are maintained within the vasculature for longer periods of time when delivered with colloids. In summary, judicious administration of crystalloid and colloid fluids together effectively raises the intravascular volume, provides replacement (crystalloid) fluid to the extravascular compartment, and helps decrease the effect the colloids have on the extravascular space.

Colloids are divided into natural and synthetic groups. Natural colloids include whole blood, plasma, lyophilized canine albumin, human serum albumin, and hemoglobin-based oxygen carriers. Synthetic colloids include gelatins, hydroxyethyl starches, and dextrans.

Dextrans
- Are glucose polymers.
- Molecular weights of 40 or 70 kDa are available.
- 40- or 70-kDa dextrans remain in intravascular compartment for 3 or 5 hours, respectively.
- Increasing doses have negative effects on hemostasis.
- Examples include dextran 40 and dextran 70.

Gelatins
- Are derived from bovine collagen.
- Molecular weights between 30 and 35 kDa are available.
- Remain in vasculature for 1 to 2 hours.
- Have known association with hypersensitivity reactions.

TABLE 4-7	Selection of Fluids for Certain Diseases					
CONDITION		**SERUM**				**FLUID OF CHOICE**
	NA+	**CL−**	**K+**	**HCO₃−**	**VOLUME**	
Diarrhea	D	D	D	D	D	Plasma-Lyte A + KCl Lactated Ringer's + KCl Normosol-R
Pyloric obstruction	D	D	D	I	D	0.9% NaCl
Dehydration	I	I	N	N/D	D	Plasma-Lyte A + KCl Lactated Ringer's 0.9% NaCl Normosol-R
Congestive heart failure	N/D	N/D	N	N	I	0.45% NaCl + 2.5% dextrose 5% dextrose
End-stage liver disease	N/I	N/I	D	D	I	Plasma-Lyte A + KCl 0.45% NaCl + 2.5% dextrose + KCl
Acute renal failure						Plasma-Lyte A Normosol R Lactated Ringer's 0.9% NaCl
Oliguria	I	I	I	D	I	0.9% NaCl
Polyuria	D	D	N/D	D	D	Plasma-Lyte A Lactated Ringer's + KCl Normosol-R
Chronic renal failure	N/D	N/D	N	D	N/D	Lactated Ringer's solution Plasma-Lyte A 0.9% NaCl
Adrenocortical insufficiency	D	D	I	N/D	D	0.9% NaCl
Diabetic ketoacidosis	D	D	N/D	D	D	0.9% NaCl (±KCl)

D, Decreased; *I,* increased; *N,* normal.

- Have no daily volume limit.
- Examples of gelatin products include the following:
  - Urea cross-linked (Polygeline)
  - Modified liquid gelatins (Gelofusine)
  - Oxypolygelatines (Gelifundol)

Hydroxyethyl Starches (HES) (Figure 4-7)

- Are high polymer glucose particles.
- Have molecular weights between 70 and 670 kDa.
- Differentiated by number of hydroxyethyl groups substituted per unit of glucose.
- Daily limit of 20-50 ml/kg depending on which HES is used.
- Cause prolonged coagulation times.

- Molecular weight solutions <200 kDa are associated with decreased capillary permeability.
- Examples of commonly used HES:
  - Hetastarch (Hespan)
  - Pentastarch (Pentaspan)
  - Tetrastarch (Voluven)

Contraindications

Colloids have been reported to increase coagulation times, cause histamine release in cats, and cause anaphylactic type reactions in some patients. To date, the benefits of colloid use have outweighed the risks, and colloids have been a popular choice in the emergency and critical care setting, particularly for resuscitation of hypovolemic animals. Recently, studies have suggested

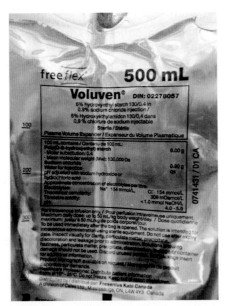

FIGURE 4-7 Synthetic colloids are effective volume expanders and are used in conjunction with crystalloids in resuscitation of hypovolemic patients.

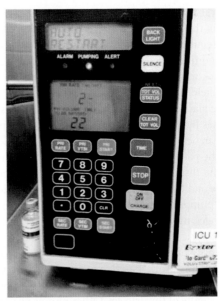

FIGURE 4-8 Infusion pumps may be used in veterinary patients to contribute to the safe administration of fluid therapy.

that the use of low molecular weight hydroxyethyl starches in patients with sepsis is less safe than previously believed. Critically ill and septic human patients that received HES had higher mortality and were more likely to undergo renal replacement therapy (RRT), to require blood transfusion, and/or to develop acute kidney injury (AKI). As of November 2013, the U.S. Food and Drug Administration has made recommendations to avoid the use of HES in this patient group and has published guidelines for patient and clinician use. Hespan 6% in NaCl, Hetastarch, Hextend, and Voluven are currently FDA-approved HES solutions for treatment and prevention of hypovolemia. There are still indications for use of HES solutions in veterinary patients. It needs to be determined if the veterinary community will follow the recommendations regarding HES use in septic human patients. More veterinary-related research is required.

DELIVERY SYSTEMS

Many veterinary hospitals use fluid infusion pumps to administer fluid and drug therapies in hospitalized patients (Figure 4-8). This equipment is not available in all hospitals and other methods of delivery and measurement are required. Administering fluids by gravity

flow is still a common practice and the technician must be aware of how flow rates are maintained using this method.

In a gravity feed system, fluids are kept in an elevated position above the patient, and gravity forces the fluids into the body. The drip rate is adjusted manually using the regulator on the fluid line. A timing measure should be affixed to the line so that dosing accuracy can be assessed regularly. Fluid rates can fluctuate when a gravity feed system is in use. Location of the catheter and patient positioning can influence the flow rate. It is important to monitor very closely for these reasons. Dial-A-Flows are devices attached to the fluid lines and can be adjusted depending on what rate is needed.

Gravity administration systems present a particular challenge with small patients. Since fluid rates can fluctuate based on patient position, a flow rate that appears to be appropriate may suddenly be increased or a fluid bolus delivered if the animal repositions the limb in which the intravenous catheter is located. Volume overload is a serious complication associated with this type of fluid delivery. Buretrols increase the margin of safety in small patients. A buretrol can be filled with a maximum of 1 to 2 hours' worth of fluids to avoid accidental volume overload.

Several types of fluid delivery systems are available for use in the veterinary practice. Fluid delivery systems help to regulate the flow of the solution and total volume of fluid administered to the patient. Elastomeric devices are used commonly for home infusion therapies in the human field but are applicable in the veterinary field. They are plastic bulb type containers that administer the fluid rates by changing the diameter of the tubing. The device can be attached to the patient using a harness and allows the patient to move without the restraint of fluid lines. The disadvantage is the number of limited sizes available and the ability to adjust rates. Two basic types of fluid pumps are available: (1) volumetric pumps and (2) syringe pumps (Box 4-1).

Volumetric pumps can be programmed to deliver any quantity of fluids over a determined period of time. These systems work based on the calculated volume (diameter) of the administration set; the pumps work independently of the drip set. Other pumps use a photo-electric eye to count the drops as they are being administered. These pumps are adjusted on a drop per minute basis. The sensor is placed on the drip chamber; calculations must be made to determine the appropriate drop rate to obtain the proper fluid dose over time.

Syringe pumps are hand-held mechanical devices that use a syringe with a measured volume of solution to administer fluid. They are most often used when administering medications to very small animals, when administering medications that are required to be given over a period of time, or when administering blood products. Syringe pumps are usually compatible with a number of different-sized disposable syringes. Settings for these devices allow accurate administration of small volumes over a long period of time (Figure 4-9). Syringe pumps can be programmed to infuse single doses over a preset amount of time, or to infuse fluids at a constant rate. Rates can be selected using different units, or according to the type of fluid or drug they are infusing.

Many fluid pumps used in veterinary hospitals are reconditioned and refurbished human units. Some are electronic units or battery operated. Fluid delivery is accurate but complications can arise because of operator error if the pump is loaded incorrectly, or the infusion rate and volume are programmed incorrectly. It is highly recommended to continue to mark bags and buretrols every 2 hours to monitor fluid delivery since the pumps can malfunction. This can be done by placing a piece of tape alongside the numbers located on the bag/buretrol. The time is written on the tape at the level of the fluid when the fluid checks are completed (Figure 4-10).

Fluid pumps can be specific to the IV fluid lines produced by the same manufacturers. When reconditioned or refurbished units are purchased, the owner's manual must be reviewed for compatibility with the brands of IV lines. The veterinary technician must read and follow all operating instructions.

COMPLICATIONS OF FLUID THERAPY

The technician plays a vital role in monitoring fluid therapy patients. Hourly evaluation of the patient is required throughout the duration of intravenous fluid delivery. At each treatment time, the technician should ensure that the animal is receiving the fluid type and additive prescribed on the flowsheet and verify that the fluid rate on the pump/dial a flow/drip set matches that of the fluid therapy orders. Nonprescribed alterations in fluid rates or fluid types put the patient at risk for a host of complications.

Persistent clinical signs of volume deficit suggest that the current fluid therapy plan is not reaching therapeutic goals. See Table 4-8 for clinical signs associated with volume depletion.

VOLUME OVERLOAD

This is a potential complication for any patient receiving fluid therapy. Causes can include subclinical heart disease or iatrogenic, overzealous administration. **Volume overload** has the following clinical signs:

- **Peripheral edema**—Subtle changes are most obvious in the hock area.
- **Cough**—If the patient has not previously been noted to have a cough, the technician should consider whether a new cough is associated with fluid administration.
- **Increased respiratory rate**—Thoracic auscultation is necessary for further evaluation. Are there moist lung sounds/crackles/wheezes?
- **Serous nasal discharge**—A small amount may be normal in some dogs but new or increased discharge may be associated with current fluid therapy.
- **Restlessness**—The cause of restlessness can be difficult to identify but volume overload should be considered.
- **Vomiting or diarrhea.**

BOX 4-1	Technical Tip: Regulating Fluid Rates

The following equations can be used to calculate drip rates for accurate fluid administration. These rates are also calculated to ensure proper functioning of fluid rate monitors and pumps.

Choosing the Fluid Delivery Set for Accurate Fluid Administration

Animals receiving 60 ml/hr or less need a buretrol and mini-drip set (60 drops/ml). Animals receiving more than 60 ml/hr need a regular drip set (10 drops/ml).

Types of Sets Available

Mine – drip set (60 drops/ml)* Regular drip set (10 drops/ml)*

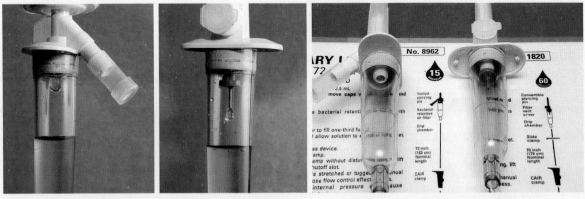

From Thomas JA, Lerche P: *Anesthesia and analgesia for veterinary technicians,* ed 4, St Louis, 2011, Mosby.

Calculating the Rate with Total Volume To Be Administered over a Specific Number of Hours

Rate (drops/min) = Drops/ml calibrated* ÷ 60 (minutes/hour) ×
Total volume to be administered ÷ Total hours of infusion

Seconds/drop = 60 ÷ Rate

Example: 400 ml is needed over a 6-hour period of time

(10 ÷ 60) × (400 ÷ 6) = 11 drops/min

60 ÷ 11 = 5 seconds/drop

Calculating the Rate with ml/hr To Be Administered

Rate (drops/minute) = ml/hr × drops/ml calibrated*
÷ 60 (minutes/hour)

Seconds/drop = 60 ÷ Rate

Example: 40 ml/hr to be administered

40 × 60 ÷ 60 = 40 drops/min

60 ÷ 40 = 1.5 seconds/drop

*Drops per milliliter are calibrated for each individual set. This information is on the package of the fluid administration sets.

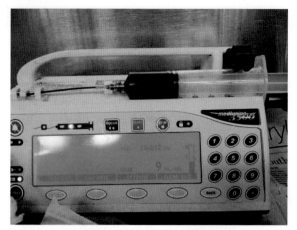

FIGURE 4-9 Syringe drivers are used for administration of small volumes of fluid, medications, or blood products.

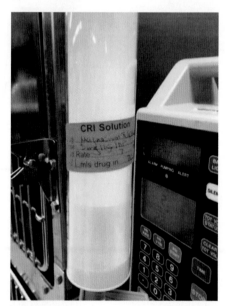

FIGURE 4-10 A buretrol is helpful in avoiding accidental administration of large fluid volumes to small patients. Additive labels are important criteria of fluid therapy. All fluids must be labeled at all times to ensure patient safety.

TABLE 4-8	Clinical Signs of Extracellular Fluid Volume Depletion and Overload	
DEPLETION		**OVERLOAD**
Pale, dry mucous membranes		Serous nasal discharge
Poor skin elasticity		Subcutaneous edema
Reduced urine output		Increased urine output with normal kidney function
Microcardia on thoracic radiographs		Ascites
Sunken orbits		Chemosis
Cool distal extremities		Exophthalmos
Slow capillary refill time		Restlessness, coughing
Weak rapid pulse		Increased respiration rate
Increased temperature		Vomiting

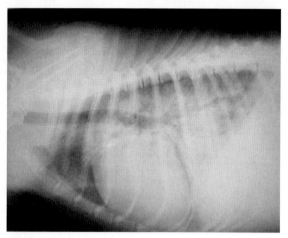

FIGURE 4-11 Pulmonary edema secondary to fluid overflow in a cat.

- **Pulmonary edema or pleural effusion**—Thoracic auscultation is recommended in any patient with new or increased respiratory rate or effort because volume load can lead to severe respiratory compromise if not treated promptly (Figure 4-11).

- **Radiographs**—Required to confirm the cause of tachypnea.

Technicians involved in administering fluids must understand the basic principles of fluid therapy, be familiar with the characteristics of the fluids being infused, and understand the patient-specific goals of fluid therapy. Diligent patient monitoring allows the technician to troubleshoot effectively, safely deliver intravenous fluids, and contribute significantly to the convalescence of veterinary patients.

SCENARIO

Purpose: To establish confidence in calculations pertaining to fluid therapy and its safe administration.

Scenario

A 3.5-year-old MN Persian is admitted to the hospital. The owner reports that the cat has been vomiting for the past 3 days and she does not believe he has been eating during that time. His stool was normal until last night, at which point he developed profuse watery diarrhea. Initial assessment reveals the following vital signs:

- Temperature 37.0° C (98.6° F)
- Heart rate 240 bpm
- Respiratory rate 40 breaths/min
- MM pink, tacky; CRT 2-3 sec
- Femoral pulse palpable
- Skin tent prolonged

Questions

1. What is this cat's hydration status?
2. Via which route will you administer fluids?
3. What volume of fluid would you give in the first 24 hours of fluid resuscitation?

Discussion

1. The cat is estimated to be 7% dehydrated based on the fact that it is tachycardic, has tacky mucous membranes, a prolonged skin tent.
2. IV fluids would be most appropriated for this cat as its clinical signs are not likely to resolve quickly enough to make any other route safe or practical.
3. The cat would receive 552 ml of fluid in the first 24 hours based on the following:
   Fluid deficit in ml = 4.6 x 0.07 x 1000 = 322 mls (volume deficit)
   Maintenance requirements in ml = 4.6 x 50 ml/kg/day = 230 mls
   Maintenance + deficit = volume to be delivered in first 24 hrs = 552

MEDICAL MATH EXERCISE

A 35-kg German shepherd diagnosed with hemorrhagic diarrhea (HGE) needs a 20 ml/kg bolus of Plasma-Lyte in 20 minutes and then started on a 1.5 times requested maintenance rate of 60 ml/kg/day.

   a. How many milliliters of Plasma-Lyte will you bolus?
   b. What fluid rate will you deliver the bolus?
   c. What is the maintenance rate?
   d. What will be the rate of fluids per hour?

REFERENCES

DiBartola S, Bateman S: Introduction to fluid therapy. In DiBartola S, editor: *Fluid, electrolyte, and acid-base disorders*, ed 3, St Louis, 2006, Saunders, pp 325–344.

Donohoe C: Patient monitoring. In *Fluid therapy for veterinary technicians and nurses*, West Sussex, 2012, Wiley Blackwell, pp 107–134.

Mazzaferro E, Powell L: Fluid therapy for the emergent small animal patient, *Vet Clin Small Anim* 43:721–734, 2013.

Mensack S: Fluid therapy: options and rational administration, *Vet Clin Small Anim* 38:575–586, 2008.

Morrison C, Carrick M, Norman M, et al.: Hypotensive resuscitation strategy reduces transfusion requirements and severe postoperative coagulopathy in trauma patients with hemorrhagic shock: preliminary results of a randomized controlled trial, *J Trauma* 70(3):652–663, 2011.

Novak L, Shackford SR, Bourguignon P, et al.: Comparison of standard and alternative prehospital resuscitation in uncontrolled hemorrhagic shock and head injury, *J Trauma* 47:834–844, 1999.

Silverstein D, Aldrich J, Haskins S: Assessment of changes in blood volume in response to resuscitative fluid administration in dogs, *J Vet Emerg Crit Care* 15(3):185–192, 2005.

Tobin J, Dutton R, Pittet J, et al.: Hypotensive resuscitation in a head-injured multi-trauma patient, *J Crit Care*, 2013. Accessed at http://dx.doi.org/10.1016/j.jcrc.2013.11.017.

Wellman M, DiBartola S, Kohn C: Applied physiology of body fluids in dogs and cats. In *Fluid, electrolyte, and acid-base disorders in small animal practice*, St Louis, 2006, Saunders, pp 3–26.

CHAPTER OUTLINE

Whole Blood and Components
Whole Blood
Packed Red Blood Cells
Plasma Components
Platelets
Blood Sources
Blood Collection
Anticoagulant-Preservative Solutions
Blood Collection Systems
Blood Collection Techniques
Processing and Storage
Leukoreduction
Storage Lesions
Blood Administration

Blood Compatibility
Component Preparation
Administration Volume
Administration Routes
Administration Rates
Blood Filters and Transfusion Methods
Transfusion Reactions
Alternate Transfusion Products and Methods
Hemoglobin-Based Oxygen Carrier Solutions
Xenotransfusion
Autotransfusion

LEARNING OBJECTIVES

After studying this chapter, you will be able to:

- Understand the concepts in component transfusion therapy and gain knowledge on blood product administration.
- Learn basic blood banking, involving donor selection, blood collection, processing, and storage.
- Learn methods of blood compatibility testing and gain knowledge in transfusion complications.
- Become familiar with alternative transfusion methods and products.

The first recorded animal-to-animal transfusion was performed in the 1600s as an experiment in blood transfusions for human medical application. Much knowledge has been gained since then, and as a result of the increased specialization in veterinary medicine, the demand for blood products has risen dramatically. These specialties (i.e., emergency medicine, critical care, oncologic medicine) have created a need for knowledge and expertise in veterinary **transfusion medicine.** The importance of transfusion education for veterinarians, veterinary technicians, and students continues to unfold. Education is clearly the link to ensuring the overall quality of all aspects of **blood banking** and transfusion services.

KEY TERMS

Blood administration
Blood banking
Component therapy
Transfusion complications
Transfusion medicine

A safe and adequate supply of blood components for transfusion is invaluable. The American Association of Blood Banks has established acceptable standards for the collection, processing, storage, distribution, and administration of human blood and blood components. Each blood bank and transfusion service strictly follows these standards, as well as certain legal requirements of local, state, and federal governments (most importantly, those of the Food and Drug Administration). Strict compliance with these standards reflects a commitment to providing quality products and appropriate care for patients receiving transfusion support. Although government organizations play less of a role in ensuring quality practices in veterinary medicine, the industry is striving to adhere to similar standards. To that end, the industry is always more aware of evidence-based practices, building on past efforts of associations such as the Association of Veterinary Hematology and Transfusion Medicine to uphold standards.

WHOLE BLOOD AND COMPONENTS

Blood is made up of two portions: (1) a cellular portion and (2) the plasma, which acts as a carrier medium for the cells, proteins, gases, nutrients, vitamins, and waste products. With the availability of variable speed, temperature-controlled centrifuges and the advent of plastic storage bags with integral tubing for collection, processing, and administration, specific blood component therapy is possible. Whole blood (WB) can be stored or processed into one or more of the following components: red blood cells (RBCs), platelets, and plasma. Plasma can be processed into plasma protein concentrates called cryoprecipitate (CRYO) and cryosupernatant. Serum albumin and immunoglobulins are commercially manufactured for therapy as well. Blood components permit specific replacement therapy for specific disorders, reduce the number of transfusion reactions as a result of diminished exposure to foreign material, and decrease the fluid volume and the amount of time needed to transfuse. Additionally, appropriate therapeutic use of blood components increases the number of patients who benefit from this limited resource.

Employment of **component therapy**—or targeted, purposeful replacement of components only when required by the patient—will bring the most benefit for the risk of transfusion. Each component of blood has a specific role or function in the body. Certain disease states require replacement of one or any combination of these components. The component or components chosen will depend on the crisis at hand.

WHOLE BLOOD

Initial collection yields fresh whole blood (FWB) and is defined as blood stored at room temperature for up to 8 hours after collection. FWB provides RBCs, white blood cells (WBCs), functional platelets, plasma proteins, and coagulation factors. Certain components in blood are more fragile than others and will become less effective with time and changes in ambient temperature. To achieve full benefit of all components when needed, FWB should be administered immediately after collection.

Although specific component therapy may be safer, WB transfusions still have their use in patients requiring multiple components. In some clinics, FWB may be the only option offered, if components are not banked or separated in-house. FWB is used in actively bleeding, anemic animals with thrombocytopenia or thrombopathia (requiring RBCs and platelets), anemia with coagulation factor deficits (requiring RBCs and hemostatic proteins), and massive hemorrhage (rapid loss of all components). A patient with massive, uncontrolled hemorrhage may require a *massive transfusion,* which is traditionally defined as replacement of blood approaching or exceeding one total blood volume within a 24-hour period. More modern definitions indicate replacement of more than half the total blood volume in 4 hours. In cases of severe hemorrhage, administration of all components is observed to result in better patient survival when compared to replacement of only RBCs.

After collection, WB must be processed into components or (at the least) refrigerated at 1° C to 6° C within 8 hours. After 24-hour storage of WB, platelet function is lost and the concentration of labile coagulation factors decreases (factor V and factor VIII). The product is then defined as *stored WB* and provides RBCs, the more stable coagulation factors, and other plasma proteins (i.e., albumin, globulins). The length of time a unit of WB can be stored under refrigeration depends on the anticoagulant-preservative solution (APS) used in collection. With the advantages in the use of blood components well documented in human and veterinary medicine, as well as the improved availability of these products as a result of commercial blood banks, the use of stored WB is no longer considered the treatment of choice. Stored WB may be considered in patients that require oxygen-carrying support, coagulation factors, or intravascular volume expansion, only after careful consideration of risks in transfusing unnecessary antigenic material.

The use of WB, fresh or stored, is not recommended in severe chronic anemia. Chronically anemic patients may have a reduced red cell mass but have compensated over time by increasing their plasma volume to meet their total blood volume. Administration of WB may expose these patients to the risk of volume overload, leading to transfusion-associated circulatory overload, especially in patients with preexisting cardiac disease or renal compromise.

PACKED RED BLOOD CELLS

Packed red blood cells (PRBCs) can be harvested from a unit of WB after centrifugation at 4° C and stored at 1° C to 6° C for durations dependent on the anticoagulant preservative solution used. PRBCs are used primarily to provide oxygen-carrying capacity for patients showing signs of hypoxia attributable to the deficiency in circulating RBC mass. Decreased red cell mass can result from increased blood loss (surgical or traumatic hemorrhaging, coagulopathy, or parasitism), increased RBC destruction (immune-mediated, toxicities, oxidative damage, or mechanical damage), or reduced RBC production (decreased erythropoietin production or response, nutritional deficiencies, and bone marrow dysfunction). Anemia is discussed in more detail in Chapter 16: Hematologic Emergencies.

"Transfusion triggers" or "transfusion thresholds" have been suggested in which a patient's need for an RBC transfusion would be determined by lab values assessing anemia (packed cell volume [PCV], hematocrit [HCT], or hemoglobin [Hb] level).

> *TECHNICIAN NOTE* However, basing decisions to transfuse solely on these lab values is not recommended, and clinical assessment of the patient is important to prevent unnecessary transfusions.

Clinical signs, such as weakness, dulled mentation, or collapsing, and compensatory signs, such as tachycardia and increased respiratory rate and effort without a suspect cause aside from anemia, serve as a reason for red cell transfusions. With that said, a PCV of less than 20% (Hb level of less than 7 g/dl) is very likely to result in clinical signs of anemia. Increased serum lactate levels can be a good indicator of tissue hypoxia from inadequate oxygen-carrying capacity, given that perfusion is not impaired. Human studies observe reduced transfusion-associated complication rates, mortality, cardiac morbidity, and hospital stay length when "restrictive" transfusion thresholds (Hb level lower than 7 to 8 g/dl) are compared to "liberal" thresholds (transfusions given at Hb concentrations >10 g/dl). The importance of evaluating a patient's need for RBC transfusions primarily based on clinical signs aided by laboratory parameters to minimize unnecessary risks still remains.

> *TECHNICIAN NOTE* "Treat the patient, not the number."

Although it seems logical that blood loss should be replaced with WB, replacing blood volume with crystalloid or synthetic colloid solutions and utilizing PRBCs when oxygen-carrying capacity is in question are often adequate therapy for the majority of acutely bleeding patients. Transfusion of PRBCs is not recommended in patients who are well compensated for their anemia (e.g., chronic renal failure).

In addition to provision of oxygen carrying capacity, RBC transfusions have a couple of less recognized benefits. Evidence supports better hemostasis in patients with a higher HCT, independent of platelet counts. The mechanism behind this phenomenon is currently under investigation, but could be related to RBCs stimulating thromboxane production by platelets, ADP release from RBCs acting as platelet agonists, displacement of platelets by RBCs towards the endothelium promoting platelet adhesion, and reduction of free nitric oxide (an inhibitor of platelet adhesion and aggregation) through binding to Hb. RBC transfusions can also provide available iron for anemia caused by iron deficiency, making RBC transfusions an excellent treatment option for iron deficiency anemia by providing oxygen-carrying capacity and building blocks for new hemoglobin.

PLASMA COMPONENTS

In addition to water and electrolytes, plasma contains hemostatic proteins, albumin, immunoglobulins, and some other proteins. Coagulation factors (factors II, VII, IX, X, XI, and XII), coagulation cofactors (factors V and VIII), and von Willebrand factor (vWF) in plasma play vital roles in coagulation. Plasma also contains anticoagulation proteins such as antithrombin, protein C, and protein S. Fibrinolytic/antifibrinolytic proteins such as plasminogen, antiplasmin, and plasminogen activator inhibitor-1 are also present. Albumin is a natural colloid that produces oncotic pressure and serves many other functions. Immunoglobulins have shown some promise in its use for immune suppression. Another protein of interest is α-macroglobulins, which are observed to be depleted in patients with severe pancreatitis, though benefit of transfusion for this protein remains to be proven.

Fresh Frozen Plasma

Plasma is primarily used for its coagulation factor value; it does not contain functional platelets. Most coagulation proteins are stable at 1° C to 6° C, with the exception of factors V and VIII. To maintain adequate levels of all factors, plasma is harvested from a unit of WB and frozen at −18° C or colder within 8 to 24 hours from the time of initial collection (Walton et al, 2014). This product is then labeled as *fresh frozen plasma* (FFP) and will retain its coagulation factor efficacy for 12 months provided it is maintained at the appropriate temperature. FFP can be used to treat most coagulation factor deficiencies (e.g., disseminated intravascular coagulation, liver disease, anticoagulant rodenticide toxicity, hereditary coagulopathies) and potentially other conditions (e.g., acute pancreatitis). FFP is not recommended for use as a blood volume expander or for protein replacement in animals with hypoproteinemia.

Frozen and Liquid Plasma

Plasma may be separated from a unit of WB any time during storage (through its expiration date). When stored at −18° C or colder after harvesting, the component is called *FP* and may be kept for up to 5 years from the date of initial WB collection. Additionally, if FFP is not used within 12 months, then it can be relabeled as *frozen plasma* (FP) and stored for an additional 4 years. If plasma is not frozen, then it is called *liquid plasma* (LP) and has a shelf life not exceeding 5 days after the expiration date of the WB from which it was harvested.

FP and LP may have varying levels of the more stable coagulation factors, as well as albumin; however, FP and LP do not contain functional platelets or the labile coagulation factors V and VIII. FP and LP can be used

to treat stable clotting factor deficiencies and certain cases of acute hypoproteinemia (i.e., parvoviral enteritis). If animals severely or chronically protein deficient are chosen to be treated with plasma, large volumes are required to have a measurable effect in managing the acute effects of hypoproteinemia (i.e., pulmonary edema, pleural effusion). The primary cause of acute effects of hypoproteinemia is hypoalbuminemia, or low serum albumin level. Hypoalbuminemia may result from protein losing enteropathy or nephropathy, septic peritonitis, trauma, burns, and any other pathologies causing protein loss. The dose required for this particular use is 20 to 25 ml/kg to achieve an increase of 0.5 g/dl in plasma albumin level. For example, a 25-kg patient with an albumin level of 1.0 g/dl will require 1000 to 1250 ml of plasma to regain a low normal plasma albumin level of 2.0 g/dl. In addition, this does not take into account ongoing loss from the patient's pathology, which adds to required plasma volume. Use of plasma in this manner will pose a higher transfusion-related complication risk, be an inefficient use of plasma, and will be at a significant cost to the owners. Serum albumin concentrate is a better source of albumin. Synthetic colloid solutions should be considered because they are readily available and more effective in increasing colloid osmotic pressure. As with FFP, FP and LP are not recommended for use as a blood volume expander.

Cryoprecipitate and Cryosupernatant

CRYO is the cold-insoluble portion of plasma that precipitates after FFP has been slowly thawed at 1° C to 6° C (i.e., refrigerator). The precipitated material separated by centrifugation contains concentrated amounts of von Willebrand's factor, factor VIII, fibrinogen, and fibronectin (factor XIII). After production, CRYO can be frozen at −18° C or colder and has a shelf life of 1 year from the original date of WB collection. CRYO can be used in patients with possible or diagnosed von Willebrand's disease, hemophilia A, or fibrinogen deficiency. Advantage in its use over FFP is the provision of a therapeutic level of these factors with a small volume transfusion, reducing the risk of intravascular volume overload. Each unit of CRYO contains approximately 25 to 50 ml of plasma.

The plasma separated from the cryoprecipitate is called cryosupernatant (may also be referred to as cryopoor plasma), containing remaining factors and proteins (II, V, VII, IX, X, XI, XII, albumin, immunoglobulins).

It is useful in treating specific factor deficiencies like hemophilia B (factor IX deficiency) and vitamin K antagonism (factor II, VII, IX, and X deficiency) such as anticoagulant rodenticide toxicity. Cryosupernatant can be used as a source of albumin, though the same hesitations for use of plasma for albumin supplementation still apply. Cryosupernatant can be stored for 1 year, frozen.

Albumin

Albumin serves in the vasculature to provide colloid osmotic pressure (accounts for approximately 80% of serum oncotic pressure), functioning to retain blood volume. Clinical manifestations of hypoalbuminemia include pulmonary and other types of edema attributable to fluid effusion from decreased colloid osmotic pressure, and compromised perfusion due to lowered intravascular volume. Albumin plays a role in regulating coagulation by mediating thromboxane A_2 (a prothrombotic) levels. Hypoalbuminemia leads to increased thromboxane A_2 levels, contributing to a hypercoagulable state. Albumin also functions as a carrier for chemicals, drugs, and hormones, as well as scavengers of toxins and free radicals.

Albumin may be considered for use in protein-losing enteropathy, protein-losing nephropathy, hepatic dysfunction, peritonitis, polytrauma, pancreatitis, burn injury, heat-induced illness, and any other causes of hypoalbuminemia. Albumin transfusions are considered when hypoalbuminemia (albumin <2.0 g/dl) is thought to be leading to edema, hypotension, and compromised perfusion, with other methods (crystalloid, synthetic colloid, vasopressors, and treatment of underlying cause) being unsuccessful in providing proper colloid osmotic pressure or perfusion.

Human serum albumin (HSA) has been used in canine patients with hypoalbuminemia. However, these infusions have a significant chance of an immunologic reaction because human albumin differs from canine albumin by 20% of its amino acid sequence. Previous sensitization to human albumin and subsequent acute hypersensitivity reactions are especially a concern when repeat doses are necessary. Type III hypersensitivity reactions after HSA administration leading to vasculitis have been reported as well (Powell et al, 2013).

Canine-specific albumin has recently been produced as a commercial product, observed to increase serum albumin levels in the recipients with a low chance of immunologic complications. The most recent published study indicated albumin administration in dogs with septic peritonitis to have improved albumin level, Doppler blood pressure values, and colloid osmotic pressure measurements, as well as a comment on the association between albumin transfusion and survival (Craft and Powell, 2012). These studies, however, do have some limitations, and a connection between an improvement in serum albumin level and ultimate survival in veterinary patients continues to be a topic under investigation. In addition, commercial supply of canine-specific albumin has seen inconsistency, making it difficult to obtain at the time of writing.

Immunoglobulins

The use of human intravenous immunoglobulin (hIVIG) has gained some attention in the veterinary field for its use as an immunosuppressant in refractory immune-mediated diseases. The original intent of research on the product was to determine efficacy in treating immunodeficiencies, but administration of IVIG was found to cause an immunosuppressive effect instead. Immune-mediated hemolytic anemia (IMHA), immune-mediated thrombocytopenia (IMT), pemphigus foliaceus or other immunologic dermatologic disorders, acute canine polyradiculoneuritis (Hischvogel et al, 2012), and sudden acquired retinal degeneration syndrome are some of the conditions IVIG has been used on with limited success (Whelan et al, 2009; Spurlock and Prittie, 2011). The immunoglobulin (Ig) content of plasma solutions is not observed to be sufficient to provide an immunosuppressive dose, and a concentrate derived via fractionation from thousands of blood donors is required. The concentrate consists mostly of biologically active IgG, though other Ig types are present. The mechanism of immunosuppression is thought to involve an inhibition of phagocytic activity of mononuclear lymphocytes (Sibley et al, 2013), inhibition of cytotoxic T-cell function, and blunting of damage caused by complement activation and proinflammatory cytokines. Adverse effects such as allergic and anaphylactic reactions, delayed hypersensitivity reaction, renal failure, hypotension, and aseptic meningitis are reported, especially with repeated administration (Spurlock and Prittie, 2011). Thrombotic consequences known to occur in human use have been reported in dogs as well, though its association to IVIG infusion (versus underlying disease) is uncertain.

PLATELETS

Platelet Concentrate Solutions

Platelet-rich plasma (PRP) is harvested from a unit of FWB that is less than 8 hours old and has not been cooled below 20° C. Refrigerated platelets do not maintain function or viability as well as platelets stored at room temperature. The PRP may be administered after centrifugation, or the platelets may be further concentrated by additional centrifugation and removal of most of the supernatant plasma, referred to as platelet concentrate (PC). A dosing of 1 platelet unit derived from a single 450 ml of FWB (typically containing 1.0×10^{11} platelets/100 ml bag for PC, 200 ml for PRP) (Guillaumin et al, 2008) donation is recommended per 10-kg body weight, and is expected to increase the platelet count by 40,000/μL (Abrams-Ogg et al, 2003). The advantage to using PRP or PC over FWB for platelet transfusion is the reduced volume required to transfuse a high concentration of platelets, decreasing the risk of fluid overload, and minimizing immunologic complications through reduction of antigenic material transfused. Disadvantages include need for specialized equipment and staff training in processing, and a reduced (80%) yield of platelets from FWB, reducing the total platelet number available to the patient. Fresh PRP and PC have a short shelf life of 5 days. Platelets cryopreserved with 6% dimethyl sulfoxide (DMSO) have been observed to provide effective hemostasis, though with reduced in vivo recovery (59%) and shortened survival time in circulation (Guillaumin et al, 2008).

The major indication for platelet transfusion is to stop severe, uncontrolled, or life-threatening bleeding in patients with decreased platelet number (thrombocytopenia), function (thrombopathia), or both. Platelet transfusions have the longest survival time and are most effective in patients with thrombocytopenia from reduced platelet production. Survival time of platelets in patients in disseminated intravascular coagulation is shorter because of consumption. In situations of platelet destruction, such as idiopathic thrombocytopenia purpura, the survival of transfused platelets is a matter of minutes rather than days; however, platelet transfusion may still be warranted if the patient is acutely bleeding into a vital structure (i.e., brain, myocardium, lungs). Patients experiencing massive hemorrhage may also require platelet support to compensate for excessive consumption during hemostasis and the dilution factor associated with volume replacement therapy. Preemptive transfusion of platelets may be considered in patients with thrombocytopenia or thrombopathia requiring life-saving procedures with anticipated hemorrhaging, although difficult because of the limited access to platelet products. A "transfusion trigger" for platelets is also uncertain, although a platelet count of greater than 10,000/μL is thought to be sufficient to prevent spontaneous bleeding, and recommendations are made in this range.

In veterinary medicine, platelet preparation is difficult in regard to the volume needed to measurably increase platelet numbers in larger breed dogs. In some patients, however, cessation of bleeding after platelet transfusion has been achieved without a measurable increase in platelet number. Because of the impracticality associated with production of this component in the required volume necessary for significant effect, as well as the specific storage requirements and short shelf life, veterinary medicine routinely treats patients with thrombocytopenia and thrombopathia (with active bleeding) with FWB through which the patient will receive both platelets and oxygen-carrying support (Table 5-1). Use of FWB for platelets eliminates the need for expensive equipment for processing and storage, but if the patient requires more than one unit of platelets for effective hemostasis, risk of volume overload and potential for immunologic reactions become more important considerations.

BLOOD SOURCES

Historically, veterinarians have relied on donor dogs or cats living within the hospital facility, or owned by hospital staff, as a source of blood for transfusion purposes. Blood was collected for immediate use, and little emphasis was placed on quality control. However, these few in-house donors became less able to meet the growing need for transfusion. Currently, several commercial animal blood banks and community-based blood donor programs have been established to help meet blood transfusion needs. These facilities supply safe and high-quality blood products that are processed according to the standards set forth by the American Association of Blood Banks. Blood banking staff also share expertise in transfusion medicine through newsletters and individual case consultation requests. Purchasing products from these blood banks and maintaining an inventory within the hospital may be much more time efficient and

TABLE 5-1	Transfusion Therapy				
COMPONENT	**CONTENTS**	**INDICATIONS**	**SHELF LIFE**	**PREPARATION**	**COMMENTS**
Fresh whole blood (FWB)	Red blood cells (RBCs), plasma proteins, all coagulation factors, white blood cells (WBCs), platelets (approximate hematocrit [HCT] 40%)	Acute active hemorrhage, hypovolemic shock, thrombocytopenia or thrombopathia with active bleeding	Less than 8 hours after initial collection	Use immediately after collection (temperatures below 20° C compromise platelet viability)	Restores blood volume and oxygen-carrying capacity; may help control some microvascular bleeding in patients with thrombocytopenia/thrombopathia; ideal product in massive transfusions
Stored whole blood (WB)	RBC, plasma proteins (approximate HCT 40%)	Anemia with hypoproteinemia, hypovolemic shock	Greater than 8 hours old and up to 30 days (dependent on APS used); refrigerate at 1-6° C	Warm only if risk of hypothermia (temperatures exceeding 37° C will result in hemolysis and bacterial proliferation)	Restores blood volume and oxygen-carrying capacity; WBC and platelets not viable; factors V and VIII diminished; not recommended for chronic anemia
Packed red blood cells (PRBCs)	RBC (approximate HCT 80%), reduced plasma	Increase red cell mass in symptomatic anemia	20-37 days, dependent on APS used; refrigerate at 1-6° C	Warm only if risk of hypothermia (temperatures exceeding 37° C will result in hemolysis and bacterial proliferation); may reconstitute with 0.9% sodium chloride before administration	Same oxygen-carrying capacity as WB but less volume
PRBCs, additive solution added	RBC (approximate HCT 60%), reduced plasma, 100 ml of additive solution	Increase red cell mass in symptomatic anemia	20-37 days, depending on APS and additive solution used; refrigerate at 1-6° C	Warm only if risk of hypothermia (temperatures exceeding 37° C will result in hemolysis and bacterial proliferation); may reconstitute with 0.9% sodium chloride before administration	Additive solution extends shelf life of PRBCs by improving storage environment; reduces viscosity for infusion
Platelet-rich plasma (PRP)/ platelet concentrate (PC)	Platelets, few RBCs and WBCs, some plasma	Life-threatening bleeding caused by thrombocytopenia or thrombopathia	5 days at 20-24° C; constant, gentle agitation required	Should administer immediately after collection and preparation	Should not refrigerate

TABLE 5-1	Transfusion Therapy—cont'd				
COMPONENT	**CONTENTS**	**INDICATIONS**	**SHELF LIFE**	**PREPARATION**	**COMMENTS**
Fresh frozen plasma (FFP)	Plasma, albumin, all coagulation factors	Treatment of coagulation disorders/factor deficiencies, liver disease, disseminated intravascular coagulation, anticoagulant rodenticide toxicity	12 months frozen at −18° C or colder	Thaw in 37° C warm-water bath (temperatures exceeding 45° C will result in protein denaturation and bacterial proliferation)	Frozen within 8 hours after collection; no platelets; can be relabeled as *frozen plasma* (FP) after 1 year for additional 4 years; must be administered within 4 hours after thawing, or refrozen within 1 hr
FP	Plasma, albumin, stable coagulation factors	Treatment of stable coagulation factor deficiencies	5 years frozen at −18° C or colder	Thaw in 37° C warm-water bath (temperatures exceeding 37° C will result in protein denaturation and bacterial proliferation)	Frozen after more than 8 hours after collection; no platelets; can be used to treat some cases of acute hypoproteinemia (20-25 ml/kg); must be administered within 4 hours after thawing
Cryoprecipitate (CRYO)	Factor VIII, von Willebrand's factor, fibrinogen, fibronectin	Hemophilia A von Willebrand's disease, hypofibrinogenemia	12 months frozen at −18° C or colder	Thaw in 37° C warm-water bath (temperatures exceeding 37° C will result in protein denaturation and bacterial proliferation)	Must be administered within 4 hours after thawing
Cryosupernatant	Factors II, VII, IX, and X; albumin	Vitamin K dependent coagulation factor deficiency	12 months frozen at −18° C or colder	Thaw in 37° C warm-water bath (temperatures exceeding 37° C will result in protein denaturation and bacterial proliferation)	Can be used to treat some cases of acute hypoproteinemia (20-25 ml/kg); must be administered within 4 hours after thawing

cost-effective than maintaining in-house donors and likely provides more specific products to treat specific disorders.

Large blood banks obtain their supplies from closed donor colonies or volunteer donor programs. Each approach has advantages and disadvantages. Animals rescued from terminal situations (i.e., retired racing dogs, dogs given or claimed by the Society for the Prevention of Cruelty to Animals) may support closed donor colonies. These animals are given a second chance at life and are adopted into homes after a predetermined stay at the blood bank facility. An unknown medical history is the biggest disadvantage in securing donors from these sources. Blood banks employing specific pathogen-free donor colonies will not encounter issues of unknown medical history, though this is a rare practice.

Other blood banks have opted to establish volunteer donor programs to meet the transfusion needs of the profession. Recruitment of donors is accomplished through employees' personal pets, healthy client-owned animals, breeders, and organized dog clubs. Client education concerning the importance of blood product availability and the need for blood donors is instrumental in establishing a donor pool. Informed and educated pet owners are valuable assets to this type of program. Most are willing to volunteer their pets for periodic blood donation (i.e., three to four times a year) once they understand the need for blood products and the elements of the donation process. Comparable to those who volunteer to help human blood donor programs, these pet owners are motivated by altruism. Nevertheless, potential donors may carry illnesses that could possibly affect the safety of the donation process and the safety and quality of the blood products, thereby further compromising patients, or both.

> **TECHNICIAN NOTE** For this reason, it is important to verify donor health status through an extensive medical history, physical examination, and appropriate laboratory testing, all of which are performed on the day of the donation.

Canine donors must meet specific requirements before being accepted into the program (Box 5-1). Donors must be a minimum of 1 year of age and weigh at least 25 kg to allow for the collection of a full unit (i.e., 450 ml ± 10%). Collection of 19 ml/kg (475 ml for 25 kg) of blood does not incur a clinically significant decrease in blood pressure (Couto and Iazbik, 2005). While donations every 3 to 4 weeks may be possible with diligent monitoring for need of nutritional supplementation, allowing a minimum of 6 to 8 weeks in between blood donations is currently recommended (if not longer) to prevent risks in affecting active lifestyles of many volunteer donors and to prevent owner dissatisfaction. Donors should be healthy; should have a current vaccination status for distemper, hepatitis, parainfluenza, parvovirus, and rabies; and should not be on medication at the time of donation (excluding heartworm and ectoparasite preventative). Because every donor program should strive for canine blood donations without sedation, good temperament is required for successful donations.

BOX 5-1 | Canine Donor Requirements

Donors meeting the following criteria can safely donate 19 ml/kg of blood every 6 to 8 weeks:
- Between the age of 1 and 8 years
- Body weight greater than 25 kg
- In good general health
- Current on vaccinations
- Maintained on heartworm and ectoparasite preventatives
- Not currently taking any drugs aside from those listed previously
- Screened free of bloodborne pathogens
- Have never received a blood transfusion
- Conformation and suitable jugular vasculature for repeated venipuncture
- A good temperament, being able to stay still through a donation
- Blood type desired by the bank
- A committed owner

> **TECHNICIAN NOTE** Care in creating a positive donation experience through positive reinforcement and minimizing stress is vital. On an annual basis, a complete blood count, serum biochemistry profile, and testing for geographically specific infectious agents (e.g., *Ehrlichia canis*, *Babesia canis*) should be performed (Table 5-2). Before each donation, donor HCT (≥40%) or hemoglobin (≥13 g/dl) level is checked. Previous exposure to foreign blood will eliminate the animal from becoming a donor because of potential sensitization and development of alloantibodies, making previous transfusions an exclusion criterion.

In the past, pregnancies have been theorized to be a cause for alloantibody formation through fetal and maternal blood exposure, leading to sensitization. A study reinforced a lack of development of pregnancy-induced alloantibodies, supporting safety in dogs with prior history of pregnancy to become donors (Blais et al, 2009). However, a donor that is currently pregnant should not donate until well after the neonates are weaned. Although each donor should be evaluated as an individual, most dogs are retired from the blood donor program by the age of 8 years.

Blood types are genetic markers on the surface of RBCs, specific to each species, and antigenic. A set of

TABLE 5-2	Canine Infectious Disease Screening	
DISEASE	**DISEASE AGENT**	**SCREENING**
Babesiosis	*B. canis, B. gibsoni*	Recommended
Leishmaniasis	*L. donovani*	Recommended
Ehrlichiosis	*E. canis, E. ewingii, E. chaffeenis*	Recommended conditional
Brucellosis	*B. canis*	Recommended
Anaplasmosis	*A. phagocytophilum, A. platys*	Conditional
Neorickettsiosis	*N. risticii, N. helminthica*	Conditional
Trypanosomiasis	*T. cruzi*	Conditional
Bartonellosis	*B. vinsonii*	Conditional
Lyme	*B. burgdorferi*	Not recommended
Rocky Mountain spotted fever	*R. rickettsia*	Not recommended

From Wardrop et al: Canine and feline blood donor screening for infectious disease, *J Vet Intern Med* 19:135-142, 2005.

blood types of two or more alleles makes up a blood group system. More than 12 blood group systems have been described in dogs, 6 of which belong to the dog erythrocyte antigen (DEA) nomenclature. The current nomenclature lists each system as the DEA followed by a number (DEA 1, 3, 4, 5, 6, 7, 8). Each DEA antigen is located on a separate genetic locus, and can coexist on red cell surfaces. Each locus consists of a positive or null phenotype (e.g., DEA 1 positive, 3 negative, 4 positive, 5 negative), with decimals being used for different positive alleles resulting in distinct surface antigens.

> **TECHNICIAN NOTE** The DEA 1 system had been thought to have three subtypes—DEA 1, DEA 1.2, and DEA 1.3—though recent evidence is suggestive of these subtypes being varying levels of expression of the same antigen (i.e., DEA 1 strong, normal, weak, and very weak) (Canard et al, 2013). In light of this evidence, the rest of this chapter will refer to what is traditionally known as DEA 1.1 as DEA 1. A dog's DEA status is denoted by the DEA with positive antigens (e.g., DEA 1, 4, 7 for dogs positive only in DEA 1, 4, and 7). An additional blood group antigen called Dal has also been identified, first found lacking in expression in some Dalmatians.

Five additional antigens are described in the literature. Very limited surveys on the frequency of canine blood types have been reported (Table 5-3). Some blood types are rare (e.g., DEA 3), whereas others are more common (DEA 4). A full understanding of erythrocyte antigens is outside the scope of this text, and interested readers are encouraged to pursue further literature in hematology (Day and Cohn, 2012; Weiss and Wardrup, 2010).

Clinically, the most severe antigen-antibody reaction is observed with the DEA 1 antigen. *Significant naturally occurring alloantibodies are not seen in the dog;* therefore antigen-antibody reactions are not likely to occur on initial transfusion. However, dogs that are DEA 1 negative can develop alloantibodies to DEA 1 from a mismatched first transfusion. These anti-DEA 1 antibodies can develop within as few as 4 days from initial transfusion and can potentially destroy the donor's RBCs, ultimately minimizing the benefits of the transfusion. However, a previously sensitized DEA 1–negative dog can experience an acute hemolytic transfusion reaction after transfusion of DEA 1–positive blood. Transfusion reactions may also occur after a previously transfused (and now sensitized) dog receives blood that is mismatched for any red cell antigen other than DEA 1. These reactions may occur with a second transfusion as early as 4 days after sensitization. For example, a previously sensitized DEA 4–negative dog experienced an acute hemolytic transfusion reaction while receiving DEA 4–positive blood. Despite the variety of identified and unidentified blood types and the limited availability of compatibility testing in clinical practice, transfusion reactions are rarely reported (transfusion complications are discussed further later in the chapter).

TABLE 5-3	Blood Type Frequencies in Dogs			
BLOOD GROUP	**ALPHABETICAL NOMENCLATURE**	**PHENOTYPES**	**PREVALENCE**	**NATURAL ANTIBODY**
DEA 1	A	1, 1.2, 1.3, null*	62%, 2%, 0.1%	<2%
DEA 3	B	3, null	5%	8%-15%
DEA 4	C	4, null	98%	Rare
DEA 5	D	5, null	15%	10%
DEA 6	E	6, null	96%	Unknown
DEA 7	F	7, 7^I, null	40%-55%	10%-40%
DEA 8	Tr	8, null	20%-40%	Unknown
Dal	N/A	Dal, null	99%	Rare

From Hale A: Canine blood groups and blood typing. In Day MJ, Kohn B, editors: *BSAVA manual of canine and feline haematology and transfusion medicine,* ed 2, Gloucester, 2012, BSAVA, pp 280-283.
*NOTE: Nomenclature may change to Strong, Normal, Weak, Very weak, and Null.

Because of the strong antigenicity of DEA 1, typing of donors for DEA 1 is strongly recommended. Simple in-practice blood-typing kits are commercially available to classify dogs as DEA 1 negative or positive. Card agglutination, immunochromatographic cartridge, and gel column blood typing kits are available on the market, each observed to be accurate (>90%) in determination of DEA 1 status (Seth et al, 2012).

TECHNICIAN NOTE   The immunochromatographic cartridge test (Figure 5-1) is recommended because of its ability to type through auto-agglutination, ease of interpretation, and wide availability. Blood from a DEA 1–negative donor can be given to DEA 1–negative and DEA 1–positive patients. Dogs positive for the DEA 1 antigen can be accepted into the donor pool, as long as recipients are typed before administration, with DEA 1–positive blood being given only to patients positive for DEA 1 (see Table 5-3).

Donors should ideally be more extensively tested by commercial laboratories for other DEA types, allowing inclusion of donors with the least antigenic blood (negative for all testable DEA except 4, which has 98% prevalence). At the time of writing, extensive typing through laboratory services gives minimal information, because antisera used for typing are unavailable for all but DEA 1, 4, and 7. These laboratories may also provide testing for existing alloantibodies, indicating previous exposure to red cell antigens. Blood banks should strive to keep donors with blood types DEA 4 positive (RBCs

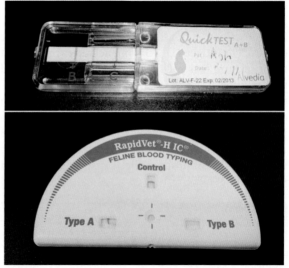

FIGURE 5-1 (Top) Immunochromatographic cartridge manufactured by Alvedia, showing a rare type AB cat. Canine blood typing kits in similar form are available. **(Bottom)** Another immunochromatographic cartridge manufactured by DMS Laboratories.

positive for DEA 4 only) or DEA 1, 4 positive (RBCs positive for DEA 1 and 4 only) without serum alloantibodies to minimize chances of complications, though testing only for DEA 1 may be opted because of expense and a lack of ability to test many DEAs.

The approach to the feline donor is much more complicated than with its canine counterpart. At present, few commercial feline blood banks exist. In addition, volunteer programs for cats hold many risks. Although dogs will donate blood voluntarily, the majority of cats must be sedated for blood donation purposes. The legal ramifications associated with sedating personal pets for blood donation are significant and warrant careful consideration. Another concern is that cats can harbor infectious agents more readily than dogs. For this reason, only 100% indoor cats should be used.

Feline donors have similar requirements to dogs (Box 5-2). Feline blood donors should be young, good-natured adults between the age of 1 and 8 years. They should be large and lean, weighing at least 5 kg to allow for collection of a 50-ml unit of blood. Blood collection

BOX 5-2 | **Feline Donor Requirements**

Donors meeting the following criteria can safely donate 11 ml/kg of blood every 6 to 8 weeks:
- Between the age of 1 and 8 years
- Body weight greater than 5 kg
- In good general health
- Current on vaccinations
- Maintained on ectoparasite preventatives
- Not currently taking any drugs aside from those previously listed
- Screened free of bloodborne pathogens
- Have never received a blood transfusion
- Conformation and suitable jugular vasculature for repeated venipuncture
- A good temperament, without being overly stressed from donation process
- Kept indoors and have no contact with outdoor cats
- A committed owner

under inhalant anesthesia or sedation of 50 ml in cats 4 to 8 kg was observed to have varying effects on blood pressure, with mean arterial pressure (MAP) in some dropping below 60 mm Hg (Iazbik et al, 2007; Morrison et al, 2007). Because of this, a collection volume of less than 11 ml/kg is recommended. Good health can be verified through a medical history, physical examination, and routine laboratory testing. Donors should have current vaccination status for rhinotracheitis, calicivirus, panleukopenia, and rabies. Annual laboratory screening includes complete blood count, serum biochemistry profile, and infectious pathogens such as feline leukemia virus, feline immunodeficiency virus, *Mycoplasma haemofelis,* and *M. haemominutum* (Table 5-4). Before each donation, donor HCT (≥35%) or hemoglobin (≥11 g/dl) level is checked.

One blood group system recognized in the cat is the AB system. It contains three blood types: (1) A, (2) B, and (3) the extremely rare AB. The majority of domestic short hair and domestic long hair cats have the most common type A blood. Many purebred cats (and some domestic short hair cats) have been identified with type B blood. The proportion of type A and B varies not only among the different breeds but also geographically. The rare type AB blood has both the A and the B antigen on the red cell surface. The *Mik* antigen system is also recognized as separately occurring from the AB system, through investigation of the observation of AB system matched transfusions leading to an acute hemolytic transfusion reaction (Weinstein et al, 2007).

TABLE 5-4 | **Feline Infectious Disease Screen**

DISEASE	DISEASE AGENT	SCREENING
Feline leukemia virus	Feline leukemia virus	Recommended
Feline immunodeficiency virus	Feline immunodeficiency virus	Recommended
Hemoplasmosis	M. haemofelis, M. haemominutum	Recommended
Bartonellosis	B. henselae, B. clarridgeiae, B. cholera	Recommended conditional
Cytauxzoonosis	C. felis	Conditional
Ehrlichiosis	E. canis-like	Conditional
Anaplasmosis	A. phagocytophilum	Conditional
Neorickettsiosis	N. risticii	Conditional
Feline infectious peritonitis	Feline enteric coronavirus	Not recommended
Toxoplasmosis	T. gondii	Not recommended

From Wardrop et al: Canine and feline blood donor screening for infectious disease, *J Vet Intern Med* 19:135-142, 2005.

Cats differ from dogs in that naturally occurring alloantibodies against the other blood group are present at significant levels. Cats with type B blood have high titers of naturally occurring anti-A alloantibodies, whereas type A cats have low titers of anti-B alloantibodies. These alloantibodies can cause two serious problems:

Transfusion reactions—Cats with rare type B blood can experience potentially fatal reactions if they are given a transfusion of type A blood. Type A cats receiving type B blood may not exhibit clinical signs associated with an acute adverse reaction; however, the half-life of the type B cells will be short and the transfusion ineffective.

Neonatal isoerythrolysis—If a queen with type B blood is bred to a tom with type A blood and produces kittens with type A blood, then the antibodies in the colostrum of the queen are acquired by the kitten through passive transfer and will destroy type A RBCs, leading to anemia and jaundice.

When administering type B blood to a type A cat, an obvious clinical reaction may not occur; however, the transfused red cells have a half-life of approximately 2 days. Ultimately, this has no positive effect on the patient. In administering type A blood to a type B cat, the red cell survival can be minutes to hours with severe clinical (sometimes fatal) signs. Administration of a small amount of blood to test for incompatibility is not an acceptable procedure. Life-threatening acute hemolytic transfusion reactions can be observed with administration of as little as 1 ml of AB-incompatible blood. These reactions can be avoided by typing donors and patients. Blood-typing kits similar to those used in dogs are also commercially available (see Figure 5-1).

Because of the presence of naturally occurring alloantibodies, no universal blood type exists in the cat. All feline blood donors and recipients must be blood typed, and only type-specific blood should be administered. A blood crossmatch (BCM) should also be performed to ensure blood compatibility. The extremely rare blood type AB cat lacks anti-A and anti-B alloantibodies and can be safely transfused with type A or B blood if type AB blood is not available. However, alloantibodies in the plasma of type A and B blood may cause a hemolytic transfusion reaction due to the presence of anti-A or anti-B antibodies. Because of this, type A PRBC is preferable to be used in type AB cats, as the anti-B antibodies occur at a lower titer in type A blood, and

using PRBC minimizes the amount of plasma containing anti-B antibodies being transfused.

BLOOD COLLECTION

Quality should be the primary goal in the collection, processing, storage, and administration of all blood products. At each step, practices preventing or delaying adverse changes to blood constituents as well as minimizing bacterial contamination and proliferation are critical.

ANTICOAGULANT-PRESERVATIVE SOLUTIONS

Several anticoagulants, anticoagulant-preservative solutions (APSs), and additive solutions (ASs) are available for blood collection for transfusion purposes. The primary goal of preservative solutions is to maintain red cell viability during storage, lengthening the survival of red cells post-transfusion. According to the American Association of Blood Banks standards, 75% of transfused RBCs must survive for 24 hours after infusion for the transfusion to be considered acceptable and successful. The longer cells are stored, the more their viability decreases. Predetermined storage times are based on studies that have investigated adverse biochemical changes that take place during red cell storage. These alterations, referred to as the *storage lesion,* include such things as a decrease in pH and 2,3-diphosphoglycerate level (2,3-diphosphoglycerate loss occurs only in dogs), an increase in the percentage of hemolysis, and an increase in ammonia level within the blood product (storage lesions are discussed in more detail later). All of these changes ultimately lead to a loss of red cell function and decreased viability post-transfusion. Each APS is made of differing combinations of citrate (the anticoagulant) and nutrients such as dextrose, adenine, or mannitol. Nutrients are often added in the form of ASs when PRBCs are processed, extending the shelf life further. A ratio of citrate-based APS to blood of 1.4:10 (1 ml of APS to 7.14 ml of blood) is considered optimal for anticoagulation. Red cell shelf life will vary with the APS and AS used (Table 5-5).

BLOOD COLLECTION SYSTEMS

WB is most often collected into commercially available plastic bags (Fenwal Inc., Lake Zurich, IL; Terumo Medical

TABLE 5-5	Red Cell Shelf Life of Canine Red Blood Cells	
ANTICOAGULANT-PRESERVATIVE SOLUTION (APS)	**ADDITIVE SOLUTION (AS)**	**RED CELL SHELF LIFE IN DAYS**
Acid citrate dextrose (ACD)	None	21*
Citrate phosphate dextrose Adenine 1 (CPDA-1)	None	20†
Citrate phosphate dextrose (CPD)	None	21*
CPD	AS-1 (Adsol)	37†
CPD	AS-5 (Optisol)	35†
Citrate phosphate 2 dextrose (CP2D)	None	21*
CP2D	AS-3 (Nutricel)	35†

*Extrapolated from human data.
†Based on veterinary literature and evidence on PRBCs.

Corp, Somerset, NJ). These sterile bags are considered "closed" collection systems in that they allow for collection, processing, and storage of blood and blood components without exposure to the environment, diminishing the risk of bacterial contamination to the product. These systems are available in a variety of configurations that will determine blood component preparation and storage. They all meet human blood banking standards and have been tested successfully in veterinary medicine.

A single blood collection bag is used for the collection of WB when it is to be administered as WB. This system consists of a main collection bag containing APS and integral tubing with a 16-gauge needle attached. A single blood collection bag is not recommended for component preparation because the bag must be entered to harvest components, risking environmental exposure and potential bacterial contamination. If the bag is entered, the system is considered "open," and the product must be used within 24 hours. Other collection systems consist of a primary collection bag containing APS and one, two, or three satellite bags intended for component preparation (Figure 5-2, A). One of the satellite bags may contain 100 to 110 ml of an additive solution used for red cell reconstitution after plasma removal. Additive solutions (i.e., saline, dextrose, adenine) extend PRBC storage time.

In the dog, blood may be collected using the human blood collection bags; however, the size of these systems prohibits their use in cats. Currently, smaller closed collection systems are not commercially available. In addition, blood component preparation is difficult because of the small volume of blood with which to work. Recommendations have been made to use the 450-ml blood collection system used in humans and dogs by expressing a majority of the APS from the main collection pack into a satellite container via integral tubing. The remainder of the APS in the collection tubing will likely be appropriate for 1 unit of WB (e.g., 40 to 50 ml), though this should be confirmed for the manufactured bag used by the blood bank (1 ml of APS/7.14 ml of blood). Using this approach to blood collection maintains a closed system. Because of the size of both the collection bag and the collection line and its attached needle (16 gauge), justifying this method may be difficult.

Because of the lack of commercially prepared closed blood collection systems for cats, collecting blood for separation and processing without risking contamination has been difficult. By modifying current blood collection protocols, the Penn Animal Blood Bank has developed a closed collection system for small blood volumes (20 to 50 ml) by using commercially available blood collection products. All connections are established and sterility is maintained by using a tube-welding instrument. Tube welders are not easily affordable by many practices, and the blood banking community still lacks options for closed collection system for cats.

Semiclosed systems consisting of an assembly of a 19-gauge butterfly catheter, three-way stopcock, 60-ml syringe, and a single or multiple 100-ml blood collection bag with injection ports sterilized for addition of APS (7.5 ml to collect 52.5 ml for a total of 60 ml) immediately before collection have been developed for blood collection in cats (Figure 5-3, A). This setup is technically an open system because the connections are not seamless and addition of APS through the injection port has the potential to compromise the sterility. The stock of APS has potential in harboring contaminants depending on technique employed and frequency in extracting necessary portions. Much care and precaution must be

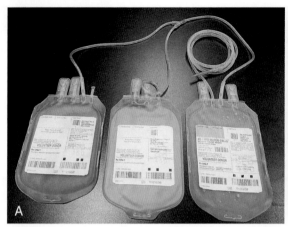

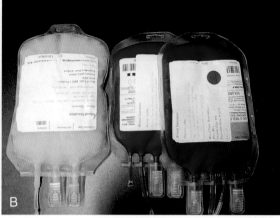

FIGURE 5-2 A, Blood collection bag with multiple satellites. **B,** Finished product. A single donation was separated into plasma and two PRBC packs.

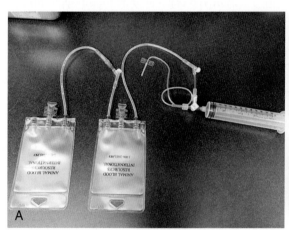

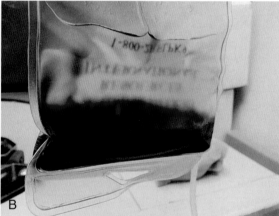

FIGURE 5-3 A, Semiclosed feline blood collection system. **B,** Feline WB after centrifugation. A clear separation between plasma and cellular components is seen.

taken in ensuring maintenance of sterility during collection, and quality control by periodically culturing blood collected in this manner is recommended, especially in the case of blood storage and processing.

BLOOD COLLECTION TECHNIQUES
Canine Blood Collection

The term blood "donation" implies a voluntary giving of the blood. In reality, our donors, at least initially, are volunteered by their owners to donate blood and usually require restraint. However, many of our canine donors will tolerate donating without sedation, and with gentle handling and proper training will learn to willingly donate. Blood donation will become a pleasant and routine

experience. A quiet, secluded room should be set aside, equipped with appropriate supplies (Box 5-3), and regularly used as the donation room.

> **TECHNICIAN NOTE** Effort should be made to habituate the donor to the room, providing ample praise and treats, creating a pleasant donation process. The collection process will require two to three people (one person for restraint, one person for the venipuncture, and an optional person to handle items surrounding the collection). The involvement of the owner should be gauged on an individual basis because the owner's presence may comfort or amplify anxiety.

| BOX 5-3 | Supplies and Equipment for Canine Blood Collection |

All equipment and supplies used for the blood collection should be gathered ahead of time and set up in the room before the donation process is started. The following is a list of materials needed:

- 450-ml blood collection bag (with appropriate satellites for desired blood product)
- Gram scale
- Scrub
- Atraumatic blood tubing clamp (or hemostat with IV tubing covers)
- Blood tubing stripper
- Thermal sealer (or aluminum sealing rings)
- Treats
- Vacuum chamber*
- Suction machine*

*Blood collection with a vacuum chamber setup is utilized by many blood banks to facilitate the collection of blood. These items are optional.

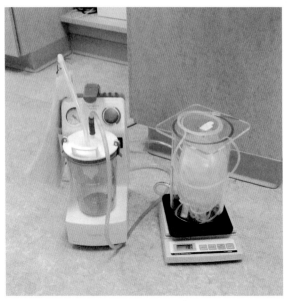

FIGURE 5-4 A vacuum collection system.

One method of collection involves the plastic bag collection system being placed within a vacuum chamber and blood withdrawal facilitated by establishing negative pressure (Figure 5-4). The blood collection bag is hung from a hook on the chamber lid. The collection line with attached needle is brought through a notch between the cylinder and lid, and a hemostat is clamped on the line distal to the needle. A vacuum source is connected via tubing to an inlet in the chamber. The chamber is placed on a scale, the scale is turned to zero, and the suction is adjusted to less than 3 inches of mercury. The needle is inserted into the jugular vein, the hemostat is removed, and blood flows into the collection line to the bag as the scale measures the grams of blood collected (1 ml of WB weighs approximately 1.06 g). When the desired amount is collected (i.e., 405 to 495 ml or 429 to 525 g), the hemostat is clamped on the line, the needle is removed, and pressure is applied to the collection site. Another method of collection involves the donor being placed on a surface higher than the blood collection system to use gravity in assisting the collection through establishment of a pressure gradient. The blood collection bag is placed on a gram scale on the ground, the scale is turned to zero, and the rest of the collection process is the same as that in vacuum-assisted collection.

The advantages of vacuum-assisted collection include faster blood collection times and the donors' ability to stay sitting up on the ground during collection to potentially eliminate stresses of being restrained on a table. The disadvantage would include the potential for the suction machine to increase stress (though many acclimate quickly) and financial investment. Comparatively, gravity-assisted collection requires restraining of the donor on an elevated surface and may increase the collection time; however, blood collection can still be completed within several minutes, thereby eliminating the financial requirement. There is no difference in the occurrence of postdonation hematomas seen (Conversy et al, 2013). The availability of a vacuum-assisted collection system will allow flexibility in tailoring collection methods to the least stressful way for the donor and accustomed to by the staff, maximizing chances of a successful collection. Successful collection depends on many factors (e.g., animal restraint, venipuncture technique, vacuum pressure). After collection, the WB unit can be used immediately, stored as WB, or processed into components and stored according to established blood banking protocols.

The venipuncture site should be monitored until hemostasis is achieved. Donors typically will be able to get up and walk around the donation room. Complications such as hypotension, bruising or extravasation, and irritation of the area clipped and prepped may occur. Food and water should be offered. Donors should be restricted from exercise for at least 24 hours and avoid pressure being placed on the jugular with neck leads.

Feline Blood Collection

Feline blood is typically collected under sedation with a semiclosed system such as that described previously. Varying sedation protocols are utilized involving opioids, benzodiazepines, α_2-agonists, and dissociatives, and sometimes protocols involve anesthetics like propofol or inhalants. Sedation protocols should consider potentials of harm to the donor, minimizing chances of hypotension, provide analgesia for the venipuncture, and allow for a smooth and swift recovery. Avoidance of hypotension is a concern during blood collection. Careful monitoring of the donor is essential, because hypotension can be encountered despite all precautions, particularly in the feline donor. Many institutions routinely administer intravenous or subcutaneous isotonic crystalloid solution at a dose of two to three times the volume of blood drawn to feline blood donors immediately after donation. Others only treat the donors if symptoms of hypotension occur. To avoid hypotension, the donor's hydration status at time of donation should be adequate and the target collection volume should not exceed recommended amounts (19 ml/kg for dogs, 11 ml/kg for cats).

Ideally, a quiet, secluded room should be set aside and regularly used as the donation room (Box 5-4). Quick access to emergency supplies and equipment should be available in case of adverse anesthetic events. The collection process will require at least two people (one person for monitoring and positioning as needed, one person for the venipuncture). During collection, the syringes should be gently inverted to allow for mixing of blood and anticoagulant, preventing clot formation. After collection, blood can be transferred from the syringes through the three-way stopcock into the attached sterile bag to be used immediately, stored as WB, or processed into components provided quality control is performed.

After donation, the donor should be monitored until full recovery. Complications such as hypotension, bruising or extravasation, and irritation of the area clipped and prepped may occur. Perfusion parameters such as heart rate (HR), mucous membranes/capillary refill time (MM/CRT), and pulse quality should be monitored. If fluid replacement was not provided before this point,

---

BOX 5-4	Supplies and Equipment for Feline Blood Collection

All equipment and supplies used for the blood collection should be gathered ahead of time and set up in the room before the donation process is started. The following is a list of materials needed:
- Feline blood collection bag system
  - Custom-made closed collection system *or*
  - Preassembled and sterilized "semi-closed" commercial set *or*
  - 60-ml syringe, 3-way stopcock, 19-gauge butterfly, feline donor bag
- Scrub
- Blood tubing stripper
- Thermal sealer (or aluminum sealing rings)
- Blood pressure monitor
- Oxygen line and mask*
- Endotracheal tube and laryngoscope*

*Oxygen support if called for in the practice's sedation protocol, and preparedness for adverse events during donation is important.

---

subcutaneous infusion of crystalloids is recommended to be given before the effects of sedation dissipate. Food and water should be offered once the donor has recovered from the sedation. If the donor is donating as frequently as every 3 to 4 weeks, oral iron supplementation is recommended.

PROCESSING AND STORAGE

The centrifuge rotor size, speed, and duration of spin are the critical variables in preparing components by centrifugation. Each individual centrifuge must be calibrated for optimal speed and specific time of spin for each component, and thus published protocols may vary slightly. The technician can harvest PRBCs from WB (fresh or stored) by centrifuging the unit with a relative centrifugal force (RCF) of $4000\text{-}5000 \times g$ at $4°$ C for 5 to 10 minutes for canine blood, and at $3000\text{-}4000 \times g$ at $4°$ C for 5 to 10 minutes for feline blood. If a refrigerated centrifuge is not available, then the RBCs may be allowed to separate from refrigerated WB by sedimentation over a period of time. Unfortunately, the process of natural sedimentation decreases the volume of plasma that can be removed and increases the chance of red cell contamination to the final product. After separation has occurred, as much plasma as possible is removed with a plasma extractor. The resulting

PRBCs should then be reconstituted with a nutrient additive solution before storage to maintain the cells in a healthier environment. The use of additive solutions allows for increased plasma yield and extended storage time. In addition, reconstitution of the cells will result in a HCT of 60% to 70%, reducing the viscosity of the PRBCs. If an additive solution is not used, enough plasma should be left in the unit to maintain a HCT not exceeding 80%. Removal of more plasma will lead to insufficient nutrients in solution to support storage. If an additive solution was not used at the time of processing, then PRBCs can be reconstituted with approximately 100 ml of 0.9% sodium chloride before administration to reduce viscosity. Only isotonic saline should be used to dilute blood components, because nonisotonic fluids may cause red cell damage (e.g., dextrose 5% in water) and calcium-containing fluids may initiate blood coagulation (e.g., lactated Ringer's solution). The technician should remember that PRBCs can be refrigerated at 1° C to 6° C, with storage time defined by the anticoagulant-preservative or additive solution used in collection and processing. If the red cells were separated in a system that was open at any time, then the product must be used within 24 hours.

Fresh plasma will provide plasma proteins and coagulation factors; it does not contain viable platelets. The same value is retained for up to 1 year if fresh plasma is frozen at −18° C or less within 8 hours from the time of collection. Because of this, if plasma is harvested from a unit of WB more than 8 hours after collection, the product is traditionally labeled as *FP*. However, a recent study observed an adequate level of coagulation factors in plasma separated after 24 hours of storage, indicating more flexibility in the timing of FFP processing than previously thought (Walton et al, 2014). Both canine and feline FFP can be refrozen as FFP within 1 hour of thawing, with no significant changes in hemostatic qualities (Yaxley et al, 2010). However, the practice of repeatedly thawing and refreezing FFP to extract small portions for therapeutic use is not recommended because this likely will cause unit contamination and the effect of repeated thaw-freeze cycles on hemostatic quality is uncertain.

CRYO is harvested from a unit of FFP that has been allowed to thaw slowly at 1° C to 6° C for approximately 12 to 18 hours. The slushy plasma is centrifuged at 5000 × g at 4° C for 5 to 7 minutes. The supernatant plasma is expressed using a plasma extractor into a satellite bag, labeled as cryosupernatant and refrozen at −18° C with an expiration date of 1 year. The white foamy precipitate left behind (mostly adhered to the bag) in 10 to 15 ml of LP is labeled as CRYO and refrozen at −18° C with a shelf life of 12 months. In the case of blood collection specifically for creation of cryoprecipitate, a dose of desmopressin at 6 mcg/kg IV diluted in 15 ml of normal saline administered 30 to 60 minutes before donation can increase the expression of vWF, increasing the quality of cryoprecipitate (Johnstone, 1999).

PRP is harvested from FWB centrifuged at $1000 \times g$ for 4 minutes or at $2000\text{-}2500 \times g$ for 2.5-3 minutes at 20° C to 24° C. A slower speed, referred to as a "light spin," and a warmer temperature allow viable platelets to clump above the buffy coat. The WB should not be cooled below 20° C before the PRP is removed, and the separation must occur within 8 hours from the time of collection. The plasma should be extracted to approximately 1 cm above the RBC border to prevent contamination of the PRP with RBC and leukocytes. Platelets can be further concentrated by additional centrifugation of the PRP at $2000 \times g$ for 10 minutes at 20° C to 24° C. After centrifugation, the platelet-poor plasma is expressed into an attached satellite bag and the remaining PC allowed to rest undisturbed for approximately 1 hour, allowing platelets to disaggregate. Manual agitation of the platelet pellets may be necessary to ensure even resuspension of the platelets. Platelets prepared in this manner are observed to produce a yield of 74% with a mean value of 8×10^{10} platelets (Abrams-Ogg, 1993). PRP and PC can be stored at room temperature for 5 days under constant agitation before platelet function is significantly decreased (Allyson and Abrams-Ogg, 1997). Cryopreserved PC is commercially available, though shows decreased posttransfusion function and survival time.

The shelf life of blood components is determined by the type of system used for blood collection; the APS used; the time between collection, processing, and storage; and the temperature and conditions under which products are stored. It is critical that appropriate temperatures are consistently maintained to secure the quality of both red cell and plasma products. Refrigerators and freezers for blood component storage should be dedicated for this purpose, and evaluation of their temperatures should be performed daily. Commercially available blood refrigerators and freezers are built to continuously monitor and record temperature, with audible alarm systems that activate before blood products reach unacceptable temperatures.

LEUKOREDUCTION

Leukoreduction, the act of utilizing a filter to remove white blood cells from collected blood, has been a topic of interest, because removal of WBCs from transfusion products should reduce cytokine accumulation during storage and immunogenic potential. These leukocyte reduction filters have been observed to effectively remove leukocytes while maintaining in vivo viability of RBCs in canine blood (Brownlee et al, 2000). Removal is most effective when collected blood is filtered after being cooled to 4° C and should be performed prestorage (WB filtered before centrifugation), observed to cause reduced inflammatory effects in dogs upon transfusion (McMichael et al, 2010). Leukoreduction in veterinary practice is currently rare because of expense, although filters are more affordable than previous years. In the case of feline blood, leukoreduction is currently not practical because the filter retains a significant volume of blood, reducing the total transfusion volume drastically.

STORAGE LESIONS

Current practices in blood banking involve the usage of APS and additive nutrient solution that are labeled for 42 days of storage.

> *TECHNICIAN NOTE*   More recent evidence gathered over the past decade indicates stored red blood cells have impaired RBC survival and reduced efficacy as an oxygen carrier, and even incite adverse effects in the recipient causing mortality and morbidity. These changes are seen as early as 7 to 14 days into storage, and involve a collection of biochemical, biomechanical, and oxidative changes to the RBC and storage solution, all collectively referred to as "storage lesions."

Mature RBCs lack mitochondria and rely on glycolysis for ATP production, leading to a lowered pH of the suspension fluid. ATP production is reduced by the acidic environment, and combined with depletion, leads to decreased RBC membrane integrity. Lowered pH also affects 2,3-diphosphoglycerate (2,3-DPG) levels, reducing hemoglobin's effectiveness as oxygen carriers, though this effect is reversible and not significant in cats. Hemoglobin in longer stored RBC products contains free hemoglobin and microparticles that scavenge nitrous oxide (NO) upon transfusion and cause a vasoconstrictive effect impairing blood flow, stimulate coagulation, induce oxidative damage, and cause proinflammatory effects. Microparticles, which are vesicles that have budded off of cellular components, induce proinflammatory and procoagulant effects. Stored RBCs show morphologic changes to echinocytes and spheroechinocytes leading to a loss of deformability and impairment in normal flow through capillaries. Oxidative damage leads to increased hemolysis and methemoglobin formation, decreasing viable RBC count and oxygen-carrying capacity.

There are many complicated mechanisms at play during RBC storage. To summarize the effects, storage lesions can lead to impaired RBC survival, reduce the efficacy of RBCs as oxygen carriers, and induce adverse effects such as arrhythmias, thrombosis, systemic inflammation, transfusion-related acute lung injury (TRALI), acute respiratory distress syndrome (ARDS), hypotension, and multiple organ dysfunctions. These changes occur as early as 7-14 days into storage, making supplying our patients with safe transfusion products a realistic challenge. Storage lesions and their clinical impact is a topic of ongoing investigation while blood banks strive to balance provision of fresher products and minimizing wasting of blood.

BLOOD ADMINISTRATION

BLOOD COMPATIBILITY

Pretransfusion testing is necessary to ensure the best possible results of a blood transfusion. Compatibility testing includes testing of the donor, selection of appropriate donor units based on the patient's blood type, and blood crossmatch (BCM). Although pretransfusion testing will help to determine incompatibility between the donor and recipient, normal survival of transfused cells in the patient's circulation cannot be guaranteed. Blood samples for initial testing should be collected from all patients before infusion of any donor blood products.

Blood Types

Ideally, all canine blood donors and all recipients should be blood typed for DEA 1 before a transfusion. The erythrocyte antigen DEA 1 is very antigenic and responsible for most blood incompatibilities in dogs. An immunochromatographic blood-typing kit is commercially available to classify dogs as DEA 1 positive or negative. The assay is based on immuno-chromatography, using a porous strip impregnated with antibodies in two locations. In the initial sample area, red cells with the target antigens form immune complexes with antibodies that are labeled with a chromatographic substance such as colloidal gold or selenium. The red cells then pass through the detection area with antibodies fixed in place, which stops the migration of the red cells by attaching to them. This results in a colored band as the indicator for the blood type if positive, and a lack of a band if negative. Immunochromatographic tests have the advantage that they can filter agglutinated cells, allowing for blood type determination even when autoagglutination is present.

Another assay is based on the agglutination reaction that occurs when erythrocytes that contain DEA 1 antigen on their surface membranes interact with a murine monoclonal antibody specific to DEA 1. DEA 1 negative blood can be given to DEA 1 negative and DEA 1 positive patients. DEA 1 positive blood can only be given to patients positive for DEA 1. In an emergency situation, or with specific medical conditions that preclude conclusive typing (e.g., autoagglutination in a patient with immune-mediated hemolytic anemia when using agglutination card tests), DEA 4 positive (negative for all testable DEA, including DEA 1) or DEA 1 negative blood should be used to avoid sensitization to the DEA 1 antigen.

Blood-typing kits similar to those used in dogs are available for cats. Type A blood should be given to type A cats because administration of type B blood will result in mild reactions and delayed hemolytic reactions. Type B blood should be given to type B cats because administration of type A blood will result in a severe, acute hemolytic transfusion reaction and anaphylaxis.

When using card agglutination tests, samples need to be evaluated for autoagglutination. If macroscopic autoagglutination exists, then washing RBCs three times with phosphate-buffered saline (see BCM procedure following) may eliminate the problem; otherwise, blood typing cannot be performed.

Blood Crossmatch

A BCM is performed to detect serologic incompatibility by identifying antibodies in donor or recipient plasma against recipient or donor RBCs. A BCM is divided into two parts: (1) the major crossmatch consists of mixing the patient's plasma with the donor's RBCs; (2) the minor crossmatch consists of mixing the donor's plasma with the patient's RBCs. Of the two tests, the major BCM is much more important in determining survival of the transfused RBCs.

For first-time transfusions in dogs, the necessity for a crossmatch is often debated because of the lack of naturally occurring antibodies for DEA 1 and the unlikelihood of an obvious incompatibility reaction. However, if there is any uncertainty in the transfusion history or in dogs that have received RBC transfusions more than 4 days previously, a crossmatch should be performed before performing RBC transfusions. Because cats have naturally occurring alloantibodies and may experience a severe reaction to their first transfusion, a BCM should be performed before any blood transfusion if blood typing is not available. A BCM is recommended even for the first transfusion since positive crossmatch results are possible even when blood is matched through the AB system because of antigens such as *Mik*. As with dogs, feline patients that have received RBC transfusions more than 4 to 7 days previously should be crossmatched before receiving any additional RBC transfusions (Box 5-5).

An autocontrol with recipient RBCs and plasma is included, because some recipients may have autoagglutination interfering with the BCM. If the patient control is positive (i.e., agglutination is present), then one cannot draw conclusions about blood compatibility between patient and donors. Any hemolysis, agglutination, or both in the major or minor BCM (but not the control) indicates an incompatibility and the need to choose a new donor. The minor BCM should be compatible in dogs but is of lesser importance in that canine donor plasma should not contain significant antibodies. Feline patients must be given type-specific plasma products because of the presence of naturally occurring alloantibodies.

Because a traditional test tube crossmatch method may take longer than desired in an emergency situation, the slide method may be utilized for a less sensitive, but swifter result (see Box 5-5). More recently, an immunochromatographic crossmatch kit for canines has been released on the market (Alvedia LabTEST XM®, Limonest), reducing the subjectivity in interpretation. A compatible BCM does not prevent sensitization or delayed transfusion reactions; it simply indicates that at the present time no antibodies against the RBCs are detected.

BOX 5-5 | Procedure for Blood Crossmatch

Test Tube Crossmatch (40 min–1 hr)
1. Collect blood into a (EDTA) tube from the recipient and possible donor or donors (or obtain anticoagulated blood from the aliquots on the blood bag).
2. Centrifuge (1000 × g for 5 minutes) to separate plasma from red blood cells (RBCs), remove plasma from each sample with a pipette, and transfer the plasma to clean, labeled glass or plastic tubes. Note any hemolysis.
3. Wash RBCs three times with normal saline.
    a. Add 4 to 5 ml of normal saline.
    b. Mix well.
    c. Centrifuge 1 to 2 minutes.
    d. Remove saline, leaving a pellet of RBCs at bottom of tube.
4. Resuspend with normal saline to make a 3% to 5% RBC suspension. (Add 0.2 ml of RBCs and 4.8 ml of normal saline to a glass or plastic tube.)
5. Prepare (for each donor) four tubes labeled donor control, major, minor, and recipient control. Add to each tube 2 drops (50 µL) of plasma and 1 drop (25 µL) of RBC suspension as follows:
    a. Donor control – donor plasma + donor RBCs
    b. Major – recipient plasma + donor RBCs
    c. Minor – donor plasma + recipient RBCs
    d. Recipient control – recipient plasma + recipient RBCs
6. Mix gently and incubate for 15 to 20 minutes at 37° C in a warm-water bath.
7. Centrifuge for 15 seconds at 1000 × g.
8. Examine supernatant for hemolysis.

9. During the gentle resuspension of the pellet of RBCs (by tapping the tube), examine for macroscopic agglutination and classify as 1+ (fine), 2+ (small), 3+ (large), or 4+ (one large agglutinate).
10. If macroscopic agglutination is not seen, observe a sample on a slide with a microscope for agglutination.
11. If there is agglutination on the recipient control, autoagglutination is occurring and a reliable crossmatch cannot be performed. If there is agglutination on the donor control, the blood should not be used, and if a fresh collection, the donor should be evaluated.

Slide Method (20–30 min)
1. Collect blood into a (EDTA) tube from the recipient and possible donor or donors (or obtain anticoagulated blood from the aliquots on the blood bag).
2. Centrifuge (1000 × g for 5 minutes) to separate plasma from red blood cells (RBCs), remove plasma from each sample with a pipette, and transfer the plasma to clean, labeled glass or plastic tubes. Note any hemolysis.
3. Prepare (for each donor) four glass slides labeled donor control, major, minor, and recipient control. Add to each slide 2 drops of plasma and 1 drop of RBCs as follows and mix together:
    a. Donor control – donor plasma + donor RBCs
    b. Major – recipient plasma + donor RBCs
    c. Minor – donor plasma + recipient RBCs
    d. Recipient control – recipient plasma + recipient RBCs
4. Mix gently by rocking the slide back and forth and observe for macroscopic agglutination for 2 minutes. If no agglutination is seen, examine for microscopic agglutination.

COMPONENT PREPARATION

Properly administered cold blood will not increase the chance of a transfusion reaction; however, large amounts of cold blood given at a rapid rate can induce hypothermia leading to cardiac arrhythmias and coagulopathy. Routine warming of red cell products is not recommended because it may increase RBC fragility and promote growth of microorganisms. Exceptions are made in neonates, hypothermic patients, and patients receiving massive transfusions.

Several types of blood warmers are commercially available. Actively warming the blood bag before administration or allowing it to sit at room temperature has little to no effect. If active warming is employed, the temperature should not exceed 37° C to 42° C, and the unit is placed in a plastic bag before being placed in the blood warmer. RBC products brought to room temperature and re-refrigerated should be used within 24 hours according to AABB standards.

> **TECHNICIAN NOTE** If warming is employed, using in-line fluid warmers positioned very close to the patient (<2.5 cm) is required to prevent equilibration to room temperature before the blood reaches the patient (Chiang et al, 2011; Lee et al, 2014).

Frozen plasma products should also be thawed in a 37° C warm-water bath, or commercial plasma thawer. Allowing frozen plasma to sit at room temperature for several minutes before it is placed in the warm-water bath may help prevent cracking of the bag. The plasma is placed in a plastic bag before positioning it in warm-water bath so that leaks can be easily detected. Once thawed, products should remain at 37° C for no longer than 15 minutes to minimize the degradation of certain coagulation factors. No plasma product should be exposed to temperatures exceeding 45° C to avoid denaturation and loss of protein function (Isaacs et al, 2004). FFP can be refrozen if within 1 hour of thawing, without a significant loss in hemostatic function. Warming red cell products or thawing plasma products in a microwave oven is not recommended.

ADMINISTRATION VOLUME

The aim of transfusion in the patient with anemia is not to return the packed cell volume to normal values but instead to meet oxygen demands and correct the clinical signs. The volume of blood administered depends on the onset and degree of anemia, clinical status of the patient, and body weight of the patient. Various methods of RBC dosing are found in literature, and one method was recently found to be accurate in predicting PCV increase in dogs when dosing RBC products (Box 5-6). In more urgent need for transfusions, an average dose of 10 ml/kg of PRBCs or 20 ml/kg of WB may be administered, followed by a reevaluation of clinical signs. A similar feline formula has not yet been studied, and a general guideline of 2 ml/kg of WB or 1 ml/kg of PRBCs for a 1% PCV rise is followed. Anemic cats generally receive 1 unit of WB or PRBCs and are reevaluated for clinical signs.

Plasma products to treat coagulation factor deficiency related coagulopathy (FFP, FP, cryosupernatant) are generally transfused at 10-12 ml/kg and the patient reevaluated. Plasma transfusions for hypoproteinemia are possible, but are not recommended. Very high volumes are required (20-25 ml/kg for a 0.5 g/dl increase in serum albumin), leading to increased risk of immunologic reactions and volume overload. Clinical evaluation of the patient after the transfusion will determine whether further blood product support is necessary.

ADMINISTRATION ROUTES

Blood and blood components can be administered via the intravenous or intraosseous route. Intravenous is obviously the most effective route because the infused RBCs or

---

BOX 5-6   RBC Dosing Formula

Canine

1. $VT = 90 \, ml \times BW \, (kg) \times \dfrac{Desired \, PCV - Patient \, PCV}{PCV}$

2. $VT = 2 \, ml \times Desired \, PCV \, rise \times BW \, (kg)$

3. $VT = 1.5 \, ml \times Desired \, PCV \, rise \times BW \, (kg)$

4. $VT = 1 \, ml \times Desired \, PCV \, rise \times BW \, (kg)$

where VT is the volume to be transfused.

Formula 1: Suitable for all RBC products, but requires knowledge of PCV of the RBC product
Formula 2: Most suitable for PRBCs with PCV of 80% (no additive solution)
Formula 3: Most suitable for PRBCs with PCV of 60% (additive solution added)
Formula 4: Most suitable for WB, with PCV typically ≈45%

From Short JL, Diehl S, Seshadri R et al: Accuracy of formulas used to predict post-transfusion packed cell volume rise in anemic dogs, *J Vet Emerg Crit Care* 22:428-434, 2012.

---

plasma products are immediately available to the general circulation. Use of catheters in the extremities is more suitable in patients with coagulopathies, while jugular catheters or central lines can allow for use of larger catheters and accommodate a faster transfusion rate. Theoretical concerns exist when rapid transfusions of cold or longer stored RBCs with elevated potassium levels are administered through a central line inducing arrhythmias, and proper monitoring is warranted. The intraosseous route is used in neonates and small patients when vascular access is difficult or unsuccessful. When delivering blood products intraosseously, infused cells and proteins are available to the general circulation within minutes. The most common sites for intraosseous catheter placement are the trochanteric fossa of the femur, the wing of the ilium, and the shaft of the humerus. Care should be taken in the placement of these catheters because of the increased risk of osteomyelitis.

ADMINISTRATION RATES

Administration rates are variable. For example, a patient with massive hemorrhage may require a more rapid transfusion than a normovolemic patient with chronic anemia. Blood should not be administered at a rate exceeding 22 ml/kg/hr; however, rate is less critical in a hypovolemic animal than in a normovolemic animal where circulatory overload is a potential problem. Animals with cardiac compromise cannot tolerate high infusion rates and a rate of 4 ml/kg/hr should not be exceeded.

It is recommended that blood components always be infused slowly (e.g., 0.25 to 1 ml/kg/hr) for the first 10 to 15 minutes while the technician closely observes the animal for signs of an acute transfusion reaction. The blood product should then be infused as quickly as will be tolerated, but infusion should not take longer than 4 hours to minimize RBC dysfunction and potential for bacterial proliferation. Before infusion, baseline values of attitude, rectal temperature, pulse rate and quality, respiratory rate and character, mucous membrane color, capillary refill time, hematocrit (HCT), total plasma protein, and plasma and urine color should be monitored. The majority of these parameters should be checked every 30 minutes during transfusion and evaluated routinely after the transfusion to ensure the desired effect has been achieved.

BLOOD FILTERS AND TRANSFUSION METHODS

All blood products should be filtered to help prevent thromboembolic complications. Standard blood infusion sets have in-line filters with a pore size of approximately 170 to 260 µm. A filter of this size will trap cells, cellular debris, and coagulated protein. Trapped debris combined with room temperature conditions may promote proliferation of any bacteria that may be present; therefore blood infusion sets may be used for several units of blood products or for a maximum time of 4 hours. Microaggregate filter systems with a pore size of 18 to 40 µm may be used for low-volume transfusion (i.e., <50 ml of WB, <25 ml of PRBCs or plasma). Concerns surrounding the use of microaggregate filters with canine transfusions exist, possibly leading to RBC survival time of less than 1 day when used with a syringe pump (McDevitt et al, 2011). Because of this, RBC transfusions in dogs are performed with more caution, avoiding use of microaggregate filters when possible. Use of these filters in transfusion of cat RBCs does not seem to affect RBC survival time (Heikes and Ruaux, 2013).

The use of mechanical pumps for RBC transfusions is known to cause a degree of hemolysis depending on storage time, flow rates, and viscosity, and reduced RBC survival time post-transfusion (McDevitt et al, 2011).

The use of infusion pumps designed for IV fluid infusion and the effect on veterinary blood products have not been thoroughly evaluated, and consulting with the manufacturer is recommended. Limited data suggest the use of volumetric fluid pumps to cause variable reduction in RBC survival time, while RBCs transfused with gravity flow maximize RBC survival. In a life-threatening reduction of oxygen-carrying capacity requiring immediate, rapid transfusions, pressurizing the blood bag is acceptable, because the patient benefit from immediate replacement of RBCs and hemoglobin far exceeds the concern of hemolysis of a portion of the RBCs and reduced survival time (though a pressure beyond 300 mm Hg has chances of breaking open bag seams).

TRANSFUSION REACTIONS

Animals should be carefully monitored for any adverse reactions during and for several weeks after transfusion. Transfusion reactions can be classified as immunologic or nonimmunologic in origin.

Allergic reactions are classified as type I hypersensitivity immunologic reactions. In these reactions, immunoglobulin E antibodies bound to mast cells are activated by introduced antigens, inducing degranulation and release of inflammatory mediators (such as histamine and leukotrienes), and trigger localized or generalized inflammation, leading to mild symptoms of vomiting, diarrhea, fever, urticaria, pruritus, or facial swelling (Figure 5-5). Mild symptoms are treated by stopping the transfusion to

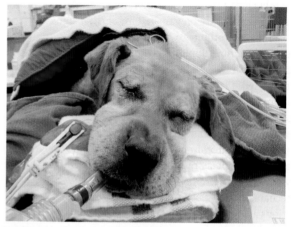

FIGURE 5-5 Type I hypersensitivity reaction and facial swelling from a plasma transfusion on a patient with pulmonary hemorrhage from anticoagulant rodenticide toxicity.

prevent further introduction of antigens, antihistamines, and supportive care. In severe cases, anaphylaxis results from a massive release of mediators, causing hemodynamic collapse and shock. Anaphylaxis is treated by stopping the transfusion and administering glucocorticoids for their antiinflammatory effects, initiating IV fluid resuscitation and, potentially, vasopressors. Epinephrine may also be warranted. Type I hypersensitivity reactions can occur with any blood component, and are only one example of transfusion complications.

Transfusion complication rates are variable and can be immunologic or nonimmunologic. Hemolytic transfusion reaction (HTR), like allergic reactions, is another immunologic response, and can have acute or delayed onset. The existence of IgG and IgM antibodies against mismatched RBC antigens (corresponding to blood types) results in type II hypersensitivity reactions, causing intravascular or extravascular hemolysis of transfused red blood cells (RBCs).

Acute hemolytic transfusion reactions (AHTRs) occur when a patient already has significant levels of antibodies before a transfusion, as with type B felines receiving type A blood or dogs that have had previous transfusions of mismatched blood. Previous exposure and sensitization of the immune system will lead to acquired antibodies reaching significant levels approximately 4+ days after exposure. These antibodies lead to severe AHTR upon second exposure, as with DEA 1 negative canines receiving DEA 1 positive blood for a second time. AHTR can be accompanied by severe type I hypersensitivity-related hemodynamic collapse, further compromising oxygen delivery. AHTR results in fever, salivation, vomiting, diarrhea, disseminated intravascular coagulation, and consequences of hemoglobin release leading to severe hemoglobinemia and hemoglobinuria with intravascular hemolysis. Treatment for AHTR consists of providing cardiovascular support with fluid therapy and vasopressors as needed, suppressing inflammation with glucocorticoids, and providing supportive care. Delayed hemolytic transfusion reactions (DHTRs) can be asymptomatic or manifest as a precipitous drop in PCV with clinical signs of anemia days to weeks post-transfusion, and they are accompanied by hyperbilirubinemia and bilirubinuria when clearance mechanisms are overwhelmed. Hemolytic transfusion reactions are largely avoidable by proper blood type matching and crossmatching before transfusions.

Febrile nonhemolytic transfusion reactions (FNHTRs) are believed to be immune responses to leukocyte antigens and cytokines accumulated during storage, and cause fever, nausea, and vomiting. Leukoreduction, or filtering of leukocytes out of blood products, seems to reduce the incidences of FNHTR. Leukoreduction is not commonly performed in the veterinary field because of the cost of leukoreduction filters.

A few other immunologic complications of interest exist. Transfusion-related acute lung injury (TRALI) is characterized as an acute onset of dyspnea and hypoxemia with diffuse pulmonary infiltrates without signs of circulatory overload. The pathophysiologic mechanism of TRALI is not completely understood, though it seems to involve coupling inflammatory disease and blood transfusions. Transfusion-related acute lung injury is treated by supporting respiratory function through oxygen supplementation and mechanical ventilation, if required.

Transfusion-related immunomodulation (TRIM) is characterized as immunosuppression following blood component transfusion, leading to increased hospital-acquired infection rates. Serum sickness, or type III hypersensitivity reactions, occurs weeks after transfusion and is caused by immune complex deposition in lymph nodes, joints, kidneys, vessel walls, and onto blood cells themselves. Fever, erythema, edema, urticaria, neutropenia, lymph node enlargement, joint swelling, and proteinuria may result, each requiring appropriate therapy.

Nonimmunologic complications typically arise from physiologic consequences of blood component contents and infectious agents. The most common and significant nonimmunologic complication is transfusion-associated circulatory overload (TACO). Any component transfusion adds to patient blood volume, increasing the hydrostatic pressure exerted on vessel walls. Especially when larger volume transfusions are performed on patients with cardiovascular disease or positive fluid balance, edema results, which most commonly occurs in the lungs. Clinical signs of respiratory distress, coughing, hypertension, jugular venous distention, and cyanosis may be seen. Transfusion-associated circulatory overload is managed by stopping the transfusion, implementing diuretic therapy, and providing supplemental oxygen (if hypoxemia results from pulmonary edema). The patient's cardiovascular status and fluid balance should always be assessed before determining the required volume and administration rate to minimize risks of TACO.

Any type of trauma to the RBCs will potentially cause hemolysis: (1) overheating RBC products (also will cause protein denaturation and may increase bacterial growth during infusion), (2) freezing RBC products, (3) mixing RBC products with nonisotonic solutions causing cellular damage, (4) warming and then rechilling blood products, and (5) collecting or infusing blood through infusion pumps and small needles or catheters.

Bacterial pyrogens and sepsis can be a complication of improperly collected and stored blood. Dark-brown to black supernatant plasma in stored blood indicates digested hemoglobin from bacterial growth. Any blood with discolored supernatant should be immediately discarded. Transfusion of components contaminated with bacteria may lead to sepsis and other signs of bloodstream infections. Patients experiencing this complication will most often mount a febrile response 15 to 20 minutes from the start of infusion.

Citrate intoxication may occur when the citrate/blood volume ratio is disproportionate or in massively transfused patients, particularly in patients with liver dysfunction. Common clinical signs include involuntary muscle tremors, cardiac arrhythmias, and decreased cardiac output. This compromised state can be confirmed by obtaining ionized serum calcium level. If citrate toxicity is in question, then blood administration should be discontinued and calcium gluconate administered. Ammonia accumulation in stored blood products can result in hyperammonemia in patients with hepatic failure, and result in neurologic symptoms of ataxia, head pressing, circling, and seizures. Hypothermia can occur when large amounts of cold blood products are transfused, with various consequences (though routine warming of blood products is not recommended).

> **TECHNICIAN NOTE** Technicians play a major role in detecting signs of complications early. Heart rate, respiratory rate and effort, mucous membrane color, capillary refill time, blood pressure, mentation, and signs of nausea, vomiting, and edema should be monitored frequently during the first 30 to 60 minutes (every 5 to15 minutes), and continued less frequently for the rest of the transfusion (every 30 to 60 minutes). A dedicated technician utilizing transfusion monitoring forms should objectively track parameters and have a checklist for important points before, during, and after transfusions.

Although many transfusion complications manifest with nonspecific signs such as fever, vomiting, and diarrhea, subtle changes in parameters like heart rate, respiratory character, blood pressure, and mentation should alert the technician to stop the transfusion and consult the veterinarian for further treatment, based on these patient symptoms. By having a thorough knowledge of transfusion-related complications, technicians will be able to act swiftly, anticipating the needs of patients, and contributing to the best possible patient outcomes.

ALTERNATE TRANSFUSION PRODUCTS AND METHODS

HEMOGLOBIN-BASED OXYGEN CARRIER SOLUTIONS

The hemoglobin-based oxygen carrier solution (HBOC) Oxyglobin® (hemoglobin glutamer 200, OPK Biotech) is an acellular, bovine origin, polymerized hemoglobin solution intended for use in providing oxygen-carrying capacity. HBOC solutions have an advantage over RBC products in their acellular nature, eliminating the need for RBC antigen–based compatibility testing. HBOC facilitates better oxygen delivery than native hemoglobin, and has a long shelf life (3 years for Oxyglobin). The solution has a higher colloid osmotic pressure, which can be beneficial in hypovolemic or hypotensive patients, but poses a higher risk of fluid overload in normovolemic patients or patients with cardiac disease. HBOCs can be useful as an "oxygen bridge" to supplement oxygen-carrying capacity while a suitable RBC match is found or underlying cause is treated (half-life of 15 to 20 hours) and as a nonimmunogenic oxygen carrier for patients with a high risk of immunologic complications (immune-mediated hemolytic anemia, highly alloimmunized patients from repeated transfusions). A typical transfusion monitoring protocol is warranted, because immunologic complications are not out of question, and fluid overload is a concern. Supply of HBOCs over the years has been inconsistent, and the veterinary community awaits consistent commercial supply of this RBC substitute.

XENOTRANSFUSION

Maintaining a large number of type B (or type AB, though demand is rare) feline donors has been a challenge for many blood banks. One method of providing oxygen-carrying capacity to type B feline patients without available compatible blood is the practice of xenotransfusion. Xenotransfusion is the act of transfusing blood from a member of one species to a member of a different species. Canine blood has been occasionally used to provide oxygen-carrying capacity for feline patients. Cats do not have naturally occurring antibodies against dog erythrocyte antigens, with first exposure leading to sensitization and a delayed hemolytic transfusion reaction 4 to 7 days later. Subsequent transfusions administered more than 4 to 6 days after exposure result in anaphylaxis. For this same reason, canine transfusions without blood type matching are discouraged; considering xenotransfusion as a readily available option is discouraged.

> **TECHNICIAN NOTE** Xenotransfusion is justifiable if the patient will die without a transfusion and no other option is available, including compatible blood source or RBC substitutes. Veterinary professions must educate the owners of the risks associated with this therapy and only used as last resort since not recommended.

AUTOTRANSFUSION

Autotransfusion is the act of removing blood from a patient and administering it back into the patient's circulation. In emergency medicine, the blood is collected out of a body cavity where hemorrhage has occurred.

> **TECHNICIAN NOTE** Autotransfusion eliminates the concerns of blood type incompatibilities and can provide life-saving oxygen-carrying capacity when blood product supply is low.

Salvaged blood may be transfused with a syringe or fluid bag, utilizing blood administration filters. Addition of anticoagulants is unnecessary because blood pooled in body cavities has typically consumed coagulation factors and has undergone fibrinolysis. Concerns with autotransfusion lie in potential contaminants to the blood such as bacteria, malignant cells, and thrombi, as well as the potential to induce coagulopathies and systemic inflammation. Good case selection and ready-made autotransfusion kits will help alleviate demands on the blood bank.

REFERENCES AND FURTHER READINGS

Abrams-Ogg AC: Triggers for prophylactic use of platelet transfusions and optimal platelet dosing in thrombocytopenic dogs and cats, *Vet Clin North Am Small Anim Pract* 33:1401–1418, 1993.

Abrams-Ogg AC, Kruth SA, Carter RF, et al.: Preparation and transfusion of canine platelet concentrates, *Am J Vet Res* 54:635–642, 2003.

Abrams-Ogg AC, Schneider A: Principles of canine and feline blood collection, processing, and storage. In *Schalm's veterinary hematology*, ed 6, Ames, Iowa, 2010, Wiley-Blackwell, pp 731–737.

Allyson K, Abrams-Ogg AC, Johnstone IB: Room temperature storage and cryopreservation of canine platelet concentrates, *Am J Vet Res* 58:1338–1347, 1997.

Blais MC, Rozanski EA, Hale AS, et al.: Lack of evidence of pregnancy-induced alloantibodies in dogs, *J Vet Intern Med* 23:462–465, 2009.

Brownlee L, Wardrop KJ, Sellon RK, et al.: Use of a prestorage leukoreduction filter effectively removes leukocytes from canine whole blood while preserving red blood cell viability, *J Vet Intern Med* 14:412–417, 2000.

Canard B, Barthélémy A, Felix N, et al.: Stability of DEA1+ antigen expression and production of allo-antibodies after transfusion in dogs. A preliminary study, In *Proc 19th Int Vet Emerg Crit Care Symp* 814, 2013.

Chiang V, Hopper K, Mellma MS: In vitro evaluation of the efficacy of a veterinary dry heat fluid warmer, *J Vet Emerg Crit Care* 21:639–647, 2011.

Conversy B, Blais MC, Carioto L, et al.: Comparison of gravity collection versus suction collection for transfusion purposes in dogs, *J Am Anim Hosp Assoc* 49:301–308, 2013.

Couto CG, Iazbik MC: Effects of blood donation on arterial blood pressure in retired racing Greyhounds, *J Vet Intern Med* 19:845–848, 2005.

Craft EM, Powell LL: The use of canine-specific albumin in dogs with septic peritonitis, *J Vet Emerg Crit Care* 22:631–639, 2012.

Day MJ, Kohn B: *BSAVA manual of canine and feline haematology and transfusion medicine*, ed 2, Gloucester, 2012, British Small Animal Veterinary Association.

Feldman BF, Sink CA, Burton DL, editors: *Practical transfusion medicine for the small animal practitioner*, Jackson, Wyo, 2004, Teton New Media.

Guillaumin J, Jandrey KE, Norris JW, et al.: Assessment of a dimethyl sulfoxide-stabilized frozen canine platelet concentrate, *Am J Vet Res* 69:1580–1586, 2008.

Heikes BW, Ruaux CG: Effect of syringe and aggregate filter administration on survival of transfused autologous fresh feline red blood cells, *J Vet Emerg Crit Care*, 2013. (Epub ahead of print).

Hischvogel K, Jurina K, Steinberg TA, et al.: Clinical course of acute canine polyradiculoneuritis following treatment with human IV immunoglobulin, *J Am Anim Hosp Assoc* 48:299–309, 2012.

Iazbik MC, Gomez Ochoa P, Westendorf N, et al.: Effects of blood collection for transfusion on arterial blood pressure, heart rate, and PCV in cats, *J Vet Intern Med* 21:1181–1184, 2007.

Isaacs MS, Scheuermaier KD, Levy BL, et al.: In vitro effects of thawing fresh-frozen plasma at various temperatures, *Clin Appl Thromb Hemost* 10:143–146, 2004.

Johnstone IB: Desmopressin enhances the binding of plasma von Willebrand factor to collagen in plasmas from normal dogs and dogs with type I von Willebrand's disease, *Can Vet J* 40:645–648, 1999.

Lee RA, Millard HA, Weil AB, et al.: In vitro evaluation of three intravenous fluid line warmers, *J Am Vet Med Assoc* 244:1423–1428, 2014.

McDevitt RI, Ruaux CG, Baltzer WI: Influence of transfusion technique on survival of autologous red blood cells in the dog, *J Vet Emerg Crit Care* 21:209–216, 2011.

McMichael MA, Smith SA, Galligan A, et al.: Effect of leukore-duction on transfusion-induced inflammation in dogs, *J Vet Intern Med* 24:1131–1137, 2010.

Morrison JA, Lauer SK, Baldwin CJ, et al.: Evaluation of the use of subcutaneous implantable vascular access ports in feline blood donors, *J Am Vet Med Assoc* 230:855–861, 2007.

Powell C, Thompson L, Murtaugh RJ: Type III hypersensitivity reaction with immune complex deposition in 2 critically ill dogs administered human serum albumin, *J Vet Emerg Crit Care* 23:598–604, 2013.

Seth M, Jackson KV, Winzelberg S, et al.: Comparison of gel column, card, and cartridge techniques for dog erythrocyte antigen 1.1 blood typing, *Am J Vet Res* 73:213–219, 2012.

Sibley TA, Miller MM, Fogle JE: Human intravenous immuno-globulin (hIVIG) inhibits anti-CD32 antibody binding to canine DH82 cells and canine monocytes in vitro, *Vet Immunol Immunopathol* 151:229–234, 2013.

Spurlock NK, Prittie JE: A review of current indications, adverse effects, and administration recommendations for intravenous immunoglobulin, *J Vet Emerg Crit Care* 21:471–483, 2011.

Walton JE, Hale AS, Brooks MB, et al.: Coagulation factor and hemostatic protein content of canine plasma after storage of whole blood at ambient temperature, *J Vet Intern Med* 28:571–575, 2014.

Wardrop KJ, Owen TJ, Meyers KM: Evaluation of an additive solution for preservation of canine red blood cells, *J Vet Intern Med* 8:253–257, 1994.

Wardrop KJ, Tucker RL, Mugnai K: Evaluation of canine red blood cells stored in a saline, adenine, and glucose solution for 35 days, *J Vet intern Med* 11:5–8, 1997.

Weinstein NM, Blais MC, Harris K, et al.: A newly recognized blood group in domestic shorthair cats: the *Mik* red cell anti-gen, *J Vet Intern Med* 21:287–292, 2007.

Weiss DJ, Wardrop KJ: *Schalm's veterinary hematology,* ed 6, Ames, Iowa, 2010, Wiley-Blackwell.

Whelan ME, O'Toole TE, Chan DL, et al.: Use of human im-munoglobulin in addition to glucocorticoids for the initial treatment of dogs with immune-mediated hemolytic anemia, *J Vet Emerg Crit Care* 19:158–164, 2009.

Yaxley PE, Beal MW, Jutkowitz LA, et al.: Comparative stability of canine and feline hemostatic proteins in freeze-thaw-cycled fresh frozen plasma, *J Vet Emerg Crit Care* 20:472–478, 2010.

SCENARIO

Purpose: To provide the veterinary technician with the opportunity to build or strengthen his/her knowledge on component therapy and execute veterinarian orders on administration.

Stage: Emergency clinic is considered a level II facility and has an in-house blood bank storing blood products purchased from commercial blood banks. You have access to PRBCs, FFP, cryoprecipitate, synthetic colloids, and isotonic crystalloids. There are hospital-approved donors to call if FWB is needed.

Scenario

Consider the following patients:

Patient 1: A 3-year-old female Vizsla weighing 27.1 kg walks into the hospital, having difficulty breathing and coughing some blood, and bruising is seen on the abdomen. Upon examination she is found to be tachycardic (HR 140 beats/min), tachypneic (RR 56 breaths/min) with increased effort, lungs auscult harsh with some crackles, mucous membrane (MM) is pink with a capillary refill time (CRT) of less than 1 second. Pulse quality is normal. Initial blood work shows packed cell volume (PCV) of 40%, platelet count of 248,000/µL, PT/PTT is prolonged. Thorac-ic radiographs show signs of pulmonary edema. The patient is hospitalized for respiratory support, and the owner calls later and informs you the neighbors have placed some rat bait in their yard.

Patient 2: A 14-year-old female DSH weighing 3.1 kg is brought to the hospital because she has been lethargic at home. Upon examination she is found to be tachycardic (HR 200 beats/min), slightly tachypneic (RR 40 breaths/min) with in-creased effort in breathing; lungs auscult clear. Her MM is pale with a hint of pink, and CRT is 1-2 sec. Pulses feel normal. Initial blood work shows her PCV is 11%, TP is 5.8 g/dl. She has been on subcutaneous fluid therapy at home for chronic kidney disease.

Patient 3: A 5-year-old male King Charles spaniel weighing 8.8 kg is brought in after having progressively liquid and bloody diarrhea for 2 days, and has been hospitalized and received IV fluid therapy for 24 hours. Upon reassessment this morning, his HR is 160 beats/min, RR 32 breaths/min, MM pale pink, CRT of 2+ seconds. Skin turgor is fast with a gelatinous consistency. Blood work today shows PCV of 32%, TP of 3.6 g/dl, and serum albumin of 1.3 g/dl.

Patient 4: A 4-year-old male mix breed dog is rushed in after being stabbed repeatedly in the chest and abdomen by a neighbor, reportedly in self-defense. The dog is estimated to weigh 35 kg. The patient is visibly bleeding out of his abdominal wounds, and is barely conscious. Two peripheral IV catheters are quickly placed while the open wounds are bandaged and reduction of the bleeding is attempted.

Delivery
- Present all cases to the staff.
- Initial discussion: Allow **10-20 minutes** for the staff to reviews the cases, and make recommendations about the blood products that are indicated for use.
- Have staff explain their rationale.
- Follow-up discussion: Provide an administration order (typically in the form of *"Give X ml of [chosen product] at Y ml/hr for the first 15 minutes and then the rest over Z hours"*) that agrees with your hospital protocols, and have the staff describe the plan.

Questions
- Initial discussion
  - What is the patient's problem, and what is its likely cause?
  - Discuss the blood products that are suitable for use, if any. Explain why they may be used.
  - Discuss any alternative blood product that may be used, and explain why the alternative is less optimal (if applicable).
- Follow-up discussion
  - What compatibility testing should be performed, if any?
  - What supplies will you need?
  - How will the blood product be prepared for transfusion?
  - What are the initial rate and target rate of administration?
- What parameters should be monitored during transfusion, and are there any to which there should be paid special attention?

Key Teaching Points
- Provides veterinary technicians the opportunity to review indications of blood components.
- Provides the opportunity to consider alternatives if the supply is limited, and understand additional risks.
- Veterinary technician can practice devising a realistic plan based on hospital transfusion protocols.

References
- Table 5-1 in chapter text provides a summary of blood component content, indications, and preparation.

MEDICAL MATH EXERCISE

A donor is receiving desmopressin for cryoprecipitate preparation. The donor's order states: *Give 6 mcg/kg of desmopressin diluted to a total of 15 ml with saline IV.*

The concentration of desmopressin is 0.1 mg/ml. The donor weighs 30 kg.

1. How many micrograms of desmopressin do you need?
2. How many milliliters of stock desmopressin do you need?

6

Nutritional Support for the Critically Ill Patient

Daniel L. Chan

KEY TERMS

Enteral nutrition
Feeding tubes
Malnutrition
Nutritional assessment
Parenteral nutrition

CHAPTER OUTLINE

Nutritional Assessment
Goals of Nutritional Support
  Nutritional Plan
  Calculating Nutritional
    Requirements

Role of the Veterinary Technician
Enteral Nutrition
Parenteral Nutrition
Monitoring and Reassessment
Summary

LEARNING OBJECTIVES

After studying this chapter, you will be able to:

- Understand the important role nutrition plays in the recovery phase of many conditions in small animals
- Be able to list and describe the consequences of malnutrition but also of over-feeding
- Be able to describe the various forms of nutritional support that can be used in small animal practice and list the advantages and disadvantages of each option
- Understand how a nutritional plan is tailored to the needs of a patient, how the plan is executed, and how to monitor the patient receiving nutritional support

There are a number of reasons for critically ill animals to be at high risk for becoming malnourished. Moreover, critically ill animals undergo several metabolic alterations that further increase this risk. During periods of nutrient deprivation, a healthy animal will primarily use fat stores for energy. However, sick or traumatized patients will catabolize lean muscle first rather than fat when they are not provided with sufficient calories. This loss of lean tissue reduces the animal's strength, compromises immune function and wound healing, and likely negatively impacts overall survival, although this is difficult to prove. The risk of **malnutrition** primarily relates to inadequate food intake because it is not uncommon for inappetence to be one of the main clinical problems in animals requiring medical care. Animals are presented for loss of appetite, an inability to eat or tolerate feedings, persistent vomiting, or diarrhea that accompanies many disease processes. Because malnutrition can occur quickly in these animals, it is vital that we identify animals at risk for malnutrition, and initiate early nutritional support for these patients. The first step of nutritional support is to identify the most appropriate route for nutrition—either enteral (using the gastrointestinal tract) or parenteral (intravenous, IV) nutrition if oral intake is not adequate. The goals of nutritional support are to treat malnutrition when present and, just as important, to prevent malnutrition in patients at risk. Whenever possible, the enteral route should be used because it is the safest, most convenient, and most physiologically sound method of nutritional support. However, when patients are unable to tolerate enteral feeding or unable to use nutrients administered enterally, parenteral nutrition (PN) should be considered. Ensuring the successful nutritional management of critically ill patients involves selecting the right patient, making an appropriate nutritional assessment, and implementing a feasible nutritional plan.

NUTRITIONAL ASSESSMENT

As with any medical intervention, risks of complications are always possible. Minimizing such risks depends on patient selection and patient assessment. The first step in formulating a nutritional strategy involves making a systematic evaluation of the patient, referred to as a **nutritional assessment**. Nutritional assessment identifies malnourished patients who require immediate nutritional support and also identifies patients at risk for developing malnutrition in which nutritional support will help to prevent malnutrition. This process of nutritional assessment has recently been formalized into a Nutritional Assessment Checklist (Figure 6-1) that has been promoted as part of a Nutrition Toolkit made available by the World Small Animal Veterinary Association's WSAVA's Global Nutrition Committee (www.wsava.org/nutrition-toolkit).

Indicators of overt malnutrition include recent weight loss of at least 10% of body weight, poor hair coat quality, muscle wasting, and signs of poor wound healing. However, these abnormalities are not specific to malnutrition and are not present early in the process. In addition, fluid shifts may mask weight loss in critically ill patients. Factors that predispose a patient to malnutrition include anorexia lasting longer than 3 days, serious underlying disease (e.g., trauma, sepsis, peritonitis, pancreatitis, gastrointestinal surgery), and large protein losses (e.g., protracted vomiting, diarrhea, draining wounds). Nutritional assessment also identifies factors

that can affect the nutritional plan, such as cardiovascular instability, electrolyte abnormalities, hyperglycemia, and hypertriglyceridemia, as well as concurrent conditions, such as kidney or hepatic disease that will influence the nutritional plan (e.g., require reduction in protein or phosphorous content). Appropriate laboratory analysis (i.e., serum biochemistry) should be performed in all patients to assess these parameters. Before implementation of any nutritional plan, the patient must be cardiovascularly stable, with major electrolyte, fluid, and acid-base abnormalities corrected.

An important aspect of nutritional assessment involves determination of a body condition score (BCS). Various systems have been proposed, and each of these systems seeks to qualitatively assess whether an animal is emaciated, thin, in ideal body condition, overweight, or obese. These systems incorporate both a visual and a tactile assessment of the animal's body, paying careful attention to abdomen, ribs, pelvic bony prominences, and tail/head. The most commonly used systems implement either five or nine categories. Neither system is superior; the most important point is that the veterinary team within a practice should adopt one of these systems and use it consistently. The entire veterinary staff should use BCS in every assessment of both healthy and hospitalized patients. By consistently using the BCS, one can effectively communicate the progression of an animal's body condition during the course of a disease and recovery. The WSAVA's Nutrition Toolkit also includes noncommercially branded BCS charts that can be used to train both staff and clients. To communicate which BCS system is being used, the BCS should reflect the scale being used. For example, a dog that is in ideal body condition should be listed as 3/5 or 5/9, depending on the system being used. This will eliminate any confusion.

GOALS OF NUTRITIONAL SUPPORT

Even in patients with severe malnutrition, the immediate goals of therapy should focus on resuscitation, stabilization, and identification of the primary disease process. As steps are made to address the primary problems, formulation of a nutritional plan should strive to prevent (or correct) overt nutritional deficiencies and imbalances. By providing adequate energy substrates, protein, essential fatty acids, and micronutrients, the staff ensures that the animal's body will support wound healing, immune function, and tissue repair. A major goal of nutritional

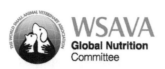
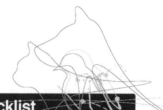

Nutritional Assessment Checklist

To be completed by the pet owner. Please answer the following questions about your pet:

Pet's name: _____   Species/breed: _____   Age: _____

Owner's name: _____   Date form completed: _____

1 How active is your pet?	Very active ☐	Moderately active ☐	Not very active ☐
2 How would you describe your pet's weight?	Overweight ☐	Ideal weight ☐	Underweight ☐
3 Where does your pet spend most of the time	Indoor ☐	Outdoor ☐	Indoor & Outdoor ☐

Please list below the brands and product names (if applicable) and amounts of ALL foods, treats, snacks, dental hygiene products, rawhides and any other foods that your pet is currently eating, including foods used to administer medications:

Food	Form	*Amount	Number	Fed since
Examples:				
• Purina Cat Chow	dry	½ cup	2x/day	Jan 2010
• 90% lean hamburger	pan-fried	3 oz (85 grams)	1x/week	May 2011
• Milk Bone medium	dry	2	3/day	Aug 2012
• Greenies Salmon Dental	treat	2	daily	Jan 2013

*If you feed by volume, what size measuring device do you use? _____
*If you feed tinned/canned food, what size tins/cans? _____

4 Do you give any dietary supplements to your pet (for example: vitamins, glucosamine, fatty acids, or any other supplements)?   **No** ☐   **Yes** ☐

If yes, please list brands and amounts:_____

To be completed by the health care team:

Has the diet history form been reviewed?   **No** ☐   If not, please review the diet history form   **Yes** ☐   If yes, please continue:

Current body weight: _____   Ideal body weight: _____

Current body condition score* _____/9   or _____/5   *Refer to the body condition scoring chart

Muscle Condition Score: normal ☐   mild wasting ☐   moderate wasting ☐   severe wasting ☐

Screening evaluation checklist
Pets that are healthy and without risk factors need no additional extended evaluation

Nutritional screening risk factors (extended evaluation is OPTIONAL)	Check ✓ if present
Extremely low or high activity level	☐
Multiple pets in a household	☐
Gestation	☐
Lactation	☐
Growth period	☐
Age of >7 years	☐
Nutritional screening risk factors (extended evaluation is MANDATORY)	
History of altered gastrointestinal function (e.g., vomiting, diarrhea, nausea, flatulence, constipation)	☐
Previous or ongoing medical conditions / disease	☐
Currently receiving medications and/or dietary supplements	☐
Unconventional diet (e.g., raw, homemade, vegetarian, unfamiliar)	☐
Snacks, treats, table food > 10% of total calories	☐
Inadequate or inappropriate housing	☐
Physical examination	
Body condition score less than 4 or greater than 5 (on 9-pt scale)	☐
Muscle condition score: Mild, moderate, or severe muscle wasting	☐
Unexplained weight change	☐
Dental abnormalities or disease	☐
Poor skin or hair coat	☐
New medical conditions / disease	☐

NO CHECKED ITEM(S) ON THIS PAGE? The Nutrional Assessment is complete
CHECKED ITEM(S) ON THIS PAGE? Continue on the next page

wsava.org

FIGURE 6-1 WSAVA Nutritional Assessment Checklist used to aid in assessing the risk for developing malnutrition and need for nutritional support. This checklist is part of the Global Nutrition Committee Toolkit, which is being reproduced in its entirety. The Global Nutrition Committee Toolkit is provided courtesy of the World Small Animal Veterinary Association. (From World Small Animal Veterinary Association Global Nutrition Committee. Accessed at www.wsava.org/nutrition-toolkit.)

Extended evaluation checklist

Changes in food intake or behavior

a. Amount eaten: increased ☐ decreased ☐
b. Chewing: normal ☐ abnormal ☐
c. Swallowing: normal ☐ abnormal ☐
d. Nausea: yes ☐ no ☐
e. Vomiting: yes ☐ no ☐
f. Regurgitation: yes ☐ no ☐

Condition of the integument

a. Easily-plucked hair: yes ☐ no ☐
b. Thin skin: yes ☐ no ☐
c. Dry or scaly skin: yes ☐ no ☐

Abnormalities in serum chemistry profile

a. Glucose: low ☐ normal ☐ high ☐
b. Albumin: low ☐ normal ☐ high ☐
c. Total protein: low ☐ normal ☐ high ☐
d. Electrolytes:
low _____
high _____
e. Urea: low ☐ normal ☐ high ☐
f. Creatinine: low ☐ normal ☐ high ☐
g. Total T4: low ☐ normal ☐ high ☐

Abnormalities in complete blood count

a. Anemia: yes ☐ no ☐
b. Lymphopenia: yes ☐ no ☐

Other _____
_____
_____

Abnormalities on fecal flotation / smear / culture: _____
_____

Abnormalities on urinalysis: _____

Abnormalities on other diagnostic tests: _____
_____

Provide the following recommendation(s):

Change in the caloric intake recommended? No ☐ Yes ☐ If yes, calculate:
Current caloric intake** _____ kcal or kJ/day
**Refer to information obtained from the diet history form.
Recommended caloric intake*** _____ kcal or kJ/day
*** Refer to the calorie requirement form.

Change in the diet recommended? No ☐ Yes ☐ If yes, describe:
New diet recommended _____

Change in the feeding management recommended? No ☐ Yes ☐ If yes, describe:
Amount per serving _____ cups _____ cans _____ grams
Number of servings per day _____
Treat(s) (if applicable); amount(s) and number(s) per day _____
Be sure to specifically discuss **table foods**, **supplements**, and **medication administration** with the owner.

Change of environmental factors recommended? (i.e., issues with multiple pets, other food providers and sources, extent of enrichment, activity of pet, environmental stressors)

No ☐
Yes ☐ Describe: _____

Recommendations for monitoring given to the client?
(i.e., BW, BCS, MCS, food intake, appetite, gastrointestinal clinical signs, activity, overall appearance)
No ☐
Yes ☐ If yes, please describe: _____

Did client purchase the recommended food? No ☐ Yes ☐
Educational information or tools dispensed? No ☐ Yes ☐

wsava.org

FIGURE 6-1, cont'd WSAVA Nutritional Assessment Checklist used to aid in assessing the risk for developing malnutrition and need for nutritional support.

support is to minimize metabolic derangements and catabolism of lean body tissue. During hospitalization, restoration of previous healthy body weight is *not* a priority, because weight restoration will only occur when the animal is recovering from a state of critical illness. The goal of nutritional support during hospitalization is to prevent further losses to lean tissue and to provide energy and nutrients required for healing. With these principles in mind, it is prudent to provide nutritional support in a conservative and gradual manner with frequent reassessment.

NUTRITIONAL PLAN

Proper diagnosis and treatment of the underlying disease is the key to the success of nutritional support. Based on the nutritional assessment, a plan is formulated to meet the patient's energy and other nutritional requirements and, at the same time, address any concurrent condition or conditions requiring adjustments to the nutritional plan. The anticipated duration of nutritional support, which will largely depend on clinical familiarity with the specific disease process and sound clinical judgment, should be estimated and factored into the plan. For each patient, the best route of nutrition should be determined—**enteral nutrition** versus **parenteral nutrition**. This decision should be based on the underlying disease and the patient's clinical signs. Whenever possible, the enteral route should be considered first. If enteral feedings are not tolerated or the gastrointestinal tract must be bypassed, then PN should be considered. Nutritional support should be introduced gradually and reach target levels in 48 to 72 hours.

CALCULATING NUTRITIONAL REQUIREMENTS

The patient's resting energy requirement (RER) is the number of calories required for maintaining homeostasis while the animal rests quietly. A common way to calculate the RER is use the following formula:

$$RER = 70 \times (\text{body weight in kilograms})^{0.75}$$

For animals weighing between 2 and 30 kg, the following linear formula gives a good approximation of energy needs:

$$RER = (30 \times \text{body weight in kilograms}) + 70$$

Traditionally, the RER was then multiplied by an illness factor between 1.0 and 1.5 to account for increases

in metabolism associated with different conditions and injuries. Recently, less emphasis has been placed on these subjective illness factors, and current recommendations are to use more conservative energy estimates (i.e., to forgo the use of illness factors) to avoid overfeeding. Overfeeding can result in metabolic and gastrointestinal complications, hepatic dysfunction, increased carbon dioxide production, and weakened respiratory muscles. Of the metabolic complications, the development of hyperglycemia is most common in veterinary patients.

Currently, the RER is used as an initial estimate of a critically ill patient's energy requirements. It should be emphasized that these general guidelines should be used as starting points, and animals receiving nutritional support should be closely monitored for tolerance of nutritional interventions. Continual decline in body weight or body condition should prompt the clinician to reassess and perhaps modify the nutritional plan (e.g., increase the number of calories provided by 25%).

ROLE OF THE VETERINARY TECHNICIAN

The technical staff is absolutely crucial in providing nutritional support. Because technical staff spend the most contact time with patients, they are best suited in identifying patients in need of nutritional support, using the nutritional plan, and assisting in placement of feeding tubes, placement of catheters for PN, and monitoring the patient for complications. In most practices, the technical staff should be empowered to assist clinicians in formulating the nutritional plan for a patient and help assess the response to treatment. The next few sections are devoted to the role of technical staff in the provision of the different types of nutritional support.

ENTERAL NUTRITION

As previously mentioned, the enteral route of nutritional support is usually preferable. Enteral nutrition is safer and less expensive than PN, and it helps to maintain intestinal structure and function. Enteral nutrition includes all forms of oral feeding (e.g., hand feeding, syringe feeding) and tube feedings (e.g., nasoesophageal [NE], esophagostomy [E], gastrostomy [G], jejunostomy [J] feeding tubes). Even with the use of **feeding tubes**, patients can easily be discharged for home care with good owner compliance. Most feeding tube complications include tube occlusion and localized irritation at the tube exit site. More serious complications include infection at the exit site or, rarely, complete tube dislodgment and peritonitis if the tube was a G or J tube. Staff can avoid feeding tube complications by using the appropriate tube, making proper food selections, and preparing and carefully monitoring clients (encouraging pet owners to follow home care guidelines and watch for potential problems).

Assisted feedings (either by hand or by syringe) are usually ineffective in providing adequate amounts of calories. Nevertheless, these techniques are important in two ways. First, assisted feeding can aid in assessing whether the patient's gastrointestinal tract can tolerate feedings. Should the patient vomit after assisted feeding, consideration should be given for PN. Second, assisted feeding can help determine when a patient's appetite is improving. Appetite stimulants such as cyproheptadine or mirtazapine are usually not very effective when given to completely anorectic patients; however, they can stimulate animals to eat more consistently when they are beginning to eat on their own but are not yet eating sufficiently.

The important point to remember with syringe feeding is that it should never be a stressful event. If the animal resists or objects to syringe feeding, then placement of a feeding tube should be considered. Should a patient begin to associate eating with a stressful situation, the animal may develop a food aversion that further complicates nutritional support (this is especially true in cats). Another important point is that syringe feeding should never be done to a patient that is dyspneic or with compromised ability to protect its airways (e.g., patients without a gag reflex or laryngeal paralysis), because the risk for aspiration is too great.

If a feeding tube is required for nutritional support, the next step is selecting the type of feeding tube to be used (Table 6-1). Feeding tubes commonly used in dogs and cats include NE, E, and G tubes. Although described, the use of J tubes in general practice is still uncommon. The veterinary technician can play a major role in the placement of such tubes, because placement techniques often require more than one person. Moreover, the staff can be extremely helpful in setting up and preparing the tubes and patients for these procedures. Once the desired feeding tube is placed, radiography should be used to confirm satisfactory tube placement.

NE tubes are very easy to place and require very little sedation. Application of local anesthetics to nasal mucosa and proper lubrication of the tube can improve the animal's tolerance for such a tube placement. However, NE tubes have disadvantages. First, only liquid diets can be used, and these diets are usually only 1 kcal/ml; therefore administering an adequate amount of calories to the patient is difficult. Second, this tube usually

TABLE 6-1	Feeding Tube Selection		
FEEDING TUBE	**DURATION**	**ADVANTAGES**	**DISADVANTAGES**
Nasoesophageal (NE tube)	Short term (<5 days)	Inexpensive Easy to place No anesthesia required	Requires liquid diet Some animals will not eat with NE tube in place
Esophagostomy (E tube)	Long term	Inexpensive Easy to place Can use calorically dense diets	Requires anesthesia Cellulitis can occur if tube is removed early
Gastrostomy (G tube)* Percutaneous endoscopically guided (PEG) surgically placed	Long term Long term	Easy to place Can use calorically dense diets Can use calorically dense diets	Requires anesthesia Requires endoscope Requires anesthesia and laparotomy
Jejunostomy (J tube)	Long term	Bypasses stomach and pancreas Can be used in patients with pancreatitis	Requires anesthesia and laparotomy For all in-hospital use Requires continuous rate infusion Requires liquid diet Peritonitis can occur if tube is removed

*For all the G tubes, peritonitis is a possible complication if the tube leaks or is removed early.

requires placement of an Elizabethan collar to prevent removal by the animal; therefore placement is not well tolerated. Feeding via NE tubes should be limited for very short-term use or in particularly unstable animals that cannot tolerate anesthesia. In some animals, bolus feedings of liquid diets through NE tubes elicit nausea and vomiting. A useful strategy in such cases is to attempt NE feedings via a slow continuous infusion with a syringe or infusion pump. The technician should start with 1 to 2 ml/hour infusions and increase gradually until the caloric goals are met.

E tubes are much more versatile and can be used for effective nutritional support. Placement requires a brief period of anesthesia; the technique is easily mastered and allows feeding for prolonged periods of time. The technique for placement is detailed in Box 6-1 and a step-by-step procedure is also described. Both the tube and the feedings are well tolerated by patients, and most clients can become adept at this feeding method. Flushing of the tube with water after each use will prevent clogging. Oral liquid medications can also be administered via the E tube; however, crushed and dissolved medications should not be administered via the E tube because of the high likelihood of clogging of the tube. In the event of clogging of the tube, one may dislodge the obstruction with warm water by applying pressure and suction with a syringe. Other methods include infusing a carbonated beverage or a solution of pancreatic enzyme and sodium bicarbonate. Feedings should be done using gently warmed foods and performed over a 10- to 15-minute period.

Surgically placed G tubes and percutaneous endoscopically placed gastrostomy (PEG) tubes require more involved procedures using anesthesia and special equipment. These types of tubes are more appropriate for long-term nutritional support. Cases in which G or PEG tubes may be indicated include severe esophageal dysfunction (e.g., megaesophagus, severe esophagitis, esophageal stricture, esophageal or pharyngeal neoplasia) or protracted debilitating diseases (e.g., end-stage chronic renal failure). Special kits for these tubes are commercially available (Figure 6-2). These larger tubes allow for feeding of "blenderized" diets that could not be administered via NE or E tubes. The exit site for the G or PEG tube should be frequently assessed (for signs of infection) and appropriately managed. Feeding

BOX 6-1	Esophagostomy Tube Placement

1. Proper placement of an esophagostomy (E) tube requires the distal tip to be placed in the distal esophagus or into the stomach. This may require premeasuring the tube. Rather than cutting the distal tip and creating a sharp edge, the exit side hole should be elongated using a small blade.

2. The patient should be anesthetized and preferably intubated.

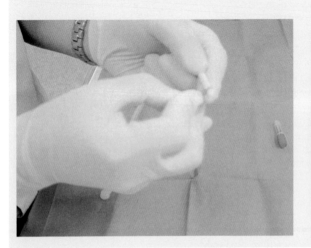

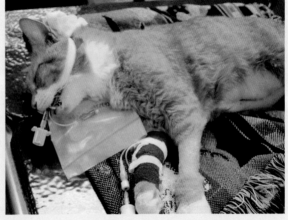

BOX 6-1 | Esophagostomy Tube Placement—cont'd

3. While in right lateral recumbency, the left side of the neck should be clipped and a routine surgical scrub performed.

5. The tip of the Rochester-Carmalt is then pushed dorsally, pushing the esophagus toward the skin.

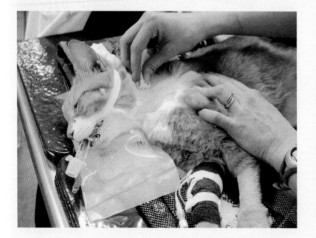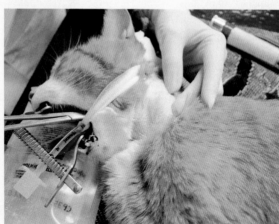

4. A curved Rochester-Carmalt forceps is placed into the mouth and down the esophagus to the midcervical region. The jugular vein should be identified and avoided.

6. The tip of the Rochester-Carmalt is palpated over the skin to confirm its location, and an incision is made through the skin and into the esophagus. The mucosa of the esophagus is relatively more difficult to incise than the skin.

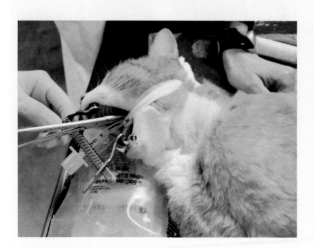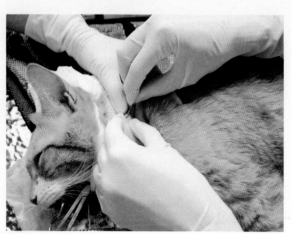

Continued

BOX 6-1 | Esophagostomy Tube Placement—cont'd

7. The tip of the instrument is then forced through the incision.

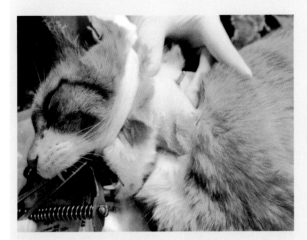

8. The incision can be slightly enlarged with the scalpel blade to allow opening of the tips of the Rochester-Carmalt and placement of the E tube within the tips.

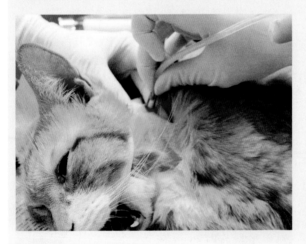

9. The Rochester-Carmalt is then clamped closed and pulled from the oral cavity.

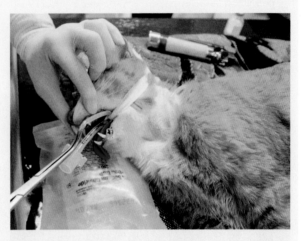

10. The tips of the Rochester-Carmalt should be disengaged and the tip of the E tube curled back into the mouth and fed into the esophagus.

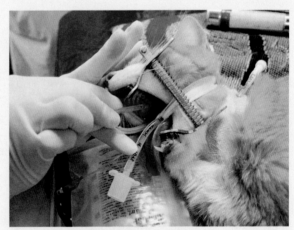

BOX 6-1 | Esophagostomy Tube Placement—cont'd

11. As the curled tube is pushed into the esophagus, the proximal end is gently pulled simultaneously. This will result in a subtle "flip" as the tube is redirected within the esophagus. The tube should easily slide back and forth a few millimeters, confirming that the tube has straightened.

13. The incision site should be briefly rescrubbed before a purse-string suture is placed to secure the tube in place.

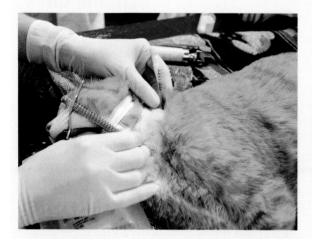

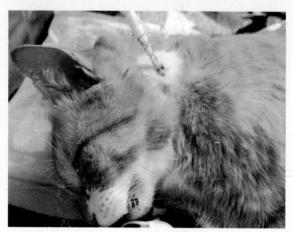

12. The clinician should visually inspect the oropharynx to confirm that the tube is no longer present within the oropharynx.

14. The tube is further secured in place with a "Chinese finger trap" suture around the tube.

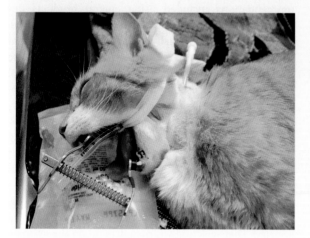

Continued

BOX 6-1 Esophagostomy Tube Placement—cont'd

15. A light wrap is applied to the neck.

16. Correct placement should be confirmed with either radiography or fluoroscopy.

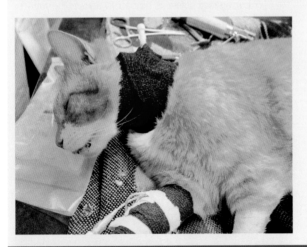

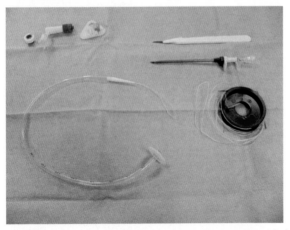

FIGURE 6-2 Placement of percutaneous endoscopically-guided gastrostomy (PEG) tube has been made easier with availability of all-inclusive kits that include the gastrostomy tube, trocar introducer, suture, scalpel blade, anchors and adaptors.

through a G or PEG tube should never cause the patient discomfort. Should discomfort occur, the tube should be immediately evaluated for correct placement. These tubes could be replaced by more cosmetic (and often costly) low-profile feeding tubes if the G or PEG tube is to be used for more than a couple of months. The only advantage of these tubes is that they are largely inconspicuous and may be less easily dislodged.

In cases in which the patient undergoes abdominal surgery and reason exists to bypass the upper gastrointestinal (GI) tract (i.e., severe necrotizing pancreatitis, pancreatic abscesses or masses, or duodenal resections), a J tube may be placed. This will allow jejunal feedings while the upper GI tract heals. Although previous recommendations included using enteral products designed for humans, the use of veterinary liquid diets, such as CliniCare, is usually well tolerated. It is vital that patients with J tubes be carefully monitored, because leakage or displacement usually results in peritonitis. Care must also be used in properly labeling J tubes, because critically ill patients typically have other concurrent IV and urinary catheters that can be confused with the J tube, resulting in serious consequences. Feeding through J tubes should be administered as continuous infusions via pumps rather than bolus feeding, which may be associated with nausea or pain.

Based on the type of feeding tube chosen and the disease process being treated, an appropriate diet should be selected. Diet selection will also depend on the animal's clinical parameters and laboratory results (Box 6-2). The amount of food is then calculated, and a specific feeding plan is devised. Generally, NE, E, and G tube feedings are administered every 4 to 6 hours, and feeding tubes should be flushed with 5 to 10 ml of water after each feeding to minimize clogging of the tube. By the time of

BOX 6-2	Worksheet for Calculating Enteral Nutrition*

1. Resting energy requirement (RER):
   RER = 70 × (current body weight in kilograms)$^{0.75}$
   or, for animals weighing between 2 and 35 kg:
   RER = (30 × current body weight in kilograms) +
   70 = ___ kcal required/day
2. Product selected _____
   Contains _____ kcal/ml
3. Total volume to be administered per day:
   $\frac{\text{kcal required/day}}{\text{kcal/ml in diet}}$ = ___ ml/day
4. Administration schedule:
   One half of total requirement on day 1 = ___ ml/day
   Total requirement on day 2 = ___ ml/day
5. Feedings per day:
   Divide total daily volume into 4 to 6 feedings (depending on duration of anorexia, patient tolerance) = ___
   feedings/day
6. Calculate volume per feeding
   $\frac{\text{Total ml/day}}{\text{Number of feedings/day}}$ = ___ ml/feeding (day 1)
   = ___ ml/feeding (day 2)

Diet Options
Esophagostomy (E) and gastrostomy (G) tubes
Hill's a/d (canned)
- Supplies 1.3 kcal/ml straight from can but needs to be diluted for tubes
- 1 can + 50 ml of water = 1.0 kcal/ml
- 1 can + 25 ml of water = 1.1 kcal/ml (for larger tubes)

Royal Canin low-fat canine diet (canned)
- When a low-fat enteral diet is required
- 1 can blenderized with 360 ml of water, then strained = 0.8 kcal/ml

Nasoesophageal (NE) and jejunostomy (J) tubes
Veterinary liquid diets
- CliniCare canine/feline liquid diet (1.0 kcal/ml)
- CliniCare RF feline liquid diet (reduced protein formula –1.0 kcal/ml)
- Human enteral products

*Be sure to adjust the animal's IV fluids accordingly.
NOTE: Most human liquid diets provide 1.0 kcal/ml but do not meet canine or feline requirements (and must be supplemented).

discharge, however, the number of feedings should be reduced to three to four times per day to facilitate owner compliance.

For E and G tubes, a volume of 5 to 10 ml/kg per individual feeding is generally well tolerated (may vary with the individual patient). In patients that are generally healthy but cannot consume food orally (e.g., jaw fracture), larger volumes of food per feeding (15 to 20 ml/kg) may be tolerated. Because enteral diets are mainly composed of water (most canned food is >75% water), the amount of fluids administered parenterally should be adjusted accordingly to avoid volume overload. Prevention of premature removal of tubes can be accomplished using an Elizabethan collar and wrapping the tube securely. Care should be taken to avoid wrapping the tube too tightly (doing so could lead to patient discomfort and possibly compromise ventilation).

PARENTERAL NUTRITION

PN is more expensive than enteral nutrition and currently only available for hospitalized animals. Indications for PN include vomiting, severe malabsorptive disorders, and severe ileus. The terminology used to describe the use of PN in veterinary patients has evolved, and so it is worth reviewing the terminology. Total parenteral nutrition (TPN) was previously defined as the provision of all of the patient's protein, calorie, and micronutrient requirements intravenously, whereas partial parenteral nutrition (PPN) was defined as the provision of only a part of this requirement (typically 40% to 70% of the energy requirement). More recently, there has been a shift away from describing PN in terms of "meeting energy and nutrient requirements" because they remain largely unknown in animals, and so recent recommendations emphasize categorizing PN by the mode of delivery such that PN delivered into a central vein is described as 'central PN' and PN delivered into a peripheral vein is described as 'peripheral PN.' For the purposes of this chapter, 'PPN' will refer to peripheral PN.

Because PPN only provides a portion of the patient's RER, it is only intended for short-term use in a nondebilitated patient with average nutritional requirements. Regardless of the exact form of PN, IV nutrition requires a dedicated catheter that is placed using aseptic technique. Once PN is initiated, the catheter should no longer be used for administration of IV medications or collection of blood (it should only be used to administer PN). Long catheters composed of silicone, polyurethane, or polytetrafluoroethylene are recommended for use with PN to reduce the risk of thrombophlebitis. Multi-lumen catheters are often recommended for PN because they can remain in place for longer periods of time (as compared with normal jugular catheters) and provide other ports for blood sampling and administration of additional fluids and IV medications. Most PN solutions are composed of a carbohydrate source (dextrose or glycerol), a protein source (amino acids), and a fat source (lipids). Vitamins and trace metals can also be added.

The need to administer certain PN solutions via central veins relates to the osmolarity and pH of the solution. PPN, on the other hand, is formulated so that it can be administered through a peripheral catheter because of its lower osmolarity (usually <1000 mOsm/L). Formulation of PN solutions requires special equipment and training; therefore it is best obtained from a local human hospital or human home healthcare companies. Usually an order provides 3 to 5 days of PN for a patient and should be stored in the refrigerator. Each bag of PN holds a 1-day amount of solution and should be administered via constant rate infusion over 24 hours. Cyclical PN (i.e., providing PN during certain hours of the day and discontinuing it at night) is discouraged, because it increases the likelihood of catheter contamination. If the practice cannot provide 24-hour care, then consideration should be made to refer the case to another facility.

After 24 hours, a new bag of PN must be used (first allowing it to warm to room temperature), with fresh setups and IV lines. Bags, lines, and catheters should always be handled aseptically. Once a patient is started on PN, the system should be maintained as a closed system (no medications are to be injected either into the bag or into the line, and the lines should not be disconnected during walks or diagnostic procedures). The technician should simply disengage the line from the infusion pump and carry the bag and line with the patient while adjusting the drip flow regulator to a slow drip. Doing this will prevent the catheter from becoming occluded and avoid backflow of blood into the line. Should the line or bag ever be compromised (e.g., chewed lines, dis-

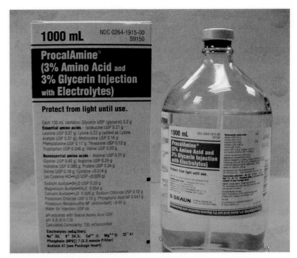

FIGURE 6-3 In facilities in which parenteral nutrition is not individually compounded, ready-made combination products containing amino acid and glucose are a convenient and practical method for delivery of nutritional support in patients that cannot be fed enterally.

lodged catheters, inadvertent disconnection), the entire setup (including the bag) should be discarded and a new setup and bag should be hung.

As an alternative, there are commercially available, ready-to-use preparations of glucose and amino acids for peripheral use; however, these formulations provide approximately less than 50% of required calories (when administered at maintenance fluid rate), and they should only be used for short-term or in conjunction with enteral nutrition. One such product is ProcalAmine (McGraw), which is a 3% amino acid solution and 3% glycerol (carbohydrate source). This product (Figure 6-3), which contains approximately 25 mEq/L of potassium chloride, is administered at normal fluid maintenance rates (limited because of the inclusion of maintenance potassium concentrations), either via a central or via a peripheral IV catheter, and provides 245 kcal/L of solution administered. A protocol for setting up a patient on such a solution is provided in Box 6-3. As with enteral nutrition, PN should be instituted gradually over 48 to 72 hours. Animals receiving PN should have their catheters and lines checked daily, and these procedures must be handled with aseptic technique to avoid contamination. It is important to adjust other IV fluids accordingly for the amount of fluid being administered to avoid fluid volume overload.

BOX 6-3	Calculations for Setting Up Peripheral Parenteral Nutrition Using ProcalAmine® (3% Glycerol, 3% Amino Acid Solution)

1. Calculate resting energy requirement (RER):

   RER = 70 × (current body weight in kg)$^{0.75}$

   or for animals weighing between 2 and 30 kg:

   RER = (30 × current body weight in kg) + 70

   RER = ___ kcal/day

2. Select target protein level and calculate protein required:

PROTEIN LEVEL	CANINE (G/100 KCAL)	FELINE (G/100 KCAL)
Standard	4	6
Reduced	2-3	3-4
Increased (excessive protein losses)	6	7-8

   (RER ÷ 100) × ___ g/100 kcal protein level = ___ g of protein required/day

3. Calculate rate of ProcalAmine required:

   ProcalAmine is a 3% amino acid solution; thus it has 0.03 g of protein/ml

   PPN rate requird = ___ g of protein/day ÷ 0.03 g of protein/ml ÷ 24 hours = ___ ml/hr or PPN

Make sure this rate of infusion is acceptable for this patient.

4. Calculate proportion of RER provided at this rate:

   ProcalAmine has 0.25 kcal/ml of energy

   Energy provided by PPN = 0.25 kcal/ml × ___ ml/hr of PPN × 24 hr = ___ kcal/day

   Proportion of energy from PPN = ___ PPN energy ÷ ___ RER × 100 = ___ %

5. Calculate rate of glucose infusion at calculated PPN rate:

   ProcalAmine has 3% glycerol (dextrose equivalent) (i.e., 30 mg/ml)

   Glucose infusion rate = ___ ml/hr PPN ÷ 60 min × 30 mg/ml ÷ kg body weight = ___ mg/kg/min glucose

Glucose infusion rate should not exceed 4 mg/kg/min because it may cause hyperglycemia. May need to decrease infusion rate and recalculate.

MONITORING AND REASSESSMENT

Body weight should be monitored daily when providing enteral nutrition or PN. However, the team should take into account fluid shifts in evaluating changes in body weight. For this reason, assessment of BCS is important as well. The use of the RER as the patient's caloric requirement is merely a starting point. The number of calories provided may need to be increased to keep up with the patient's changing needs (typically by 25% if well tolerated). In patients unable to tolerate the prescribed amounts, the clinician should consider reducing amounts of enteral feedings and supplementing the nutritional plan with PPN.

Possible complications of enteral nutrition include mechanical complications such as clogging of the tube or early tube removal. Metabolic complications include electrolyte disturbances, hyperglycemia, volume overload, and gastrointestinal signs (e.g., vomiting, diarrhea, cramping, bloating). In critically ill patients receiving enteral nutritional support, the team must also be vigilant for the development of aspiration pneumonia. Monitoring parameters for patients receiving enteral nutrition include body weight, serum concentrations of electrolytes, tube patency, appearance of tube exit site, gastrointestinal signs (e.g., vomiting, regurgitation, diarrhea), and signs of volume overload or aspiration pneumonia.

Possible complications with PN include sepsis, mechanical complications of the catheter and lines, thrombophlebitis, and metabolic disturbances such as hyperglycemia, electrolyte shifts, hyperammonemia, and hypertriglyceridemia. Avoiding serious consequences of complications associated with PN requires early identification of problems and prompts action. Frequent monitoring of vital signs, catheter exit sites, and routine biochemistry panels may alert the staff to developing problems. If the patient may have a catheter infection, then PN should be discontinued and discarded and the catheter removed and cultured. The development of persistent hyperglycemia during nutritional support may require an adjustment to the nutritional plan (e.g., decreasing dextrose content in PN) or administration of regular insulin and, therefore, will necessitate more vigilant monitoring.

With continual reassessment, the team can determine when to transition the patient from assisted feeding to voluntary consumption of food. The discontinuation of nutritional support should only begin when the patient can consume approximately its RER without much coaxing. In patients receiving central PN, transitioning to enteral nutrition should occur over the course of at least 12 to 24 hours, depending on patient tolerance of enteral nutrition.

SUMMARY

Although critically ill patients are often not regarded as in urgent need of nutritional support (given their more pressing problems), the severity of their injuries, their altered metabolic condition, and the necessity of frequent fasting place these patients at high risk of becoming malnourished during hospitalization. Proper identification of these patients and careful planning and execution of a nutrition plan can be key factors to successful recovery. Therefore the inclusion of the technical staff in the formulation and administration of nutritional support to critically ill patients is absolutely essential.

PRODUCTS LISTED

NE tube: Feeding tube, Professional Medical Product Inc., Greenwood, SC.

E tube: Esophagostomy tube, Smiths Medical PM, Inc., Veterinary, WI.

Low-profile G tube: Corflo-Cubby low-profile gastrostomy device, VIASYS Healthcare Medsystems, Wheeling, IL.

J tube: Enteral feeding tube, VIASYS Healthcare Medsystems, Wheeling, IL.

CliniCare canine and feline liquid diet, Abbott Animal Health, Abbott Park, IL.

CliniCare feline RF liquid diet, Abbott Animal Health, Abbott Park, IL.

ProcalAmine, McGraw Inc., Irvine, CA.

SUGGESTED READINGS

Buffington T, Holloway C, Abood A: Clinical dietetics. In Buffington T, Holloway C, Abood S, editors: *Manual of veterinary dietetics*, St Louis, 2004, Saunders, pp 49–141.

Chan DL: Nutritional requirements of the critically ill patient, *Clin Tech Small Anim Pract* 19:1–5, 2004.

Chan DL: Nutrition in critical care. In Bonagura JD, Twedt DC, editors: *Kirk's current veterinary therapy*, ed 15, St Louis, 2014, Saunders, pp 38–43.

Chan DL, et al.: Retrospective evaluation of partial parenteral nutrition in dogs and cats, *J Vet Intern Med* 16:440–445, 2002.

Freeman LM, Chan DL: Parenteral and enteral nutrition, *Compend Stand Care Emerg Crit Care* 3:1–7, 2001.

Gajanayake I, Wylie CE, Chan DL: Clinical experience using a lipid-free, ready-made parenteral nutrition solution in dogs: 70 cases (2006-2012), *J Vet Emerg Crit Care* 23:305–313, 2013.

Jensen K, Chan DL: Nutritional management of acute pancreatitis in dogs and cats, *J Vet Emerg Crit Care* 24:50–240, 2014.

Marks SL: Nasoesophageal, esophagostomy, and gastrostomy tube placement techniques. In Ettinger S, Feldman E, editors: *Textbook of veterinary internal medicine*, ed 6, St Louis, 2005, Elsevier, pp 329–335.

Michel KE: Interventional nutrition for the critical care patient: optimal diets, *Clin Tech Small Animal Pract* 13:204–210, 1998.

Reuter JD, et al.: Use of total parenteral nutrition in dogs: 209 cases (1988-1995), *J Vet Emerg Crit Care* 8:201–213, 1998.

Zsombor-Murray E, Freeman LM: Peripheral parenteral nutrition, *Compend Contin Educ Pract Vet* 21:512–523, 1999.

SCENARIOS

DEVISING A NUTRITIONAL PLAN

Purpose: To provide the veterinary technician with the opportunity to work through clinical situations where animals may require nutritional support.

Stage: Veterinary hospital is considered a moderate level facility with at least 2 veterinary technicians on every shift, 24 hr a day, 7 days a week.

Scenarios

Monday morning after a busy weekend with a number of admissions.

Patient 1: A 3-year-old female Cocker spaniel is presented for 2 days of vomiting, lethargy, and inappetence. The dog has excessive salivation and vomits greenish fluid during examination. Dog has obvious discomfort on abdominal palpation. Dog weighs 13 kg and has body condition score of 6/9. Blood is collected for serum biochemistry and a SNAP cPL (canine pancreas-specific lipase) test. Blood is grossly lipemic, the SNAP cPL result is "abnormal," and the provisional diagnosis of acute pancreatitis is made.

Patient 2: A 10-year-old female DSH cat is presented for a 5-day history of vomiting, lethargy. The cat has reportedly stopped eating 10 days ago. The cat has lost 12% of body weight since last examined and is now 3.5 kg and has body condition score of 3/9. The cat is icteric, dehydrated, and weak with depressed mentation and signs of nausea. Laboratory findings include high bilirubin concentration, increased alkaline phosphate, and ALT activities. Ultrasonographic findings include an enlarged, hyperechoeic liver with rounded edges. The cat is provisionally diagnosed with hepatic lipidosis.

Patient 3: A 7-year-old male Labrador retriever presents for severe chronic vomiting (>5 times a day for past 2 weeks). The dog has lost 10% of body weight in past month. The dog weighs 23 kg and has body condition score of 4/9. Ultrasonographic examination does not reveal intestinal foreign body but does show diffuse thickening of the bowel and enlarged mesenteric lymph nodes. A fine-needle aspirate of one of the mesenteric lymph nodes confirms intestinal lymphoma. The plan is to initiate an aggressive protocol of chemotherapy.

Delivery

- Write case ideas on separate sheets.
- Staff reviews case details and has **3-5 minutes** to review each case.
- Questions following case evaluations are answered.
- Discussion should continue without goal being to find the right answer.

Questions

- For each patient, perform a nutritional assessment and state whether the animal is in need of nutritional support.
- For patients requiring nutritional support, select the best route or form of nutritional support and describe the best strategy for addressing nutritional needs.
- For each patient, what would need to be completed before initiating nutritional support?
- What complications may arise with the chosen form of nutritional support for each patient?

Key Teaching Points

- Provides veterinary technicians opportunity to assess nutritional status of patients and determine patients in most urgent need of nutritional support.
- Provides veterinary technicians opportunity to discuss most appropriate strategies for nutritional support in different case scenarios.
- Allows discussion of modes of nutritional support available at the hospital.
- Allows veterinary technicians to participate and contribute to nutritional plans of patients and anticipate possible complications associated with different modes of nutritional support.

Discussion

Patient 1: This patient does not have obvious signs of malnutrition but is at moderate risk of becoming malnourished. Since acute pancreatitis can resolve with supportive care and the patient can resume eating within 3 days, the dog may not need special nutritional support. However, acute pancreatitis is no longer considered a condition where enteral nutrition is contraindicated. If the dog's nausea and abdominal pain are controlled, the dog may be offered enteral nutrition. The diet should be easily digestible and be of low fat content. The initiation of feeding can begin as soon as nausea and pain are controlled. If the dog does not eat voluntarily, a feeding tube should be considered. Since the pancreatitis may resolve in a few days, a nasoesophageal feeding tube may be sufficient. However, in some cases esophagostomy feeding tubes may be required. Possible complications with enteral nutrition include vomiting, aspiration pneumonia, and inflammation/infection of feeding tube stoma sites.

Patient 2: This cat already has signs of malnutrition, and the prolonged state of starvation makes nutritional support a high priority. The cat's condition does require investigation and stabilization before nutritional support is initiated. The cat's fluid, electrolyte, and acid-base status should be addressed before nutritional

Continued

support is provided. Cats with hepatic lipidosis may have hepatic encephalopathy and this must be investigated before making a nutritional plan. If vomiting and nausea can be controlled, the enteral route of feeding is preferred. An esophagostomy tube is most commonly used in cats with hepatic lipidosis. Because this is a surgical procedure, a cat's coagulation times should be checked and addressed before a tube can be placed. If encephalopathy is a concern, the amount of protein in the diet may be reduced and medical therapy for encephalopathy should be initiated. Complications associated with feeding cats with hepatic lipidosis include vomiting, worsening of encephalopathy, and inflammation or infection at the feeding tube stoma site.

Patient 3: This patient does have overt signs of malnutrition and also has a high risk of having a prolonged period of gastrointestinal dysfunction. A significant portion of the intestines is affected, and return to normal function may take several weeks to months. Since this dog will unlikely tolerate any form of enteral nutrition in the short term, and the patient is already malnourished, a plan to support this dog with parenteral nutrition is indicated. Before formulating parenteral nutrition, a full biochemistry panel is required to evaluate liver and kidney function as well as electrolyte balance. A dedicated catheter, preferably a central vein, for delivery of parenteral nutrition should be placed. Complications associated with parenteral nutrition include mechanical, infectious, and metabolic complications; therefore patients receiving parenteral nutrition require frequent and close monitoring.

MEDICAL MATH EXERCISE

A 4-kg cat is only eating half a pouch of food a day while hospitalized. Each food pouch contains 120 kcal.

1. How much of the cat's resting energy requirement are currently being met?
2. How many pouches of food should this cat consume to meet 100% of RER?

7 Oxygen Therapy Techniques

Andrea M. Steele

CHAPTER OUTLINE

Definitions/Acronyms
How to Assess the Need for Oxygen
How to Assess Oxygen Levels
How to Deliver Oxygen
  Flow-by Oxygen
  Mask Oxygen
  Oxygen Hood/Cage

Nasal Cannula
Naso-Oxygen Catheter
Transtracheal Oxygen Catheter
Hyperbaric Oxygen Therapy
Oxygen Toxicity
Conclusion

LEARNING OBJECTIVES

After studying this chapter, you will be able to:
- Understand various methods of oxygen supplementation.
- Understand methods to assess oxygenation and oxygen supplementation.

The ability to provide oxygen is vitally important in a veterinary hospital. Oxygen is required to assist the patient's respiration during anesthesia and to carry inhalant anesthetic drugs. It may be used in the preoperative phase before induction to minimize the negative effects of induction drugs. It is frequently required postoperatively for at-risk patients (such as brachycephalic patients, high ASA status patients, and geriatric patients) to provide support during the recovery period.

In an emergency setting, oxygen therapy is used during the emergent period to assist with stabilizing both respiratory and nonrespiratory emergency patients. In the critical care setting, oxygen may be used therapeutically over hours, days, or even weeks while an animal is hospitalized.

For all of these reasons, oxygen is a requirement for **all** veterinary hospitals, and levels of oxygen in cylinders must be assessed frequently to ensure that the hospital will maintain the proper supply. It is imperative that this be part of standard inventory assessment, as with other medications and supplies.

Oxygen must be provided during general anesthesia with an intubated or masked patient for the duration of the procedure. In the emergent or critical care setting, oxygen is delivered based on the needs of the patient. It is an important aspect of the veterinary technician's job to understand the patient's clinical signs and be able to interpret monitors and blood gas results in order to determine the need for oxygen. Of course, the veterinarian is responsible for the "prescription" of oxygen; however, assessing the need for increased or possibly decreased oxygen support is often the technician's responsibility.

DEFINITIONS/ACRONYMS

Hypoxemia is defined as a partial pressure of oxygen in the arterial blood (PaO_2) of less than 80 mm Hg. Severe hypoxemia is <60 mm Hg.
SpO_2 is the percent of hemoglobin saturated with oxygen.
PaO_2 is the partial pressure of oxygen in the *arterial* blood.
PvO_2 is the partial pressure of oxygen in the *venous* blood.
FiO_2 is the fraction of inspired oxygen (i.e., room air = 21% or 0.21).
P/F ratio is the PaO_2/FiO_2 ratio (i.e., $100/0.21 = \approx500$).

HOW TO ASSESS THE NEED FOR OXYGEN

The need for supplemental oxygen can be assessed from many different behaviors, clinical signs, and vital signs and through the use of different monitors and laboratory values. There is a more thorough discussion of respiratory assessment in Chapter 18: Respiratory Emergencies. It is important to remember that with respect to oxygenation, behavior and postural changes are as important as vital signs in assessing need. A patient that is sleeping comfortably, curled in a ball, and with a relatively low respiratory rate is likely not hypoxemic, and may benefit more from a hands-off approach rather than waking for a full assessment. On the other hand, the patient with respiratory disease that is restless, cannot lie down, and is panting is having difficulties and intervention is necessary. This patient needs a full assessment. Finally, the respiratory patient that is suddenly laterally recumbent, with increased respiratory rate and effort, is severely compromised, and may arrest. The technician should immediately notify the veterinarian of this situation and prepare for emergency interventions including resuscitation.

HOW TO ASSESS OXYGEN LEVELS

The **pulse oximeter** is an invaluable tool that will provide a measure of the percent saturation of hemoglobin with oxygen. Many clinics do not have access to blood gas analysis, yet own a pulse oximeter. Although a pulse oximeter is not infallible, this tool, combined with assessment of the clinical picture of the patient, will allow the veterinary team to assess the degree of respiratory compromise of the patient. A patient that is breathing normally and has a normal heart rate, normal vital signs, and normal behavior yet has a pulse oximeter reading of 90% may not be hypoxemic, and you should verify the pulse oximeter reading. There are only a few reasons for obtaining a falsely elevated reading; however, a falsely decreased reading is very common. Repositioning the probe or moistening the mucous membranes will ensure there is a good signal. If the percentage is consistent in other locations, or increases when oxygen is provided, the value is accurate. In addition, all pulse oximeters have a method of indicating signal strength, displayed either as: (1) a waveform (a plethysmograph), (2) a red/yellow/green LED light that changes color as the signal strength changes, or (3) as an audible signal that changes tone as signal strength increases or decreases. It is important to note that pulse oximetry gives information on oxygenation only, and does not provide any information about ventilation. For more information on the theory and interpretation of pulse oximetry, known as the **oxyhemoglobin** dissociation curve, please see Box 7-1.

Arterial blood gases (ABGs) are the gold standard method of measuring oxygen levels in the blood. Although technically more demanding, more invasive, and more expensive than pulse oximetry measurements, ABGs provide substantially more information, including oxygenation, ventilation ($PaCO_2$), and metabolic status. ABGs can be used in conjunction with pulse oximetry to calibrate the SpO_2 range that is acceptable for the patient. This can minimize the use of ABG measurements to a few times a day, reducing time and, in the absence of an arterial line, discomfort to the patient. Venous blood gases (VBGs) can be used to monitor CO_2 levels in the venous blood ($PvCO_2$), which are typically 5 mm Hg higher than $PaCO_2$ values. Because VBGs are much easier to obtain, they are a perfectly acceptable

BOX 7-1	Oxyhemoglobin Dissociation Curve

The pulse oximeter uses LED lights of varying wavelengths in order to differentiate between the proportion of oxyhemoglobin vs. deoxyhemoglobin in the blood. Oxyhemoglobin and **deoxyhemoglobin** absorb light of different frequencies, and a photodetector in the sensor measures the amount of light transmitted through the tissue. Pulse oximetry requires pulsatile (arterial) blood flow.

Limitations of pulse oximetry include motion, poor perfusion, stray light, presence of dysfunctional hemoglobins (such as carboxyhemoglobin, methemoglobin), and pigmented skin/mucous membranes.

Understanding the relationship between SpO_2 (as measured on the pulse oximeter) and PaO_2 (as measured on a blood gas) will allow the technician to use the pulse oximeter to titrate oxygen to meet demand. This relationship is demonstrated with the oxyhemoglobin dissociation curve, which is shown in Figure 7-1. The curve is a sigmoid curve, indicating that the relationship between SpO_2 and PaO_2 is nonlinear. Note that the curve becomes horizontal at approximately a PaO_2 of 100 mm Hg and SpO_2 of 100%, although it begins to flatten at approximately 80 mm Hg. Extrapolating the SpO_2 at a PaO_2 of 80 mm Hg to the curve (red line) gives a SpO_2 of approximately 94%. This indicates that for a patient to be considered normohypoxemic, the patient must have a SpO_2 of >94%. Below this number, the patient is likely hypoxemic. This is not an exact science, because the curve is susceptible to changes in temperature and CO_2 levels, changes in pH, and changes in metabolic rate. Once the curve flattens, we have much less indication of where the PaO_2 may actually lie.

The ratio of PaO_2/FiO_2 (P/F ratio) is important in understanding oxygen supplementation. The normal P/F ratio should be ≈500, meaning absolute perfect lung function. On room air, this would equate to a PaO_2 of ≈100 mm Hg divided by the FiO_2 of 21% (100/0.21), which equals 476 mm Hg. Another way to look at this is to multiply the FiO_2 (in %) by 5 to get the expected PaO_2 (in mm Hg) for a normal patient. Therefore, a patient breathing 100% oxygen would expect to have a PaO_2 of 500 mm Hg.

A patient under anesthesia, breathing 100% oxygen, should have a pulse oximeter reading of 100%, equivalent to a reading of >300 mm Hg for PaO_2. As stated previously, a perfectly normal patient would expect to have a PaO_2 on an arterial blood gas of 500 mm Hg,

while breathing 100% oxygen. Based on properties of the oxyhemoglobin dissociation curve, when the pulse oximeter reads 100%, we do not know if the PaO_2 is 300 or 500 mm Hg. Most anesthetists become concerned when the pulse oximeter reading drops to 98%, because this means that the patient has fallen to between somewhere between 100 and 300 mm Hg for PaO_2. This could indicate a functional lung problem such as severe atelectasis, or something more unexpected such as a pneumothorax, pulmonary thromboembolism, or pulmonary edema. Although a patient at 98% is not hypoxemic, the relative "return" on the inspired oxygen is quite poor, indicating that there is a problem that needs to be addressed.

For a patient that is being monitored in the ICU on room air, a SpO_2 >93% indicates the patient should be saturating adequately. This represents the point on the curve that corresponds to approximately 80 mm Hg for PaO_2 (below which is termed hypoxemia). There are several factors that cause the curve to shift to the right, or to the left. It is important to realize that while for most patients, 93% on the pulse oximeter *should* be acceptable, because of the potential for shifts in the curve, it is important to add a small buffer. Most criticalists agree that to maintain sufficient PaO_2, pulse oximeter readings should be approximately 94% to 95%, in order to be confident that the patient is not hypoxemic. This number, in addition to the clinical status of the patient (HR, respiratory rate, work/pattern of breathing, mucous membrane color, and behavior) should be used to determine if the patient needs oxygen supplementation.

When a patient is receiving supplemental oxygen, the goal is not to have a SpO_2 of 100%. As in the case of the aforementioned anesthesia example, 100% on a pulse oximeter means that the patient's PaO_2 is somewhere between 300 and 500 mm Hg. Is this necessary? Indeed, it is not. The clinical signs of hypoxemia should be reversed at a PaO_2 of approximately 80 mm Hg. The patient does not really NEED more than that. This is equivalent to approximately 93% on the pulse oximeter. Using the guideline of providing oxygen so that the patient maintains between 94% and 95% ensures that the patient stays above a PaO_2 of 80 mm Hg, and likely less than 100 mm Hg. This makes the use of a pulse oximeter a useful, yet somewhat inexact method of "titrating" oxygen.

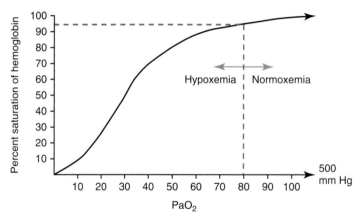

FIGURE 7-1 Oxyhemoglobin dissociation curve.

means of monitoring ventilation; however, they do not assess oxygenation.

HOW TO DELIVER OXYGEN

Oxygen in a veterinary clinic is normally provided in pressurized tanks, which provide 2000 PSI. A regulator is attached to the tank, which will reduce the delivery pressure to 50 PSI to work with anesthetic machines and other medical equipment. In many cases, single or multiple oxygen tanks are connected to pipes, which deliver the oxygen to anesthetic machines in the surgery and treatment areas. In some cases, clinics may also have outlets or dropdowns throughout the hospital that allow connection of a flowmeter. In the absence of flow meters, a tank and regulator may need to be set at cage side to provide oxygen to critical patients. It is important to adhere to all workplace safety guidelines in your locale for the storage, movement, and use of compressed gases.

Many clinics are now choosing oxygen condensors or concentrators to provide oxygen. These are machines that take room air, and extract the oxygen, producing ~90% pure oxygen. These units are quite useful, although they are limited in the pressure they can provide, and the flow rate. Most models provide oxygen at a pressure of only 5-10 PSI, which is not sufficient for use with a ventilator, and some anesthetic machines may alarm with that low an inlet pressure. Flow rate is commonly only up to 5 L/min or up to 10 L/min depending on the model chosen. These are important considerations if planning to choose one of these machines. Tank oxygen must always be available as a backup, in the event of a condenser failure.

Oxygen delivery can be a challenge in veterinary patients. Choosing the best method for the individual patient is very important. Some patients may find certain delivery methods particularly stressful, and this can impact their response to therapy. Oxygen supplementation can take many forms, and it is important to explore various modalities to offer the best choices for both the clinic and the patient. Table 7-1 lists the necessary equipment for different types of oxygen supplementation.

The most common methods of oxygen delivery in veterinary patients are listed in the following sections.

FLOW-BY OXYGEN

Flow-by delivery of oxygen is the most simple method of oxygen delivery, and is surprisingly effective and well tolerated by sick patients (Figure 7-2). It is estimated that flow rates need to be 100 to 150 ml/kg/min to reach approximately 40% FiO_2. Many patients will resent these high flow rates blasting into their faces. For recumbent patients, this method works very well. Patients that constantly avoid the flow are probably not the best candidates for this method.

MASK OXYGEN

Masks can be used in two manners: First, with the diaphragm on, the mask can be placed on the face. This method works well on a recumbent, minimally responsive patient, but remember that the mask must be connected to a circle or Bain system for CO_2 to escape. Do not use this method when delivering oxygen via a direct O_2 line from a wall flowmeter, or from the fresh gas outlet on the anesthesia machine. Mask O_2 is most frequently used for preoxygenation before induction of

TABLE 7-1	Equipment Required for Various Oxygen Supplementation Methods
METHOD	**EQUIPMENT**
Common to **all** methods	Oxygen source (tank or oxygen converter) Flowmeter delivering up to 15 L/min
Flow-by oxygen	Oxygen supply tubing or anesthetic circuit Recommended: sterile humidifier system (reusable or disposable)
Mask oxygen	Oxygen supply tubing or anesthetic circuit Oxygen mask, with or without diaphragm
Oxygen hood	Oxygen supply tubing or anesthetic circuit Oxygen hood Recommended: oxygen analyzer to determine FiO_2 Recommended: sterile humidifier system (reusable or disposable)
E-collar oxygen hood	Oxygen supply tubing E-collar (large size for the patient that extends comfortably past the nose) Plastic food wrap and tape Recommended: oxygen analyzer to determine FiO_2 Recommended: sterile humidifier system (reusable or disposable)
Oxygen cage	Oxygen supply source Oxygen cage (retrofit or stand-alone)
Nasal cannula	Sterile humidifier system (reusable or disposable) 6-25 feet of oxygen supply tubing (¼ inch) if additional length necessary Appropriate size nasal cannulas White tape Optional: topical anesthetic drops (prilocaine)
Nasal oxygen catheter	Sterile humidifier system (reusable or disposable) 6-25 feet of oxygen supply tubing (¼ inch) 6, 8, or 10Fr nasal catheter (human) or equivalent size PVC or red rubber feeding tube Topical anesthetic drops (proparacaine) and lidocaine 2% jelly as a lubricant Adapter to connect to oxygen supply line (McGyver alert!)

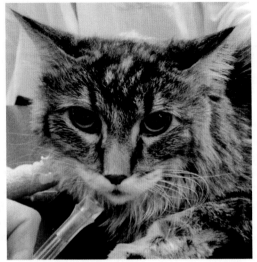

FIGURE 7-2 Flow-by oxygen provided with an O_2 line.

anesthesia. A tight-fitting mask is likely to be very stressful for a dyspneic patient, and therefore may not be the best choice. A second method is to use the mask with the diaphragm removed. This works very well to "funnel" the oxygen towards the patient's nose, and also reduces the oxygen "blast" to the face by diffusing the flow over a larger area. This is generally well tolerated if the mask is not forced on the patient's face, but rather used to direct oxygen to the face. Because this system is not sealed, oxygen can be delivered directly from a wall oxygen outlet, without a circle or Bain circuit, since CO_2 will be flushed from the open mask.

OXYGEN HOOD/CAGE

This is a method of providing an oxygen-rich environment in which the patient's entire body, or head and neck alone, may be involved. An oxygen cage has the added benefit of being temperature and humidity controlled, and many models also extract CO_2 (usually with soda

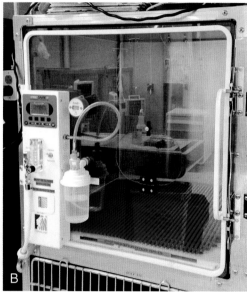
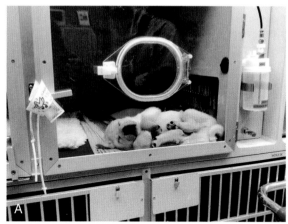

FIGURE 7-3 A, A fully integrated, stand-alone oxygen cage with heating, cooling, and humidifying and dehumidifying functions. **B,** An example of a retrofit style oxygen cage that can be custom made to fit an existing cage.

lime). Desired FiO_2 values can often be dialed in to the machine, and an O_2 demand value offers precise control over the FiO_2, much like a thermostat. Oxygen cages can be stand-alone, fully integrated units (Figure 7-3, *A*) or retrofit units (Figure 7-3, *B*) that are fitted onto existing cages. The less advantageous side of these machines is that some models can be costly, and they are often very noisy units. Many clinics purchase refurbished or retired oxygen incubators from human neonatal intensive care units (NICUs). These also work great and adjust for temperature, humidity, and FiO_2. The only caution with these units is to ensure that the inside is safe for your patient. It may be necessary to make adjustments to the floor of the incubator to ensure a mobile patient cannot be trapped between the bed (which is usually attached) and the walls of the incubator. Babies, typically in incubators, are too young to be mobile, whereas the veterinary patient may be very mobile. Oxygen cages have a few disadvantages: (1) the high oxygen flow rates required to meet the desired FiO_2 can be costly; (2) opening of the cage/incubator will result in a rapid decrease in FiO_2; and (3) the nature of the cage requires the caregivers to be very "hands-off."

Oxygen hoods are very low tech, and rely on high oxygen flow to flush CO_2 out of vents on the side (Figure 7-4). These can be very cost-effective as far as equipment costs, but they do use a lot of oxygen at high flow rates;

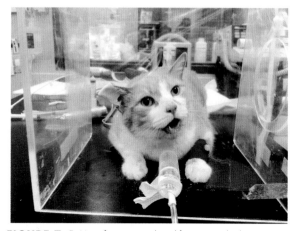

FIGURE 7-4 Use of an oxygen hood for a severely dyspneic cat.

thus, running them can be expensive. The advantages outweigh the disadvantages however, as they tend to be very well tolerated, and allow for performing treatments, physical exams, and other procedures, while keeping the patient's head in the oxygen.

These units can be custom-made or manufactured at a local plexiglass shop. A simple oxygen hood may be created using an Elizabethan collar, with the front covered in clear plastic wrap. The top fourth is left uncovered to allow CO_2 to escape. An oxygen tube is introduced at the back of the collar, and a flow rate of 5 to

10 L/min is used. All oxygen hoods have the risk of increased CO_2 production and overheating. It is important to have adequate ventilation to ensure CO_2 can escape, as well as high enough flow rates to ensure that CO_2 and heat are dispersed. Panting dogs are often not good candidates for an oxygen hood because they will not allow heat dispersion. A thermometer placed under the hood can help to ensure the temperature is being monitored closely. Oxygen and/or CO_2 analyzers can also be used to closely monitor FiO_2 and CO_2 levels in the hood.

Cats especially like oxygen hoods, because they can offer hiding places within their cages. For added privacy for the stable, but oxygen-dependent kitty, a cover can be placed partially over the hood. Cats frequently sleep within the hood, emerge to use the litter box and nibble their food, and then return to the hood. Dogs, on the other hand, find hoods confining, and rarely choose to enter them.

Oxygen hoods and cages are particularly useful during the emergent phase when a patient needs oxygen supplementation but is resistant to flow-by, mask, or more invasive methods. Sedation, when used, will be more effective when the patient is less stressed; and, therefore, giving an injection and then placing the patient in the cage or hood will allow the animal to relax and become sedate while enjoying the benefits of increased oxygen flow. This technique often makes the respiratory patient easier to stabilize.

NASAL CANNULA

Nasal cannulas are frequently referred to as nasal "prongs." Cannulas work very well on brachycephalic breeds because the space between the nostrils is relatively wide, although they are also effective on most types of dogs, and often cats. They are available in adult, pediatric, and neonatal sizes. The appropriate size must be chosen for the patient, because the distance between prongs must match the distance between the nares to be comfortable and easy to maintain. Sometimes cutting some of the length off the prongs makes the cannulas more tolerable. A piece of white tape, used to make the lines attached to the prongs into a sharper curve, will allow the prongs to sit more naturally on the patient's face (Figure 7-5). Patients usually do not like high flow rates through prongs, because the flow hitting the mucosa can be irritating and cause the patient to sneeze or try to remove the prongs. Instilling local anesthetic drops (proparacaine 0.5%) may make the prongs more

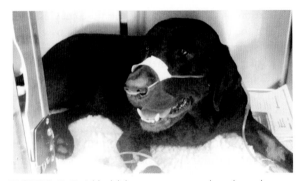

FIGURE 7-5 A black lab receiving oxygen through nasal prongs.

tolerable. Prongs are perfect in the emergent phase to give oxygen quickly, and also make the hands of helpers more available.

An added benefit of nasal cannulas is they are also sold with end-tidal CO_2 monitoring capabilities for sidestream $EtCO_2$ analyzers. One limb provides oxygen to one of the prongs, whereas the other side attaches to an $EtCO_2$ monitor. This allows for provision of oxygen while also monitoring ventilation.

NASO-OXYGEN CATHETER

This is a tube that is placed into the nasal cavity, nasopharynx, or even the trachea of the patient. This is the most invasive means of oxygen supplementation but works well for patients requiring longer term oxygen, or in facilities where judicious use of oxygen is important (for example, a clinic that does not have an oxygen manifold system, and requires changing of oxygen tanks frequently). The oxygen catheter is a very efficient means of delivering oxygen, and typically gives a high FiO_2 of 40% to 60%, with a relatively low flow rate. Flow rates of 50 to 100 ml/kg/min are generally well tolerated. Bilateral catheters may be placed, with possible flow rates between the two catheters up to 200 ml/kg/min. Oxygen should be humidified with sterile water to protect the nasal mucosa.

Complications associated with nasal insufflation include gastric distention (typically with high flow rates) and epistaxis.

Naso-oxygen catheters are contraindicated in patients with known coagulation disorders, because there is a high risk of bleeding during placement attributable to the vascularity of the mucosa. If significant epistaxis does occur, instillation of a few drops of a 1:100,000 diluted epinephrine solution (diluted epinephrine) and

application of ice on the top of the nose may assist in slowing the hemorrhage, and should be discussed with your veterinarian.

Most frequently, a catheter is placed into the nasal cavity; however, for dogs that tend to mouth-breathe (such as brachycephalics), placing the catheter deeper into the nasopharynx may offer the most benefit. This is referred to as a nasopharyngeal oxygen catheter. Occasionally, a patient may benefit from administration of oxygen directly into the trachea, in which case the catheter is passed even further, into the trachea. This is referred to as a nasotracheal oxygen catheter, and requires more expertise for its placement. This is rarely used in veterinary medicine, because these catheters are generally poorly tolerated and can lead to increased risk of aspiration pneumonia.

Human nasal catheters are dedicated polyvinyl chloride (PVC) tubes with multiple fenestrations at the end to disperse the main flow of oxygen to reduce nasal irritation. True nasal catheters are available in sizes from 6 French (6Fr) to 16Fr. Small dogs and cats can usually accommodate a 6Fr tube; medium sized dogs, 8Fr; and large dogs, a 10Fr or 12Fr catheter. Frequently, in veterinary medicine, feeding tubes (PVC or red rubber) are used in place of the human catheters. Caution should be used to minimize flow rates, since the lack of additional fenestrations will cause oxygen to blast at a high flow forcefully onto the nasal mucosa (Figure 7-6). Typically a 5Fr or 6Fr catheter can accommodate up to 1 to 2 L/min, while a 10Fr catheter can be increased up to 5 L/min flow rate. Factors such as tube diameter, length, patient size, placement site, and flow rate all contribute to determine the maximum FiO_2 that can be achieved. Using too high a flow rate not only will be uncomfortable for the patient but also will result in a high-pitched whistling noise in the delivery system and increase the risk of rupture of the humidifier chamber as a result of the increased pressure. The deeper the catheter is placed, the higher the flow rate it can accommodate, and thus the higher the FiO_2 that can be achieved. Placement of naso-oxygen catheters is discussed in Box 2-2.

TRANSTRACHEAL OXYGEN CATHETER

A transtracheal oxygen catheter is used to administer oxygen directly into the trachea of the emergent patient. The same catheter types used for nasal oxygen delivery can be used for transtracheal oxygen, although silicone catheters are best for this purpose

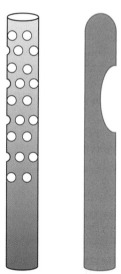

FIGURE 7-6 Comparison of a true human nasal catheter with a red rubber catheter frequently substituted in veterinary patients. Although both are effective, note the numerous fenestrations and open end of the nasal catheter, compared to the single opening in the red rubber catheter. The nasal catheter acts to disperse the energy of the oxygen flow over a larger area, and thus reduces the risk of mucosal irritation.

because silicone is softer, less irritating, and less damaging to the tracheal mucosa. With high flow rates, "whip injury" to the tracheal mucosa from the catheter is possible; thus the softer and more pliable catheters may cause less damage. These devices are placed surgically using a scalpel or large-bore needle. The area between the fourth and fifth cartilaginous ring is prepared and anesthetized locally, and a puncture slightly larger than the catheter is made in this space. The catheter is advanced into the trachea so that its tip is directly above the carina. The proximal end of the catheter is connected to the oxygen source tube and the flow is directed to approximately 3 L/min. The flow rate is determined by the animal's minute ventilation. If the animal's breathing is deep and rapid, higher flow rates may be necessary. It is important to realize that this method cannot be used in place of a tracheostomy with upper airway obstruction. Although it will provide oxygen, the patient will not be able to exhale through the tube, and therefore will not be able to ventilate the lungs when there is a total obstruction. A transtracheal catheter may be irritating to the patient and cause the patient to cough, which may hinder its effectiveness.

Equipment
Appropriate size and type of tube for patient
Permanent marker
Proparacaine drops
Lidocaine jelly (2%) to use as lubricant (nonsterile)
Suture (nonabsorbable) ± waterproof white tape ± instant glue

A traditional naso-oxygen catheter is placed by measuring from the nose to the medial or lateral canthus of the eye, where a mark is placed on the tube with permanent marker. For a nasopharyngeal catheter, measurement should be made to the vertical ramus of the mandible. The patient should be restrained with the nose pointed towards the ceiling, and the person performing the procedure should instill local anesthetic drops (such as proparacaine ophthalmic drops) into the nares. With one hand around the muzzle, the tube is inserted into the chosen nostril by directing the catheter ventromedially. The tube is advanced gently, but quickly, and there should be little resistance. The tube is advanced to the mark made on the tube and then advanced 1 or 2 more centimeters, to ensure that the catheter is not in the dorsal meatus. If it continues to advance easily, you are assured the tube is entering the nasal cavity, and the tube can then be pulled back to the measured mark. If the tube will not advance beyond the mark on the tube, suspect that it is located in the dorsal meatus, in which case it needs to be pulled out and redirected. There is an increased risk of bleeding in the dorsal meatus, and the patient will not receive a very high FiO_2. Proper placement is demonstrated in Figure 7-7. The catheter can be affixed using cyanoacrylate glue (instant glue), a finger-trap suture pattern, or tape wings and suture. If using glue, please ensure that only the tiniest of drops are used to minimize hair loss on the face. The catheter should be sutured or glued at the junction of the nose and the skin, and then may be affixed along the side of the face, below the eye, or curved upward and affixed between the eyes. An Elizabethan collar may need to be placed to ensure that the catheter is not removed by the patient.

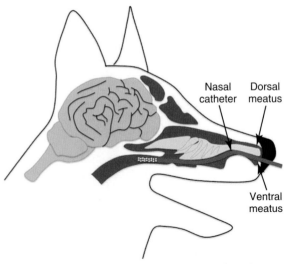

FIGURE 7-7 Illustration of the nasal passages of the dog, and correct placement of a nasal catheter in the ventral meatus.

is not humidified for long periods of time can result in drying and irritation of the mucous membranes, or if in an oxygen hood or cage, can cause dryness of the eyes and conjunctivae. Humidifiers can be single-use disposable units or reusable units that should be emptied, sterilized, and refilled frequently (Figure 7-8).

> **TECHNICIAN NOTE** When choosing an oxygen supplementation method, consider stress versus function, and choose the most appropriate method for your patient.

HYPERBARIC OXYGEN THERAPY

Hyperbaric oxygen therapy (HBOT) is becoming more common in veterinary clinics, due to financing arrangements and more research into the uses of HBOT. The principle is to use increased atmospheric pressure (>760 mm Hg normal sea level barometric pressure) to allow more dissolved oxygen in the blood. It has shown more indications for treatment of wounds, severe burns, and infections, rather than respiratory distress. This is the ultimate "hands off" therapy, because a pressurized chamber cannot simply be opened in order to deal with a patient that is having difficulties; it must undergo depressurization first. Placing an unstable patient in this type of environment may be less than ideal.

Any prolonged oxygen supplementation should use humidified oxygen. An oxygen humidifier is a bubble chamber of sterile water that attaches to a flowmeter. The oxygen bubbles through the water, increasing the oxygen's humidity before delivery. Using oxygen that

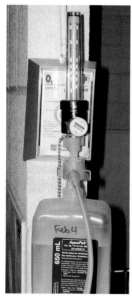

FIGURE 7-8 Example of a commercial, single-use, oxygen humidifier filled with sterile water.

One final note regarding oxygen supplementation methods, such as flow-by, mask (to a degree), nasal cannulas, and nasal catheters, is that the patient is also breathing surrounding ambient air. The oxygen concentration coming from the oxygen source is 100%; however, because it is not providing 100% of the patient's tidal volume with the oxygen flow, the actual FiO_2 level reaching the patient's trachea is diluted by the room air (21% O_2) surrounding the patient. The actual FiO_2 level will depend on the patient's tidal volume and respiratory rate and the flow of oxygen in liters per minute.

OXYGEN TOXICITY

Oxygen is a drug and like any drug can have negative consequences when overdosed or used inappropriately. Oxygen toxicity is a real complication of oxygen "overdose." In the emergent phase, any patient that would benefit from oxygen should be given oxygen as needed. This phase will last less than 2 hours on average, and monitoring the amount of oxygen given is not as important at this stage. A patient under general anesthesia will be breathing 100% O_2 through the endotracheal tube for the duration of the surgery. Oxygen toxicity becomes more of a concern with patients receiving oxygen

supplementation in an intensive care unit (ICU) environment, rather than during anesthesia induction.

Once a patient is noted to require long-term oxygen therapy, the amount of oxygen given must be carefully monitored, or "titrated." It is not appropriate to simply keep a patient at a level of oxygen because the patient "appears to be doing well." The goal is ultimately to send the patient home, and in most cases this cannot be achieved without removing the oxygen supplementation.

Oxygen starts to cause damage after about 6 hours, although the signs are typically not observable until much later. This first phase is called the initiation phase, and occurs during the first 24 to 72 hours on 100% oxygen. This phase is associated with reactive oxygen species (ROS), which directly damage the pulmonary epithelium. ROS are produced in the normal reduction of oxygen in the electron transport chain, producing adenosine triphosphate (ATP). The more oxygen that is provided, the more ROS are formed, overwhelming the body's antioxidant systems. The second stage is an inflammatory phase in which there is increased tissue permeability and pulmonary edema, and as the damage continues, fibrosis can occur.

Current recommendations are to avoid an FiO_2 value of >60% for more than 24 to 72 hours, unless absolutely necessary.

> **TECHNICIAN NOTE** Always ensure the amount of oxygen provided is consistent with the patient's needs, and not simply following a static number on the patient's order sheet. Technicians need to be involved and make recommendations for the best chance of success!

CONCLUSION

Oxygen supplementation is a commonly misunderstood or underestimated "treatment" that technicians administer on a frequent basis. Not only are there various methods of delivery but also there are many different methods in which to monitor the oxygen delivery to the patient. It is important for the technician to ask for oxygen parameters that the veterinarian will prescribe, to titrate the oxygen to effect, and to avoid overdosing.

SUGGESTED READINGS

Hackett TB, Mazzaferro EM: Oxygen supplementation and respiratory sampling techniques. In *Veterinary emergency and critical care procedures*, Ames, Iowa, 2012, Wiley-Blackwell, pp 133–170.

Manning AM: Oxygen therapy and toxicity, *Vet Clin North Am* 32(6):1005–1020, 2002.

Mendelson Y: Pulse oximetry, theory and applications for non-invasive monitoring, *Clin Chem* 38/39:1601–1607, 1992.

Zimmerman ME, Hodgson DS, Bello NM: Effects of oxygen insufflation rate, respiratory rate, and tidal volume on fraction of inspired oxygen in cadaveric canine heads attached to a lung model, *Am J Vet Res* 74:1247–1251, 2013.

SCENARIO

Purpose: To provide the veterinary technician with the opportunity to build or strengthen the ability to quickly evaluate a situation faced in a typical emergency clinic.

Stage: This emergency clinic is considered a moderate level facility *(Levels are currently being determined by VECCS and may have specific information by publication)* and always has at least four staff members available including one ER clinician, two veterinary technicians, and one receptionist who also assist with animal handling when necessary. There is a back-up clinician on call to assist with surgeries.

Scenario

Sunday afternoon.

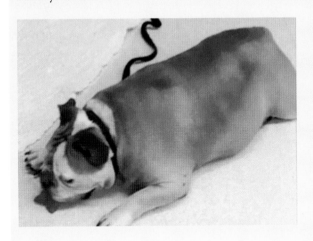

A 6-year-old English bulldog presents at the clinic on a hot, humid day. He had a long walk with his owner and then the owner noted his dog's breathing was sounding much louder than usual, and his tongue was more purple. As they continued, the bulldog refused to walk any further and collapsed on the grass, panting heavily. The owner called his wife to come pick them up, and brought the dog to the emergency clinic.

On presentation, the dog is panting heavily, and has severe stertor and stridor. His mucous membranes are very purple/blue, including his tongue. He has a very exaggerated inspiratory pull, using abdominal muscles. The dog dropped heavily on the tile floor.

Delivery

- Ask the group of technicians for "first steps" with this patient: triaging, admitting, initial interventions.
- Have them write the following on a white card:
  - Triage score
  - Whether a treatment area or exam room is needed
  - First initial interventions

Questions

- Why did they choose the triage score?
- What was the single most concerning parameter/clinical sign they were seeing?
- Discuss whether the patient was stable enough to go to an exam room, vs the treatment room.
  - If they decided the patient could wait in an exam room, have them justify their answer.
  - If they decided the patient should go to the treatment room, have them justify their answer (e.g., oxygen source, emergency supplies).
- Discuss emergency interventions. What should be the first intervention?
  - Oxygen supplementation
  - IV catheter
  - Sedation
  - Temperature/active cooling
  - All of the above
- Discuss oxygen supplementation.
  - What method might be best?
  - Will the bulldog need long-term oxygen supplementation?
  - Consider equipment the clinic has on hand; discuss if other oxygen supplementation equipment should be ordered.

Continued

SCENARIO—cont'd

Key Teaching Points

- Provides veterinary technicians the opportunity to review hospital procedures and guidelines on how to approach emergency receiving.
- Provides an opportunity to discuss as a group, in a low-stress situation, how others would handle the same situation.
- All discussion should be nonjudgmental and constructive and ensure that all sides are addressed. For example, the technician who decides the patient is stable enough to go to the exam room with the owner may feel that the stress of removing the patient from the owner may cause him to decompensate quickly. The technician feels it would be advisable for the veterinarian to assess the patient first. This is a valid point; however, the oxygen equipment, emergency intubation, cooling supplies, and access to emergency drugs may be preferable in this situation. The veterinarian can be called to assess the patient immediately.

- Some clinic policies allow owners to remain at their pet's side in the treatment area. This is a good opportunity to remind all technicians of your hospital policy on clients in the back office, or discuss if a change in policy is indicated in certain situations.

MEDICAL MATH EXERCISE

A patient is breathing 50% oxygen in an oxygen cage. An arterial blood gas measurement shows his PaO_2 is 72 mm Hg. What is his P/F ratio?

- a. 72
- b. 144
- c. 36
- d. 50

8 Mechanical Ventilation

Andrea M. Steele

CHAPTER OUTLINE

Important Terms
Indications for Mechanical
  Ventilation
Mechanical Ventilation Strategies
  According to Disease Type
Placing the Patient on the Ventilator
Nursing Considerations for Long-
  Term Ventilator Patients

Monitoring of the Ventilator Patient
Maintenance of the Ventilator
  Patient
Troubleshooting
Weaning from the Ventilator
Summary

KEY TERMS

FiO_2
Frequency
Minute volume
Peak inspiratory pressure
Positive end-expiratory
  pressure
Pressure support
Respiratory failure
Tidal volume
Ventilation
Weaning

LEARNING OBJECTIVES

After studying this chapter, you will be able to:

- Understand the difference between anesthesia ventilation and critical care ventilation.
- Understand the criteria for ventilation and recognize impending respiratory failure.
- Understand the nursing care required for critical ventilation patients.

In veterinary medicine, ventilators are primarily used in two fields: anesthesia and critical care medicine. Anesthesia ventilators are becoming more and more common in veterinary practices, while critical care ventilators are generally reserved for specialty referral hospitals.

Mechanical **ventilation** is the act of assisting or fully controlling respiration of a patient with positive pressure, either with a manual hand-held device or with a mechanical device. Most are referred to as "positive pressure ventilators" because they push air/oxygen into the lungs with pressure. Negative pressure ventilators also exist, which assist breathing by generating negative pressure around the patient, resulting in decreased intrathoracic pressure, and inspiration. These machines were commonly referred to as "Iron Lungs," and were common in the polio era. Although they can still be found today, they are generally not used in veterinary medicine.

Mechanical ventilation of an anesthetized patient may be performed for many reasons. A sigh, often given at 5- to 10-minute intervals, is a type of positive pressure ventilation, albeit intermittent rather than continuous. This is most often performed using the rebreathing bag of the anesthetic machine, to provide a longer, and deeper-than-normal, breath to reduce atelectasis. "Hand-bagging" is similar to a sigh, but is more continuous for a short period of time. This may be performed in the absence of a mechanical ventilator for various reasons, such as if a patient becomes too deeply (and the inhalant is turned off) or too lightly anesthetized (and the inhalant is turned up) or if a patient is apneic. Hand-bagging is often used to ventilate a critical patient during transfer to a critical care facility, and is also used during CPR. An Ambu-bag (Figure 8-1) may be used instead of an anesthetic machine rebreathing bag, when a patient is being bagged with oxygen alone.

Many veterinary clinics now own mechanical ventilators that attach to or are integrated into their anesthetic machine. These ventilators are driven by fresh gas flow, and may or may not have some electrical connection and controls. Most modern machines have a bellows or piston system that delivers each breath. Each cycle of the ventilator pushes fresh gas and inhalant into the patient's lungs, up to a set maximum pressure. Generally, these ventilators are volume controlled, and pressure limited. They are quick and easy to set up, either from the start of anesthesia or during anesthesia if the anesthetist notices hypoventilation or other ventilatory concerns. A major drawback to most of these units is the inability to reduce oxygen concentration, unless a blender valve has been installed. Although this is usually not a concern for an anesthetized patient, it does become a concern if a patient requires long-term ventilation. With a blender valve, these types of ventilators are frequently used for longer-term

ventilation, although most successfully for the category of patients that are unable to ventilate due to neuromuscular disease or injury, versus those with injured lungs.

Ventilation of critical patients is very different from ventilation of most anesthetic patients, and will be the main focus of this chapter. In general, a critical patient may require long-term ventilation, which may be hours to days or even weeks. Patients may require ventilation for many reasons, but the primary reasons are they cannot ventilate (move CO_2 out of the lungs) or they cannot oxygenate sufficiently, even with supplementation. A critical care ventilator is a machine that can handle lung pathology or maintain normal lungs without harm, and do so over a long period of time.

Critical care ventilators are usually microprocessor controlled and have oxygen mixing capabilities through the use of either medical air or a built-in compressor, so that a precise FiO_2 (fraction of inspired oxygen) can be dialed into the machine. These ventilators also have the ability to select peak end-expiratory pressure, peak inspiratory pressure, and inspiration to expiration ratio, among other more advanced settings. These settings will be explained further. Critical care ventilators also have the ability to deliver mandatory volume (volume to deliver is dialed into the machine) or mandatory pressure (deliver a maximum pressure to provide a variable tidal volume). These ventilators offer several different modes, which allow for complete or partial control of breathing, or simply assisted breaths, where a little pressure support is given to spontaneous breaths. There are numerous factors involved in choosing an appropriate mode, which will vary depending on clinician and patient.

IMPORTANT TERMS

Tidal volume (TV) is the volume delivered per breath. Depending on the mode of ventilation (pressure controlled versus volume controlled), the TV may be a number that is dialed into the machine, or it may be related to the pressure setting. For example, in the pressure controlled mode, the pressure setting may be 20 cm H_2O; the resulting TV becomes the volume the ventilator can deliver up to that pressure. The variability of the TV is a factor of the compliance of the lungs (elasticity), the level of anesthesia, and the presence of pleural fluid or air.

Frequency (F) is the number of breaths per minute. In mandatory ventilation, this is the number of mandatory breaths per minute. In settings such as synchronized

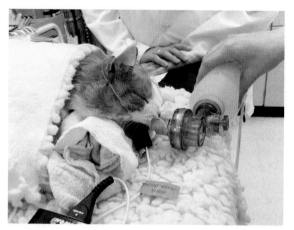

FIGURE 8-1 A cat that has been rapidly intubated, because of severe respiratory distress, is hand-bagged using an Ambu bag device.

intermittent mandatory ventilation (SIMV), or assist control, the patient can breathe "on top" of these mandatory breaths, and therefore there may be both a spontaneous frequency and a mandatory frequency displayed. This is the number of breaths either triggered by the patient or caused by breathing between mandatory breaths.

Minute volume (MV) is the volume delivered over 1 minute. This is the frequency multiplied by the tidal volume *(F × TV)* and is usually expressed in liters per minute.

FiO$_2$ is the fraction of inspired oxygen delivered. Generally on critical care units, this is a number that can be dialed into the machine. Both medical air (or a compressor) and oxygen are used to "mix" oxygen to the exact FiO$_2$ value.

Peak inspiratory pressure (PIP): Patients with pulmonary disease often have more friable lungs than healthy patients and thus can tolerate far lower tidal volume and pressure settings than patients with normal lungs. For example, typical anesthesia settings for a ventilator are 10 to 20 ml/kg for tidal volume and up to 30 cm H$_2$O for pressure (which a normal patient will rarely need). A patient with a primary lung disease will be more adequately ventilated at a tidal volume of 6 to 8 ml/kg and a higher frequency, with a maximum pressure of 30 cm H$_2$O (the difference being that because of decreased compliance and increased resistance, the patient may actually need 30 cm H$_2$O to get the desired tidal volume). The higher frequency ensures that sufficient MV is delivered, even though the tidal volumes are much smaller than would be typical for normal, healthy lungs. The pressure setting on a critical care ventilator is typically termed the peak inspiratory pressure (PIP) or peak pressure.

Positive end-expiratory pressure (PEEP) is particularly important when ventilating patients for pulmonary conditions such as acute respiratory distress syndrome (ARDS), pulmonary edema, and pneumonia. The addition of PEEP can dramatically reduce the required FiO$_2$, reduce the risk of oxygen toxicity, reduce atelectasis, and improve the overall efficiency of ventilation. PEEP can cause reduced cardiac output and should be avoided or minimized in patients with hypovolemia or unresponsive hypotension. PEEP is airway pressure that is present during exhalation, and acts to slow the expiratory phase. This can also result in a reduced ability to remove CO$_2$ from the lungs. Absolute contraindications to the use of PEEP are tension pneumothorax (but this can be treated) and barotrauma. PEEP will also increase central venous pressure. Therefore, it may be contraindicated in patients with elevated intracranial pressure

(e.g., a dog with severe pulmonary contusions *and* head trauma). The patient must be monitored closely, and the more severe problem takes precedent.

INDICATIONS FOR MECHANICAL VENTILATION

Critical patients are at risk of respiratory failure from a number of causes. There are two types of **respiratory failure,** and these hinge on the physiology of gas transport in the lungs. The two types are hypoxemic respiratory failure and hypercapnic respiratory failure. Table 8-1 summarizes the two types.

Typically, hypoxemic respiratory failure is associated with severe lung parenchymal and/or interstitial disease, or diseases affecting the lung blood supply. Oxygen supplementation in mild cases of these types of diseases will often be sufficient to support PaO$_2$; however, in severe cases, increasing the FiO$_2$ will not prevent hypoxia. In the end stages, respiratory effort causes fatigue, and there is often a concurrent increase in PaCO$_2$ as ventilation becomes less effective.

Hypercapnic respiratory failure is associated with diseases that affect ventilation, such as neurologic derangements and airway disease (e.g., asthma and chronic obstructive pulmonary disorder [COPD], in which the patient is not able to sufficiently ventilate the lungs); and while the lung tissue at the alveolar level is essentially normal, there is an increase in the PaCO$_2$ value because carbon dioxide cannot be removed from the lungs. In cases of neuromuscular disease with weak respiratory muscles, the patient will compensate by using

TABLE 8-1	Categories of Respiratory Failure	
ACUTE HYPOXEMIC RESPIRATORY FAILURE		**ACUTE HYPERCAPNIC RESPIRATORY FAILURE**
Low PaO$_2$, low to normal PaCO$_2$ (early phases)		Low PaO$_2$, elevated PaCO$_2$
Associated with: • ARDS • Pneumonia • Pulmonary edema • Pulmonary thromboembolism		Associated with: • CNS disorders • Neuromuscular disease • Airway disease • Musculoskeletal disease
"Abnormal Lung"		"Normal Lung"
Increasing FiO$_2$ has little effect		Increasing FiO$_2$ will reverse hypoxemia

accessory muscles (mostly abdominal) to move air, thus increasing the respiratory effort. Respiration becomes an active process, using excessive energy, increasing oxygen demand, and causing fatigue. The patient will have difficulty regulating body temperature because of the activity of large muscle groups, and CO_2 production will be increased from increased metabolic activity, further contributing to hypercapnia. Eventually the animal will no longer be able to compensate and will begin to fatigue, and without treatment respiratory failure and death will ensue.

Based on the two types of respiratory failure, criteria for mechanical ventilation have been established and are as follows:

- Inability to remove CO_2 from the blood
  - PCO_2 continues to rise or stays elevated above expectations given the patient's work of breathing.
- Inadequate tissue oxygenation
  - PaO_2 is inadequate and cannot be elevated by supplemental oxygen.
  - PaO_2 continues to decline, despite increased FiO_2.
- Impending respiratory failure
  - The patient may be exhibiting signs of respiratory failure, such as changes in respiratory patterns or apnea.
- Increased work of breathing
  - The work of breathing is causing the patient to fatigue, and become hyperthermic or tachycardic, for example.

MECHANICAL VENTILATION STRATEGIES ACCORDING TO DISEASE TYPE

Mechanical ventilation for patients with any form of pulmonary disease is very different from ventilation for other types of disease, such as neuromuscular diseases or central nervous system (CNS) disorders. In neuromuscular or CNS diseases, the lung is functionally normal with no impairment in gas exchange. Rather, the nerves or muscles involved in breathing can become ineffective in these patients, resulting in impaired ventilation.

TECHNICIAN NOTE Ventilating paralyzed patients differs from ventilating patients with primary lung disease, because the former usually do not require high oxygen levels and can be ventilated with regular rates and volumes.

BOX 8-1	Conditions That Often Require Mechanical Ventilation

Primary Pulmonary Disorders
- Pneumonia (aspiration/bacterial/fungal)
- Pulmonary contusions
- Smoke inhalation
- Pulmonary edema (noncardiogenic or cardiogenic)

Nonpulmonary Disorders
- Systemic inflammatory response syndrome (SIRS; initiating acute respiratory distress syndrome [ARDS])
- Sepsis
- Respiratory paralysis

These patients may need to have ventilatory support for several days to even weeks before they are able to completely breathe on their own. Essentially the goal in these types of cases is to ventilate without causing harm, and maintain body condition through physiotherapy and nutrition.

Ventilation is an invasive procedure that may leave a patient at risk of developing a nosocomial infection such as a pneumonia, or can cause lung trauma, atelectasis, and other issues.

In patients with severe pulmonary disease requiring ventilation, issues of lung compliance, lung resistance, barotrauma, oxygen toxicity, and secretions all combine to make ventilation much more difficult and frustrating. Compounding this may be systemic illness in the patient, requiring use of vasopressors and/or inotropes for pressure support. Heavy sedation to general anesthesia is usually required for these patients, increasing the level of care necessary for their maintenance. Nutritional needs must be evaluated and met, through either enteral or parenteral means. Patients can be on a ventilator for several days or longer and often experience rapid changes in condition that require continual adjustments in ventilator settings. Box 8-1 summarizes common conditions requiring mechanical ventilation.

PLACING THE PATIENT ON THE VENTILATOR

Placing a patient onto a ventilator is one of the most critical periods and requires intense focus and preparation on the part of the veterinary team. Often, this is a stepwise procedure, where the patient is rapidly intubated as a result of respiratory distress and then hand-bagged, while a discussion with the owner ensues about ventilation and a plan is made. During this time, it is important that the team assemble the needed supplies, injectable anesthetics, and monitoring equipment.

> **TECHNICIAN NOTE** In most cases a patient will be endotracheally intubated initially, and this should be performed as aseptically as possible, using sterile gloves, a disinfected laryngoscope, sterile lubricant, and a sterile endotracheal (ET) tube.

In some cases, such as in airway trauma, a patient may have had a tracheostomy tube placed, in which case this will be attached to the ventilator. Some clinicians may prefer to transition a long-term ventilator patient to a tracheostomy tube once the patient is stabilized, since it can allow the patient to be lightened considerably from anesthesia. In some cases, a patient may even be able to eat and drink while being ventilated (Figure 8-2). This is most common with neuromuscular conditions.

> **TECHNICIAN NOTE** Designating at least one technician to monitor the patient during the transition to the ventilator is paramount. Many patients arrest during this transition, and the quicker a change in the patient is noted, the more likely CPR may be successful. Since these patients are not usually fully instrumented until they are on the ventilator, it is important that a technician is palpating a pulse continually during this period and noting any change in rate or pulse quality.

The first hour after placing the patient on the ventilator is also critical. This is the time when the clinician is trying to determine appropriate ventilator settings and/or mode, and it is not unusual to have very increased $PaCO_2$ and very low PaO_2 readings during this time. Consequently, blood gases may need to be run every 5 to 10 minutes in the beginning, and therefore it is important to have an arterial line placed as quickly as possible. In addition, trying to instrument the patient with various monitors will be performed in the first few minutes.

Ideally, a central venous line with multi-lumens will also be placed in a ventilator patient, because numerous injectable drugs will need to be given, many with incompatibilities within the fluid line. This does not need to be performed immediately, but can usually wait until the patient is more stable. Consider placing an additional

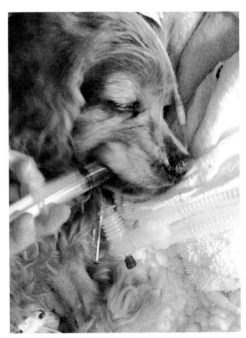

FIGURE 8-2 An example of a dog on a ventilator with a tracheostomy tube, accepting water via syringe.

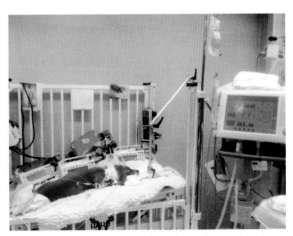

FIGURE 8-3 Keep the area of ventilation clear and readily accessible by ventilating in a crib, or on a stretcher.

peripheral intravenous catheter for the short term to assist with drug administration.

It is important that the area where a patient is being ventilated be well organized and readily accessible. Removing cage doors or using a crib with sides that can drop will allow the best access to the patient (Figure 8-3). Many institutions will ventilate patients on a stretcher.

NURSING CONSIDERATIONS FOR LONG-TERM VENTILATOR PATIENTS

There are numerous skills and tasks required to maintain a ventilator patient, and also to avoid complications. These can be divided into two categories: monitoring and maintenance.

MONITORING OF THE VENTILATOR PATIENT

Most ventilator patients are heavily sedated or fully anesthetized using injectable anesthetics. Protocols will vary among facilities, but are usually a combination of two to three drugs such as propofol, diazepam or midazolam, dexmedetomidine, ketamine, fentanyl, or others. Each drug is chosen based on the individual patient and the patient's disease state, and to minimize the negative effects of each drug. Each drug should be administered in such a way that it can be rapidly adjusted, preferably via syringe pump or buretrol. Note that a standard "cocktail" recipe that might work well for a typical anesthetic patient may not work well for a ventilator patient. Generally these patients are not subjected to surgical stimuli; however, they may react to noise in a busy ICU environment, such as slamming cage doors and barking dogs. They need to be anesthetized sufficiently to maintain an ET tube, but do not need to be very deeply anesthetized.

> **TECHNICIAN NOTE** Keep in mind that little things like using earplugs or covering the eyes with a towel can help to reduce the amount of anesthetic needed.

As with any anesthetized patient, monitoring is very important to ensure success. The anesthetized patient's condition may change moment to moment, and require interventions. It is very possible to ventilate a dead patient, and without appropriate monitoring, it could be some time before this is noticed. For that reason, a ventilator patient requires a 1:1 patient to technician ratio, with a technician literally at their bedside for the duration of the ventilation.

> **TECHNICIAN NOTE** Staffing should be increased whenever a ventilator patient presents to ensure that sufficient assistance is on hand.

Typical monitoring of a ventilator patient includes continuous electrocardiography (ECG), direct arterial blood pressure, end-tidal CO_2, pulse oximetry, and arterial blood gases. Hands-on monitoring includes assessing palpebral reflex and jaw tone and performing digital palpation of pulses. With the lack of stimuli, ventilator patients are notorious for becoming too deep in their anesthetic plane, and this constant monitoring will allow the technician to respond rapidly. Alternatively, when kept at a fairly light anesthetic plane, ventilator patients are known to extubate themselves by reacting to a loud noise or painful stimuli suddenly. Careful titration of the injectable anesthetics is paramount to avoiding patients that are both too deeply and too lightly anesthetized. Keep in mind a small bolus of injectable anesthetic, such as propofol or ketamine, may assist with certain procedures, and avoid a patient waking.

> **TECHNICIAN NOTE** Ensure that at all times an induction dose of an injectable anesthetic is in a syringe at the cageside, in case of sudden awakening.

Other monitoring of a ventilator patient includes examining ventilation parameters. Generally, this is performed hourly, where parameters such as Mode, FiO_2, PIP, PEEP, I:E ratio, Frequency, TV, and MV are all recorded, and any changes (dialed in or patient driven) are noted. This can be done on a flowsheet at the cageside, or even directly into a spreadsheet on a computer or tablet, and helps to show trends in ventilation as the patient improves, or perhaps worsens, which allows the clinician to make informed decisions.

MAINTENANCE OF THE VENTILATOR PATIENT

There are numerous techniques that can be employed both to keep the patient comfortable as well as to ensure that the patient does not acquire ventilator-associated pneumonia or other complications.

Some of the simplest techniques involve patient positioning, and ensuring the patient is adequately padded to maintain skin integrity. The patient should be kept clean and dry at all times, and the bedding should be changed at least daily, or as it becomes soiled. It is important for the technician to visually inspect the patient's skin frequently to identify decubital ulcers in the early stages.

When moving a ventilator patient, especially one that is systemically ill and very critical, it is important to avoid making sudden changes in body positioning.

> **TECHNICIAN NOTE** Flipping a patient from lateral to lateral in one big move may cause a sudden change in hemodynamic status and ventilation/perfusion in the lungs, causing a sudden decompensation and, possibly, even death.

Changing position slowly in these patients is ideal; therefore, if the patient is in the lateral position, it is best to slowly start to move the patient towards sternal, possibly propping the patient up with additional bedding or foam wedges until sternal position is reached. Depending on the patient's condition, this can take place over a few minutes, or in extremely ill patients, a half hour or more may be needed. Keeping a close eye on heart rate (HR) and blood pressure measurements as well as SpO_2 and $EtCO_2$ values will help guide you in this process. Ideally, big movements should be performed only when it is necessary, when there are a sufficient number of staff, and when a clinician is available.

Many patients will do well being ventilated in sternal recumbency, and therefore gentle flipping of the hips and movement of the forelimbs will help to maintain patient comfort. Use of foam wedges, troughs, or other positioning aids will help to keep the patient in the desired position.

> **TECHNICIAN NOTE** Often patients will give cues that they are getting uncomfortable; they may start taking more spontaneous breaths or move their limbs slightly, or their heart rates may start to increase. Shifting their position when this happens may allow them to fall back to sleep more easily.

Ventilation is a highly invasive procedure, and ensuring cleanliness of those handling the patient, as well as the patient, is paramount. All persons handling the patient must ensure that they are handwashing adequately, and ideally, whenever handling the mouth or endotracheal tube, personnel should wear examination gloves in addition to performing handwashing.

Mouth care is an important part of ventilator patient maintenance, and is performed at a minimum of every 8 hours. Protocols are varied, and range from using sterile saline alone to using an oral mouth rinse with chlorhexidine. Regardless of the solution used at your facility, the goal is to clean the mouth and pharyngeal area thoroughly to minimize both secretions and bacteria. Ventilator-associated pneumonia (VAP) has been associated with colonization of the mouth and subsequently tracking of the bacteria on the outside of the ET tube with gastrointestinal (GI) bacteria. Mouth care should be performed with sterile solutions, sterile sponge forceps, and sterile gauze squares; all surfaces of the mouth should be wiped, including all surfaces of the tongue and cheeks, palate, and deeper to the pharyngeal area, and noting any pockets of mucus that may be accumulating (Figure 8-4, *A*, *B*). The use of a disinfected laryngoscope will allow for easy visualization of the larynx and help to avoid trauma while the area is thoroughly cleaned. Using a glycerin-based dry mouth solution after mouth care can help to maintain moisture in the mouth.

Some patients, such as those with pneumonia, will be highly productive of respiratory secretions, causing mucus accumulation in the airways and ET tube that can inhibit adequate ventilation. Edema fluid will cause problems as well. Occasionally these patients will need airway suctioning, which should be performed using a closed suction technique that is built into the ventilator circuit. Preoxygenating before performing suction is important, since ventilation will be reduced while suctioning. Most modern ventilators have an automatic setting to increase the FiO_2 for a period of 3 minutes before suctioning, and for a few minutes afterwards. It is important to always keep the suction tube moving, and rather than activating the suction continuously, using an intermittent technique will assist in preventing trauma to the airways.

The ET tube should only be replaced when necessary, after suctioning has failed to fully open the tube. Every time the tube is changed, there is an opportunity for bacteria to be introduced into the airways. Sterile technique should be used with each change, and similarly to suctioning, preoxygenation should be performed first. A full suction of the mouth and around the ET tube is a great idea if you have time to prepare for reintubation. It is important to have multiple hands available during a tube change, because this is a critical period.

Airway humidity is a concern in ventilated patients because we are bypassing the nasal passages, which normally humidify the air an animal breathes. In-line humidifiers are available for most modern ventilators

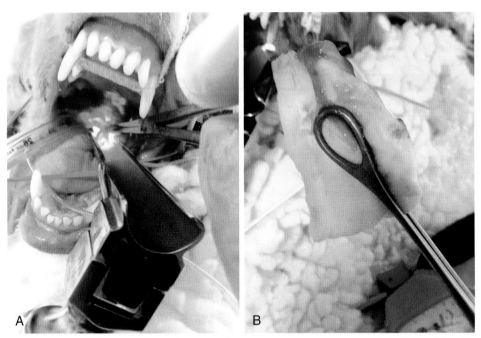

FIGURE 8-4 A, Example of mouth care performed on a ventilated patient. It is important to reach the back of the pharyngeal area to remove mucus that tracks from the nasopharynx. **B,** Gauze that has been used to clean the pharyngeal area.

that allow for warm-water vapor to be directly added to the circuit. This will also help to keep the patient warm. In the absence of a humidifier, a heat and moisture exchanger (HME) should be attached to the patient between the wye-connector and the ET tube. The HME absorbs heat and moisture that are exhaled, and essentially warms and humidifies air as it is inhaled.

Other maintenance considerations include frequent eye lubrication (at least every 4 hours) and physiotherapy of limbs to maintain flexibility. A urinary catheter should be placed both to maintain cleanliness and to quantify urine output. IV and urinary catheter care should be performed routinely per hospital protocol.

TROUBLESHOOTING

Mechanical ventilation is an advanced modality that requires keen observation skills and an understanding of what alarms may indicate. It is of the utmost importance that alarms are individualized for the patient, in order that they can notify the technician and clinician as early as possible about a problem. Alarm settings such as low or high TV, low or high MV, leak, low or high PIP,

and apnea must be set at the beginning of ventilation, and will typically be set to within ±10% of the current settings.

Alarms should never be silenced repeatedly and ignored, or adjusted so they are not as frequent, without a thorough investigation of both the patient and the machine. Problems can and will develop, and in retrospect, it may be noted that there were changes in the ventilation status of the patient. Always think about what the alarm could mean, and ask for assistance if unable to understand the alarm's significance.

Mucus can coat and begin to dry on the inside of the ET tube, and slowly occlude the lumen of the tube. This can result in slow changes to PIP or ventilator circuit resistance, which if not addressed quickly can lead to a full occlusion. Suctioning as frequently as necessary or changing the ET tube will help to alleviate this problem. As always, it is better to change the tube while everything is still working, albeit less efficiently, rather than have to react in an emergency situation caused by a tube occlusion.

Tube disconnections, airway leaks, and pneumothorax (PIP high) are examples of common alarm situations that must be corrected.

WEANING FROM THE VENTILATOR

As the ventilator patient improves, there will come a time when the clinician decides that the patient should be removed from the ventilator. Rather than this being a sudden decision, the patient will enter the **"weaning"** phase, which can last 24 hours or more. The duration of ventilation is often indicative of the length of time the patient will need to wean from the ventilator completely. The respiratory muscles begin to weaken almost immediately with ventilation, and need time to rebuild to full strength.

Criteria have been established in human medicine for assessment of weaning readiness. These include:

1. The original problem that required the patient to be ventilated has resolved sufficiently.
2. Measurable parameters (such as PaO_2, PaO_2/FiO_2 ratio, hemodynamic stability, and reduction in PEEP) have improved and stabilized.
3. The patient is able to take spontaneous breaths.

As stated, weaning is a gradual process, and in some ways begins when the patient is first placed on the ventilator. In fact, the goal during ventilation is to always provide the *minimum* ventilation necessary, and therefore always be reducing FiO_2 (usually in 5% increments) as PaO_2 improves, reducing peak pressure as TV improves and so on. The clinician will often leave orders for adjustment of ventilator settings based on current blood gas values and other parameters.

As the patient shows signs of improvement, the clinician will challenge the patient with spontaneous breathing trials. This does not mean putting the patient into a complete spontaneous mode, but again transitioning the patient to pressure support ventilation, which allows the patient to determine the frequency of breaths, but with the addition of pressure to help the patient complete each breath. Patients often have difficulty maintaining adequate MV for long periods of time because of weakened respiratory muscles, and start to fatigue. **Pressure support** will assist each breath, and the amount of support can be reduced as the patient strengthens. The pressure support period may last hours to even days, again depending on the duration of ventilation. It is important to watch the patient's work of breathing, and note if the patient is using excessive accessory muscles to breathe. Temperature and PCO_2 should be monitored closely.

Once the pressure support has been reduced to approximately 5 mm Hg, the only benefit to the pressure support is assisting the patient in overcoming the resistance in the ventilator tubing itself. If all parameters remain stable at this point, it is likely time to remove the ventilator. Disconnection is often accomplished by maintaining heavy sedation and the endotracheal tube to allow for rapid reconnection if necessary. If the patient has a tracheostomy tube, the patient can be awakened with the tracheostomy tube in place.

Oftentimes, weaning may be successful for a period of time, but then the patient begins to tire. In these cases, the patient may need to be reestablished on the ventilator for some time with pressure support, before trying to wean again. This is much easier to accomplish when the patient has a tracheostomy tube in place, rather than inducing and reintubating the patient each time.

SUMMARY

Ventilator cases are challenging for any veterinary technician. It is important to have an understanding of strategies of ventilation, goals of ventilation, and, most importantly, familiarity with the practice ventilator. The nursing care of these patients is very intense, but very rewarding when successful. These cases are not for the feint of heart, but are the favorite of many technicians who have enquiring minds and a desire to learn!

REFERENCES

Burkitt-Creedon JM, Davis H: *Advanced monitoring and procedures for small animal emergency and critical care*, Hoboken, NJ, 2012, Wiley-Blackwell.
Cairo JM: *Pilbeam's mechanical ventilation*, ed 5, Elsevier, 2012.
King L, editor: *Textbook of respiratory disease of the dog and cat*, St. Louis, 2004, Elsevier.
Silverstein DC, Hopper K: *Small animal critical care medicine*, St. Louis, 2014, Elsevier.
West JB: *Respiratory physiology*, ed 9, Baltimore, 2012, Lippincott Williams & Wilkins.
Wingfield WM, Raffe M: *The veterinary ICU book*, Jackson, WY, 2002, Teton New Media.

SCENARIO

Purpose: To provide the veterinary technician with the opportunity to build or strengthen the ability to quickly evaluate a situation faced in a typical emergency clinic.
Stage: Emergency clinic is considered a moderate level facility *(levels are currently being determined by VECCS and may have specific information by publication)* and always has at least four staff members available, including one ER clinician, two veterinary technicians, and one receptionist who also assist with animal handling when necessary. There is a back-up clinician on call to assist with surgeries.

Scenario: Saturday night

A 20-kg, 5-month-old Bernese mountain dog presents at the emergency clinic following electrocution from chewing on an extension cord. The owners noted that the circuit breaker tripped quickly, but the puppy did receive a big shock. They quickly examined him, and found burns in his mouth and on the pads of his front left foot. On the drive to the emergency clinic, they noted the puppy had become quiet and started to breathe heavily.

Upon presentation, the puppy was laterally recumbent, and in obvious respiratory distress. The primary survey revealed an increased respiratory rate and marked respiratory effort, tachycardia, pale and slightly cyanotic mucous membranes, and dull mentation. The triage technician recognized a dog that required immediate interventions, asked the owners if she could take him to the treatment area, and immediately called the veterinarian to the back.

Oxygen was provided immediately via flow-by, and an IV catheter was placed. The secondary survey was performed, and found a HR of 190 bpm, RR 72 rpm, and pulses weak and thready; auscultation revealed bilateral pulmonary crackles in the dorsal lung fields, no heart murmur. SpO_2 was 91% without oxygen. With oxygen, SpO_2 increased to 96%, and HR and RR decreased slightly.

Radiographs showed diffuse pulmonary edema in the dorsal lung fields, a normal heart size, and intact diaphragm. A diagnosis of noncardiogenic pulmonary edema (NCPE) secondary to electrocution was made by the veterinarian. NCPE typically resolves with supportive care, in 24 to 48 hr. The patient was admitted for oxygen therapy and monitoring.

A nasal catheter was placed in the right nostril, and oxygen was titrated to need using the pulse oximeter (the clinic does not have arterial blood gas capability). The veterinarian requested SpO_2 be monitored hourly, or as needed, and oxygen flow rate be adjusted to keep the dog at 95% to 96%.

The technician monitoring the dog notices that the dog is having increased respiratory effort. He has been receiving 3 L/min oxygen, and was at last check saturating at 95%. She decides to check again and is surprised to see that his saturation has decreased to 92%. She increases his O_2 flow rate to 5 L, and reminds herself to check again in 10 minutes. In 10 minutes, she notes that there is no decrease in respiratory effort and, in fact, the dog looks worse. He is lying with his head and neck extended, with tremendous abdominal effort, and appears to be "gasping." His HR is back to 200 bpm, RR 100 rpm, and he is visibly cyanotic. She immediately calls the veterinarian.

The veterinarian arrives and instantly realizes that the technician is correct and that the patient has decompensated further. He orders a propofol induction, intubation, and hand-bagging (the clinic does not have a ventilator).

Delivery

Ask the team to discuss in detail the induction, intubation, and hand-bagging of this patient.

Consider

1. Dose of propofol needed
2. How to keep puppy asleep following induction
3. Intubation issues, such as size of tube, laryngoscope
4. Use of Ambu bag vs anesthetic bag
5. Rate of ventilation
6. Consider suction if pulmonary edema fluid fills tube. No suction? Consider "dumping" the patient by raising hind end and lowering front end to encourage drainage.
7. The dog is intubated and the technician is bagging. What should be done next?
8. Decision is made to transfer. How will this be performed?
   a. Supplies needed
   b. Technician or veterinarian for transfer (bagging will have to continue)
   c. Pet transfer service an option?

MEDICAL MATH EXERCISE

A patient is being ventilated with a TV of 300 ml, at 32 breaths/min, with a PIP of 10 cm H_2O. What is the minute volume?

   a. 10 L/min
   b. 3 L/min
   c. 300 ml/min
   d. 3.2 L/min

9 Pain Assessment and Treatment

Nancy Shaffran

CHAPTER OUTLINE

Physiology of Pain
Assessment and Recognition
  What Does Pain Look Like?
  When and How Should Pain Be
    Treated?
Pain Relief
  Nonpharmacologic Interventions
  Analgesic Drugs
  Drug Options
Pure (Full) Agonists
  Morphine Sulfate
  Oxymorphone
  Hydromorphone
  Fentanyl Citrate
Mixed Agonist and Antagonist
  Opioids
  Butorphanol Tartrate
  Buprenorphine
Antagonists
  Local and Regional Anesthetics

Topical Analgesia
Local Infiltration
  Dental Nerve Blocks
  Joint Space
  Peritoneal Space
  Pleural Space
Alpha$_2$ Agonists
Alpha$_2$ Antagonist Reversal
Constant Rate Infusion (CRI)
  Morphine
  Hydromorphone
  Fentanyl
  Lidocaine
  Ketamine
  Dexmedetomidine
Epidural Anesthesia and Analgesia
Monitoring Drug Effects
Pain Management Checklist

LEARNING OBJECTIVES

After studying this chapter, you will be able to:

- Define pain.
- Introduce different options for pain management.
- Provide information on how to determine if a patient is painful.
- Define constant rate of infusion and discuss how to calculate and administer aconstant rate infusion.

Philosophers and scientists have long debated the issues of animal **pain**. Until recently, practical pain treatment in veterinary patients has not been adequately addressed. This oversight may have resulted from the following erroneous beliefs:
- Animals do not experience pain.
- Pain may be experienced but not in a way that is detrimental to an animal's well-being or that warrants treatment.

- Signs of pain are too subjective to be assessed.
- Pain is good because it limits activity.
- **Analgesia** is bad because of adverse side effects or because it interferes with the ability to accurately monitor patients.

The veterinary community now recognizes that animals experience pain and that pain must be managed for optimum health. The emerging specialty of veterinary critical care has brought greater attention to pain management. Although their analgesic needs are likely greater than the needs of stable patients, critically ill patients present unique challenges in pain recognition and choice of treatment. Choosing the correct analgesic therapy requires an understanding of the pharmacokinetics of a wide range of drugs, as well as the level or type of pain associated with various conditions. Failure to adequately manage pain in a critically ill patient lessens the chance of recovery and can result in shock and even death.

Aside from the pain associated with their illness or condition, critically ill and injured patients are subjected to numerous painful treatments and diagnostic procedures. The commitment to treat critically ill animals must include alleviating or minimizing their pain throughout the hospitalization period and beyond.

Patients that are critically ill are likely to be in pain and in need of treatment; however, because of their fragile condition, these animals may be less able to express their needs than the average, healthy animal. It has been suggested that these animals inspire less affection and greater detachment from caregivers than do healthier animals with "personality," which is thought to diminish the attention paid to their pain needs. However, one might argue that to some caregivers, critically ill patients inspire greater compassion in response to an increased perception of helplessness. Regardless, critical patients require more "intuitive" pain management because many of the common behavioral components of pain scoring are minimized.

The ambiguity in pain management rests largely in the subjective nature of pain assessment. Veterinary pain assessment is based solely on the ability to recognize often subtle, varying signs and symptoms of nonverbal patients. The study of pain in nonverbal patients (i.e., human neonates, infants, animals) is fairly recent. As incredible as it seems, the first human work examining pain manifestations in preverbal children was conducted in 1986. This research showed that healthy full-term newborns display painful distress in response to tissue damage. Crying, body movements, avoidant behaviors, and facial expressions were described as manifestations of pain in neonatal patients. Despite these acknowledgments, neonates were not routinely treated for pain for nearly 10 more years. The inability to distinguish pain from other stress, the extreme subjectivity of assessment, and persistent argument about the existence of neonatal pain confounded clinicians' efforts. Even now, human neonatal pain assessment and management remains an area of research, growth, and ethical debate.

In veterinary medicine, the issue is further confounded by several factors. First, a natural variation exists in the experience and display of pain between species, breeds, and individual animals. Veterinary technicians are expected to recognize pain in cats, dogs, and other small companion animals. There may appear to be very little similarity between a cat that sleeps curled in the back of its cage, avoiding movement or contact, and a crying, restless dog; however, both animals may be exhibiting signs of pain. Even within species, breed variations are strong. It has become customary to discriminate between perceived stoic and weak animals. Animals that do not display overt signs of pain are praised for their fortitude. Patients that show excessive signs of pain are assumed to be weak. Collies and borzois, for example, are stereotyped as fragile and without strong will to survive grave illness. Conversely, Labradors and pit bulls seem to be oblivious to pain and able to survive where other dogs might not. Tech Note: Although the specifics are arguable, most veterinary professionals probably have preconceived ideas about breed predisposition and ability to handle pain, stress, and illness. Some actual differences may exist in breed pain threshold and response; however, it is dangerous to make general assumptions about pain rather than to consider each patient individually.

Second, veterinary technicians often make assumptions about which procedures are most painful. For example, most would agree that a thoracotomy is a painful procedure, whereas an ovariohysterectomy is considered by many to be mildly to moderately painful. An examination of how these conclusions were reached is useful. No valid reason exists to make generalizations about procedures other than to assume that all invasive surgical or nonsurgical procedures are likely to cause some degree of pain. Each patient must be evaluated. Ultimately, pain treatment often is determined arbitrarily, based on a combination of limited information, subjective assessment, and personal beliefs. One can best approach a scientific and humane course of pain assessment and treatment by studying the physiology of pain, how pain is manifested in nonverbal patients, and when and how pain should be treated.

PHYSIOLOGY OF PAIN

Pain has a physiologic explanation. Pain receptors, called *nociceptors,* in the nervous system are stimulated by noxious events. The stimulus may be chemical, mechanical, or thermal. For example, chemical injury is often caused by substances such as prostaglandins and histamines produced in response to inflammation. Once a painful stimulus reaches a nociceptor cell, the information is transmitted to the brain via the spinal cord and the pain response begins. This includes the release of endogenous opioid endorphins, which function as natural analgesia. Often, in both chronic and acute situations, the level of pain exceeds the body's ability to provide relief. Acute pain is of severe, sudden onset that overwhelms endogenous analgesic mechanisms. Acute pain is the predominant concern among critically ill patients.

Chronic pain is prolonged and persistent; the body becomes habituated to nervous system responses and no longer provides adequate endogenous pain control. Regardless of whether pain is acute or chronic in nature, untreated pain can result in long-term changes in the nervous system that lead to persistent nonresponsive neuropathic pain states.

ASSESSMENT AND RECOGNITION

WHAT DOES PAIN LOOK LIKE?

IIn 1992, in an effort to form an initial consensus on what animal pain looks like, several hundred veterinary personnel from four leading veterinary institutions were surveyed. The survey was a simple form asking the participant to list all criteria he or she used to determine whether a patient was experiencing pain. The results were tabulated and categorized by frequency of response and subcategorized by professional group (i.e., technician, clinician). The top responses, in order of frequency, were vocalization, increased heart rate, increased respiratory rate, restlessness, increased body temperature, increased blood pressure (BP), abnormal

posturing, inappetence (lack of appetite), aggression, unwillingness to move, frequent changes in position, facial expression, trembling, depression, and insomnia. Also mentioned but less statistically significant were anxiety; nausea; pupillary enlargement; licking, chewing, or staring at site; poor mucous membrane color; salivation; decreased carbon dioxide; and head pressing.

More than 50% of all participants cited "known painful condition or procedure" as a reason to treat for pain. Listed criteria other than physical manifestations were the presence of one or more of the preceding signs without other attributable cause, intuition, and responsiveness to pain medication.

These findings are similar to those found in human neonates and infants, although more attention has been paid to their facial expressions and measured hormonal responses. Increased heart rate and respiratory rate, vocalization, and increased body movements are listed among the top pain manifestations in both human and veterinary patients. Several things become clear from this study. Various types of veterinary personnel have similar criteria for evaluating pain in their patients. This means that agreement exists regarding what pain looks like, although it is not necessarily scientifically conclusive. It is also clear that the list of manifestations is extensive and at times contradictory (e.g., unwillingness to move, frequent position changes). The following signs and symptoms, in the absence of any other reasonable explanation, are reasons to suspect that the animal is in pain and consider treatment. The reader should note that although the following are the most commonly described signs, they are by no means the only indicators of pain in veterinary patients:

- Increased heart rate
- Increased respiratory rate
- Increased blood pressure (BP)
- Increased temperature
- Vocalization
- Inability to rest or sleep
- Trembling
- Inappetence
- Changes in normal posture or movement
- Chewing or licking at painful site

Interestingly, although all of these signs are still considered potentially indicative of painfulness, the current leading signs of pain in small animals are more easily recognized as changes in normal behavior and body posture/position, especially in cats. Tech Note: It is probably safe to assume that any behavioral change not attributable to another known cause is likely to be an indication of pain in patients with past or present tissue injury.

WHEN AND HOW SHOULD PAIN BE TREATED?

In humans, scientific data support beneficial aspects of pain: it limits further aggravating activity, causes homeostatic regulating hormone release, and motivates the patient to seek medical attention. In small animals, these benefits are considerably less relevant and pain is considered detrimental in most cases. It has also been demonstrated that severe acute pain can have the following deleterious physiologic effects:

- Neuroendocrine responses (e.g., excessive release of pituitary, adrenal, and pancreatic hormones), possibly resulting in nutritional, growth, development, and healing disturbances, as well as immunosuppression
- Cardiovascular compromise (increased arterial BP, heart rate, and intracranial pressure and decreased perfusion)
- Increased respiratory rate accompanied by decreased partial pressure of oxygen or dyspnea
- Coagulopathies (e.g., thrombotic events, increased platelet reactivity, disseminated intravascular coagulation)
- Complications associated with long-term recumbency caused by pain or depression
- Poor nutritional intake and hypoproteinemia, resulting in slow healing

Pain should always be treated to inhibit its deleterious effects, although many analgesics are not benign and carry some risk of potential complications. Fear of side effects from analgesic drugs precludes their use in many cases. The most common arguments for withholding analgesia are as follows:

- Pain medication may cause cardiovascular compromise in fragile patients.
- Sedation may inhibit movement and lead to respiratory complications.
- Anesthetics and analgesics may mask signs of progress or regression, complicating evaluation of patient status. Cardiovascular monitoring may be obscured by sedation.
- Pain is self-protective (i.e., animals limit their own activity to minimize pain, and eliminating pain allows the patient to do further damage).
- Pain control measures may result in longer hospital stays and higher costs.

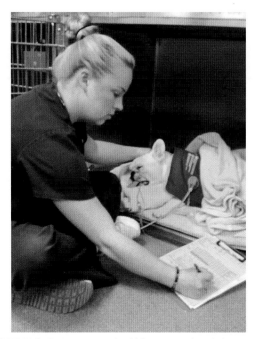

FIGURE 9-1 Pain status should be assessed and documented frequently during the recovery period.

It is always in the best interest of the patient to alleviate pain; therefore, these concerns must be addressed without withholding analgesia. The expected changes in heart rate, respiration, BP, and mentation that accompany analgesic use must be understood and baseline assessments should be made before initiation of treatment. After treatment, follow-up assessments should be made at regular intervals (Figure 9-1). More frequent cardiovascular monitoring may be needed in patients being treated for severe pain. Pain treatment may result in diminished activity and a slower return to normal body functions (e.g., eating, drinking, walking), but these effects may be less detrimental than the recovery delays associated with persistent pain.

PAIN RELIEF

NONPHARMACOLOGIC INTERVENTIONS

Before pain medication is administered, every effort should be made to provide nonpharmacologic comfort to the patient. Differentiating between physical pain and other types of stress is the first step in assessment. Stress responses to boredom, thirst, anxiety, and the need to

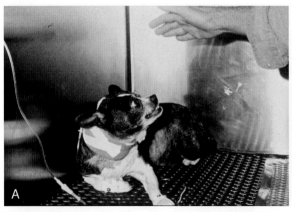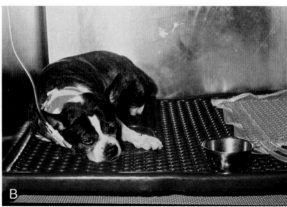

FIGURE 9-2 A, Painful postoperative foreign body removal Boston Terrier show cage aggression before treatment with hydromorphone. **B,** Painful postoperative foreign body removal in Boston terrier from panel A. Patient is now sleeping comfortably after treatment with hydromorphone.

urinate or defecate can mimic the signs of pain. All these stressors must be addressed before one can determine whether the patient needs medication. In some cases, these efforts may obviate further treatment; but even when pain medication is administered, these comfort needs must be addressed continually.

Providing comfort includes attention to physical surroundings and perceived psychologic needs. It should not be assumed that the patient will automatically assume a comfortable position. Tech Note: The patient may need to be placed in a position that reduces pressure on painful areas, facilitates adequate ventilation, and promotes sleep. Bedding, padding, and pillows can be used to provide additional support. Reducing light and sound can also encourage rest or sleep.

Assessing the patient's emotional needs may be more difficult because of the great variation in individual response to pain and stress. The critical care technician must become adept at recognizing the unique needs of each patient. Gentle stroking and calming speech can be potent means of easing stress. When distraction seems more effective, the animal can be placed in an active area with many visual and auditory stimuli. In some cases, owner visits are very comforting to the patient. In others, the patient becomes too agitated by the visit or the apparent benefits are negated by the response to the departure of the owner (Figure 9-2, *A-B*). Patient comfort can also be improved by reducing painful events. Because many nursing interventions entail painful procedures (e.g., injections, venipuncture, catheter placement, suturing), increasing technical proficiency

helps prevent pain. Tech Note: Organizing treatments efficiently to reduce the total number of disturbances is another nonmedical pain reduction intervention.

Once the patient's physical and emotional needs have been addressed, the patient's comfort is reassessed. The following questions should be asked:

- Is the patient at an acceptable comfort level?
- Is it possible that the clinical signs are manifestations of pain?
- Are there any contraindications to giving pain medications?
- Can the patient be supported through any adverse effects of drug administration?
- What is the appropriate (safe and effective) medication for the patient?
- Which nonpharmacologic pain reducers, such as cold therapy (Figure 9-3), can be considered?

It is common practice in human and veterinary medicine for nurses or technicians to assess pain status and administer appropriately ordered analgesia by continually revisiting these questions (Figure 9-4, *A-B*).

ANALGESIC DRUGS

The options for analgesia are increasing as more is understood about pain processing. Choosing the correct analgesic therapy involves understanding the pharmacokinetics of a wide range of drugs and the levels or type of pain associated with various conditions (Box 9-1).

Great individual variation in human responsiveness to drugs has been recognized. In other words, the same drug can produce vastly different results in different

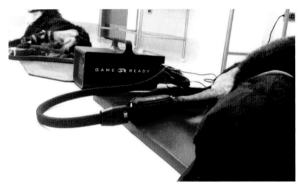

FIGURE 9-3 The Game-Ready™ circulates ice water through various size sleeves that can fit over a patient's limb, or pads that can cool larger areas. (Courtesy Dr. Kristian Ash.)

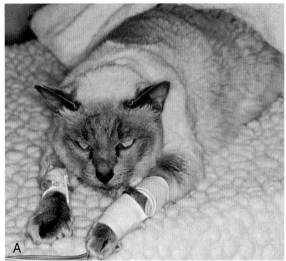

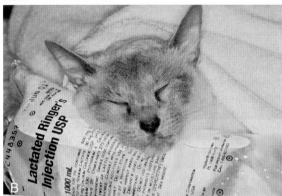

FIGURE 9-4 A, Painful pyometra Siamese before buprenorphine administration. **B,** Painful pyometra Siamese from panel *a* after buprenorphine administration.

BOX 9-1	How to Calculate a Constant Rate Infusion*

Calculating a CRI

What you need to know to begin:

- Dose of drug to be delivered (e.g., 3 mcg/kg/min or 0.18 mg/kg/hr)
- Patient's body weight in kilograms
- Fluid rate in milliliters per hour
- Fluid bag size
- Drug concentration

For dosages given in mg/kg/hr

Step 1: Set up equation based on dosage: mg/kg/hr = mg to add to bag.

Step 2: Replace hash marks with time signs: mg × kg × hr = mg to add to bag.

Step 3: Enter known information dose and weight.

Step 4: Solve for hours: fluid bag size ÷ hourly rate = number of hours bag will last.

Step 5: Solve equation: mg × kg × hr = mg to add to bag.

Step 6: Calculate drug volume and add to bag: desired mg ÷ concentration in mg/ml = number of ml to add.

For dosages given in mcg/kg/min†

Step 1: Set up equation based on dosage: mcg/kg/min = mcg to add to bag.

Step 2: Replace hash marks with time signs: mcg × kg × min = mcg to add to bag.

Step 3: Enter known information dose and weight.

Step 4: Solve for hours: fluid bag size ÷ hourly rate = number of hours bag will last.

Step 5: Solve for minutes: number of hr above × 60 min/hr.

Step 6: Solve equation: mcg × kg × min = mcg to add to bag.

Step 7: Convert mcg to mg: divide answer by 1000.

Step 8: Calculate drug volume and add to bag: desired mg ÷ concentration in mg/ml = ml to add.

*A controlled rate infusion pump is required since the rate of drug delivery must be precisely controlled. This can be a syringe pump, cassette pump, or rotary pump.

†NOTE: Two extra steps are required and shown in boldface type.

patients. These differences are partly a result of individual genetic differences, as well as a result of the nonphysiologic factors that influence any pain state: anxiety, fear, sense of control, ethnocultural background, and meaning of the pain state to the patient. This phenomenon appears to hold true for animals as well. Individual personality, breed traits, and the psychologic states of fear and anxiety all seem to play a role in the animal's perception of pain and response to treatment. This is one reason protocols for treating pain in veterinary patients have been difficult to develop. Ultimately, pain relief is the only true measure of successful treatment. The following information is meant as a guide to forming an initial treatment plan.

DRUG OPTIONS
Nonsteroidal Antiinflammatory Drugs
Nonsteroidal **antiinflammatory** drugs (NSAIDs) remain the most widely used analgesics in the treatment of chronic inflammatory pain. However, NSAIDs are also extremely effective in managing acute pain, especially when used preemptively (i.e., before tissue injury). Most surgical patients will require more than just NSAIDs to manage their perioperative pain, but many patients can be weaned to NSAIDs alone as the pain diminishes. NSAIDs are convenient to administer, are inexpensive, and provide long-lasting pain relief.

In the past NSAIDs were referred to as *antiprostaglandins*. Actually, NSAIDs do not directly inhibit prostaglandins but rather inhibit cyclooxygenase (COX), which synthesizes prostaglandin. Two types of COX exist: type 1 (COX-1) and type 2 (COX-2). NSAIDs have an effect on both types of COX. COX-2 gives rise to the group of prostaglandins that mediate the inflammatory response associated with pain; therefore COX-2 inhibition reduces inflammation, the desired effect of treatment with NSAIDs. However, COX-1 gives rise to the group of prostaglandins that maintain platelet function and gastrointestinal mucosal integrity; therefore the main disadvantage of extended NSAID administration is COX-1 inhibition resulting in mucosal sloughing, gastrointestinal (GI) ulceration, and bleeding. Non–COX-specific NSAIDs commonly used in the past include aspirin, phenylbutazone, and flunixin meglumine and have produced both pain relief and expected unwanted side effects. Ideally, NSAID therapy should be directed at selectively inhibiting COX-2

while sparing COX-1, thereby reducing inflammation while eliminating many negative effects. The newer NSAIDS are COX-2 selective but have varying inhibition of COX-2 versus COX-1. Recently the COX-2 enzyme has been shown to have very important effects in restoration of GI and renal health in the face of ulceration and hypotension, respectively. This new finding has cast doubt on the optimum ratio of COX-1 versus COX-2 inhibition. The role of COX-2 in maintenance of glomerular filtration rate in states of hypotension has led many people to stop using NSAIDs preemptively. Managing hypotension (monitoring blood pressure and providing intravenous [IV] fluids as needed) during surgery is critical for a host of reasons and doing so likely enables the safe and efficacious use of NSAIDs before surgery. To date, real-world data are the most reliable predictors of safety in this important class of drugs.

Opioids
Opioids are the most commonly used analgesics in hospitalized critically ill or injured patients because of their efficacy, rapid onset of action, and safety. The efficacy of various opioids is determined by the specific receptors in the brain and spinal cord where they exert effect. Relevant opioid receptors are classified as μ, κ, and Σ. μ receptors are chiefly responsible for analgesia; κ receptors are chiefly responsible for sedation. Both can cause some degree of respiratory depression. Σ receptors are less clinically relevant and are thought to be responsible for the adverse effects of opioid administration (e.g., dysphoria, excitement, restlessness, anxiety). Opioid drugs are classified as **agonists** (meaning that they stimulate the opioid receptors) or **antagonists** (meaning that they block particular opioid receptors). Partial agonists stimulate specific receptors but to a lesser extent than full agonists. In addition, mixed agonist and antagonist opioids stimulate some receptors while blocking others. In general, full agonists are the most potent opioids but also have the most severe adverse side effects. Side effects include vomiting, constipation, excitement, bradycardia, and panting. In humans the most severe side effect is respiratory depression, but this effect is rarely observed in veterinary patients. Pure antagonists reverse the narcotic properties of agonists. The availability of opioid antagonists makes opioid use safe because the drug effects can be removed rapidly. Mixed agonist and antagonist and partial agonist

opioids can provide reasonably good analgesia without many of the deleterious side effects of pure agonists. Opioids are metabolized by the liver and excreted via the kidneys; they should be used with some caution in patients with renal or hepatic disease. Ultimately, the type of opioid is chosen on the basis of the degree of analgesia needed and the specific needs or limitations of the individual patient.

PURE (FULL) AGONISTS

The most commonly used pure agonists in North America are morphine, oxymorphone, hydromorphone, and fentanyl.

MORPHINE SULFATE

Morphine is the gold standard for pure opioid agonists. All other drugs in this class are compared with morphine in terms of potency, efficacy, duration of action, and cost. Morphine is commonly used to provide maximal analgesia and sedation. Its relatively low cost and similar efficacy make it preferential over other opioids in some cases. However, it has additional side effects (particularly systemic hypotension, histamine release, and vomiting) that make it less desirable in many instances. Cats are particularly sensitive to morphine; therefore, lower doses are used in the cat. In addition, morphine has been shown to cause hyperthermia in cats. The typical dose for dogs is 0.5 to 2.2 mg/kg subcutaneously (SQ) or intramuscularly (IM) and 0.1 to 0.5 mg/kg IV, slowly. Cats typically receive 0.1 to 0.5 mg/kg (SQ) or IM.

OXYMORPHONE

Oxymorphone has a potency approximately 10 times greater than that of morphine and has moderate duration (4 to 6 hours). Oxymorphone may cause less respiratory depression and gastrointestinal stimulation than morphine. Some patients experience dysphoria, which may include vocalization, panting, and sensory hypersensitivity. The cost of oxymorphone also may be prohibitive. The typical dose is 0.05 to 0.1 mg/kg IV or IM.

HYDROMORPHONE

Hydromorphone shares similar characteristics with oxymorphone and has been more widely used with great success in veterinary medicine. The cost is higher than morphine but lower than oxymorphone. Typical doses are 0.1 to 0.2 mg/kg SQ, IM in the dog, and 0.05 to 0.1 mg/kg subcutSQ, IM in the cat. As with morphine, hydromorphone has been shown to cause hyperthermia in a majority of cats. It is not uncommon for animals to experience one episode of vomiting shortly after administration of hydromorphone if they are not painful at that time (e.g., pre-elective surgery).

FENTANYL CITRATE

Fentanyl is an extremely potent synthetic opioid with rapid onset but very short duration of action when administered IV bolus or IM and is therefore best delivered by constant rate infusion (CRI). Fentanyl is an excellent choice for managing severe surgical pain, especially in cardiovascularly compromised patients because it has minimal side effects compared to other opioids in this class.

Fentanyl is available as a transdermal adhesive patch of varying concentration to deliver 12.5, 25, 75, or 100 μg/hr for long-term (3 days) analgesia; however, it is difficult to establish consistent blood levels of fentanyl from this route of administration.

The onset of action of a transdermal fentanyl patch is between 12 and 24 hours, so supplemental analgesia is recommended during the initial treatment period. Concurrent use of mixed agonist and antagonist opioids reverses the effects of the fentanyl patch and should be avoided.

Recently, a topical transdermal fentanyl formulation has been licensed in the United States. Recuvyra® is a 50 mg/ml concentrated solution that is placed directly on the skin between the shoulder blades. It is licensed for 4 days of analgesia, and recommended for postoperative orthopedic and soft tissue surgeries. It is important to note that children must be isolated from the dog for 72 hours postapplication. While only available in the United States for a short time, Recuvyra has been available in Europe for several years. Veterinarians must take a brief on-line course on the safe handling and administration of the drug before ordering.

MIXED AGONIST AND ANTAGONIST OPIOIDS

Mixed agonist and antagonist opioids provide analgesia at some opioid receptors while inhibiting or decreasing stimulation at the μ receptors. Their action results in diminished analgesia and decreased side effects. These drugs partially reverse pure agonists by blocking action at the μ receptors.

BUTORPHANOL TARTRATE

Butorphanol is a κ agonist and a μ antagonist. The overall effectiveness of butorphanol as an analgesic is questionable because of its mild effects and short duration of action. Although the analgesic effects are thought to last only 45 minutes to 1 hour, butorphanol does appear to provide reasonable sedation for about 2 hours. It is expensive compared with morphine but has a significantly lower associated incidence of vomiting and dysphoria. Butorphanol is used in patients experiencing mild to moderate pain. It is available in oral and injectable forms. The typical dose is 0.2 to 0.8 mg/kg SQ/IM or 0.1 to 0.4 mg/kg IV in the dog and 0.1 to 0.4 mg/kg SQ/IM or 0.5 to 0.2 mg/kg IV in the cat.

BUPRENORPHINE

Buprenorphine is a partial μ agonist that is 30 times more potent than morphine and of longer duration because of its slow dissociation from receptors. Its best use is in dogs with moderate pain and in cats with moderate-to-severe pain. Buprenorphine is readily absorbed across mucous membranes in the feline, allowing for transmucosal administration in the cat. The typical dose is 0.01 to 0.03 mg/kg SQ, IM, or IV in the dog or cat. Cats can receive the same dose via the buccal mucosa. Duration of action is directly linked to dose. Higher doses may be required for a single dose to provide 8 hours of analgesia.

ANTAGONISTS

Opioid agonist analgesia, sedation, and side effects can be reversed rapidly with antagonists such as naloxone hydrochloride. Antagonists work by blocking opioid action at the μ receptors. Onset of reversal occurs within 1 to 2 minutes of IV administration and can last for 1 to 4 hours. Treatment can be repeated when reversing narcotics with a longer duration. The typical dose is 2 μg/kg IV. A more gentle reversal can be accomplished by diluting naloxone and administering slowly IV to effect. A dilution of 0.1 to 0.5 ml of naloxone, in 10 ml of saline, can be administered in 1-ml increments, every few minutes, allowing the technician to remove only the unwanted effects (dysphoria), without removing analgesic effects. NOTE: This is never done in an emergency; in this case, a full dose is administered.

LOCAL AND REGIONAL ANESTHETICS

Applying analgesia directly to nerve endings before they are stimulated can provide preemptive pain control while reducing or eliminating the need for systemic drugs. Local anesthetics work by disrupting neural information transmission by axons at the treatment site. Blocking neuronal activity also results in an expected loss of sensation and sometimes affects motor function. This loss of motor control is not seen with systemic analgesia. Local anesthesia should be used with caution in patients who are at risk for self-injury, such as those who have undergone orthopedic surgery.

Lidocaine, the most widely used local anesthetic, takes effect in 3 to 5 minutes and is effective for 60 to 90 minutes. The duration of lidocaine can be extended by combination with a 1:200,000 dilution of epinephrine, which causes local vasoconstriction. Epinephrine should *never* be used when vasoconstriction is undesirable such as in circumferential limb blocks. Bupivacaine has a longer onset of action (15 to 20 minutes), but its anesthetic and analgesic effects can last 3 to 6 hours. Bupivacaine is not effective as a topical analgesic, but it is an excellent choice for local infiltration.

Lidocaine, bupivacaine, and other drugs from this class are relatively safe when correctly administered. Most cases of toxicity in small animals occur as a result of accidental overdose or inadvertent IV administration. Signs of toxicity include seizures, coma, neurotoxicity, and cardiovascular collapse. Local anesthetics can directly damage tissues and cause allergic reactions or methemoglobinemia.

TOPICAL ANALGESIA

Applying topical analgesia to the surface skin or mucosa can reduce pain associated with minor procedures such as wound suturing, venipuncture, arterial puncture, or nasal cannulization. Solutions of lidocaine, bupivacaine, tetracaine, and epinephrine can be used alone or in various combinations to desensitize the application site. Gauze pads soaked with solutions can be applied directly to the site. Alternatively, several commercially prepared topical anesthetic creams and jellies can be applied as a thick paste. Regardless of application method, 20 to 30 minutes of direct contact time is needed to ensure effective analgesia.

LOCAL INFILTRATION

Injecting lidocaine or bupivacaine into local tissue can reduce pain associated with various painful procedures. This technique is useful for arterial catheter placement, thoracocentesis, abdominocentesis, and bone marrow sampling. The entry area is infiltrated with small amounts of anesthetic. Pain reduction is expected at 5 to 10 minutes after injection.

DENTAL NERVE BLOCKS

The entire muzzle can be anesthetized by blocking the infraorbital and mandibular foramina. This relatively simple technique is quite effective for dental extractions, oral mass removal, fracture repair, mandibulectomy, maxillectomy, and nasal biopsy.

JOINT SPACE

Effective analgesia before and during orthopedic surgery has been achieved by injecting local anesthetics directly into the joint space. Intraarticular morphine has also been shown to reduce joint pain. It has been suggested that applying a tourniquet above the joint for 10 minutes after injection greatly enhances drug efficacy.

PERITONEAL SPACE

Patients with abdominal pain, generally from abdominal surgery or acute pancreatitis, may benefit by local anesthetic infusion. The anesthetic must be delivered in fairly large volumes of saline to provide maximum intraperitoneal surface contact. Risks of the increase in abdominal pressure must be weighed against the benefit of analgesia.

PLEURAL SPACE

Interpleural bupivacaine infusion after thoracotomy surgery may have some analgesic benefit. Bupivacaine (1.5 to 2 mg/kg) is injected via an indwelling chest tube into the pleural space. Analgesia is thought to occur by direct blocking of the intercostal nerves. For maximum coverage, the patient should be positioned with the affected side down for 10 minutes after the injection to allow gravity to direct analgesic toward the pain site. The possibility of systemic drug absorption through the pleural tissue should be considered.

ALPHA$_2$ AGONISTS

Alpha$_2$ (α_2) agonists inhibit release of the excitatory neurotransmitter norepinephrine to produce analgesia and sedation. Alpha$_2$ agonists are short-duration analgesics and can be rapidly reversed with α_2-antagonists. This characteristic makes these drugs suitable for procedures requiring short-term restraint and analgesia as well as for surgical premedication. Alpha$_2$ agonists may bind to the same receptors as opioids and act synergistically with them. Opioid duration of action can be significantly increased if given concurrently with an α_2 agonist. Alpha$_2$ agonists can have profound effects on the cardiovascular and nervous systems, and using low doses will minimize these effects. Bradycardia and vomiting are the most common side effects with α_2 agonists. Patients receiving α_2 agonists should be heart healthy.

Xylazine, medetomidine (Domitor), and most recently dexmedetomidine (Dexdomitor) are α_2 agonists widely used in veterinary medicine. Aside from the label indications, there are a variety of ways described to utilize this drug class; as a pre-med, rough recovery rescue, and ongoing management of in-hospital pain and anxiety. Dexmedetomidine combinations are also extremely effective in cats for a variety of surgical and nonsurgical procedures.

Dexmedetomidine is labeled as a sole agent to facilitate clinical examinations, clinical procedures, and minor surgical procedures. A list of minor procedures that require sedation might include radiographs, bandage changes, cleaning ears that are not extremely painful, suturing of minor lacerations, or removal of foreign bodies from noses or ears. It is labeled similarly for use as a sedative in cats. Dexmedetomidine is also labeled as a single agent premedicant but is most frequently used off label in combination with opioids. One of the great advantages of using dexmedetomidine as a premedicant is a significant reduction (50% to 70%) in induction agent and gas inhalant. Another common use of dexmedetomidine is as a "rescue" drug for patients that are experiencing difficult recovery following anesthesia. Whether caused by pain, stress, or residual effects of anesthesia, postoperative dysphoria causes tremendous physiological stress and deleterious effects that include tachycardia, hypertension, cardiac arrhythmias, ventilation abnormalities (e.g. tachypnea with decreased tidal volume), cortisol release (which impairs proper healing), a predisposition for gastrointestinal (GI) ileus and ulceration, etc... This level of stress can cause severe problems in patients with cardiovascular or respiratory compromise. Therefore, post-operative excitement should be treated regardless of the cause. Dexmedetomidine is extremely effective at a micro dose of 1-2micrograms per kg IV in both dogs and cats to provide approximately 30 minutes of sedation, minor pain relief and potentiation of opioids.

Patients who require repeated rescue doses of dexmedetomidine can be placed on low dose (1-2micrograms/kg/hr) constant rate infusion (CRI) for continued sedation and analgesia. In addition, CRIs of dexmedetomidine are commonly used in human patients including children who are agitated in hospital, resistant to ventilators or in narcotic withdrawal. Similar success is reported in veterinary patients in intensive care units particularly in anxious breeds.

ALPHA₂ ANTAGONIST REVERSAL

One of the benefits of α_2 agonists is their ability to be reversed with α_2 antagonists. Antisedan® (atipamezole) is most commonly used to reverse dexmedetomidine. Atipamezole is the safest of all of the reversal agents because it works almost exclusively by simply displacing Dexmedetomidine from the α_2 receptors so that the nerve function can return to normal. Atipamezole has little actual drug effect of its own whereas older reversal agents, like yohimbine and tolazoline, cause both a displacement of the drug at the receptor and CNS stimulation, which causes unwanted side-effects. Furthermore, atipamezole has a long duration of action (longer than dexmedetomidine) and the animal will not 're-sedate' as often occurs with the older, shorter acting α_2 antagonists. After administration of atipamezole, patients usually awaken in about 5 to 10 minutes and are able to stand or walk in less than 10 minutes. Atipamezole rapidly reverses all physiologic effects of dexmedetomidine to 80% of baseline levels within 15 minutes.

CONSTANT RATE INFUSION (CRI)

Constant rate infusion allows continuous low-dose administration of various analgesics. Optimally CRIs are established before tissue damage (i.e., preoperatively) and run for at least 6 to 12 hours postoperatively. CRI analgesia is also quite effective in the management of hospitalized patients with preexisting or persistent medical pain. Overall dose of analgesia is typically lowered when administered by this method. Many agents can be delivered as a CRI, but the most commonly used agents are local anesthetic (lidocaine), opioids (morphine, hydromorphone, or fentanyl), N-methyl-d-aspartate antagonists (NMDA) (ketamine), and α_2 agonists (dexmedetomidine) Regardless of the drug, a loading dose is typically given immediately before beginning a CRI. These drugs can be used as single agents or in combination with one another.

Tech Note: It is important for the technician to be continually monitoring the dose of analgesic, compared to the clinical picture of the patient. Obtaining standing orders for dose ranges is ideal, because then the technician can titrate the dose within the range, based on what he or she is observing in the patient. It is not uncommon when using longer acting drugs, such as hydromorphone, to have to adjust the dose since it has been observed to frequently cause dysphoria after several hours. Since hydromorphone can last 4 to 6 hours, often the drug is accumulating in the system after prolonged use. Adjustments frequently need to be made to keep the patient at a good plane of analgesia.

MORPHINE

The main advantage of administering opioids by CRI is the avoidance of peaks and valleys typically seen with opioid bolus dosing. A lower dose of morphine can be used in a CRI than in bolus dosing, which can reduce the unwanted side effects of morphine such as dysphoria or panting. Morphine CRI is useful to manage any severe pain and can be safely combined with ketamine, lidocaine, or both.

The CRI dose for morphine is:

Dogs: 0.2 to 0.5 mg/kg **slow** IV loading bolus followed by 0.1 to 0.3 mg/kg/hr CRI
Cats: 0.05 to 0.1 mg/kg IV loading bolus followed by 0.025 to 0.2 mg/kg/hr CRI

HYDROMORPHONE

Hydromorphone has similar properties to morphine.
CRI dose is:

0.01 to 0.05 mg/kg/hr (dog and cat)

FENTANYL

Fentanyl is a full opioid agonist with similar analgesic properties but markedly less side effects compared to morphine. Other advantages of fentanyl over morphine include rapid onset of action, short half-life, and safety in cardiovascularly unstable patients. The major disadvantage is that fentanyl is considerably more expensive. Studies on fentanyl CRI in dogs have identified that the half-life of fentanyl increases when used as a CRI.

The CRI dose for fentanyl is:

Dog: 2 to 5 mcg/kg IV loading dose followed by 5 to 20 mcg/kg/hr CRI intraoperatively

2 to 6 mcg/kg/hr CRI for pain management in the ICU

Cats: 1 to 2 mcg/kg IV loading dose followed by 5 to 20 mcg/kg/hr CRI

2 to 6 mcg/kg/hr CRI for pain management in the ICU

LIDOCAINE

Lidocaine is a local anesthetic that provides excellent systemic analgesia when delivered intravenously. Lidocaine is safe for use in patients with GI disturbances, and therefore a good choice for analgesia in patients with gastric dilation volvulus or other similar disorders. Lidocaine seems to also provide benefit for patients undergoing procedures with excessive nerve trauma such as complicated back surgeries or limb amputations. IV lidocaine is extremely short acting and can be discontinued without residual effect almost immediately. Lidocaine CRI should be discontinued if the patient shows signs of toxicity including muscle tremors, seizures, nausea, or vomiting.

The CRI dose for lidocaine is:

Dog: 2 mg/kg IV followed by 20 to 50 mcg/kg/min

Lidocaine CRI doses are reported for cats, but typically lidocaine is not recommended for use in cats because of the potential for severe cardiotoxic effects.

KETAMINE

Ketamine is a dissociative anesthetic and an NMDA antagonist. Stimulation of NMDA receptors in the spinal cord results in firing of neurons that transmit pain signals. Prolonged bombardment of these receptors that occurs with intense surgical pain or long-term chronic pain results in amplification of the signals and increased excitability of the spinal neurons (hyperalgesia) *Allodynia* (nonpainful stimuli perceived as painful by the spinal cord neurons) follows. This phenomenon, collectively called *windup,* is most evident in the postoperative period once the patient has regained consciousness or in patients that present with existing severe pain. The NMDA receptor antagonist ketamine given as an intraoperative CRI binds at these CNS receptors and prevents windup. Because of its mechanism of action, ketamine is best used to manage neuropathic types of pain, particularly when the pain has been long standing and the patient

has not responded well to other analgesics. Ketamine should be always be given in combination with an opioid, and both can be delivered in the same infusion.

The CRI dose for ketamine is:

Dog and cat: 0.5 mg/kg IV loading bolus, followed by 10 *mcg/kg/min* CRI during surgery and 2 mcg/kg/min (or a dose range of 0.1 to 1.0 mg/kg/hr) for 24 hours after surgery

DEXMEDETOMIDINE

Dexmedetomidine can also be used to manage dogs and cats that display anxious, painful, or dysphoric behaviors. It can be used as a sole agent or in combination with any of the other analgesic agents.

The CRI dosage for dexmedetomidine is:

Dog and cat: 1 to 3 mcg/kg/hr

Tables 9-1 and 9-2 provide common CRI dosages of various drugs used in veterinary pain management.

Adjunctive and Adjuvant Analgesics

In addition to the classic analgesic agents, medications with other indications can be used to help manage pain. These drugs are referred to as *adjunctive analgesics* and come from many separate classes of pharmacologic compounds. *Adjuvant analgesics* are agents that can enhance analgesic drugs when co-administered but have few or no analgesic properties when given alone. The following are examples of adjunctive and adjuvant analgesics:

- Tranquilizers (phenothiazines, benzodiazepines) alter an animal's response to pain and can provide muscle relaxation. These drugs also reduce anxiety and fear, both of which can exacerbate pain.
- NMDA receptor antagonists (ketamine, amantadine) can enhance analgesia by blocking sensitization of neurons in the spinal cord and are especially useful for managing chronic or acute neuropathic or windup pain.
- Corticosteroids (prednisolone) have powerful antiinflammatory and immunosuppressive effects, "dampening the fires" of acute inflammation.
- Anticonvulsants (gabapentin, pregabalin) play an extremely important role in reducing neuropathic pain and central sensitization in severely painful patients. Gabapentin has become increasingly popular in both human and veterinary medicine as the first choice in patients whose pain does not respond to conventional therapies especially where nerve involvement is presumed.

TABLE 9-1	Dosages for Constant Rate Infusions (CRIs) Used in Cats			
DRUG	**LOADING DOSE**	**CRI DOSE**	**QUICK CALCULATION†**	**COMMENTS**
Morphine (M)*	0.10 mg/kg IM	0.03 mg/kg/hr (0.5 mcg/kg/min)	Add 15 mg to 500 ml of fluid and run at 1 ml/kg/hr	Cat may need light sedation; can be combined with K and/or L.
Hydromorphone (H)	0.025 mg/kg IV	0.01 mg/kg/hr	Add 5 mg to 500 ml of fluid and run at 1 ml/kg/hr	May cause hyperthermia; can be combined with K and/or L.
Fentanyl (F)	0.001-0.003 mg/kg IM or IV (1-3 mcg/kg IV)	2-5 mcg/kg/hr (0.03-0.08 mcg/kg/min) postop 5-20 mcg/kg/hr (0.08-0.3 mcg/ kg/min) intraop	For 5 mcg/kg/hr, add 2.5 mg to 500 ml of fluid and run at 1 ml/kg/hr	2.5 mg = 50 ml of F; remove 50 ml of LRS before adding F; can be combined with K and/or L.
Methadone	0.1-0.2 mg/kg IV	0.12 mg/kg/hr	Add 60 mg to 500 ml of fluid and run at 1 ml/kg/hr	May cause sedation; can be combined with K and/or L.
Butorphanol	0.1 mg/kg IV	0.1-0.2 mg/kg/hr	Add 50 mg to 500 ml of fluid and run at 1 ml/kg/hr or 0.1 mg/kg/hr	Only moderately potent and has ceiling effect: use as part of multimodal protocol.
Ketamine (K)*	0.25 mg/kg IV	0.12-0.6 mg/kg/hr (2-10 mcg/kg/min)	Add 60 mg to 500 ml of fluid and run at 1 ml/kg/hr or 0.12 mg/kg/hr	Generally combined with opioids; may cause dysphoria.
Lidocaine (L)	0.25 mg/kg IV	1.5 mg/kg/hr (25 mcg/kg/min) Some sources recommend no more than 10 mcg/kg/min in cats	Add 750 mg to 500 ml of fluid and run at 1 ml/kg/hr 10 mcg/kg/min would be 300 mg of lidocaine in 500 ml of fluid with a rate of 1 ml/kg/hr	750 mg = 37.5 ml; remove 37.5 ml of LRS before adding L; can be combined with opioid and/or K. **Lidocaine MAY be contraindicated in the cat because of cardiovascular effects.**
Medetomidine (Med) or dexmedetomidine (D)	Med: 1-5 mcg/kg D: 1-2 mcg/kg Can be IV or IM May not be necessary	0.001-0.004 mg/kg/hr Med (1-4 mcg/kg/hr) 0.0005-0.002 mg/kg/hr D	Add 500 mcg of Med or 250 mcg of D (0.5 ml of either) to 500 ml of fluid and run at 1-4 ml/kg/hr	Provides analgesia and light sedation. Excellent addition to opioid CRI, or can be administered as solo drug CRI.
Morphine*/ ketamine*	M: 0.10 mg/kg IM K: 0.25 mg/kg IV	0.03 mg/kg/hr M and 0.12 mg/kg/hr K	Add 15 mg of M and 60 mg of K to 500 ml of fluid and run at 1 ml/kg/hr	Can be administered up to 3 ml/kg/hr but dysphoria MAY occur. Can substitute F or methadone for M.
Morphine/ ketamine/lidocaine (MLK)	M: 0.10 mg/kg IM K: 0.25 mg/kg IV L: 0.25 mg/kg IV	0.03 mg/kg/hr M, 0.12 mg/kg/hr K; 1.5 mg/kg/hr L	Add 15 mg of M, 60 mg of K, and 750 mg (or 300 mg) of L to 500 ml of fluid and run at 1 ml/kg/hr	Can substitute H, F, or methadone for M.

*Credit: Dr. Tammy Grubb.

†Any of the drug amounts in the bag of fluids can be decreased and the fluids administered at a higher rate if necessary. For example, for morphine, ketamine, and morphine/ketamine infusions, 7.5 mg of morphine and 30 mg of ketamine can be used and the CRI can be administered at 2 ml/kg/hr if more fluids are needed.

TABLE 9-2	Dosages for Constant Rate Infusions (CRIs) Used in Dogs			
DRUG	**LOADING DOSE**	**CRI DOSE†**	**QUICK CALCULATION**	**COMMENTS**
Morphine (M)*	0.5 mg/kg IM (or 0.25 mg/kg **slowly** IV)	0.12-0.3 mg/kg/hr (2.0-3.3 mcg/kg/min)	Add 60 mg to 500 ml of fluid and run at 1 ml/kg/hr or 0.12 mg/kg/hr	MAY cause sedation; can be combined with K and/or L.
Hydromorphone (H)	0.05-0.1 mg/kg IV	0.01-0.05 mg/kg/hr	Add 5-24 mg to 500 ml of fluid and run at 1 ml/kg/hr	MAY cause sedation; can be combined with K and/or L.
Fentanyl (F)	0.001-0.003 mg/kg IM or IV (1-3 mcg/kg IV)	2-10 mcg/kg/hr (0.03-0.2 mcg/kg/min) postop 3-40 mcg/kg/hr (0.05-0.7 mcg/kg/min intraop)	For 5 mcg/kg/hr, add 2.5 mg to 500 ml of fluid and run at 1 ml/kg/hr	2.5 mg = 50 ml of F; remove 50 ml of LRS before adding F; can be combined with K and/or L; intraop dose can be up to 20-40 mcg/kg/hr.
Methadone	0.1-0.2 mg/kg IV	0.12 mg/kg/hr	Add 60 mg to 500 ml of fluid and run at 1 ml/kg/hr	MAY cause sedation; can be combined with K and/or L.
Butorphanol	0.1 mg/kg IV	0.1-0.2 mg/kg/hr	Add 50 mg to 500 ml of fluid and run at 1 ml/kg/hr or 0.1 mg/kg/hr	Only moderately potent and has ceiling effect: use as part of multimodal protocol.
Ketamine (K)*	0.25 mg/kg IV	0.12-0.6 mg/kg/hr (2-10 mcg/kg/min)	Add 60 mg to 500 ml of fluid and run at 1 ml/kg/hr or 0.12 mg/kg/hr	Generally combined with opioids; may cause dysphoria; postop dose may be higher.
Lidocaine (L)	0.5-1.0 mg/kg IV	1.5-3.0 mg/kg/hr (25-50 mcg/kg/min)	Add 750 mg to 500 ml of fluid and run at 1 ml/kg/hr or 25 mcg/kg/min	750 mg = 37.5 ml; remove 37.5 ml of LRS before adding L; can be combined with opioid and/or K.
Medetomidine (Med) or dexmedetomidine (D)	1-5 mcg/kg Med 1-2 mcg/kg D Can be IV or IM May not be necessary	0.001-0.004 mg/kg/hr Med (1-4 mcg/kg/hr) 0.0005-0.002 mg/kg/hr D	Add 500 mcg of Med or 250 mcg of D (0.5 ml of either) to 500 ml of fluid and run at 1-4 ml/kg/hr	Provides analgesia and light sedation. Excellent addition to opioid CRI, or can be administered as solo drug CRI.
Morphine*/ ketamine*	M: 0.5 mg/kg IM K: 0.25 mg/kg IV	0.12 mg/kg/hr M and 0.12 mg/kg/hr K	Add 60 mg of M and 60 mg of K to 500 ml of fluid and run at 1 ml/kg/hr	Can be administered up to 3 ml/kg/hr but sedation or dysphoria MAY occur. Can substitute H, F, or methadone for M.
Morphine/ketamine/ lidocaine (MLK)	M: 0.5 mg/kg IM K: 0.25 mg/kg IV L: 0.5 mg/kg IV	0.12 mg/kg/hr M; 0.12 mg/kg/hr K; 1.5 mg/kg/hr L	Add 60 mg of M, 60 mg of K, and 750 mg of L to 500 ml of fluid and run at 1 ml/kg/hr	Can substitute H, F, or methadone for M. Dr. Muir's dose is 3.3 mcg/kg/min M, 50 mcg/kg/min L; 10 mcg/kg/min K.

*Credit: Dr. Tammy Grubb.

†Any of the drug amounts in the bag of fluids can be decreased and the fluids administered at a higher rate if necessary. For example, for morphine, ketamine, and morphine/ketamine infusions, 30 mg of morphine and 30 mg of ketamine can be used and the CRI administered at 2 ml/kg/hr if more fluids are needed.

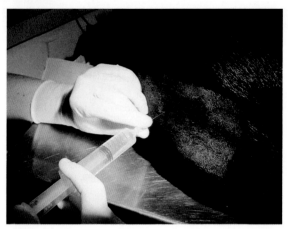

FIGURE 9-5 Single epidural injection being performed on a dog while in lateral recumbency

Typical starting dose is 5 to 10 mg/kg orally two to three times daily. Patients should be reevaluated for response frequently and dose adjustments are usually made every 5 to 7 days. Sleepiness is the side effect most commonly reported at higher doses. *Caution: Neurontin® elixir contains xylitol and may be suitable for administration to cats but not dogs.*

EPIDURAL ANESTHESIA AND ANALGESIA

Lumbosacral epidural administration of local anesthetics and analgesics is a valuable way to produce segmental anesthesia or analgesia in dogs and cats. It is an easy, safe, and effective way to alleviate pain, especially after procedures involving body parts caudal to the ribs, and should be considered an adjunct or alternative to other drug administration methods (Figure 9-5).

MONITORING DRUG EFFECTS

Perhaps the most confounding aspect of pain management is assessing pain and pain relief after treatment. The abatement or cessation of clinical signs associated with pain is the best indicator of successful treatment. Careful monitoring of cardiovascular status and mentation is vital to achieving good pain management without detrimental side effects. Effective treatment may result in cardiovascular or respiratory depression, diminished

movement, inability to eat or drink, urinary and fecal incontinence, and hypothermia. Supportive care is integral to pain management. The complications and side effects of treatment are monitored and corrected aggressively. Temperature, heart rate, pulses, respiratory rate and effort, mucous membrane color, and capillary refill time should be measured frequently. Treatment may include fluid volume and hydration support, nutritional supplementation, urinary catheterization, external warming, and even oxygen augmentation. Veterinary critical care professionals must eliminate pain and stress wherever possible and treat the adverse consequences as needed.

Parts *A* and *B* of Figure 9-6 show a widely used pain scale, developed at Colorado State University.

PAIN MANAGEMENT CHECKLIST

Veterinary technicians play a vital role in pain management. The technician is most likely to first detect signs of pain and request pain treatment. Critical care technicians can improve pain management practice in the following ways:
- Establish pain alleviation as a standard of care.
- Recognize the signs of pain.
- Respect owners' observations and assessment of pain in their pets.
- Understand and overcome the barriers to assessment and treatment.
- Be aware of known painful procedures and surgeries, and encourage preemptive and immediate postprocedure treatment.
- Reduce incidence of painful procedures by combining treatments efficiently.
- Use techniques to minimize pain (e.g., use electrocardiogram snaps instead of alligator clips; use indwelling catheters to obtain blood samples).
- Minimize pain associated with critical care techniques by improving technical skill and helping to develop new technologies that minimize pain.
- Differentiate pain from other distress such as confinement, boredom, separation from owners, insomnia, fear, and need to urinate or defecate.
- Understand the treatment options and encourage appropriate types of therapy.
- Continuously monitor the effects of various drugs in a coherent manner to evaluate treatment efficacy.
- Educate other animal caregivers about pain management issues.

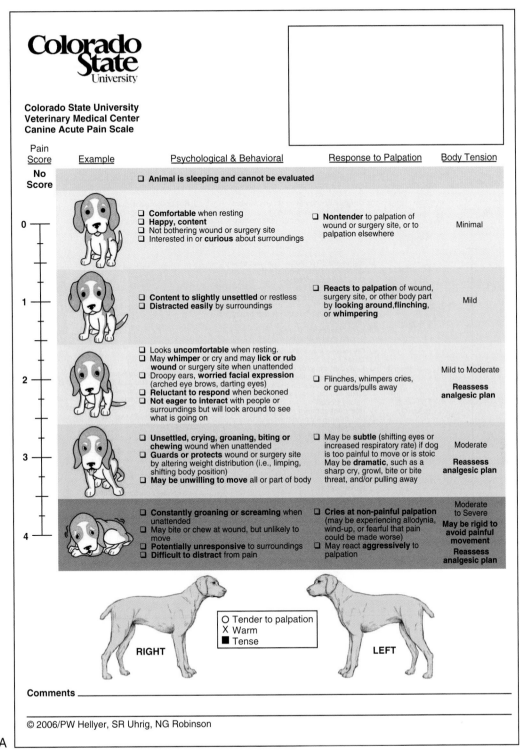

Colorado State University

Colorado State University
Veterinary Medical Center
Canine Acute Pain Scale

Pain Score	Example	Psychological & Behavioral	Response to Palpation	Body Tension
No Score		❑ **Animal is sleeping and cannot be evaluated**		
0		❑ **Comfortable** when resting ❑ **Happy, content** ❑ Not bothering wound or surgery site ❑ Interested in or **curious** about surroundings	❑ **Nontender** to palpation of wound or surgery site, or to palpation elsewhere	Minimal
1		❑ **Content to slightly unsettled** or restless ❑ **Distracted easily** by surroundings	❑ **Reacts to palpation** of wound, surgery site, or other body part by **looking around, flinching,** or **whimpering**	Mild
2		❑ Looks **uncomfortable** when resting. ❑ May **whimper** or cry and may **lick or rub wound** or surgery site when unattended ❑ Droopy ears, **worried facial expression** (arched eye brows, darting eyes) ❑ **Reluctant to respond** when beckoned ❑ **Not eager to interact** with people or surroundings but will look around to see what is going on	❑ Flinches, whimpers cries, or guards/pulls away	Mild to Moderate **Reassess analgesic plan**
3		❑ **Unsettled, crying, groaning, biting or chewing** wound when unattended ❑ **Guards or protects** wound or surgery site by altering weight distribution (i.e., limping, shifting body position) ❑ **May be unwilling to move** all or part of body	❑ May be **subtle** (shifting eyes or increased respiratory rate) if dog is too painful to move or is stoic May be **dramatic**, such as a sharp cry, growl, bite or bite threat, and/or pulling away	Moderate **Reassess analgesic plan**
4		❑ **Constantly groaning or screaming** when unattended ❑ May bite or chew at wound, but unlikely to move ❑ **Potentially unresponsive** to surroundings ❑ **Difficult to distract** from pain	❑ **Cries at non-painful palpation** (may be experiencing allodynia, wind-up, or fearful that pain could be made worse) ❑ May react **aggressively** to palpation	Moderate to Severe **May be rigid to avoid painful movement** **Reassess analgesic plan**

RIGHT   O Tender to palpation
                  X Warm
                  ■ Tense   **LEFT**

Comments _____

© 2006/PW Hellyer, SR Uhrig, NG Robinson

A

FIGURE 9-6 Pain scales used to assess acute pain levels in dogs **(A)** and cats **(B)**. (From Colorado State University, 2006; accessed at www.csuanimalcancercenter.org/assets/files/csu_acute_pain_scale_canine.pdf.)

Continued

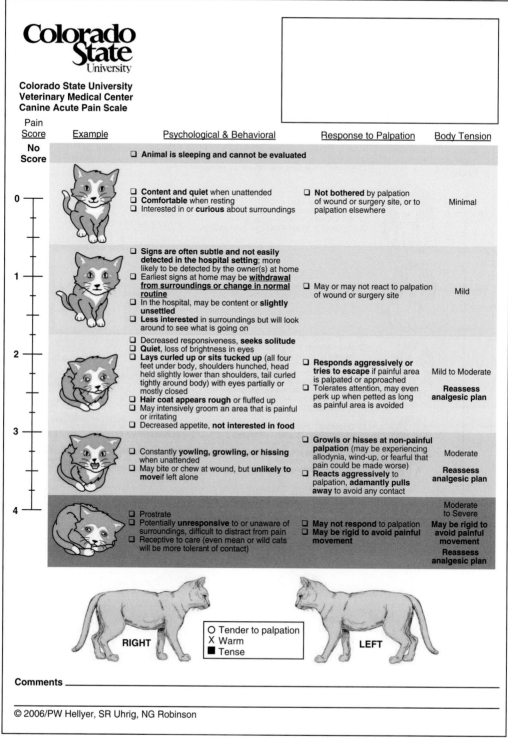

Colorado State University

**Colorado State University
Veterinary Medical Center
Canine Acute Pain Scale**

Pain Score	Example	Psychological & Behavioral	Response to Palpation	Body Tension
No Score		❑ **Animal is sleeping and cannot be evaluated**		
0		❑ **Content and quiet** when unattended ❑ **Comfortable** when resting ❑ Interested in or **curious** about surroundings	❑ **Not bothered** by palpation of wound or surgery site, or to palpation elsewhere	Minimal
1		❑ **Signs are often subtle and not easily detected in the hospital setting**; more likely to be detected by the owner(s) at home ❑ Earliest signs at home may be **withdrawal from surroundings or change in normal routine** ❑ In the hospital, may be content or **slightly unsettled** ❑ **Less interested** in surroundings but will look around to see what is going on	❑ May or may not react to palpation of wound or surgery site	Mild
2		❑ Decreased responsiveness, **seeks solitude** ❑ **Quiet**, loss of brightness in eyes ❑ **Lays curled up or sits tucked up** (all four feet under body, shoulders hunched, head held slightly lower than shoulders, tail curled tightly around body) with eyes partially or mostly closed ❑ **Hair coat appears rough** or fluffed up ❑ May intensively groom an area that is painful or irritating ❑ Decreased appetite, **not interested in food**	❑ **Responds aggressively or tries to escape** if painful area is palpated or approached ❑ Tolerates attention, may even perk up when petted as long as painful area is avoided	Mild to Moderate **Reassess analgesic plan**
3		❑ Constantly **yowling, growling, or hissing** when unattended ❑ May bite or chew at wound, but **unlikely to move** if left alone	❑ **Growls or hisses at non-painful palpation** (may be experiencing allodynia, wind-up, or fearful that pain could be made worse) ❑ **Reacts aggressively to** palpation, **adamantly pulls away** to avoid any contact	Moderate **Reassess analgesic plan**
4		❑ Prostrate ❑ Potentially **unresponsive** to or unaware of surroundings, difficult to distract from pain ❑ Receptive to care (even mean or wild cats will be more tolerant of contact)	❑ **May not respond** to palpation ❑ **May be rigid to avoid painful movement**	Moderate to Severe May be rigid to avoid painful movement **Reassess analgesic plan**

RIGHT   O Tender to palpation
X Warm
■ Tense   **LEFT**

Comments _____

© 2006/PW Hellyer, SR Uhrig, NG Robinson

B

FIGURE 9-6, cont'd Pain scales used to assess acute pain levels in dogs **(A)** and cats **(B)**.

SUGGESTED READINGS

Broome ME, Tanzillo H: Differentiating between pain and agitation in premature neonates, *J Perinat Neonatal Nurs* 4(1):53, 1990.

Craig KKD, et al.: Pain in the preterm neonate: behavioral and physiological indices, *Pain* 52:287, 1993.

Hellyer PW: Management of acute and surgical pain, *Semin Vet Surg Small Anim* 12(2), 1997.

Hellyer PW, Robertson SA, Fails AD: Pain and its management. In Tranquilli WJ, Thurmon JC, Grimm KA, editors: *Lumb and Jones' veterinary anesthesia and analgesia*, ed 4, Ames, Iowa, 2007, Blackwell, pp XX-XX.

Lamont LA, Mathews KA: In Tranquilli WJ, Thurmon JC, Grimm KA, editors: *Lumb and Jones' veterinary anesthesia and analgesia*, ed 4, Ames, Iowa, 2007, Elsevier Publishing, pp 241–271.

Lamont LA, Tranquilli WJ, Grimm KA: Physiology of pain, *Vet Clin North Am* 30(4):703–723, 2000.

Mathews KA: *Lifelearn. Veterinary emergency and critical care manual*, Ontario, 1996, Eden Mills.

Muir WW: Physiology and pathophysiology of pain. In Gaynor JS, Muir WW, editors: *Handbook of veterinary pain management*, ed 2, St Louis, 2009, Elsevier, pp 13–41.

Papich MG: Principles of analgesic drug therapy, *Semin Vet Med Surg (Small Anim)* 12:2, 1997.

Pascoe PJ: Local and regional anesthesia and analgesia, *Semin Vet Med Surg (Small Anim)* 12:2, 1997.

Rollin BE: *The unheeded cry*, New York, 1989, Oxford University Press.

Sackman JE: Pain management. In McCurnin DM, editor: *Clinical textbook for veterinary technicians*, Philadelphia, 1994, WB Saunders.

Short CE, Van Poznak A: *Animal pain*, New York, 1992, Churchill Livingstone.

Skarda R: Local and regional anesthetic and analgesic techniques: dogs. In Thurmon J, Tranquilli W, Benson G, editors: *Lumb & Jones' veterinary anesthesia*, ed 3, Baltimore, 1996, Williams & Wilkins.

Stein R: . Available at www.BASG.org, 2013.

Stevens BJ, Johnson CC, Grunau RV: Issues of assessment of pain and discomfort in neonates, *J Obstet Gynecol Neonatal Nurs* 24(9):849–855, 1995.

Tranquilli WJ, Grimm KA, Lamont LA: *Pain management for the small animal practitioner*, ed 2, Jackson, 2004, Wyo. Teton New Media.

Tyler DC, Krane EJ: Pediatric pain, *Adv Pain Res Ther*, 432, 1990.

Websites of Interest: International Academy of Veterinary Pain Management www.ivapm.org.

SCENARIO

Purpose: The veterinary technician needs opportunities to develop critical thinking skills in regards to pain management. The following scenarios will encourage the reader to be creative in his or her approach.

Stage: Hospital is a Level II emergency and critical care practice that also provides elective orthopedic surgeries 1 day/week. Fluid pumps are available for average case load and syringe pump availability limited with only 4 in working condition.

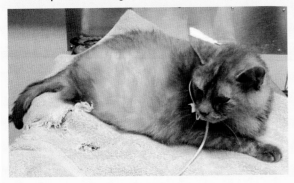

14-yr-old cat with pancreatitis is being examined: T, 99.7° F; HR, 220 bpm; RR, 42 breaths/min. Her cage is located in the center of the room in a top cage with a postoperative dog recovering from tibial plateau leveling osteotomy (TPLO) located in the cage beneath her. The dog is whining and occasionally hitting the side of the cage when trying to reposition itself.

Questions

- Which body postures may indicate pain?
- What is the primary source of pain?
- What drug modalities would you consider to alleviate the discomfort?
- What is the dose? What is the rate of infusion?
- How would you administer the drug?
- What would you avoid at this time?
- What other things could be done outside of medical management to alleviate discomfort?

Continued

SCENARIOS—cont'd

Discussion

This cat is likely to be experiencing severe abdominal pain attributable to pancreatitis. The fear and anxiety associated with hospitalization exacerbated by the dog caged beneath her will increase her distress. She should be moved to a more quiet location and provided with a safe environment including an open box with bedding. Pain management should include- opioids such as buprenorphine at a minimum dose of 0.03 mg/kg. If her pain/distress continues, she may benefit by addition of CRI of ketamine and/or dexmedetomidine. Recent investigation suggests that off label use of Cerenia® (Zoetis Animal Health) may provide additional pain relief in cats with pancreatitis.

Delivery

- Complete a review of drugs and equipment the hospital has available to meet pain management requirements.
- Use of pain scale considered.
- Photos of patients with their vitals and current condition are provided.
- Staff reviews photos and history for 3-5 minutes.
- Questions following case scenarios are asked.

- Discussion includes creating a plan for each patient involving use of medical management and other treatment modalities including position of patient, padding, physical therapy, or warming or cooling devices. Alternative therapies including acupuncture, massage, and passive range of motion (PROM) are also considered.

Key Teaching Points

- Provides the veterinary technician opportunities to use observation skills.
- Challenges the veterinary technician to use critical thinking skills on how to address different types of pain.
- Helps determine how to proceed with providing additional pain management techniques and therapies.
- Challenges the veterinary technician to be creative in how the pain management is delivered outside of medical management.

Other Resources

Pain management scale developed by Colorado State University: www.csuanimalcancercenter.org/assets/files/csu_acute_pain_scale_feline.pdf www.csuanimalcancercenter.org/assets/files/csu_acute_pain_scale_canine.pdf.

MEDICAL MATH EXERCISE

A 20-kg shepherd mix is admitted for forelimb amputation surgery. The dog is to receive a 30 mcg/kg/min infusion of lidocaine to help prevent severe nerve pain during and after surgery. The rate of fluids will be 40 ml/hr. How much 2% lidocaine will you add to a 1-L bag?

10 Anesthesia in the Critically Ill or Injured Patient

Jennifer J. Devey

CHAPTER OUTLINE

Introduction
Goals for Success
Preanesthetic Stabilization
Preanesthetic Preparedness
Setting Up for Major Surgery
Drugs
  Balanced Anesthesia
  Goals of Anesthesia
Analgesics, Local Anesthetics, and Preanesthetic Agents
  Analgesia
  Local or Regional Anesthesia
  Epidural Analgesia and Anesthesia
  Premedication
  Induction
  Alfaxalone
  Dexmedetomidine
  Etomidate
  Ketamine and Benzodiazepine
  Propofol
  Inhalants
Neuromuscular Blocking Agents
  Depolarizing Muscle Blocking Agents
  Nondepolarizing Neuromuscular Blocking Agents
  Monitoring with Neuromuscular Blocking Agents
Intubation
  Intubating a Patient with a Possible Airway Disruption
  Intubating a Patient with Upper Airway Swelling or Obstruction
Maintaining a Patient Under General Anesthesia
Controlled Ventilation
Monitoring
  Blood Pressure
Electrocardiography
Pulse Oximetry
  Pleth Variability Index (PVI)
  Capnometry
Supportive Measures Needed During Anesthesia
  Temperature Conservation and Preventing Hypothermia
  Fluid Support
Anesthetic Emergencies and Complications
Recovering the Patient

KEY TERMS

Analgesia
Balanced anesthesia
Capnography
Neuromuscular blockers
Positive pressure ventilation
PVI (Pleth variability index)

LEARNING OBJECTIVES

After studying this chapter, you will be able to:

- Learn the information that is required to make a plan to anesthetize a critical patient.
- Learn the pros and cons of different anesthetic drugs.
- Learn how to optimize monitoring in critical patients that are anesthetized.
- Learn how to minimize complications during recovery.

INTRODUCTION

Anesthesia is defined as the loss of sensation, especially related to pain, that is often delivered in order for painful procedures to be performed. The goal of general anesthesia is to provide a state of reversible unconsciousness, with adequate analgesia and muscle relaxation, in such a way that it does not jeopardize the patient's overall health. Delivering safe anesthesia to a critically ill small animal patient is one of the most important, and often one of the most challenging and stressful, tasks for a technician. In many emergency situations the technician must be both the anesthetist and the circulating nurse in the operating room. Although it is often necessary for the technician to have this dual role, it is not recommended because critically ill or unstable patients demand the undivided attention of an anesthetist.

The old adage of "there is no safe anesthesia just safe anesthetists" holds especially true for the critically ill or injured patient. It would be ideal to be able to stabilize all patients before anesthetizing them; however, some patients cannot be stabilized without surgery. The patient that cannot breathe because of a diaphragmatic hernia, the patient that has a gunshot wound and a severe hemoabdomen that is continuing to bleed, and the patient with septic peritonitis are all examples of animals that require surgery even though they are unstable and high risk. The technician must be familiar not only with anesthetic agents and their use but also with invasive and noninvasive means of monitoring critical patients. These patients may have little in the way of reserves, and the anesthetist must understand not only respiratory and cardiovascular physiology but also the pathophysiology of the disease process. Only in this manner can anesthesia be provided safely and the patient supported effectively.

Some patients may need anesthesia as they arrive in the emergency department; some of them may need surgery within the first few minutes or a few hours after arrival. This chapter attempts to provide an overview of anesthesia for this group of critically ill or injured patients. The focus will be on balanced anesthesia, which involves the administration of multiple drugs to the patient, each given for a specific purpose. It is assumed that the reader has a basic understanding of anesthetic equipment, anesthetic drugs, and basic monitoring. The reader is referred to general anesthesia texts for these specifics (Bednarski et al, 2011; Miller et al, 2009; Muir, 2012; Tranquilli et al, 2007).

GOALS FOR SUCCESS

Maintaining the ABCs of airway, breathing, and circulation is as important in the anesthetized patient as in the awake patient. Almost all anesthetic agents are respiratory and cardiovascular depressants.

TECHNICIAN NOTE The goal should be to ensure that, despite administration of drugs, the patient's respiratory and cardiovascular parameters remain as close to normal as possible.

Whereas the normal healthy patient often has enough reserves to draw upon to tolerate adverse effects of general anesthesia, the critically ill or injured patient may not. Acidosis related to poor perfusion and hypoventilation can be particularly detrimental and can cause significant abnormalities in the function of enzyme systems, cardiac function, and coagulation. Hypothermia can have similar adverse effects and every attempt should be made to prevent this from occurring.

The patient must have a patent airway and must be oxygenating and ventilating well. Hypoventilation is extremely common secondary to the underlying disease process as well as the administration of anesthetic drugs, and assisted ventilation is always indicated, preferably with the use of a mechanical ventilator.

Preload, blood pressure (BP), and heart rhythm should remain as close to normal as possible. Cardiac output (or the amount of blood that is carrying oxygen [O_2] to the peripheral tissues) depends on preload and cardiac contractility. Decreased preload can result from inadequate circulating volume, vasodilation, or a combination of the two. Tachycardia should be avoided because it shortens diastolic time, which may lead to inadequate filling of the ventricles, increased myocardial O_2 demands, and less time for the delivery of oxygen to the heart muscle via the coronary vessels. Irregular rhythms may indicate poor coordination of the heart muscle as it contracts, which can also negatively impact cardiac output.

Hemoglobin levels should not be allowed to drop to less than 7 to 9 g/dl (packed cell volume of 21% to 27%) in the acutely anemic patient in order to ensure sufficient oxygen delivery to the tissues (Hebert et al, 1999). High hemoglobin levels should be avoided to decrease the likelihood of "sludging."

Electrolytes should be maintained in as normal a range as possible to ensure good muscle function. The patient should have adequate oncotic pressure (albumin) to ensure sufficient circulating blood volume.

All patients must have a complete physical examination. The technician and the veterinarian need a baseline of physical parameters from which to work. Only in this manner can early changes in the patient's status be noted. The focus on the physical examination will vary somewhat depending on the patient's reason for presentation, and close communication must occur between the veterinarian and the technician in regard to the underlying disease, injury, and anesthetic concerns.

> **TECHNICIAN NOTE** A preanesthetic exam should always include a complete physical exam including all five vital signs (temperature, pulse rate, respiratory rate, BP, and pain) (Lynch, 2001).

Measurement of preanesthetic BP is extremely valuable in gauging the animal's reserves once anesthetic drugs have been administered. If there is minimal change in the BP following induction, then the patient will be more likely to tolerate the use of inhalant anesthesia than if there is a significant decrease in BP following induction.

The patient's respiratory rate and effort is noted, and tracheal and bilateral thoracic auscultation should be assessed. This will help localize the source of any airway or respiratory disease or problem that might be encountered during intubation or anesthesia. The presence of respiratory distress, stridor (indicating at least a 75% decrease in airway diameter), or very loud airway sounds, wheezing, crackles, areas of dullness, and subcutaneous (subcut) emphysema indicates ventilatory compromise, which may be worsened under anesthesia. Guttural or sonorous noises indicate pharyngeal disease. High-pitched or stridorous sounds indicate laryngeal or tracheal disease. Lung sounds should be compared on both sides of the thorax.

Heart tones should be auscultated and central and peripheral pulses should be palpated for both strength and presence of any deficits.

> **TECHNICIAN NOTE** Jugular veins should be clipped and evaluated for distention. A flat jugular vein that does not distend with digital pressure at the thoracic inlet is consistent with hypovolemia. The jugular vein that is distended with the patient standing or sitting may indicate a pneumothorax, pericardial effusion, or right-ventricular heart failure.

The presence of abdominal distention should be noted. Distended superficial epigastric veins (Figure 10-1) suggest high intraabdominal pressure. When this patient is placed in dorsal recumbency, additional pressure may be placed on the vena cava, thus compromising venous return to the heart and potentially leading to cardiovascular collapse.

Mucous membranes should be evaluated for color, capillary refill time, and presence of petechiation. An accurate weight (in kilograms for drug doses) should be recorded whenever possible to ensure accurate drug doses are administered; however, in some patients an approximation of the weight may be all that is possible, because moving the patient to the weigh scale may compromise care.

Depending on the age of the patient and the presence of any underlying injuries or illnesses, additional preanesthetic workup may include laboratory analysis, an electrocardiogram (ECG), radiographs, an echocardiogram, and an abdominal ultrasound. It is ideal to always have as complete a database as possible but this may not be warranted in some situations or may not be financially feasible. Lab measurements ideally should include a minimum of a packed cell volume and total solids (PCV/TS), glucose, blood urea nitrogen, and

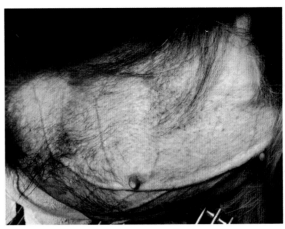

FIGURE 10-1 Distended superficial epigastric veins.

electrolytes. An albumin measurement should always be included if the patient is seriously injured because total solids/protein and albumin concentrations do not consistently correlate in the ill or injured patient and albumin level provides an indicator of the oncotic pressure. A complete blood count, chemistry panel, and urinalysis should be performed in all sick, injured, and geriatric patients and are never contraindicated in any patient.

A venous blood gas helps determine the metabolic status of the patient, provides information on tissue perfusion and ventilatory status in many patients, and ideally should be performed on all ill or injured patients. The PCO_2 value in the patient with significant perfusion abnormalities will reflect the degree of hypoperfusion. In this situation an arterial blood gas is required to assess the ventilatory status.

Coagulation parameters such as a prothrombin time (PT), activated partial thromboplastin time (aPTT) or activated clotting time (ACT), and a platelet estimate are highly recommended in critical patients. A buccal mucosal bleeding time should be performed if the breed is predisposed to von Willebrand's disease or there are any concerns about platelet function.

Thoracic radiographs are indicated in patients with a history of trauma, those with cardiorespiratory disease, and those scheduled for surgery for possible neoplasia.

> **TECHNICIAN NOTE** Critical patients can decompensate when placed into dorsal recumbency and a ventrodorsal view should not be taken if this is a concern.

A lead II electrocardiogram should ideally be assessed before anesthesia in all critical patients but especially if there is any evidence of cardiac disease or splenic disease. The presence of tall T waves (taller than one fourth the R wave amplitude) is often indicative of

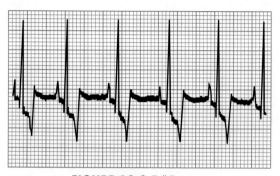

FIGURE 10-2 Tall T waves.

myocardial hypoxia (Figure 10-2). Ventricular premature complexes (VPCs) may be associated with primary cardiac disease but are also associated with splenic disease. Arrhythmias that are impacting perfusion should be treated before induction of anesthesia.

A minimum of one large-bore peripheral catheter should be placed in every anesthetized patient in case rapid volume infusion is required. Two large-bore catheters should be placed in more critical patients. A second catheter should be considered in animals with poor veins, short limbs, or other anatomic abnormalities, such as those seen in chondrodystrophic breeds, in case the primary catheter becomes nonfunctional under anesthesia.

A central line should be placed in all patients in which central venous pressure (CVP) monitoring is indicated to estimate venous volume or preload. Central lines also are useful in patients requiring infusions of hyperosmolar fluids or blood sampling intraoperatively.

An indwelling arterial catheter for direct BP monitoring and arterial blood gas determination is ideal in any critical patient.

PREANESTHETIC STABILIZATION

Every attempt should be made to stabilize the patient before anesthesia; however, in some situations anesthetizing the patient may play a role in stabilization. Patients who need O_2 should be provided with it; those with severe pulmonary edema may need diuretics. Bilateral thoracentesis usually is necessary in patients with air or fluid in the pleural space. A chest tube should be inserted in all patients with a pneumothorax when a thoracotomy is not being performed since **positive pressure ventilation** may exacerbate a pneumothorax. BP should be normalized if possible (unless hypotensive resuscitation is being performed). Venous volume should be adequate. It should be kept in mind that crystalloids are interstitial rehydrators, not intravascular volume expanders.

> **TECHNICIAN NOTE** In addition, crystalloids and synthetic colloids will dilute hemoglobin and clotting factors if given in excessive quantities. This should be avoided through the use of smaller volume resuscitation and judicious use of fresh frozen plasma or fresh whole blood.

Potentially life-threatening arrhythmias should be controlled. Body temperature should be normal, when possible.

All potentially life-threatening laboratory abnormalities should have been corrected, or should be in the process of being corrected. For example, the patient with signs of a coagulopathy should be receiving a fresh frozen plasma transfusion. The transfusion can be continued intraoperatively if the patient is not stable enough to wait for surgery until the transfusion is completed.

PREANESTHETIC PREPAREDNESS

Each patient must have an anesthetic plan. Planning helps the technician anticipate and prevent possible complications. Everything that might be needed for the anesthesia should be gathered and checked beforehand. If O_2 tanks are being used they should be checked to ensure there is an adequate supply for the anticipated length of the anesthesia. The anesthetic vaporizer should contain sufficient inhalant, the carbon dioxide absorber should be functional, the appropriate size breathing circuit and rebreathing bag should be attached, and the machine should be tested for leaks. All hoses should be in good working order. If a mechanical ventilator is being used the ventilator should be attached and parameters set for the individual patient using a test lung.

A laryngoscope with the appropriate size of Miller blade should be available along with three sizes of clear endotracheal tubes. Clear endotracheal tubes are preferred over red ones because they allow for visualization of any secretions (e.g., blood, mucus, and vomitus) that may cause an airway obstruction. In addition, clear tubes are less prone to cracking, are easier to clean, and are more flexible. If the red tubes are placed incorrectly, they may easily cause deviation of the trachea. Cuffed tubes should be placed, because ventilation cannot be effectively provided without a good seal. To help prevent iatrogenic injury to the trachea, high-volume, low-pressure cuffs should be used. The cuffs on the tubes should be checked to ensure there are no leaks. The length of the tube should be evaluated relative to the size of the patient and, if need be, premeasured to ensure it will be inserted to the level of the thoracic inlet.

TECHNICIAN NOTE Clear tubes are often very generous in length, and contribute to deadspace in the anesthesia circuit. These tubes can be cut to more appropriate lengths for the size of the patient by removing the adapter and cutting to the measured length. The cut cannot extend past the entry point for the cuff valve; therefore, it is important to note where the small tube attaches.

All monitors should be connected and working, and the appropriate fittings, adapters, and cuffs, for example, should be attached for the individual patient. Basic equipment should include an esophageal stethoscope, a BP device (preferably a Doppler ultrasonic blood flow detector so that flow and BP can be monitored), an ECG with continuous readout, a pulse oximeter, a capnometer, and a thermometer. If the patient has a chest tube, then a large syringe should be available for aspiration. Towels or blankets, warm-water circulating blankets, forced-air warmers, and fluid warmers should be available.

Planning should include consideration of patient positioning. For instance, a patient with head trauma should not be positioned with the head lower than the heart, and a patient with a diaphragmatic hernia should be positioned with the thorax higher than the abdomen. Full shoulder extension should be avoided when the patient is in dorsal recumbency whenever possible, since this compromises ventilation.

An anesthetic sheet should be used for all patients. All parameters on the monitoring sheet should be completed including vital signs, body weight, and relevant laboratory results. Standard drugs to be given in case of emergency should be available with the drug dose in milligrams, as well as the volume needed for the particular patient recorded. During an emergency, no time is available to perform these calculations. Doses should be printed or recorded on the back of the anesthetic sheet along with additional doses of induction drugs and analgesics in case the animal's plane of anesthesia needs to be adjusted. All premedication and induction drugs should be prepared. If the patient might need a constant rate infusion, such as a dopamine infusion, then it is much better to prepare the infusion in advance. Consideration should be given to the types of fluids that will need to be administered intraoperatively and fluids should be formulated, ready to be attached to the pa-

BOX 10-1	Technical Tip: Setting Up for Anesthesia

Preparing the Anesthetic Machine
Ensure sufficient oxygen (O_2) for the duration of the anesthesia with 2-4 hours additional
Ensure vaporizer filled with inhalant
Ensure carbon dioxide (CO_2) absorption granules do not need to be changed
Check all hoses for cleanliness and cracks
Ensure two sizes of rebreathing bag present
Check machine for leaks
Ensure anesthetic ventilator (if available) set up for individual to be anesthetized

Induction
Anesthetic plan
Clear, cuffed endotracheal tubes with ties and cuff-inflating syringe
Laryngoscope and appropriate-sized blade
Premedication drug(s), doses, and volumes calculated
Induction protocol doses and volumes calculated
Emergency drug doses and volumes calculated
IV fluid type and rate
Patient positioning

Monitoring Equipment
Esophageal stethoscope
Indirect BP monitor (Doppler, oscillometric) with appropriate size cuff
Capnometer
ECG with printout capability
Pulse oximeter
Thermometer

Miscellaneous Supplies
Warming blanket
Fluid and syringe pumps

---

tient. Because many of these patients require delivery of fluid volumes at precise rates, fluid pumps should be available and programmed for the appropriate fluid rates. Syringes, needles, and all medications should be present (Box 10-1).

SETTING UP FOR MAJOR SURGERY

The operating room should be kept in a constant state of readiness. Surgical packs, gowns, and gloves should be available. A warm-air or warm-water circulating blanket (or other safe, active-warming device) should be on the surgical table. The ground plate for the electrocautery device should be in place and the electrocautery unit attached. A suction canister should be in place, with a spare available. Portable suction units should be plugged into the electrical supply.

> **TECHNICIAN NOTE** Time under anesthesia must be minimized. Clipping should be done as much as possible immediately before induction of anesthesia.

Some patients with a severe hemoabdomen may be close to exsanguination, which means preparation may be limited to clipping the area of the incision followed by a quick wipe with the surgical scrub before draping. Surgeons should be gowned and gloved and instrument packs opened before induction (which should be performed in the operating room). This will allow the surgeon to enter the abdomen immediately and gain control of the hemorrhage.

DRUGS

Critically ill or injured patients will respond to analgesics, sedatives, and anesthetics differently than healthy animals for a variety of reasons (e.g., decreased volume of distribution; decreased plasma protein levels; acidosis leading to higher concentrations of the active form of the drug; decreased metabolism secondary to decreased hepatic function and hypothermia). For these reasons, doses of most anxiolytics, analgesics, and anesthetics should be reduced to 25% to 50% of normal and titrated to effect.

> **TECHNICIAN NOTE** Ideally all drugs should be given via the intravenous (IV) route, because absorption from the oral and subcutaneous (subcut) routes is unpredictable.

Intramuscular (IM) injections can also have variable uptake in patients with altered perfusion and should be given in the epaxial muscles (the muscles dorsal and lateral to the vertebrae in the region of the thoracolumbar spine), because the blood flow is more sustained to these muscles even during lower flow states. The intraosseous route of drug administration can be effective in very small patients, birds, and exotic animals.

- Be prepared with equipment, O_2, anesthetic drugs, emergency drugs, knowledge, skills, and support.
- Drugs and doses should be chosen based on the patient's age, condition, and surgery needed.
- Preemptive sedation and analgesia should be used when possible to prevent windup and to decrease the dose of induction drugs.
- Medication should always be titrated to effect.
- Rapid induction is always indicated.
- Local or regional anesthesia should be used when appropriate.
- Patients with airway or respiratory compromise should be preoxygenated.
- All patients under general anesthesia will hypoventilate and need ventilatory support.
- Monitoring is essential to prevent complications (observe, record, report, act).
- The anesthesia does not end when the surgery ends. Preoperative support must continue through the postoperative period.
- All patients need physiologic support to prevent secondary decompensation of various body systems (including the pulmonary, cardiovascular, renal, and gastrointestinal systems).

BALANCED ANESTHESIA

Balanced anesthesia involves the delivery of specific drugs for analgesia or amelioration of pain, sedation, amnesia, and muscle relaxation. Because critically ill or injured patients often need to be taken to surgery in the face of an unstable respiratory or cardiovascular system, the use of balanced anesthetic techniques becomes vital. To provide balanced anesthesia the technician must be familiar with many different drugs and their effects in the patient with altered metabolism or organ function. The critically ill animal may have no remaining reserves, so it is essential the patient receive only enough drug to achieve the analgesia and anesthesia necessary to complete the surgery.

GOALS OF ANESTHESIA

The two primary goals of anesthesia are to eliminate pain and ensure amnesia. All patients should be managed with these two goals in mind. The third goal is immobilization. Other general principles for ensuring the anesthesia is as safe as possible are outlined in Box 10-2.

ANALGESICS, LOCAL ANESTHETICS, AND PREANESTHETIC AGENTS

ANALGESIA

One of the main goals of anesthesia is to eliminate pain. Pain has detrimental effects on cardiopulmonary function, metabolism, endocrine status, and immune function. This can lead to serious physiologic effects (e.g., VPCs, hypoxia, muscle weakness, delayed tissue healing), affect the patient's well-being, and even lead to death (Anand and Hickey, 1992).

Analgesia is vital in the surgical patient because every surgical procedure causes pain. No patient is so sick that pain relief cannot be provided. Medication should be given preoperatively to prevent windup and continued intraoperatively and postoperatively. Drugs should be given on an "as needed" basis rather than on a schedule per se. Analgesia often needs to be administered intraoperatively. If the patient is responding to surgical stimuli and is deemed to perceive pain, then analgesics should be provided. Increasing the dose of an inhalant or infusing additional propofol does nothing for the pain except mask the pain, which can lead to more windup. Also, the additional drugs may worsen hypoventilation, cardiac output, and hypotension.

Whenever opioids are administered, respiration should be closely monitored. Opioids cause respiratory depression. At low doses this problem is rarely a clinically significant issue; however, this effect can be magnified when used in conjunction with inhalant anesthesia (Keating et al, 2013). Ideally, all critical patients under general anesthesia should receive ventilation, in which case respiratory depression will not be a problem. The respiratory depression seen with oxymorphone and fentanyl can be reversed with butorphanol (McCrackin et al, 1994), without decreasing the analgesic effects. Opioids decrease intracranial pressure, but the concurrent respiratory depression may lead to hypercarbia, cerebral vasodilation, and secondary intracranial hypertension. If opioids are to be used when a change in intracranial pressure is a concern, then capnometry should be closely monitored and positive pressure ventilation instituted as indicated to control the PCO_2. Opioids and inhalant anesthetics routinely are used together; however, their effects are synergistic, and the combination may lead to significant decreases in heart rate and BP. The doses of the opioid and the inhalant anesthetic must be decreased to avoid these complications. The liver metabolizes opioids, and a decrease in liver function may prolong their effect.

The choice of opioid used depends on availability and familiarity with the drug. Buprenorphine probably is the only opioid not frequently indicated in the critical patient, because it has a longer onset and duration of action, limited analgesic properties, and a high affinity for mu receptors, making it difficult to control more severe pain if the buprenorphine dose is not adequate. Butorphanol is a short-acting analgesic that clinically is most effective for treating mild soft tissue pain. It has minimal sedative and respiratory depressant effects. Because of these characteristics it is very useful in very critical patients or in patients that have not been fully cardiovascularly resuscitated. It can also be titrated effectively intraoperatively with minimal cardiorespiratory effects; however, it has a short duration of action (sometimes as short as 20 minutes) and clinically it is not as effective as other opioids, so it is less useful for treating significant soft tissue pain and musculoskeletal pain. Intermediate-acting opioids such as hydromorphone or oxymorphone are useful in patients with moderate pain. Methadone is also an extremely effective intermediate-acting opioid in dogs and cats (Warne et al, 2013). In patients with significant pain or in patients that are very critical and not tolerant of standard doses of general anesthesia, fentanyl is the best choice. Fentanyl can be given by intermittent bolus injections, but because of its short duration of effect it is best given as a constant rate infusion (CRI).

Constant rate infusions of low-dose ketamine given to effect in combination with lidocaine and an opioid provide another option for analgesia in painful patients.

Nonsteroidal antiinflammatory drugs, even the COX-2–specific drugs, are generally contraindicated in patients with hypotension or decreased tissue perfusion, those with gastrointestinal or renal disease or dysfunction, and those with thrombocytopenia or platelet dysfunction. This precludes their use in most critical patients.

LOCAL OR REGIONAL ANESTHESIA

Infiltration of nerve endings using local anesthesia is a very effective way of providing analgesia (Lukasik, 1993). Because the systemic effects of drugs used to produce local or regional anesthesia are minimal, these are relatively safe techniques to use in the compromised patient. Local or regional anesthesia can be used in combination with sedation, systemic analgesia, and anxiolysis (i.e., relief of anxiety). In the severely debilitated patient, local anesthetics in combination with systemic analgesics and sedation may be sufficient to perform the necessary surgery.

Lidocaine and bupivacaine typically are used for local, regional, or epidural anesthesia. Lidocaine can be placed directly onto the wound surface and into the skin edges to help decrease the pain associated with debridement, flushing, and suturing. Infiltration of surgical incisions with bupivacaine or lidocaine as a line block (preoperatively or postoperatively) helps to decrease the pain associated with the incision. These medications can also be infused as regional blocks, as intraarticular injections, or intrapleurally.

Local anesthetic agents also can be used intravenously at low-dose constant rate infusions to provide additional analgesia (Ortega and Cruz, 2011). It may help decrease arrhythmias and decrease the gag or cough response to intubation. Giving lidocaine also allows for a decrease in the doses of other induction agents, and it is particularly useful in patients with preexisting VPCs or in patients with possible elevated intracranial pressure. Patients receiving intravenous doses or higher doses of local anesthetic agents should be monitored closely for hypotension.

Local anesthetics are very acidic drugs and cause irritation when injected locally. This effect can be lessened by warming the solution to body temperature (Mader et al, 1994) or by adding sodium bicarbonate into the syringe with lidocaine (10% sodium bicarbonate by volume). Bupivacaine is less tolerant of alkalinization and addition of only 0.005% sodium bicarbonate by volume (0.1 ml of sodium bicarbonate in 20 ml of bupivacaine) has been recommended before precipitation occurs. Alkalinization of the local anesthetic should occur immediately before injection, because precipitation will occur with storage. If a large volume of local anesthetic is required, then it can be diluted by 50% with any fluid that has an acidic or neutral pH. By combining lidocaine and bupivacaine, the patient will benefit from the rapid onset of action of lidocaine and the long duration of effect of bupivacaine.

EPIDURAL ANALGESIA AND ANESTHESIA

Drugs administered into the epidural space can provide effective analgesia and anesthesia (Hendrix et al, 1996). When epidural analgesia is given preoperatively, there is a significant decrease in the amount of analgesia required postoperatively. Epidural anesthesia significantly lowers the requirement and may even eliminate the need for inhalant anesthesia in unstable patients. Local anesthetics such as lidocaine and bupivacaine in combination with morphine, oxymorphone, or hydromorphone typically are used for delivering epidural anesthesia (Table 10-1). Onset of action is approximately 30 to 60 minutes, and duration of effect is from 6 to 24 hours.

Placement of an epidural catheter permits supplemental dosing intraoperatively and postoperatively for anesthesia and analgesia of the thorax, abdomen, or pelvic limbs. It is easier to administer high epidural analgesia more accurately if a catheter is placed.

Potential complications of epidural anesthesia include hypotension from sympathetic blockade, respiratory depression, motor paralysis, hypothermia, urinary retention, and infections. The higher the epidural is placed, the greater the likelihood of respiratory depression and hypotension.

PREMEDICATION

Premedication involves administration of some combination of tranquilizers, sedatives, hypnotics, analgesics, and anticholinergic drugs. It decreases the doses needed for induction and maintenance anesthesia and helps ensure a smoother recovery. Many of these drugs may not be indicated in or tolerated by the critical patient; however, opioids can be used safely even in fragile patients.

Anticholinergic drugs include atropine and glycopyrrolate (see Table 10-1); these drugs are effective at reversing bradycardia secondary to increased vagal tone, decreasing airway secretions, and causing airway

TABLE 10-1	Anesthetic Drugs	
DRUG	**BOLUS DOSE***	**CONSTANT RATE INFUSION (CRI)**
Anticholinergics		
Atropine	0.02-0.04 mg/kg	
Glycopyrrolate	0.01-0.02 mg/kg	
Analgesia		
Buprenorphine	0.01-0.03 mg/kg	
Butorphanol	0.1-0.4 mg/kg	0.1-0.2 mg/kg/hr
Fentanyl	2-6 mcg/kg	2-10 mcg/kg/hr
Hydromorphone	0.05-0.1 mg/kg	0.03 mg/kg/hr
Methadone	0.1-0.4 mg/kg	
Morphine	0.1-1 mg/kg	0.05-0.1 mg/kg/hr
Oxymorphone	0.05-0.2 mg/kg	
Benzodiazepine		
Diazepam	0.1-0.5 mg/kg	
Midazolam	0.1-0.5 mg/kg	
Induction		
Alfaxalone	2 mg/kg	
Etomidate	0.5-2 mg/kg	
Ketamine	5-10 mg/kg	
Propofol	3-6 mg/kg	
Neuromuscular Blockers		
Atracurium	0.2 mg/kg load; 0.1 mg/kg redose	0.1-0.3 mg/kg/hr
Pancuronium	0.04-0.11 mg/kg	0.04 mg/kg/hr
Succinylcholine	0.22-0.44 mg/kg	0.2 mg/kg/hr

Continued

TABLE 10-1	Anesthetic Drugs—cont'd	
DRUG	**BOLUS DOSE***	**CONSTANT RATE INFUSION (CRI)**
Neuromuscular Blocker Reversal		
Atropine with edrophonium	0.01-0.02 mg/kg followed by 0.5 mg/kg IV	
Atropine with neostigmine	0.04 mg/kg followed by 0.06 mg/kg IV	
Local Anesthesia *Epidural*	If spinal or CSF decrease dose by 50%; 1 ml/10 kg to max volume of 6 ml	
Hydromorphone	0.1 mg/kg	
Morphine	0.1 mg/kg	
Oxymorphone	0.1 mg/kg	
Bupivacaine	2 mg/kg 0.5% solution (1 ml/4.5 kg)	
Lidocaine	2-4 mg/kg 2% solution (1 ml/4.5 kg)	
Intercostal Bupivacaine	2 mg/kg 0.5% solution; 0.5 ml/nerve	
Intrapleural Bupivacaine	1.5-2.0 mg/kg diluted to 1 ml/kg q6h	
Local Lidocaine	0.5-2.0 mg/kg to max 6 mg/kg with bicarbonate 1 ml per 10 ml of lidocaine	

*Doses may need to be decreased to 25-50% of standard dose in very critical patients.

dilation; however, the resulting increase in heart rate increases the myocardial O_2 demands. The increased myocardial O_2 demands may cause myocardial hypoxia and malignant arrhythmias, and anticholinergic drugs should not be given routinely to critical patients. Exceptions include those animals with high resting vagal tone when it is anticipated that surgical manipulation will lead to increased vagal tone, as well as those with significant bradycardia, significant liquid airway secretions, or increased salivation (cats being more predisposed than dogs to this side effect). If in doubt, then it is always better to administer the anticholinergic once the effects of the other administered drugs are known.

Phenothiazines, such as acepromazine, are generally indicated in critically ill or injured patients because of their vasodilatory and hypotensive side effects. These side effects can be a significant problem when normal or high doses are administered, and even low doses can cause a significant problem if the patient is not hemodynamically stable.

INDUCTION

Rapid induction to gain control of the airway always should be performed in all patients unless the animal is so fractious that rapid induction protocols are not feasible (see Table 10-1).

> *TECHNICIAN NOTE*   In the critical patient, mask or tank inductions should be avoided at all costs since struggling can increase metabolic oxygen requirements, patients may further injure themselves, and hypoxia and hypercarbia during the induction process may cause serious complications.

A laryngoscope should be used to ensure accurate intubation and to avoid laryngeal stimulation, which can increase vagal input. Once the patient is intubated the lungs should be auscultated bilaterally to ensure good breath sounds can be auscultated in all fields. The tube length should be checked; it should measure to approximately the thoracic inlet. Tubes that are inserted too far may occlude the right mainstem bronchus.

Neuroleptanalgesia implies a tranquil, dissociative, analgesic state produced by the synergism between an opioid and a tranquilizer, usually a benzodiazepine. The combination of the two drugs allows lower doses of each drug to be administered. Neuroleptanalgesia may provide anesthesia in the severely debilitated patient. In less debilitated patients, doses of inhalants can be reduced significantly. Awake intubation, or insertion of an orotracheal tube in the patient that is not unconscious, often can be performed with these combinations.

The two primary benzodiazepines used in veterinary medicine are diazepam and midazolam. Midazolam is a water-soluble benzodiazepine with similar effects to diazepam but a more consistent level of sedation and a longer half-life. Subjectively there appear to be fewer dysphoric effects with midazolam than with diazepam. This class of drug is very safe to use in most patients; caution should be exercised when using it in patients with significant liver dysfunction.

ALFAXALONE

Alfaxalone, a progesterone analog, is a synthetic neuroactive steroid that has been on the market in different forms for 45 years. It is a general anesthetic that provides excellent muscle relaxation. It has similar properties to propofol and should be used with the same caution in critical patients (Taboada and Murison, 2010). It provides rapid induction, can be used for maintenance of general anesthesia, and is associated with a rapid, smooth recovery. Some excitement has been reported on recovery, especially in cats, a side effect that seems to be absent in patients that have been premedicated. Like propofol, it does have dose-dependent respiratory depressant effects and apnea may occur postinduction, especially with rapid infusion. It also has dose-dependent cardiovascular side effects including tachycardia but the drug appears to have a wider safety margin than that for propofol (Rodriguez et al, 2012). Alfaxalone does not appear to have any analgesic properties. Heinz body formation, which can be seen with repeat dosing of propofol in cats, has not been noted with repeat dosing of alfaxalone. It is not irritating to tissues if given intramuscularly; however, because of the high volume of drug required, this route is not recommended.

DEXMEDETOMIDINE

Alpha$_2$ agonists such as xylazine, medetomidine, and dexmedetomidine are usually contraindicated in critical patients (Murrell and Hellebrekers, 2005). They cause peripheral vasoconstriction, which can lead to difficulties in monitoring blood pressure. In addition, the mucous membranes often turn cyanotic. A decrease in heart rate of up to 50% of baseline is not uncommon, and these drugs can cause atrioventricular block and ventricular premature contractions (VPCs). Dexmedetomidine can be very useful at low doses in the patient experiencing a dysphoric or painful recovery when an opioid is not sufficient; however, even at very low doses the cardiovascular effects can be significant.

ETOMIDATE

Etomidate is an imidazole derivative that is classified as a nonbarbiturate, nonnarcotic, sedative-hypnotic agent. It has poor analgesic qualities, and opioids or other means of providing analgesia should be administered if etomidate is being used. It causes mild respiratory depression but minimal change in cardiopulmonary function even in hypovolemic dogs (Sams et al, 2008). It does have mild negative inotropic effects, but they are not significant, making it a very useful drug in patients with severe cardiovascular instability. Vomiting, excitement, tremors, and apnea may be seen on induction. The neurologic signs are thought to be the result of disinhibition of subcortical neural activity and are not seizures. Etomidate decreases cerebral blood flow and metabolic O_2 requirements similar to barbiturates and can be used in patients with intracranial disease. Etomidate causes cortisol suppression for up to 6 hours after a single injection. This is of unknown significance but may be a concern in the critically ill or injured patient. Even though etomidate is metabolized in the liver, liver disease does not seem to affect its metabolism.

KETAMINE AND BENZODIAZEPINE

Ketamine in combination with a benzodiazepine such as diazepam or midazolam makes an excellent combination for induction of anesthesia in critical patients. Ketamine is a dissociative anesthetic that has good musculoskeletal analgesic properties, weak visceral analgesic qualities, and poor muscle relaxant properties. It exerts a positive inotropic effect on the myocardium and increases cardiac output, BP, pulmonary artery pressure, and CVP. For these reasons it may be contraindicated in patients with elevated left atrial pressures or pulmonary hypertension and it should be avoided in cats with hypertrophic cardiomyopathy. Because it increases myocardial O_2 demands, ketamine should be used with caution in patients with significant myocardial dysfunction. The cardiovascular effects can be prevented or diminished by concurrently administering a sedative such as a benzodiazepine.

> **TECHNICIAN NOTE** Ketamine may cause seizures, an increase in cerebral metabolic rate, an increase in intracranial pressure, and a decrease in cerebral perfusion pressure; therefore, ketamine should be used with caution in patients with intracranial disease or head trauma.

Nystagmus is common, so it is a poor choice for patients requiring ocular surgery. Ketamine increases airway secretions, and anticholinergic drugs may be indicated, especially in the cat. Intranasal ketamine and midazolam has been shown to be equally effective to intramuscular (IM) injections in inducing anesthesia in cats (Marjani et al, 2014).

PROPOFOL

Propofol is an alkylphenol classified as a nonbarbiturate, nonnarcotic, sedative-hypnotic that has poor analgesic qualities. Its advantages lie in rapid induction and recovery with no cumulative effects even after multiple doses. Disadvantages include a high rate of apnea (seen on induction) and systemic hypotension (Ilkiw et al, 1992). The hypotension is secondary to a decrease in myocardial contractility, as well as both vasodilation and venodilation. This effect is of greater significance in hypovolemic patients and propofol should be used with caution, and at low doses, in hemodynamically unstable patients. VPCs may be seen, and hypothermia is common. Tremors and opisthotonus, which may be seen, are thought to be the result of disinhibition of neural activity and are not seizures. Propofol is a good choice in patients with intracranial disease as long as they are not hypotensive, because it decreases cerebral metabolic O_2 requirements. This drug is metabolized extensively in the liver, but its effects do not appear to be prolonged in patients with significant liver dysfunction. Administration of a benzodiazepine immediately before propofol significantly decreases the dose of propofol required for induction, thus minimizing the side effects. A slow infusion of propofol over 1 to 2 minutes will also decrease the side effects.

INHALANTS

Inhalant anesthetics most commonly used include isoflurane and sevoflurane. Both inhalants cause significant dose-dependent decreases in BP and cardiac output, which could be life threatening in the critical patient (Abed et al, 2014). This is related to a combination of negative inotropic effects and vasodilatory properties because of the calcium channel–blocking effects. Injectable anesthesia is recommended when hypotension develops. Although it causes similar cardiovascular effects to isoflurane, sevoflurane sensitizes the myocardium less to the arrhythmogenic effects of catecholamines, and recovery is more rapid. Unlike sevoflurane, isoflurane is an airway irritant and has the potential to cause airway spasm. Both inhalants cause dose-related respiratory depression (centrally and as a result of direct effects on the diaphragm). Neither inhalant has any analgesic qualities, but they do provide some muscle relaxation.

NEUROMUSCULAR BLOCKING AGENTS

Neuromuscular blocking agents are very useful in the critically ill or injured patient; they help gain airway control without inducing gagging, coughing, or laryngospasm. These agents do not affect the cardiovascular system; thus the patient remains more stable under anesthesia. Good muscle relaxation is provided, which increases chest compliance and allows for more effective ventilation with lower peak inspiratory pressures (PIPs). The muscle relaxation is useful during reduction of a luxation and when treating fractures. Neuromuscular blockers do not cause any central nervous system depression.

The patient is paralyzed but aware and must receive both analgesics and sedatives or dissociative agents; however, because movement is eliminated, doses of other drugs are decreased. Since the animal is paralyzed, positive pressure ventilatory support is required. Two classes of **neuromuscular blockers** exist: (1) depolarizing and (2) nondepolarizing.

DEPOLARIZING MUSCLE BLOCKING AGENTS

Depolarizing agents act like acetylcholine at the neuromuscular junction, causing the muscle to contract. The effect is longer than that for acetylcholine, which leads to persistent contraction (muscle paralysis). Depolarizing agents are broken down by plasma cholinesterase. No antagonists are available for these drugs (see Table 10-1).

Succinylcholine is the most commonly used drug in this class. It has a rapid onset of action (within 30 to 60 seconds) and rapid recovery (within 5 to 20 minutes). Muscle fasciculations may be seen as the membranes depolarize, which can cause a transient increase in potassium levels of 0.5 to 1 mEq/L. Succinylcholine is an effective drug to use if rapid airway control is required, because of its rapid onset of action, however, it should be used with caution in patients with renal disease, severe liver dysfunction, myopathy, penetrating eye injury, or chronic debilitating disease. Succinylcholine is not recommended in patients with increased intraabdominal or increased intrathoracic pressures (e.g., tension pneumothorax, gastric dilation volvulus). Hypokalemia and hypothermia will prolong the effects of succinylcholine. Succinylcholine may cause malignant hyperthermia.

NONDEPOLARIZING NEUROMUSCULAR BLOCKING AGENTS

Nondepolarizing neuromuscular blocking agents bind to acetylcholine receptor sites at the muscle end plate, thus preventing acetylcholine from binding with the receptor sites. This prevents muscle contraction and causes a flaccid paralysis. Nondepolarizing drugs are not metabolized by cholinesterase, but anticholinesterase drugs such as edrophonium or neostigmine can antagonize them. An anticholinergic is usually administered concurrently with the reversal drug, because they may cause parasympathetic side effects such as bradycardia, salivation, miosis, and increased gastrointestinal motility. Reversal will be effective only if at least some muscle function has returned.

Atracurium is the most common nondepolarizing neuromuscular blocker used. It has a slightly longer onset of action than succinylcholine. Atracurium may not be the best first choice if rapid airway control is being attempted using just the neuromuscular blocker, because a period of time will occur when the patient cannot breathe properly but is not yet paralyzed sufficiently for intubation.

> **TECHNICIAN NOTE** A patient should never be allowed to struggle to breathe.

Atracurium is degraded by Hofmann elimination, which is spontaneous degradation that is not dependent on hepatic metabolism or renal excretion; however, its effects will be prolonged by acidosis and hypothermia.

Atracurium has an onset of action of as short as 1 minute to as long as 5 minutes and duration of effect of 20 to 45 minutes. A loading dose can be followed by repeat IV doses (using 40% of the initial dose) or a CRI. At high levels, atracurium may cause histamine release.

MONITORING WITH NEUROMUSCULAR BLOCKING AGENTS

Peripheral nerve stimulators using a train of four should be used to monitor neuromuscular blockade if available. The stimulator can be attached to the facial or ulnar nerve. If a peripheral nerve stimulator is not available, then it will be impossible to assess the depth of the block until muscle function starts to return. The patient must be artificially ventilated until good ventilatory function returns, and the patient should never be extubated until it is able to sit up. It is more difficult to monitor patients under anesthesia with neuromuscular blockade, because the normal neuromuscular reflexes are abolished. Lacrimation, salivation, slight muscle movement of the limbs or face, curling of the tip of the tongue, increased resistance to ventilation, and increased BP may be indicators that the patient is aware of its surroundings or is in pain.

> **TECHNICIAN NOTE** One of the best guides to general anesthetic depth when a neuromuscular blocker is not being used is jaw tone; it should always be present to some extent.

INTUBATION

All critical patients should be preoxygenated before induction by placing a mask over the patient's face or simply by placing a tube from an O_2 source in front of the patient's face (i.e., flow-by). The tube should be placed into the patient's mouth if it is gasping or panting. High flow rates should be used.

All patients should be intubated with the largest endotracheal tube that fits comfortably in the trachea. The anesthetist should feel comfortable intubating a patient in lateral, dorsal, and sternal recumbency. Intubating the patient in dorsal recumbency allows insertion of a tube ½ to 1 mm larger than would be placed with the patient in sternal recumbency, and it allows the patient to be intubated unassisted. To avoid aspiration, the patient should not be intubated in dorsal recumbency if the stomach is distended.

Cuffed endotracheal tubes should be placed in all patients because ventilation cannot be provided effectively without a good seal. The cuff should be inflated to provide a seal at 15 to 20 cm water pressure to a maximum of 30 cm water pressure in order to prevent damage to the trachea. If there is any concern about tracheal disease, then the cuff should be inflated to provide a seal at 10 to 12 cm water pressure. Overinflation of the cuff may lead to mucosal injury and ischemia and in the cat can lead to tracheal disruption by tearing of the trachealis dorsalis muscle (Hardie et al, 1999). Whenever the patient is turned, the endotracheal tube should be disconnected from the anesthetic machine to avoid applying torque to the tube, which may cause trauma to the trachea.

A laryngoscope should be used in all patients, and topical lidocaine (0.2 ml of 2% lidocaine per 5-kg body weight) should be used on the arytenoid cartilages if laryngospasm, gagging, or coughing on induction is undesirable. If topical lidocaine is used, then the anesthetist should wait at least 10 to 30 seconds before intubating. Atraumatic intubation is extremely important in the hypoxemic patient because stimulation of the larynx can invoke a vagally mediated bradycardia and potentially lead to vagal arrest. In the severely hypotensive patient the head should not be raised during intubation because this may decrease cerebral blood flow to the point of causing cardiorespiratory arrest. In this situation, the patient should be intubated in dorsal or lateral recumbency. If a stylet is used, care should be taken to ensure the tip does not protrude past the end of the endotracheal tube (it can cause damage to the trachea).

Once the patient is intubated and the tube is secured, the lungs should be auscultated bilaterally. Doing this allows the anesthetist to confirm that the tube is in the trachea, not the esophagus, and that the tip of the tube has not been inserted into a mainstem bronchus.

INTUBATING A PATIENT WITH A POSSIBLE AIRWAY DISRUPTION

Intubating a patient with a possible airway disruption is more complex than regular intubation. Cervical bite wounds and hanging type injuries may create a tear in the cervical trachea. Cats that have a possible trachealis

dorsalis muscle tear secondary to an overinflated endotracheal tube cuff may have a tear that starts at the midcervical or distal cervical region and ends at the bronchial bifurcation. In these patients the tube should be passed more distally than it normally would (generally to the level of the bronchial bifurcation). Artificial ventilation of this patient should be avoided until the tear is located and it is confirmed that the tube projects past the injury. If the patient must be ventilated, then it should be closely monitored for signs of a developing tension pneumomediastinum. Clinical signs include loss of Doppler blood flow sounds, hypotension, increasing difficulty in ventilation, and worsening subcutaneous emphysema.

INTUBATING A PATIENT WITH UPPER AIRWAY SWELLING OR OBSTRUCTION

Patients can present with upper airway obstructive problems secondary to trauma, neoplasia, anticoagulant rodenticide toxicities, and foreign bodies.

> **TECHNICIAN NOTE** If there is any concern that the airway will not be able to be orotracheally intubated then consideration should be given to clipping and preparing the ventral cervical region in the event a tracheostomy is required and in more severe cases an awake tracheostomy should be performed under local anesthesia (and sedation, if required) before induction.

If considerable edema exists, as in the case of the bulldog with possible laryngeal paralysis, then a single dose of fast-acting corticosteroid may help alleviate some of the swelling.

MAINTAINING A PATIENT UNDER GENERAL ANESTHESIA

Critical patients should be maintained on 100% O_2 and controlled ventilation. Metabolic O_2 requirements are approximately 5 ml/kg/min in healthy patients; however, because of the potential for leaks in the anesthetic circuit as well as a higher demand for O_2 in critical patients low-flow anesthesia should not be less than 200 to 500 ml/min. Low-flow anesthesia is ideal for the critical patient, because less moisture is lost from the airways; and because O_2 flow rates are low, less heat loss occurs.

Critically ill or injured patients under anesthesia often need modifications in their anesthetic protocols and fluid rates because they are unstable. Many of these patients will develop severe hypotension with inspired concentrations of inhalant anesthesia commonly used in healthy patients; therefore, injectable drugs are often needed intraoperatively. When patients appear to be responding to surgical stimulation, they may be perceiving pain, and analgesics should be used judiciously throughout the surgical procedure. This will allow the anesthetist to significantly lower the amount of other anesthetic agents being used. Most opioids will need to be redosed every 15 to 20 minutes. If benzodiazepines are being used, it may be necessary to redose these drugs every 15 to 20 minutes as well. In most cases subsequent doses of all drugs should be given at increasing intervals and lower amounts (usually starting at one fourth of the induction dose), because hypothermia and acidosis prolong their effects.

CONTROLLED VENTILATION

All anesthetic agents are ventilatory depressants, so ventilatory support is essential in the critical patient. This is most simply done using a mechanical ventilator (Figure 10-3); but in the absence of a ventilator, "hand-bagging" can be performed. In general, tidal volumes of 10 to 12 ml/kg (lean body weight) and a rate of 10 to 15

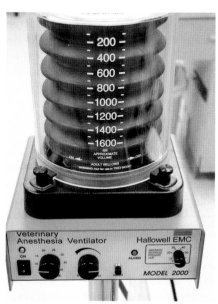

FIGURE 10-3 Hallowell 2000 ventilator.

breaths/minute should be used as starting points. PIPs should be kept below 15 cm of water whenever possible to avoid barotrauma. Tidal volumes as high as 20 ml/kg and PIPs as high as 25 cm of water may be needed. Tidal volumes are adjusted based on observation of chest movement during ventilation, lung auscultation, capnometry, blood gases if available, and BP. To avoid complications, the lowest volumes and pressures the patient will tolerate should be used.

Ventilator parameters must be adjusted according to the patient's condition. For example, patients with less compliant lungs or masses pushing on the diaphragm may require higher tidal volumes and PIPs than patients with compliant chest walls. In addition, the tubing from the anesthetic machine to the patient will absorb some of the pressure from the ventilator. If a lot of tubing is used or the tubing is compliant, then higher than expected tidal volumes and pressures may need to be used in smaller patients. The tubing becomes less of a factor in larger patients. If higher-frequency ventilation is being used, then tidal volumes can be decreased. Overventilation can lead to a decrease in preload and a secondary decrease in cardiac output and BP. Increased tidal volumes or inspiratory pressures may be needed in patients with a large amount of dead space (i.e., large amount of anesthetic tubing compared with the tidal volume), restrictive pulmonary disease, or impaired diaphragmatic movement (e.g., gastric dilation volvulus, obesity). Increases may also be required in patients restrained in dorsal recumbency with the thoracic limbs in extension, because chest wall movement will be restricted in this position.

A resuscitation bag with a reservoir and 100% O_2 should be used to ventilate the lungs of all patients during transport from the preparation area to the operating room or to radiology.

MONITORING

Monitoring the critical patient under anesthesia is vital in order to minimize morbidity. The ill or injured patient that is undergoing surgery is at risk for serious complications such as airway compromise, respiratory depression, hypercarbia, hypoxemia, arrhythmias, coagulopathy, metabolic acidosis, and even cardiac arrest. Absolute numbers are vitally important, but often the trend of change is an early indicator of whether or not the patient is beginning to decompensate.

> **TECHNICIAN NOTE** Although many pieces of equipment are available to help with monitoring the patient under anesthesia, NOTHING replaces the human being.

Patient parameters should be monitored every 5 minutes (Box 10-3). All parameters should be recorded in a permanent record that forms part of the patient's medical chart.

The anesthetist, the surgeon, and the surgical assistant must work together as a team to treat the critically ill or injured patient. Constant communication must occur among team members. For example, if the anesthetist notices that the lingual pulses do not feel very strong,

---

BOX 10-3	Recommended Monitoring Checklist for Anesthesia of the Critical Patient

Continuous monitoring by devices (numeric values and waveforms):
  Electrocardiogram (ECG), **capnography**, pulse oximetry
  Doppler blood flow (qualitative evaluation by listening to generated sounds)
  Respiratory rate and effort (by impedance), arterial and central venous pressure (CVP) (if available)
Monitoring as often as required and recorded every 5 minutes:
  Respiratory rate, heart rate, blood pressure (BP), oxygen (O_2) saturation, end-tidal carbon dioxide ($ETCO_2$)
  Pulse strength, mucous membrane color, eye position, muscle tone by estimating tone in muscles of mandible
Monitoring as often as required and recorded every 15 minutes:
  Temperature
  Fluids infused (type, rate, and running total of each), estimated blood loss (based on sponges and blood in suction reservoir)
  Urine output if catheter present
  Lung sounds and heart tones
  Stage of operation, manipulations done
Monitoring if intraoperative concerns present or surgery is longer than 2 to 3 hours:
  Packed cell volume (PCV), total solids, venous blood gas, arterial blood gas, glucose, electrolytes, albumin, coagulation parameters

---

then the surgeon should be asked to inspect internal BP (i.e., aortic pulsation). If the surgeon feels that the tissues are starting to look pale, then he or she should ask the anesthetist to check vital signs and perhaps a PCV.

Physical exam parameters provide invaluable information about the status of a patient even if machines are also being used. Respiratory rate, chest excursion, lung auscultation, and mucous membrane color can be used to assess the respiratory and ventilatory status of the patient. Lung auscultation can be performed transthoracically in some patients but an esophageal stethoscope is required in many patients. Esophageal stethoscopes are far more sensitive at detecting abnormal lung and heart sounds and are highly recommended. Pulse oximetry and capnometry also provide information about the respiratory and ventilatory status of the patient. Blood gases should be measured if there are any concerns with pulse oximetry or capnometry measurements. Heart rate, lingual pulse strength, capillary refill time, and jugular distention and filling should be used to assess the cardiovascular status of the patient. Lingual pulses are most effectively palpated just caudal to the rostral aspect of the frenulum. Eye position is not very useful at determining the level of anesthetic depth except when the eyes exhibit an extreme ventral strabismus. In this situation the patient generally is at far too deep a plane of anesthesia. Jaw tone also is a very imprecise method of determining the depth of the patient's anesthesia; however, some degree of jaw tone should ideally always be present. In addition, central venous pressure (or jugular distention and filling), blood pressure, and an electrocardiogram (ECG) should be used to assess the cardiovascular status of the patient. If only one monitor is available, blood pressure Doppler is preferred especially if the patient is small. If an oscillometric device is available, a Doppler is still recommended so that both the anesthetist and the surgeon can easily keep track of flow sounds and heart rates. Changes in either provide an instantaneous signal of an alteration in the status of the patient. If a urinary catheter is in place, urine production should be a minimum of 1 ml/kg/hour. If a urinary catheter is not present and abdominal surgery is being performed, the surgeon should be asked to monitor the urinary bladder for signs of urine production. This helps confirm adequate renal perfusion. Similarly, the gut can be subjectively evaluated during abdominal surgery. The intestine should be pink and moist, vessels should be easily visible, and pulsation should be easily detectable. Temperature monitoring is extremely important and should be assessed approximately every 15 minutes, or many multiparameter monitors have temperature probes that may be placed esophageally, or rectally, for continuous temperature monitoring. Fluid rates and volumes should be recorded a minimum of every 15 minutes.

BLOOD PRESSURE

Although blood pressure ideally is measured directly, in most hospitals indirect methods are used. Direct BP measurement is the gold standard but can be technically difficult in many patients. Normal values range from approximately 120 to 140 mm Hg systolic and 75 to 95 mm Hg diastolic. Systolic BP should be maintained higher than 100 mm Hg and mean arterial BP should be kept greater than 65 mm Hg to ensure adequate renal and splanchnic perfusion. Pulse palpation can be used as a crude assessment of BP but can be extremely inaccurate. Pulses of small animals, animals that are shaking or shivering, animals with significant vasoconstriction, or those that are obese can be difficult to palpate. When an artery is being palpated it is the pulse pressure that is being detected. This is the difference between the systolic and diastolic BP. Thus, a BP of 100/60 mm Hg may palpate the same as one of 150/110 mm Hg; however, each of these measurements would be treated very differently.

Indirectly, BP can be measured using Doppler ultrasonic flow detectors or oscillometric devices. Doppler devices allow blood flow, arrhythmias, and BP to be assessed. Because blood flow to a region actually may be more important than BP, Doppler devices provide an advantage over oscillometric devices. To use a Doppler flow detector an ultrasonic probe is placed over the palmar arterial arch of the forelimb or plantar arterial arch of the pelvic limb. To ensure a good signal the area should be shaved, a liberal amount of ultrasonic gel should be applied, and the probe should be taped firmly in place.

> **TECHNICIAN NOTE** A cuff with a width that is approximately 40% of the circumference is placed on the limb above the probe. Cuffs that are too large can lead to falsely low readings, and cuffs that are too small can lead to falsely elevated readings.

The cuffs should be placed below the tarsus and carpus to avoid getting readings that are falsely elevated (infrasonics). Both systolic and diastolic BPs can be fairly accurately assessed using a Doppler as long as the ear of the operator has become trained in the sounds that should be noted. Knowing diastolic BP is important in being able to calculate mean arterial BP (two-thirds diastolic pressure plus one-third systolic pressure). The diastolic pressure is more important than the systolic for ensuring good tissue perfusion.

Oscillometric devices detect pulsation of arterial flow under a pressure cuff. They provide a readout of systolic, diastolic, and mean arterial BPs as well as heart rate. They do not allow for assessment of flow, and readings tend to be inaccurate in the small patient and in the patient that is shaking or shivering. In small animals blood pressure readings may be improved by placing the cuff more proximally (around the humerus) or around the base of the tail. Whenever an oscillometric device is used the operator should ensure the heart rate on the machine matches the patient's actual heart rate; if they do not match, the pressure readings may be erroneous.

ELECTROCARDIOGRAPHY

Electrocardiographic monitoring records the electrical activity of the heart only, and the presence of normal complexes does not necessarily indicate normal cardiac function. Trends in the frequency and severity of any arrhythmias as well as response to antiarrhythmic therapy can be monitored. Waveform alterations such as changes in the ST segment and elevation in the T wave amplitude to more than one quarter of the R wave amplitude can be used to determine the possible presence of myocardial hypoxia/ischemia. Abnormalities in the conduction system consistent with myocardial disease, as well as pericardial effusion, frequently can be determined.

PULSE OXIMETRY

Pulse oximetry measures the saturation of hemoglobin, which correlates with oxygen content in the blood. A probe, which emits red and infrared light, is attached to the patient. Saturated hemoglobin absorbs more infrared light than desaturated hemoglobin, which absorbs more red light. A photodetector receives the light signal and the percentage of saturated hemoglobin is displayed. Tongue clips provide the most accurate readings. Tongue clips will often apply sufficient pressure to the tongue to interfere with circulation and cause inaccurate readings. This can be corrected by moving the clip at regular intervals to a slightly different location on the tongue and ensuring the tongue remains moist. Poor readings will result from poor pulsatile flow, thick tissue between the light emitter and receiver, movement, pigmentation, and strong overhead fluorescent lighting. Oxygen saturation reaches 100% at an arterial pressure (PaO_2) of about 95 mm Hg. The PaO_2 should be 4.5 to 5 times the fraction of inspired oxygen (FiO_2). Therefore with an FiO_2 of 1 (100% O_2, which is the concentration commonly given during anesthesia), the PaO_2 should be 450 to 500 mm Hg. The SaO_2 will read 100% from a PaO_2 of 500 mm Hg to below about 95 mm Hg. This makes SpO_2 a very inaccurate means of monitoring oxygenation in the patient that is receiving 100% O_2 but can be a very useful monitor in the patient receiving nitrous oxide or breathing room air.

Pulse oximetry should always be monitored in an anesthetized patient once the oxygen has been discontinued and the patient is still intubated if the patient can tolerate a tongue clip. Supplemental oxygen should be provided if there are signs of desaturation on room air. Cyanosis, which correlates with a PaO_2 of approximately 60 mm Hg, is equivalent to an SpO_2 reading of approximately 90% to 92%.

PLETH VARIABILITY INDEX (PVI)

Plethysmography defines changes in volume and has been shown to be very useful in measuring variations in blood volume. Pulse oximetry can be used to aid in this measurement (Figure 10-4). During respiration there may be variations in the pulse waveform based on changes in preload secondary to changes in intrathoracic pressure. Significant variations in the amplitude of the pulse waveform over time—as determined by a pulse oximeter—suggest the hypotensive patient is more likely to respond to fluid therapy (Forget and de Kock, 2010). If the PVI is 20 or greater then fluids will likely help resolve the problem (Muir, 2013). Hypotensive patients without a variability in the pulse wave during respiration are less likely to be fluid responsive. PVI is most accurate when the patient is being mechanically ventilated; however, it appears to be more accurate than CVP in determining the need for fluids, even in patients that are spontaneously breathing (Yin and Ho, 2012).

CAPNOMETRY

Capnometry is a noninvasive means of assessing arterial carbon dioxide tension ($PaCO_2$) and is the only noninvasive way of assessing ventilation. A detector is inserted between the endotracheal tube and the anesthetic tubing, which is then connected to the capnometer. There are two types of capnometers: sidestream and mainstream. Mainstream monitors have an infrared detector that fits over the attachment to the endotracheal tube (Figure 10-5). Mainstream sensors are heated to avoid vapor condensation, which can lead to falsely elevated readings. Sidestream monitors have a piece of hollow tubing that is attached to the endotracheal tube fitting at one end and the capnometer at the other end. In small animals air is usually sampled at 50 or 100 ml/minute through the tubing into the machine for analysis. Moisture traps are an essential part of these devices. The tubing should always be placed in a vertical direction to avoid excess moisture accumulation and the tubing needs to be evaluated at regular intervals for moisture accumulation, which can lead to falsely elevated readings. The capnometer analyzes the carbon dioxide level in the air in the tubing and provides a digital or waveform readout as well as a numeric analysis. Waveform display always is preferred since it allows for early

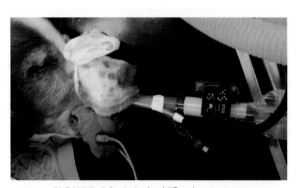

FIGURE 10-4 Radical-7® pulse oximeter.

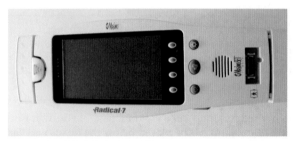

FIGURE 10-5 EMMA® mainstream capnometer.

detection of changes in ventilation, including increasing lung stiffness, chronic obstructive airway disease, and problems with the fresh gas supply (i.e., exhausted CO_2 absorber).

Assuming normal perfusion to the lungs and no airway obstruction, end-tidal carbon dioxide ($ETCO_2$) correlates with $PaCO_2$. The $ETCO_2$ levels generally will be about 3 to 5 mm lower than $PaCO_2$ because of dead space ventilation. If pulmonary blood flow is inadequate the CO_2 levels will be very subnormal (<15 to 18 mm Hg). The $ETCO_2$ generally should remain between 30 and 35 mm Hg in critical patients, although this number may need to be adjusted based on blood gas results and any underlying diseases or injuries.

SUPPORTIVE MEASURES NEEDED DURING ANESTHESIA

TEMPERATURE CONSERVATION AND PREVENTING HYPOTHERMIA

Hypothermia is a very common problem in anesthetized patients. Aggressive attempts should be made to maintain normothermia because hypothermia can lead to cardiac arrhythmias, hypotension, coagulation problems, and sluggish blood flow. Hypothermia can cause peripheral vasoconstriction leading to increased peripheral tissue acidosis secondary to anaerobic metabolism. Ventricular fibrillation and asystole may develop, starting at 28° C. Hypothermia should be avoided in a critical patient unless the patient is undergoing surgery that would benefit from induced hypothermia. Anesthetic requirements will decrease as the patient's temperature decreases.

The use of plastic wrap, bubble wrap, infrared heating lamp, warm irrigation fluids, warm IV fluids, hot-water circulating blankets, and warm-air circulating blankets can be implemented to reduce hypothermia. The patient should not be placed on a cold surface. Using warm water to perform the surgical scrub and avoiding over-wetting the patient may help. Low-flow anesthesia will help slow the development of hypothermia, and the use of a heating circuit in the patient's anesthetic tubing is an excellent way to decrease heat loss during anesthesia (Figure 10-6). Care always should be taken with any item used to supply supplemental heat to ensure it does not cause burns. All warm-water bottles and warm-water circulating blankets should be covered in a towel

before placement next to the patient to prevent burns. Fluids used to lavage body cavities or large wounds also should be warmed to body temperature.

FLUID SUPPORT

Fluid therapy is much more important for the critically ill or injured patient under anesthesia than for the healthy patient, but the endpoints are the same. The goal of fluid therapy is to maintain an adequate circulating blood volume, adequate hemoglobin levels, and adequate clotting factors. Crystalloids are redistributed primarily to the interstitium; if increased intravascular volume is required, then a combination of colloids, both synthetic and biologic, and crystalloids is indicated.

Based on normal fluid requirements, and evaporative fluid losses under anesthesia, a maintenance rate of 5 ml/kg/hr of a balanced electrolyte solution should be administered (Muir, 2013). This rate needs to be increased on the basis of blood loss. If the patient has advanced heart or liver disease, then it may be important to use a half-strength or three-quarter–strength sodium solution to avoid sodium (and thus fluid) overload.

If the patient is hypoglycemic, dextrose should be supplemented in the fluids. Dextrose supplementation should be considered in any patient if hypoglycemia during the procedure is a possibility. This includes patients with liver disease, patients with endotoxemia, and all pediatric

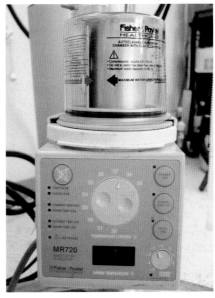

FIGURE 10-6 Fisher & Paykel MR270 anesthesia humidifier.

patients. If the patient is significantly hypokalemic, then potassium should be supplemented to help with muscle strength and cardiac function, and to avoid prolonging the effects of drugs such as neuromuscular blockers. If potassium is being supplemented then intraoperative monitoring of serum potassium levels may be indicated.

ANESTHETIC EMERGENCIES AND COMPLICATIONS

Any complications that can arise during general anesthesia of the healthy patient can occur in the critical patient under anesthesia (Table 10-2). The best treatment is prevention. The following section focuses on complications specific to critically ill or injured patients and problems that may pose more of a risk to these patients in the intraoperative or perioperative period. Hypoventilation and severe hypotension are probably the two most important complications. If these problems are left unresolved, they can lead to respiratory and cardiac arrest. If even moderate hypotension is allowed to persist for short periods of time, significant postoperative morbidity can occur.

Anesthetic drugs, central nervous system disease, airway obstruction, space-occupying intrathoracic masses, pneumothorax, severe abdominal distention (e.g., gastric dilation volvulus, severe ascites), musculoskeletal disease, obesity, and body position can all cause hypoventilation. If a ventilator is being used, then the cause may be

TABLE 10-2 Anesthetic Complications

CAUSE	DIAGNOSTIC TEST	TREATMENT
Anaphylaxis* Drug induced	Clinical signs (hypotension, facial edema)	Discontinue drug Treat for allergic reaction
Perivascular Injection Perivascular administration of drug	Clinical sign (perivascular swelling)	Dilute with saline 5-10× volume (± sodium bicarbonate)
Regurgitation/Vomiting Decreased lower esophageal sphincter (LES) tone Drug-induced	Clinical sign	Suction ± Nasal irrigation ± Lavage esophagus ± Nasogastric tube placement Extubate with cuff partially inflated
Air Embolism* Vessel or vascular sinus open to air Pneumocystogram	Severe bradycardia progressing to asystole	Position patient so that air floats to apex of heart and aspirate Consider hyperbaric oxygen (O_2)
Malignant Hyperthermia* Succinylcholine Inhalant anesthetics	Rectal temperature Electrolytes, blood gas	Provide 100% O_2 Discontinue anesthetic Active cooling Dantrolene 3 mg/kg IV
Cyanosis Lack of O_2 supply	Check O_2 tanks and flowmeter	Provide 100% O_2
Airway obstruction	Check endotracheal tube Auscult lungs[†] Auscult lungs[†]	Unkink, suction, or replace as indicated
Pulmonary failure	Auscult lungs[†] Arterial blood gas	Increase peak inspiratory pressure (PIP), respiratory rate, positive end expiratory pressure

TABLE 10-2	Anesthetic Complications—cont'd	
CAUSE	**DIAGNOSTIC TEST**	**TREATMENT**
Inadequate pulmonary circulation secondary to hypotension, pneumothorax, or pericardial tamponade	Auscult lungs[†] Check blood pressure (BP) Check jugular distention Check end-tidal carbon dioxide ($ETCO_2$)	Correct underlying cause
Lack of Thoracic Expansion		
Hypoventilation	See causes of hypoventilation below	Correct underlying cause
Barotrauma and pneumothorax	Auscult lungs Check for jugular distention Perform thoracentesis	Perform thoracentesis
Hypoventilation		
Anesthetic drugs	Check drug doses	Decrease drugs Discontinue inhalant temporarily Administer positive pressure ventilation
Airway obstruction	Check endotracheal tube and hoses	Unkink, suction, or replace as indicated
Pneumothorax	Auscult lungs Check for jugular distention Perform thoracentesis	Perform thoracentesis
Body position		Loosen limb restraints Alter position if possible
Ventilator problems (inappropriate settings, air leak, lack of O_2)	Check ventilator settings Check for air leak in cuff, hoses	Correct underlying problem
Need for Increased PIP		
Airway obstruction	Check endotracheal tube and hoses	Unkink, suction, or replace as indicated
Underlying pulmonary disease (space-occupying mass, fibrosis)	Measure arterial blood gas	Consider increasing PIP, respiratory rate, or allowing permissive hypercapnia
Barotrauma and pneumothorax	Auscult lungs Check jugular distention Perform thoracentesis	Perform thoracentesis
Decreased Oxygen Saturation Measured by Pulse Oximetry (SpO_2)		
Insufficient O_2	Check O_2 supply and flowmeter	Provide 100% O_2
Esophageal or bronchial intubation	Visualization, auscult lungs Check $ETCO_2$	Reposition tube
Obstructed endotracheal tube	Check tube	Replace tube
Poor perfusion	Check BP	Correct hypotension
Sensor malfunction	Check tongue clip Measure arterial blood gas	Reapply clip, moisten tongue Change sensor
Bronchospasm	Tachypnea Auscultation Response to treatment	Treat with bronchodilator
Aspiration pneumonia	Check oral cavity, pharynx, and endotracheal tube	Suction airway
Severe anemia	Check mucous membranes and packed cell volume (PCV)	Blood transfusion

Continued

TABLE 10-2	Anesthetic Complications—cont'd	
CAUSE	**DIAGNOSTIC TEST**	**TREATMENT**
Decreased ETCO$_2$		
Hyperventilation	Check ventilation Auscult lungs Check thoracic expansion Check pain	Correct underlying problem
Esophageal or bronchial intubation	Visualization, auscultation	Reposition tube
Obstructed endotracheal tube	Check tube	Replace tube
Poor pulmonary circulation	Check for lung overinflation Check BP	Decrease ventilation Correct hypotension
Pulmonary or pleural space disease Ventilation/perfusion mismatch	Measure arterial blood gas	Ventilate based on blood gas Treat underlying problem
Increased ETCO$_2$		
Hypoventilation	Check ventilation Auscult lungs Check thoracic expansion	Correct underlying problem
Carbon dioxide (CO$_2$) absorber not working	Check CO$_2$ absorber	Change absorber
Increased dead space	Tachypnea Check inspired CO$_2$ level Check anesthesia circuit	Increase or institute ventilation Consider neuromuscular blocker Correct underlying problem
Lung disease	History Auscult lungs Blood gas	Alter ventilation parameters Treat underlying disease
Moisture in sensor	Check sensor and tubing	Replace
Hypertension		
Underlying disease Drug induced	Systolic >180 mm Hg Diastolic >120 mm Hg	Increase dose of inhalant Consider nitroprusside
Hypotension		
Hypovolemia	Check BP Check lingual pulses	Colloid and crystalloid administration
Too deep a plane of anesthesia	Check vaporizer settings	Adjust settings
Inadequate preload from pressure on vena cava	Check underlying disease	Increase fluids Correct underlying disease
Bradycardia	Check heart rate	Increase fluids Correct underlying disease
Poor cardiac contractility	Check heart rhythm	Dobutamine infusion Antiarrhythmic drugs
Refractory vasodilation	Rule out other causes	Dopamine at vasopressor doses, norepi-nephrine if inadequate response
Peripheral vasoconstriction, hypothermia	Check temperature	Warm patient
Severe Hypotension (Arrest Pending)		
Severe hypovolemia Cardiac failure Extreme depth of anesthesia	Check BP Check heart rate and electrocardiogram (ECG) Check ETCO$_2$	Discontinue anesthetic agents Fluid resuscitation Surgeon to place pressure on cranial abdominal aorta if abdomen open Positive inotropic and vasopressor support

TABLE 10-2	Anesthetic Complications—cont'd	
CAUSE	**DIAGNOSTIC TEST**	**TREATMENT**
Bradycardia		
Too deep a plane of anesthesia	Check anesthetic depth	Decrease or discontinue drugs Administer atropine
Opioids		Atropine 0.04 mg/kg IV‡
Severe hypotension	Check BP Check heart rate and ECG Check ETCO$_2$	Discontinue anesthetic agents Fluid resuscitation Surgeon to place pressure on cranial abdominal aorta if abdomen open Positive inotropic and vasopressor support
Surgical manipulation of vagus nerve or organs innervated by vagus nerve	Check with surgeon	Decrease surgical stimulation
Tachycardia		
Pain	Check level of anesthesia/analgesia	Administer analgesics
Hypoxia	Check for airway obstruction	Unkink, suction, or replace as indicated
	Check for tension pneumothorax or mediastinum from barotrauma	Thoracentesis
Supraventricular Tachycardia		
Idiopathic heart disease Pulmonary disease Pain	Check ECG	Treat underlying problem Diltiazem Avoid beta blockers
Multifocal Ventricular Premature Contractions (VPCs), Ventricular Tachycardia		
Myocardial hypoxia (traumatic myocarditis)	Check ECG Check BP Check central venous pressure (CVP) Check electrolytes	Ensure O$_2$ being provided Ensure appropriate analgesia Ensure adequate volume Lidocaine 2 mg/kg followed by constant rate infusion (CRI) at 25-75 mcg/kg/min If unresponsive, consider procainamide 6-8 mg/kg over 5 min followed by CRI at 15-40 mcg/kg/min or magnesium sulfate at 1 mEq/kg over 30 min
Splenic disease	Check ECG Check BP Check electrolytes	As in previous section
Acidosis	Check ETCO$_2$ Check blood gas Check BP Check CVP Check electrolytes	Improve perfusion Antiarrhythmic drugs as in previous section
Sinus Arrest, Severe or Second-Degree Atrioventricular Block		
	Check ECG	Atropine 0.04 mg/kg IV‡
High CVP		
Hypervolemia	Check CVP	Diuretics Decrease or stop fluids
Pneumothorax, pneumomediastinum	Auscult lungs Check jugular distention Perform thoracentesis	Thoracentesis Centesis of mediastinal space

Continued

TABLE 10-2	Anesthetic Complications—cont'd		
CAUSE	**DIAGNOSTIC TEST**	**TREATMENT**
Sinus Arrest, Severe or Second-Degree Atrioventricular Block—cont'd		
Pericardial tamponade	Auscult heart Check ECG	Pericardiocentesis
Low CVP		
Hypovolemia	Recheck CVP Check BP	Increase fluid administration
Pallor		
Anemia	Check PCV	Blood transfusion
Hypotension	Check BP	Blood transfusion
Hypothermia and vasoconstriction	Check temperature Check ECG	Warm patient Correct arrhythmias

*Rare complication.

†Using esophageal stethoscope.

‡High-end doses of atropine (0.04 mg/kg IV) should be used because lower doses may lead to a second-degree atrioventricular block and worsening of the problem. If the patient does not respond, the clinician should consider doses up to 0.5 mg/kg IV or epinephrine to effect (beginning at 0.001 mg/kg/min).

inappropriate ventilator settings, an air leak in the system (endotracheal tube cuff, anesthetic hoses), lack of O_2 in the tank, obstruction of the airway, or resistance to lung expansion.

An observed increase in the spontaneous respiratory rate or ventilatory effort is not always the result of the patient becoming more aware; therefore, the cause of these changes should be determined before deepening the level of anesthesia, which may be disastrous. Pain and hypercarbia secondary to hypotension with inadequate pulmonary circulation, airway obstruction, or pulmonary or pleural space disease are the most common causes. Other causes of increased ventilatory rate or effort include hypoxia, opioid pant, hyperthermia, and pressure buildup in the rebreathing bag.

Pneumothorax can occur secondary to volutrauma or barotrauma from artificial ventilation. Clinical signs include hypotension, bradycardia, tachycardia, greater resistance to ventilation, cyanosis, a thoracic cage that does not deflate on expiration, loss of lung sounds on auscultation, subcutaneous emphysema, distended jugular veins, increased CVP, and decreased Doppler flow sounds. If a pneumothorax is suspected, then a thoracentesis should be performed immediately.

Hypotension generally is caused by hypovolemia or anesthetic drugs. Hypovolemia may be an actual volume deficit such as occurs with severe blood loss. It can be the result of a relative blood loss that occurs when a

patient with a large abdominal mass or a gravid uterus is placed in dorsal recumbency. The pressure on the vena cava in these patients can cause partial occlusion of the vessel. In a small percentage of patients, cardiac arrhythmias may be the cause. Primary signs of hypotension include an increasing heart rate (assuming the baroreceptor reflex has not been overridden), vasoconstriction, poor pulses, decreasing $ETCO_2$, and signs of deepening anesthesia.

Anesthetic drugs, hypoxemia, hypotension, hypothermia, acidosis, anemia, hyperthermia, toxemia, and cardiac trauma usually cause cardiac arrhythmias that appear when patients are under anesthesia. They must be identified rapidly and treated accordingly.

RECOVERING THE PATIENT

Serious problems can occur during either the induction period or the recovery period. Monitors should not be disconnected until it has been determined that the patient is truly stable and ready to be extubated or to be moved to a recovery area.

> **TECHNICIAN NOTE** Vital signs (minimum of heart rate [HR], respiratory rate [RR], and blood pressure [BP]) should continue to be recorded on the anesthetic sheet every 5 minutes until the patient is extubated.

Ventilation must be acceptable before the patient is moved to the recovery area. Before completely discontinuing assisted ventilation it should be determined that the patient can maintain an end-tidal CO_2 measurement of at most 40 mm Hg and that the capnogram indicates a normal waveform. If the patient was connected to a ventilator that permits the patient to spontaneously breathe without the ventilator being activated, then the patient's tidal volume should be assessed as being adequate before completely discontinuing assisted ventilation. Before disconnecting the oxygen completely it should be determined that the patient's pulse oximetry reading is 96% or greater on room air. If it is less than 96%, the patient should be reconnected to the oxygen to ensure the low reading is not misinformation from the probe. If the probe is functioning properly, the saturation should rapidly increase to 99%. If these actions do not then troubleshoot the problem, until an accurate reading is provided try disconnecting the animal from the oxygen again. If the pulse oximetry reading drops again to 96% and the patient is not ventilating adequately, then assisted ventilation should be provided. If the patient is ventilating adequately then the patient may need supplemental oxygen support during the recovery process. This can be provided via the anesthetic machine or by inserting a red rubber tube that is connected to an oxygen source down the endotracheal tube. Nasopharyngeal or nasotracheal oxygen support may be indicated once the patient is extubated. The endotracheal tube cuff should not be deflated until the patient is ready to be extubated since silent regurgitation is always possible during recovery. If the patient is placed in recovery with an endotracheal tube in place, the head and neck should be elevated approximately 30 degrees to help prevent aspiration if the patient silently regurgitates. The oropharynx should be examined before extubation and carefully suctioned and cleaned (along with the esophagus if a large amount of liquid is present), if there is any evidence of regurgitation.

Patients should be aggressively rewarmed if they are hypothermic, being careful to ensure burns do not occur. Vital signs, including BP, should be checked every 5 to 10 minutes until the patient is in sternal recumbency. The patient should not be left unattended until it is sternal. Fluid support should be continued as required to maintain normal CVP and urine production. Any positive inotrope, vasopressor, or antiarrhythmic drugs should be continued as required to maintain normal BP and cardiac rhythm.

Analgesia is vitally important in the postoperative period, and the patient should be given medication according to need, not just on a set schedule. Often constant rate infusions (CRIs) are required and doses may need to be reduced. A syringe pump is recommended. Regional and epidural analgesia can be repeated postoperatively as required.

These patients often have received a number of drugs and large amounts of fluids during anesthesia. Significant metabolic abnormalities may have occurred secondary to the underlying disease. Laboratory tests should be checked in the immediate postoperative period, including measurements of a minimum of a PCV, total solids, glucose, albumin, electrolytes, and venous or arterial blood gas. Abnormalities should be corrected as indicated.

REFERENCES

Abed JM, Pike FS, Clare MC, et al.: The cardiovascular effects of sevoflurane and isoflurane after premedication of healthy dogs undergoing elective surgery, *J Am Anim Hosp Assoc* 50:27–35, 2014.

Anand KJS, Phil D, Hickey PR: Halothane-morphine compared with high dose sufentanil for anesthesia and postoperative analgesia in neonatal cardiac surgery, *New Engl J Med* 326:1–9, 1992.

Bednarski R, Grimm K, Harvey R, et al.: AAHA anesthesia guidelines for dogs and cats, *J Am Anim Hosp Assoc* 47:377–385, 2011.

Forget P, de Kock LF: Goal-directed fluid management based on the pulse oximeter-derived pleth variability index reduces lactate levels and improves fluid management, *Anesth Analg* 111:910–914, 2010.

Hardie EM, Spodnick GJ, Gilson SD, et al.: Tracheal rupture in cats: 16 cases (1983-1998), *J Am Vet Med Assoc* 214:508–512, 1999.

Hebert PC, Wells G, Blajchman MA, et al.: A multicenter, randomized, controlled clinical trial of transfusion requirements in critical care, *New Engl J Med* 340:409–417, 1999.

Hendrix K, Raffe MR, Robinson EP, et al.: Epidural administration of bupivacaine, morphine or their combination for postoperative analgesia in dogs, *J Am Vet Med Assoc* 209:598–607, 1996.

Ilkiw JE, Pascoe PJ, Haskins SC, et al.: Cardiovascular and respiratory effects of propofol administration in hypovolemic dogs, *Am J Vet Res* 53:2323, 1992.

Keating SCJ, Kerr CL, Valverde A, et al.: Cardiopulmonary effects of intravenous fentanyl infusion in dogs during isoflurane anesthesia and with concurrent acepromazine or dexmedetomidine administration during anesthetic recovery, *Am J Vet Res* 74:672–682, 2013.

Lukasik V: Neuromuscular blocking drugs and the critical care patient, *JVECC* 5:99–113, 1993.

Lynch M: Pain as the fifth vital sign, *J Infus Nurs* 2:85–94, 2001.

Mader TJ, Playe SJ, Garb JL: Reducing the pain of local anesthetic infiltration: warming and buffering have a synergistic effect, *Ann Emerg Med* 23:550–554, 1994.

Marjani M, Akbarenejad V, Bagheri M: Comparison of intranasal and intramuscular ketamine-midazolam combination in cats, *Vet Anesth Analg*, 2014. http://dx.doi.org/10.1111/vaa.12183.

McCrackin MA, Harvey RC, Sackman JE, et al.: Butorphanol tartrate for partial reversal of oxymorphone-induced postoperative respiratory depression in the dog, *Vet Surg* 23:67–74, 1994.

Miller RD, Erikson LI, Fleisher LA, et al.: *Miller's anesthesia*, ed 7, Philadelphia, 2009, Elsevier.

Muir WW, Hubbell H: *Handbook of veterinary anesthesia*, ed 5, Philadelphia, 2012, Elsevier.

Muir WW: A new way to monitor and individualize your fluid therapy plan, *Vet Med*, Feb 1, 2013.

Murrell JC, Hellebrekers LJ: Medetomidine and dexmedetomidine: a review of cardiovascular effects and antinociceptive properties in dogs, *Vet Anesth Analg* 32:117–127, 2005.

Ortega M, Cruz I: Evaluation of a constant rate infusion of lidocaine for balanced anesthesia in dogs undergoing surgery, *Can Vet J* 52:856–860, 2011.

Rodriguez JM, Munez-Rascon P, Navarrette-Clavo R, et al.: Comparison of cardiopulmonary parameters after induction of anaesthesia with alphaxalone or etomidate in dogs, *Vet Anaesth Analg* 39:357–365, 2012.

Sams L, Braun C, Allman D, et al.: A comparison of the effects of propofol and etomidate on the induction of anesthesia and on cardiopulmonary parameters in dogs, *Vet Anesth Analg* 35:488–94, 2008.

Taboada FM, Murison PJ: Induction of anaesthesia with alfaxaolone or propofol before isoflurane maintenance in cats, *Vet Rec* 167:85–89, 2010.

Tranquilli WJ, Thurmon JC, Grimm KA, editors: *Lumb and Jones veterinary anesthesia and analgesia*, ed 4, Ames, Iowa, 2007, Blackwell.

Warne LN, Beths T, Holm M, et al.: Comparison of perioperative analgesic efficacy between methadone and butorphanol in cats, *J Am Vet Med Assoc* 243:844–850, 2013.

Yin JY, Ho KM: Use of plethysmographic variability index derived from Masimo® pulse oximeter to predict fluid or preload responsiveness: a systematic review and meta-analysis, *Anaesthesia* 67:777–783, 2012.

SCENARIO

Scenario

An overweight bulldog (body condition score of 7/9) has been under anesthesia for a foreign body removal. The patient is being ventilated with a Hallowell ventilator.

Questions

1. During recovery, once the ventilator is turned off, what three parameters can be assessed to determine if the patient is ventilating adequately so the dog can be moved to a recovery kennel?
2. The oxygen is disconnected during recovery and the pulse oximeter displays a saturation of 95%. Discuss what measures should be taken next.
3. If the patient needs oxygen support while it is still intubated, how can this be given?

Discussion

1.
   - Maintenance of an adequate tidal volume based on estimation from movement of the ventilator bellows
   - Maintenance of an adequate minute ventilation based on respiratory rate and estimation of movement of the ventilator bellows
   - Maintenance of an acceptable end-tidal carbon dioxide ($ETCO_2$)

2. The patient should be reconnected to oxygen. If the pulse oximeter reading improves, the patient should be left on oxygen and consideration should be given to assisting ventilation again. A trial off oxygen should be performed approximately every 5 minutes. If the pulse oximeter reading does not improve, the pulse oximeter probe should be repositioned.

3. If the patient is ventilating adequately (acceptable $ETCO_2$) but not oxygenating, supplemental oxygen should be continued using a sterile red rubber tube inserted down the endotracheal tube. Other methods may also be acceptable. An oxygen cage is less than ideal since the patient cannot be closely monitored, which is essential in this patient that is not extubated.

MEDICAL MATH EXERCISE

Patient order states: give 20 mg/kg cefazolin. The patient weighs 32 kg. The concentration of the cefazolin is 100 mg/ml.

  a. What dose in mg should be given?
  b. What dose in ml should be given?

11 Isolation Techniques in Clinical Practice

Louise O'Dwyer

CHAPTER OUTLINE

Infection Risks in Veterinary Clinics
Infection Control Programs
  Biosecurity
  Hand Hygiene
  Gloves
  Attire
  Laundry
  Personal Protective Equipment (PPE)
  Footwear
  Cleaning and Disinfection

Isolation Protocols
Isolation Facilities
  Isolation Room
  Footbaths/Footmats
  Nursing Patients Housed in Isolation
  Waste Disposal
  Improvised Isolation (In-Hospital Isolation)
  Antimicrobial Stewardship

LEARNING OBJECTIVES

After studying this chapter, you will be able to:

- Understand the importance of biosecurity within veterinary practice
- Understand what comprises appropriate personal protective equipment (PPE) for use in isolation.
- Understand the importance of cleaning and disinfection.
- Understand the importance of hand hygiene in infection control.
- Know how to implement an infection control program.
- Know how to set up and run an isolation unit.

Preventing infection is an important consideration for each critically ill patient. There is very little research currently available to guide best practice for veterinary patients; however, many resources are available from the human medical field. Veterinary infection control practices tend to be more diligently followed in situations where zoonotic diseases are under consideration (e.g., leptospirosis). Contagious animal diseases also tend to heighten awareness and prompt effective implementation of infection control practices. Critically ill veterinary patients are also at high risk for developing many **nosocomial infections** that might not otherwise be considered highly contagious (Kirby, 2009).

Human behavior in situations where there is not a perceived risk tends to veer towards nonadherence of effective infection control practices. Human and veterinary infection control practices have gained heightened attention because of the emergence of methicillin-resistant *Staphylococcus aureus* and methicillin-resistant *Staphylococcus pseudintermedius* in addition to several other multi–drug-resistant organisms in human and small animal critical care practices around the world (Weese, 2012). Research on this topic has consistently shown that effectively implemented guidelines rely on the following: the healthcare team must have common sense and knowledge of basic principles; guidelines must be suited to the local environmental conditions and problems; healthcare workers must understand the principles; the team must be effectively supported in order to achieve successful change (National Institute for Healthcare Excellence [NICE], 2012). Simply making a policy and expecting it to be enforced are unlikely to accomplish significant change. Infection control practices can be categorized into several important areas: **hand hygiene**, cleaning and disinfection of facilities and equipment, appropriate use of isolation facilities, and antibiotic use stewardship (Canadian Committee on Antibiotic Resistance [CCAR-CCRA], 2008).

INFECTION RISKS IN VETERINARY CLINICS

It is ideal that all patients presented to veterinary clinics should be evaluated to assess their infectious disease risk. This should be done by the primary veterinarian in charge of the case but may be delegated to the veterinary technician by following specific criteria that have been developed. All hospital personnel should be notified about the outpatient's signalment, history, physical findings, and/or laboratory results that are suspect of contagious disease. The team approach will ensure appropriate handling of the patient and implementation of correct cleaning and disinfection procedures of the environment.

Before patients leave the exam room or treatment area, those being admitted into veterinary clinics (day patients, overnight, or long-term) should ideally be assigned a biosecurity status, based on signalment, history, physical findings, and/or laboratory diagnostics. This will determine where the patient will be hospitalized and the order of care. The appropriate biosecurity status should be placed on the cage hospitalization sheets (see below). The veterinarian in charge of the case is responsible for the assignment of appropriate

biosecurity status. It is also the responsibility of the veterinarian to ensure that prescribed biosecurity standard operating procedures (SOPs) are instituted and followed. This responsibility may be delegated to a qualified staff member (e.g., senior veterinary technician). Deliberate deviations from protocol are discouraged but permissible when considered to be in the best interest of the patient or the safety of personnel. Justification for such deviations should be briefly noted in the patient record and initialed by the veterinarian in charge of the case.

INFECTION CONTROL PROGRAMS

All comprehensive infection control programs generally center on the following three goals: (1) decreasing the likelihood of exposing patients to infectious agents, (2) maximizing the participation of personnel in infection control activities, and (3) optimizing the efficiency of infection control procedures and policies.

Infection control measures that are effective against one agent are usually effective against others, particularly if they share common routes of transmission or have common risk factors in patients; however, it is a good practice to evaluate each potential infectious disease when creating an infectious control program. Design of infection control programs should focus on practical control plans for known problems, but it is important to not ignore the potential for newly recognized and reemerging diseases. Infectious diseases continue to emerge internationally and many are of relevance to veterinary medicine. The general strategy used in infection control protocols should be sufficiently rigorous to protect against most emerging issues, at least at a basic level. However, infection control programs should also be adequately "fluid" so that they can be modified to address new issues and they should also be reassessed on a regular basis (e.g., annually). Disinfectants being used will commonly need to be reevaluated and this may create the need for revisions to the program developed. It is important to ensure the disinfectants are clinically appropriate and proper concentrations are being used. The availability and type of disinfectants change regularly. More environmentally friendly products have been tested to be just as effective against many of the organisms found in hospital settings.

Disease transmission is one aspect of an infection control strategy or protocol that should be considered for every patient. Three elements are required for successful disease transmission: (1) a source of infection, (2) host susceptibility, (3) routes of transmission. Animal sources of infection can include endogenous microflora that are pathogenic to humans. Environmental sources of infection can include contaminated walls, floors, worktops, cages, bedding, equipment, supplies, feed, soil, and water. Host susceptibility to infection can vary greatly among the general population, with increased susceptibility seen in the unvaccinated, the very young and the elderly, those who are immunosuppressed or pregnant, or those with injuries that would allow a break in the normal defense mechanisms. These patients should also be considered when designing infection control protocols, because these patients will be highly susceptible to infections. Isolation guidelines for human medicine target the prevention of five different routes of transmission: contact transmission, droplet transmission, airborne transmission, common vehicle transmission, and vector-borne transmission (Garner, 1996).

Contact transmission is typically the most common mode of transmission and involves transmission of infectious agents to patients by staff or directly between patients. This can include the transfer of methicillin-resistant *Staphylococcus aureus* (MRSA) from a colonized person to an animal under their care, transmission of parvovirus between dogs by personnel or through ingestion of the pathogen, or transmission of an organism through puncture wounds such as needle sticks or bites.

Droplet transmission involves transmission of infectious agents in relatively large fluid droplets generated by coughing, snorting, or vocalizing. These large droplets do not remain suspended in the air for long periods nor are they transmitted long distances; therefore special air handling is not required. Transmission of bacterial agents from a coughing dog to another dog kenneled in relative proximity is an example of droplet transmission.

Airborne transmission involves agents that can be transmitted effectively in small particles (5 micrometers or smaller) that can remain suspended in air and travel greater distances. Special air handling is required to control this route of transmission. Feline influenza can be spread through a ward via the airborne route over extended distances.

Common vehicle transmission involves infection caused by contact with contaminated items such as feed bowls, leads, stethoscopes, thermometers, and other medical equipment.

Vector-borne transmission involves vectors such as mosquitoes, flies, and rodents. This may be of particular concern in some areas with reportable vector-borne diseases. These routes for **disease transmission** need to be taken into consideration whenever hospitalizing patients, and determining their biosecurity status.

BIOSECURITY

The following is a list of suggestions for infection control strategy (biosecurity):

- Tier 1 (T-1): *Patients at high risk for acquiring infections as a result of poor immune status.* Examples of T-1 patients include critically ill, immunocompromised, unvaccinated (noninfectious, young animals), or neonatal patients or those requiring long-term ICU care. Depending on the level of monitoring required, patient risk, and individual practice facilities and staff, T-1 patients may be hospitalized in the general ward areas or in the ICU. Despite generally being classified as tier 4 patients (see later) unvaccinated parvovirus patients may be placed into the ICU because they are considered immunocompromised; thus effective barrier nursing must occur and consideration must be paid to other patients housed within that ward. The risk status of the T-1 patient may be changed to tier 2 as the patient's condition improves.

- Tier 2 (T-2): *Patients with no evidence of contagious disease from the patient's history, physical examination, or laboratory results.* Examples include patients presenting following minor trauma, elective surgical procedures, and noninfectious disease work-ups. These patients must be handled after T-1 patients in order to limit the possibility of transmitting disease from patients with subclinical infections.

- Tier 3 (T-3): *Patients that have infectious diseases deemed to be mildly or moderately contagious to other patients or personnel.* Examples include patients with, or suspected of having, multi–drug-resistant bacterial infections (e.g., methicillin-resistant *Staphylococcus aureus*), those with open draining wounds, ringworm, leptospirosis, giardia, feline leukemia virus (FELV), or feline immunodeficiency virus (FIV), for example. T-3 patients are hospitalized in the general ward areas, providing appropriate personal protective equipment (PPE) is worn. If intensive care is required, cages in the ICU may be used. In the ICU, a perimeter around T-3 cases should be clearly marked on the floor when the possibility of contamination with urine or feces exists (e.g., leptospirosis, or a kennel within a kennel technique used, such as smaller kennel placed into a walk-in kennel). When housing tier 3 patients in the ICU, the risk posed to other patients in the ward, especially T-1 cases, should be considered. It is suggested that patients infected with methicillin-resistant *Staphylococcus aureus* (MRSA) should only be kenneled in isolation.

- Tier 4 (T-4): *Patients that are known or suspected to have highly contagious diseases.* Examples include viral enteritis (parvovirus, coronavirus), bacterial enteritis *(Salmonella),* infectious hepatitis, systemic canine distemper, canine influenza, bordetellosis, and acute (active) feline upper respiratory disease (*Chlamydiophila,* herpesvirus, calicivirus, reovirus). T-4 patients should be placed directly into small animal isolation, preferably without accessing other areas (i.e., wards, within the clinic). If the patient cannot be carried, a gurney should be used for transfer. Examination rooms should be clearly marked as contaminated and the veterinary staff and front desk notified so that appropriate cleaning and disinfection measures may be undertaken. T-4 patients must remain in isolation until discharged.

Additional considerations are made in regards to the environmental factors of each room including such factors as type of furniture, equipment, or floor, for example. Protocols are designed on how to specifically clean and disinfect each item and surface area. The protocols are tailored to the specific veterinary clinic and include all rooms (e.g., consulting rooms, laboratory, wards, surgery anesthesia prep areas). Details of how to clean and disinfect the walls, floors, doors, handles, switches, windows, blinds, computers, and furniture including e-desks, tables, trolleys, and machines are included (CCAR-CCRA, 2008).

HAND HYGIENE

Hand hygiene is one of the most important aspects of infection control within hospital environments, but is one of the most difficult to enforce. When questioned, most individuals indicate that their own hand hygiene practices are acceptable and are regularly performed. In fact, adherence to hospital guidelines in all appropriate situations is rarely as high as would be expected (Nakaura et al, 2012). There are numerous reasons that have been cited as contributing factors for nonadherence to hand hygiene, including guidelines that are too complex and hard to follow, personnel who are too busy, lack of education about the importance of hand hygiene, use of old habits that are too hard to change, and the concern that hand hygiene practices can cause drying and dermatitis (Nakamura et al, 2012). Hand hygiene implementation plans have to take all of these factors that may affect adherence into consideration when guidelines are developed and deployed.

Adherence to hand hygiene practices can be improved through a number of methods. It is important to include staff in product selection and choices. Personal preference and individual reaction to different products may assist in adherence because of fragrance, consistency, or interactions with skin during regular use, so ideally a range of different antimicrobial hand washes/rubs should be available. Healthcare workers must understand the importance of hand hygiene, the ramifications of poor practice, and the correct techniques that should be followed. Clearly defined and objective outcomes that are measured and reported frequently can also serve to both motivate and remind veterinary staff and promote adherence (CCAR-CCRA, 2008).

As "general" guidelines, staff should be reminded that hand washing will be practiced by all team members after handling every patient; before starting administrative or client service tasks; before and after using the bathroom; and before consumption of food or drink or use of personal hygiene products such as hand lotions or lip balms. Hands should also be washed just before leaving the practice for the day or when the healthcare worker is on a break.

GLOVES

Gloves are an important component of all barrier protocols, including an essential aspect of personal protective equipment (PPE). It is important, however, to educate hospital personnel that gloves do not replace the necessity for strict hand hygiene practices. Gloves may have small unapparent defects including holes. Hand hygiene should be performed immediately following glove removal and immediate discarding of gloves. Care should be taken to remove gloves before handling items such as pens, stethoscopes, thermometers, medical records, telephones, or door handles. Gloves are changed between all patient contacts.

ATTIRE

Staff should change into work clothing (e.g., scrub suits) in the workplace. This action should be carried out to prevent transference of microorganisms from inside and outside the workplace. Hospital personnel should change their hospital outerwear before leaving the building and related items should not be taken out of the hospital. Wearing protective outerwear home increases the risk of transmission of **pathogens** from the hospital to the household and from animals at home to hospitalized animals. Ideally, workplace clothing should remain "on site"; this means the laundry of workplace clothing should be carried out in the workplace whenever possible. If not possible, protective clothing should be carried to and from the workplace in a closed plastic bag.

Staff clothing should be visibly clean at all times. Clothing should be changed whenever it is visibly soiled or otherwise contaminated with body fluids perceived or known to pose a risk. Soiled clothing should be laundered as soon as possible. Additionally, outerwear should always be changed frequently (at least daily), because gross contamination does not need to be present for pathogen contamination to have occurred.

The *Journal for Infection Control and Hospital Epidemiology* recommends the following in regards to hospital attire:

1. Arms should be bare below the elbow (BBE). Avoid wearing wristwatches, jewelry, and ties.
2. Healthcare workers should have two white coats and have easy access to laundering items.
3. White coats should be removed before coming in contact with patients.

TECHNICIAN NOTE Wearing stethoscopes, lanyards, identification tags, and leads around the neck should be avoided wherever possible when handling animals or performing clinical tasks because they also can act as vectors for the transmission of infection.

Equipment pockets or pouches worn in addition to protective clothing must be visibly clean at all times. Separate pockets or pouches must be used in the main hospital areas and for the surgical areas. These must be laundered once weekly or as soon as they become soiled and/or contaminated.

LAUNDRY

Disposable items are preferable for use in isolation. This may not be a practical option for some clinics because of the increased cost. Linens can be a potential source of microorganisms, but these risks can be reduced with appropriate washing and drying. As mentioned, ideally all workplace clothing should be laundered on site. Ideally, a washing machine and tumble-dryer separate from those used for such items as animal bedding are used. The same protocol for laundry of bedding should be used (e.g., high-temperature wash followed by high-temperature tumble-drying). Microbial numbers on soiled linen (e.g., blankets, towels) can be significantly reduced via their dilution and the mechanical activity of washing and rinsing. Generally, linens should be laundered together (apart from uniforms, which should be washed and dried separately) using an appropriate detergent. If required, and if appropriate, disinfectants (e.g., bleach) can be added to the wash cycle, along with detergent. The hottest washing setting, ideally >70° C, should be used followed by drying in a hot tumble-dryer to promote the killing of microorganisms. If there is any doubt about the efficiency of the washing and drying facilities when dealing with some contagious diseases (e.g., parvovirus), bedding should be disposed, or not used. An additional useful item for use not only in isolation wards but also in all patient wards is a wash bag. Wash bags are water-soluble bags that dissolve on contact with warm water. All dirty linen is placed directly into these bags, which are then tied and placed directly into the washing machine, thereby reducing contamination of the environment by dirty bedding or clothing, for example (Figure 11-1).

PERSONAL PROTECTIVE EQUIPMENT (PPE)

All personnel entering an isolation area housing a potentially infectious animal, regardless of whether they plan on having direct contact with the animal, must wear appropriate PPE. At a minimum, this should

OUTSIDE

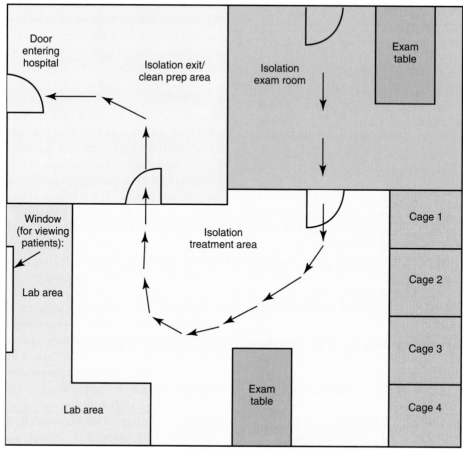

FIGURE 11-1 The use of a water-soluble laundry bag, which minimizes contamination of the environment and washing machine by contaminated linens.

consist of a clean lab coat or similar item of outerwear that is only worn in the isolation area and also disposable examination gloves. Depending on the diagnosis and the mode of transmission of the disease, shoe covers, masks, and eye protection may be required when handling an animal in isolation, but ideally a full-length, long-sleeved gown should be worn (Figure 11-2). All PPE should be discarded (if disposable) after a single use. Reusable gowns and lab coats used in isolation should be laundered after a single use. Storing/hanging and reusing a contaminated gown or lab coat inevitably lead to contamination of hands, clothing, and the environment. Therefore, when removed, these items should immediately be placed in the isolation room refuse or laundry bag; this also includes the use of gloves, which should be changed after single use with a patient. Hands must be washed immediately after gloves are removed. Eye/nose/mouth protection can potentially be reused with the same animal if they are not visibly soiled and can be consistently removed without contamination of the inside of the eyewear/mask or the immediate environment. Nose and mouth masks should only be reused by the same person. If the eyewear or mask becomes contaminated with body fluids such as urine or feces, it should be replaced with a clean article. All designated personal protective equipment must remain in the isolation room.

TECHNICIAN NOTE Properly donning and removing of PPE plays an important part in infectious disease control. The following is the recommendation provided by the Centers for Disease Control and Prevention (CDC).

Donning

- A gown, face shield or goggles, mask, and gloves are donned. The ties on the mask and gowns should be tied in the back and the glove cuffs should be positioned over the gown sleeve.

Removing

- Removing the attire occurs at the doorway before leaving the patient room. Hand hygiene facilities must be available.
- The outside front of the attire is considered contaminated.
- The inside, outside back, and ties on the mask/gowns in back are considered clean.
- Gloves are removed by grasping the inside cuff and pulling forward, being careful not to touch the outside layer of the glove.
- The mask is removed by grasping the back ties.
- The gown is removed by grasping the back ties. The gown is folded inside-out during the removal process to avoid exposure to the outside surface area.
- All items are disposed using hospital protocol.

Hand hygiene occurs immediately after removal of PPE.

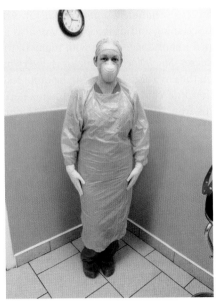

FIGURE 11-2 The minimal PPE should include a full-length, long-sleeved gown/apron; gloves; and overshoes.

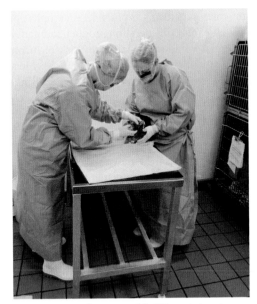

FIGURE 11-3 Staff wearing full PPE, including boots, while dealing with a patient in isolation.

FOOTWEAR

Staff footwear should have closed toes and should be able to be fully immersed in disinfectants. This will reduce the risk of injury from dropped equipment (e.g., scalpels, needles) or from scratches caused by animals and also protect staff from contact with potentially infectious substances. Designated footwear for isolation (e.g., boots or disposable shoe covers) should be worn because infectious materials are likely to have contaminated the floor, and use of the proper footwear will prevent spread of contaminants to other areas of the practice (Figure 11-3). Such footwear should be removed immediately, as soon as the contaminated area has been vacated, and should either be immediately disposed (if disposable) or be left at the entrance of the contaminated area on the "dirty" side.

CLEANING AND DISINFECTION

A second front of infection control practice is cleaning and disinfection. With the advent of methicillin-resistant *Staphylococcus aureus* (MRSA) and methicillin-resistant

Staphylococcus pseudintermedius (MRSP) in veterinary hospitals, cleaning and disinfection have also assumed heightened importance. Along with many of the infectious diseases, *Staphylococcus aureus* is a very hardy organism in the environment and can be quite resistant to desiccation in a compatible environment. Recovery of organisms from the environment has been documented months and years after becoming infected (Dancer, 2008). A dirty environment or one with a significant biofilm allows protection of the organism and facilitates the spread of infection (Dancer, 2008). Routine cleaning of contact surfaces such as door handles, light switches, computer keyboards or mice, and the undersurface of tables and other commonly touched areas that are not part of a routine cleaning must become part of the detailed cleaning and disinfecting regimen. These commonly touched but less routinely cleaned surfaces serve as a major source for the spread of zoonotic organisms such as MRSA from patients to humans and back again and must be addressed effectively in the face of any outbreak (CCAR-CCRA, 2008).

Effective cleaning and disinfection protocols address as many microorganisms as possible. A complete protocol must take into consideration product compatibilities and synergies while minimizing any risk of incompatibility or patient risk from toxic substances. Most importantly, the local "problematic" microorganisms must be considered carefully and products should be selected that deal effectively with them (CCAR-CCRA, 2008).

Cleaning

Cleaning is defined as the removal of all visible debris and is arguably the most important step in decontamination of animal environments. Even the best disinfectants will be minimally effective when used in the presence of moderate volumes of dirt and organic debris such as feces and bedding material. The presence of organic matter (e.g., dirt, debris, feces) will act as a physical barrier between disinfectants and microorganisms and provide a nutritional source for microorganisms. This results in reduced efficacy of disinfection by inactivation of many chemicals. Not only does cleaning enhance the efficacy of the disinfection process by providing optimal conditions for desired biochemical reactions, but also cleaning can actually remove a majority of microorganisms so that fewer need to be killed by disinfectants. Therefore, removal of as much organic debris as possible is required for optimal disinfection. This involves physical cleaning (including

the removal of all bedding and feces) and scrubbing of surfaces to remove adherent debris and biofilms, using hot water and detergent. Detergents should be utilized to loosen organic debris, emulsify fats, and decrease biofilm formation. The disinfectant to be used must be considered when choosing a detergent because there can be interaction between chemicals in detergents and disinfectants. Next, the detergent must be effectively rinsed from the surface, leaving no residue, because many disinfectants can be neutralized by the presence of residual detergents.

> **TECHNICIAN NOTE** Residual standing pools of water can dilute the disinfectant that is applied next. In addition, they may serve as reservoirs for replication and survival of microorganisms (CCAR-CCRA, 2008). Therefore, standing pools of water should be drained or removed before application of disinfectant.

Disinfection

Even with proper cleaning and selection of an appropriate disinfectant, disinfection errors can occur. It is critical to remember that all disinfectants do not have the same effectiveness. As with antimicrobial drugs, disinfectants have a spectrum of activity, which can be highly variable between disinfectant classes. Selection of the most appropriate disinfectant can be complex, involving a variety of factors including spectrum of activity, relative efficacy in the presence of organic debris, toxicity to animals and humans, potential damaging effects on certain surfaces, cost, and potential environmental effects (Table 11-1). There is no standard disinfectant to be used in all situations in animal facilities. When disinfectants with a narrower spectrum of activity are used as the primary disinfectant, protocols should be in place to use alternate products with a higher level of activity (e.g., in the isolation unit). There are many issues to consider when choosing a detergent and disinfectant product that are unique to each specific situation, and are best covered by reviews of these products (Hall, 2010).

The study of resistant genes to disinfectants must also be considered. Many bacteria can develop resistance to specific disinfectant classes, in a similar way to antibiotic resistance. During an outbreak situation, it may be important to consider this as one possibility of why a past successful cleaning and disinfection protocol has failed and contributed to the outbreak (Wortinger, 2011b).

TABLE 11-1	Commonly Used Disinfectants and Their Efficacy		
DISINFECTANT	**ACTIVITY OF INORGANIC DEBRIS**	**SPECTRUM**	**COMMENTS**
Hypochlorite (bleach)	Broad activity, including non-enveloped viruses *Mycobacteria* and bacterial spores at >1000 ppm (1:50 dilution of medium bleach) No activity against *Cryptosporidium*	Broad spectrum, including non-enveloped viruses and bacterial spores.	Used to disinfect clean environmental surfaces Sporicidal activity is particularly useful Efficacy decreases with increasing pH, decreasing temperature, and in the presence of ammonia and nitrogen. Varying concentrations can be used. 1:64 dilution of standard commercial bleach is most commonly used. Higher concentrations, up to 1:5 medium bleach (10,000 ppm recommended for blood spills), can be used but should be reserved for infrequent use in special situations (e.g., in isolation). Inactivated by cationic soaps/detergents, sunlight, and organic matter at low dilutions. Chlorine gas can be produced when mixed with other chemicals (acids, such as toilet descalers). Is irritating and corrosive
Quaternary ammonium compounds	Variable activity Effective against gram-negative bacteria and enveloped viruses Variable efficacy against gram-positive bacteria Limited activity against enveloped viruses No activity against bacterial spores	Variable In general, effective against gram-negative bacteria and enveloped viruses, variably effective against gram-positive bacteria, limited activity against enveloped viruses, and no activity against bacterial spores	There are differences between different types of quaternary ammonium compounds. Are commonly used primary environmental disinfectants, although the spectrum is not necessarily optimal In general, they have low toxicity. They are inactivated by anionic detergents. Some residual activity occurs after drying. Are less effective in cold temperatures and at low pH Are stable in storage Have natural detergent property
Phenols	Relatively broad spectrum of activity, with limited activity against non-enveloped viruses No activity against bacterial spores	Relatively broad spectrum, with limited activity against non-enveloped viruses and no activity against bacterial spores	Main advantage is they have better activity in organic debris. Can be irritating to skin and mucous membrane surfaces Reportedly toxic to cats. Some residual activity occurs after drying. Are noncorrosive Are highly irritant
Peroxygen/ accelerated hydrogen peroxide	Broad spectrum of activity, including bacterial spores and non-enveloped viruses Limited mycobactericidal activity	Broad spectrum, including bacterial spores and non-enveloped viruses	Is an excellent choice for routine environmental disinfection, footbaths, and environmental fogging Rapid action makes them a good choice for footbaths. Is inactivated by organic matter Has low toxicity except at high concentrations Is environmentally friendly Can be corrosive to plain steel, iron, copper, brass, bronze, vinyl, rubber, and concrete Is more expensive than most other disinfectant options Is irritating to skin and mucous membranes

Continued

TABLE 11-1	Commonly Used Disinfectants and Their Efficacy—cont'd		
DISINFECTANT	**ACTIVITY OF INORGANIC DEBRIS**	**SPECTRUM**	**COMMENTS**
Alcohols	Moderate activity No activity against non-enveloped viruses, bacterial spores	Moderate No activity against non-enveloped viruses, bacterial spores	Are not appropriate for environmental disinfection Can be used to disinfect certain medical and patient care items, but better disinfectants are available Are minimally toxic Are fast acting
Chlorhexidine gluconate	Moderate activity Limited activity against enveloped viruses Reduced activity against non-enveloped viruses, bacterial spores	Moderate Limited activity against enveloped viruses No activity against non-enveloped viruses, bacterial spores	Is inappropriate for environmental disinfection Appropriately diluted solutions are suitable for use on tissues or on materials that contact skin or mucous membranes. Is minimally toxic Bactericidal activity on skin is more rapid than that of many other compounds, including iodophors. Residual effect on skin diminishes regrowth
Povidone iodine	Moderate activity Limited activity against enveloped viruses No activity against non-enveloped viruses, bacterial spores	Moderate Limited activity against enveloped viruses No activity against non-enveloped viruses, bacterial spores	Is inappropriate for environmental disinfection Appropriately diluted solutions are suitable for use on tissues or on materials that contact skin or mucous membranes. Is minimally toxic but some people can become sensitized to skin contact Appropriate dilution is important to maximize activity.

It is critical that disinfectants are applied at the correct concentration and within the correct period of time following preparation to maximize the potential to be effective. The disinfectant solution in many circumstances should be left to dry on the surface to allow maximal killing time or effectiveness (Wortinger, 2011b). It is also important to consider that microbial responses to disinfectant exposures are not uniform. There is tremendous variation in the ability of microorganisms to tolerate cleaning and disinfection. Most enveloped viruses are easy to eliminate while protozoal oocysts, non-enveloped viruses, and bacterial spores may be difficult or impossible to kill.

> **TECHNICIAN NOTE**   In order for disinfection to be effective, a few key factors must be considered: the presence of organic debris, disinfectant concentration, temperature, and contact time. Organic matter inactivates disinfectants to varying degrees and it is important that it is removed before disinfection takes place.

Most disinfectants are available as concentrates and diluted before use. Dilution of disinfectants is an important process, and must be performed by measurement, not estimation. Excessively dilute disinfectant solutions may have little or no effect, while excessively concentrated solutions can be dangerous to use in addition to being wasteful of resources. The use of wall or hose-mounted metered dispensing units ensures that disinfectants are appropriately diluted. For some disinfectants, different concentrations may be recommended for different situations. This is especially important when stock solutions are prepared for use over time. Some disinfectants, once diluted, have a short shelf life and therefore all bottles should be clearly labeled with an expiration date. Cleaning staff must be informed of the importance of disinfectant dilution and trained in proper methods. Contact time is critical, particularly for certain disinfectants and difficult to kill microorganisms. If disinfectants are applied and immediately rinsed away, there is little chance that they can be effective. Most disinfectants require 10 to 30 minutes of contact time. Disinfection produced by chemical reactions are slowed in cold temperatures, which should be considered when determining the amount of contact time that is required. Disinfectants should never be combined because of the potential for inactivation and production of toxic gases. If spray bottles of disinfectants are used, these bottles should also be disinfected once empty, before being refilled.

> **TECHNICIAN NOTE** The nozzles/spouts of such bottles can harbor resistant microorganisms if not disinfected, and act as a source of contamination (Figure 11-4).

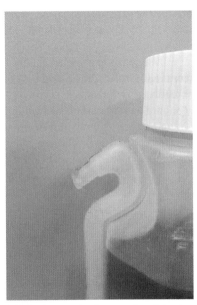

FIGURE 11-4 The nozzles/spouts of such bottles can harbor resistant bacteria.

The following need to be considered during cleaning and disinfection:
- Ensure all areas are well ventilated during disinfection.
- Gloves should always be worn when handling disinfectants; remember: some disinfectants will cause decomposition of latex gloves. For small jobs, disposable nitrile gloves should be used instead. For large jobs, heavier rubber gloves (e.g., common dishwashing gloves) can be used, but reusable gloves of this type must also be disinfected at the end of each task.
- Use of protective eye goggles is also recommended when handling disinfectants because of the splash risk.

- Always apply the selected disinfectant according to the product label, with particular attention to the following:
  - Appropriate dilution
  - Required contact time
- If patients or personnel may have direct skin contact with the surface, or if the disinfectant used may damage a particular surface, the disinfectant may need to be rinsed off with clean water after an appropriate amount of time has elapsed.
- Following disinfection, allow all surfaces to dry completely.

ISOLATION PROTOCOLS

The use of protocols within isolation is an essential part of ensuring all procedures are performed consistently by staff.

> **TECHNICIAN NOTE** Isolation protocols need to consider a variety of issues, including indicators for isolation, cleaning and disinfection protocols, protocols regarding personnel movement and barrier precautions, protocols for patient contact and movement, waste disposal, and supply stocking.

Defining methods for identifying animals that need to be isolated and establishing specific criteria for handling these animals are critical, and these methods must be properly communicated to all individuals associated with patient or facility care. Developing protocols for rapid identification of patients that represent a contagious disease hazard is critical to the success of any biosecurity program. The best isolation units are not effective if unoccupied. Specific disease and syndrome criteria for isolation should be developed to facilitate prompt isolation of appropriate individuals. Isolated animals should be physically separate from the rest of the hospital population at all times if at all possible. This means that isolation units should be designed so that animals will rarely, if ever, have to leave the unit except for those that need an emergency procedure such as surgery. Stocks, examination areas, and scales should be available. Ideally, there should be minimal contact of personnel with isolated animals and their environment. The ability to monitor patients in isolation using viewing windows or by remote electronic means (e.g., web cameras, closed-circuit video) facilitates the ability to deliver excellent patient care while minimizing risks associated with direct contact. Isolation units must be strictly managed with specific predetermined protocols in order to reliably manage the risk of transmission. Isolation protocols should be comprehensive and clearly documented in writing. Proper training of all staff, particularly lay staff who may have no background in infectious diseases and infection control, is critical.

ISOLATION FACILITIES

One important aspect of infection control practice is the isolation of patients that serve as an important risk to either humans or other patients. In most cases, isolation facilities in veterinary hospitals have been poorly designed and have often been an afterthought during construction (CCAR-CCRA, 2008). Isolation protocols and isolation facilities should be designed with two main goals in mind: the prevention of transmission of pathogens from infected animals to other animals, people, or the hospital environment; and the prevention of nosocomial infection to high-risk individuals (e.g., immunosuppressed patients). Identification of the isolation status of patients is critical. Appropriate signage should be used to make it clear to all personnel that the animal may be infectious and that additional protocols must be used.

Isolation facilities must allow isolation of individuals from one another. There also needs to be an anteroom where individuals entering the isolation space can don and remove appropriate and effective PPE or devices to protect themselves and prevent the spread of infection. Such devices, like gowns, can be perceived by healthcare workers as an impediment or inconvenience and therefore, education and monitoring of adherence are extremely important facets of an effective policy (Wortinger, 2011a). Healthcare workers should also be educated or have guidelines to consult regarding what PPE is necessary depending on the known or suspected pathogens in question (CCAR-CCRA, 2008).

ISOLATION ROOM

Isolation units should be designed so that patients do not have to leave the unit. Sufficient kennels, examination areas, and weigh scales should be available if possible. The isolation unit should be designed so that there is minimal movement of personnel and items between it and the main hospital. A changing area should ideally be present in the unit so that staff can both don and remove PPE without contaminating other areas of the hospital. Ideally, the isolation unit should be physically separated from the main hospital.

Minimal contact of personnel with infectious animals and the isolation unit is ideal, and patient access should be restricted to designated personnel. Sealed windows used as viewing sites allow for general inspection of patients without having to enter the unit. Closed-circuit television is a useful addition; this can even take the form of digital video baby monitors to allow the frequent remote monitoring and evaluation of patients without entering the unit.

The room should be well ventilated, ideally with negative airflow at appropriate rates of exchange. Solid walls or impermeable compartments should be present between kennels and runs. Drains and easy to disinfect kennels are highly recommended.

The unit should be well stocked with equipment, ideally including an oxygen supply and nebulizer, for example. Materials that cannot be cleaned and disinfected should be avoided for use in the isolation ward.

Wherever possible, equipment (including bowls, utensils, stethoscopes, pens, and thermometers, for example) should be restricted to use in isolation only. Supplies for disinfection should be ready available, along with waste containers. A dedicated drip stand and infusion pump should also be available for each patient to avoid cross-contamination. Obvious supplies for use within the isolation unit should also be available to include a selection of consumables, such as needles, IV catheters, syringes, dressings, bandages, IV fluids, routinely used medications, waste bags, and cleaning equipment. A system can be created to prevent the consumables from being contaminated if more then one patient is in the isolation unit. Individual patient packs can be created using a ziplock bag or disposable closed container that is assigned for an individual patient. Any consumable needed is placed in the sealed container, and when the patient leaves, the container with additional items is discarded. Bedding and equipment should be color coded for use in isolation only. Great care should be taken when removing contaminated material for cleaning elsewhere (e.g., laundry). Baskets/cages, leads, harnesses, and muzzles should be restricted to a single patient and laundered or thoroughly cleaned and disinfected before reuse.

A negative airflow system should ideally be in place within the isolation unit, whereby air is drawn into the isolation room, and the movement of air from the isolation room to other areas of the clinic is prevented (i.e., vented outdoors). When this is not possible, a high-efficiency particulate absorption (HEPA) air filtration system should be installed for the air being vented from the isolation room.

FOOTBATHS/FOOTMATS

Footbaths or footmats are used to decrease (but do not eliminate) microbiologic contamination of footwear. Footbaths are shallow containers containing a disinfectant solution. Footmats are spongy commercial mats covered with a durable, easy-to-clean material that can be saturated with disinfectant. In the majority of isolation units, a bactericidal footbath will be placed just inside the isolation area doorway. All practice team members must dip soles of shoes immediately before departing this area and step onto a disposable absorbent pad. Footmats can increase compliance because they are easier to use, but they are more expensive and more difficult to maintain than footbaths. Data regarding the need for and efficacy of footbaths and footmats are very limited, and there is essentially no information relating to small animal clinics specifically. It has been shown that footbaths can reduce bacterial contamination of footwear in large animal clinic settings. Although other sources of contamination have been shown to be more significant in infection transmission, footwear and floor surfaces cannot be overlooked in an infection control program in a small animal clinic, because patients so often have extensive direct contact with the floor.

Possible problems with footbath or footmat use must also be considered. Footbath or footmat use is almost invariably accompanied by spillage of disinfectant solution; this can create a slipping hazard on smooth floor surfaces, which are typically present in small animal clinics. Certain disinfectants can also damage floor surfaces and footwear with prolonged contact. Footbaths or footmats should be considered when personnel will be walking on a surface that could potentially be more contaminated than the general floor environment, and where spread of this contamination might pose a risk to patients or personnel. The most likely area where footbaths or footmats could be useful would be at the exit of an animal housing area (e.g., dog run) that contains a potentially infectious case, and where clinic personnel will be walking in and out of the potentially contaminated area. The need for routine use of footbaths or footmats in isolation areas where animals are confined in cages is questionable. If footbaths or footmats are used, selection of an appropriate disinfectant is important. The disinfectant should be effective against the specific pathogen(s) of concern, stable in solution, and effective with a relatively short contact time. Oxidizing agents such as accelerated/stabilized hydrogen peroxide and peroxygen disinfectants are ideal. The solution should be changed daily, or sooner if gross contamination of the bath/mat occurs.

NURSING PATIENTS HOUSED IN ISOLATION

Patients that are housed in isolation should not be walked or allowed to urinate or defecate in public areas or areas used by other animals. This may pose difficulty in smaller practices where a large space within the isolation area is not available. There may be occasions, however, when patients being housed in isolation must be taken elsewhere in the clinic for essential procedures such as radiographs or surgery; if at all possible, this should be done at the end of the day or when there is the least animal and personnel movement in the clinic. Moving the patient on a gurney is ideal in order to minimize the risk of contamination of the floor and clinic environment. Whenever dealing with patients, PPE should always be worn. It should be remembered that other animals should always be kept out of the immediate area while the procedure is being performed. The procedure area should be thoroughly cleaned and disinfected as soon as the procedure is completed. If radiography, for example, is being performed, the person responsible for taking the film will place radiography cassettes inside clinical waste bags to protect the item from contamination as much as is possible.

Ideally, one practice team member should be assigned each day to care for the needs of contagious patients. This staff member will be responsible for isolation unit cleaning, patient treatments, supplemental client communication, and assistance during any required procedures. The veterinary technician assigned to the patient must be informed that a patient is to be handled with this status. Practice team members who believe they have additional risk factors may inform the veterinarian in charge of the case and be excused from this responsibility. Factors such as pregnancy status, previous experience, and health risks such as immunosuppression should be considered.

WASTE DISPOSAL

All potentially infectious waste should be placed into plastic refuse bags (isolation room waste should be double-bagged) before being relocated to a specified location for biologic/clinical waste. Items that may cause offensive odors can be double-bagged in biologic/clinical waste bags and frozen until the biologic/clinical waste is collected. Items considered potentially infectious waste include body fluids or tissues from any patient that was designated as contagious or zoonotic or any item that could have come into contact with them. Any item used in the isolation area is also handled as biologic/clinical waste.

IMPROVISED ISOLATION (IN-HOSPITAL ISOLATION)

In some situations, placing potentially infectious animals in an isolation unit is not possible because of patient care issues or limitations in isolation space. In this situation, consideration needs to be given to management of higher risk patients within the general hospital environment. This scenario means it is vital to have isolation protocols available to allow for an increased level of protection. Specific criteria should be developed to determine when it is appropriate to implement these protocols. An isolation "zone" can be created around the patient's kennel by applying tape to the floor. The inside perimeter is considered contaminated. Protocols should be developed regarding the handling of animals, the kennel, and the area around the kennel. Animals that are isolated in the hospital should not leave their kennel unless they are being transported for required procedures. If movement is required, then the potential for environmental contamination can be reduced by moving the patient on a gurney. Traffic areas should be promptly cleaned and disinfected following transportation. Protective barrier clothing such as full waterproof coveralls or full-length waterproof gown, gloves, and dedicated footwear or boot covers should be worn for any contact with the patient or its environment. The area around the kennel should be considered potentially contaminated and disinfected routinely (at least three to four times per day). Disinfectant footbaths or footmats used at the edge of the "contaminated area" can reduce bacterial contamination of footwear (see Footbaths/Footmats). Patients should not be allowed contact with neighboring animals and ideally patients should not be placed in close

proximity to the isolated patient. Specific protocols should be developed for cleaning in-hospital isolation kennels, including the use of designated, specific equipment and the timing of cleaning.

ANTIMICROBIAL STEWARDSHIP

It has become increasingly important for veterinarians to be responsible stewards of the antimicrobial drugs they utilize. The use of antimicrobials in companion animal practice and not just food production circumstances will continue to be evaluated. The documented ability of certain microorganisms to share resistance genes places all antibiotic use under scrutiny (Fishman, 2006). The mechanisms of antibiotic resistance are numerous.

Designing an effective infection control strategy is multifactorial and should be planned with a specific clinic in mind. Staff training is an additional factor. New staff need to be aware of the practice protocols and existing staff should be updated with new information.

REFERENCES

Canadian Committee on Antibiotic Resistance (CCAR-CCRA): *Infection prevention and control best practices for small animal veterinary clinics*, Vancouver, British Columbia, 2008, Author.

Dancer SJ: Importance of the environment in methicillin-resistant *Staphylococcus aureus* acquisition: the case for hospital cleaning, *Lancet Infect Dis* 8(2):101–113, 2008.

Fishman N: Antimicrobial stewardship, *Am J Med* 119(6 Suppl 1): S53–61, 2006.

Garner JS: Hospital Infection Control Practices Advisory Committee: guideline for isolation precautions in hospitals, *Infect Control Hosp Epidemiol* 17:53–80, 1996.

Hall M: *The technician's role in the prevention and control of disease in the small animal hospital,* American College of Veterinary Medicine Conference Proceedings, 2010, Anaheim, Calif.

Kirby R: *Antibiotic use in the intensive care unit: challenging cases,* Western Veterinary Conference Proceedings, Las Vegas, Nev, 2009.

Nakamura RK, Tompkins E, Braasch EEL, et al.: Hand hygiene practices of veterinary support staff in small animal private practice, *J Small Animal Pract* 53, March 2012.

National Institute for Healthcare Excellence (NICE) infection prevention and control of healthcare-associated infections in primary and community care, NICE clinical guideline 139, issued March 2012. Accessed at guidance.nice.org.uk/cg139www.nice.org.uk/nicemedia/live/13684/58656/58656.pdf, Oct 8, 2013.

Weese JS: Staphylococcal control in the veterinary hospital, *Vet Dermatol* 23(4):292–298, 2012.

Wortinger A: *Zoonosis: what is all the fuss about?* Western Veterinary Conference Proceedings, 2011a, Las Vegas, Nev.

Wortinger A: *Disinfection and disease: what we need to know,* Western Veterinary Conference Proceedings, 2011b, Las Vegas, Nev.

SCENARIO

Scenario

Purpose: To introduce staff to proper handwashing techniques and provide them with an opportunity to assess efficacy of their own hand hygiene. This exercise can be performed in any facility and recommended to include in the orientation of new team members.

Items or products necessary:

As a training exercise to assess the efficacy of hand hygiene, ultraviolet (UV) fluorescent hand lotions can be used. These lotions are applied to the hands, which are then washed using the staff member's standard hand-washing technique. The hands are then examined under ultraviolet light; any remaining lotion on the hands will fluoresce, thereby demonstrating to the staff member areas that have been missed using the hand-washing technique. This will highlight the importance of technique in this important stage of infection control.

Sykes JE, Hartmann K, Lunn KF, et al: 2010 ACVIM Small animal consensus statement on leptospirosis: diagnosis, epidemiology, treatment, and prevention. *J Vet Intern Med* 25:1–13, 2011.

## CHAPTER 4

Emergency Care for Small Animals

This section discusses the importance of an organized work space in the emergency department and the types of emergencies seen in the small animal emergency facility. The technician plays a vital role in stabilizing these animals.

KEY TERMS

Acuity
Communication
Grief
Levels of severity
Preparedness
Team
Trauma-induced stress
Wellness

CHAPTER OUTLINE

**Preparation—The Readiness
  Assessment**
  Example of a Huddle
Facility
  Entrance
  Waiting Room
  Treatment Area
  The Client

Assessment of the Emergent Patient
  Triage
  Greeting the Client
  Readiness
  Approach
  Communication
  Re-Energizing

LEARNING OBJECTIVES

After studying this chapter, you will be able to:

- Provide information on how to prepare self, facility, and team to receive emergencies.
- Define and describe how to triage the emergency patient.
- Identify the systematic approach to receiving the emergent patient.
- Improve communication to be more efficient and increase patient safety.
- Recognize signs of traumatic stress and discuss treatment and preventative measures.

*Emergency **preparedness** is a team sport*

Eric Whitaker

Receiving a patient in an emergent state requires teamwork, where clearly identified roles are established. The veterinary technician involved in emergency medicine is required to play dual roles simultaneously—medical support for the pet and emotional support for the owners. Both have their own challenges but the skill set can be developed.

The hospital environment needs to embrace a shared mental model and commitment to provide each patient with a rapid response and relief of his/her emergent state. This can be accomplished only if all members of the staff feel like an integral member of the **team**. The hospital environment must include a commitment to collaboration, mutual accountability, open lines of **communication**, and recognition and professional respect in order to achieve success.

The use of protocols in the emergency setting has been strongly recommended by the Emergency Nurses Association (ENA). Their position statement includes the use of hospital-based guidelines developed for specific disease processes, to expedite care by allowing the nurses to begin specific diagnostic tests or procedures before being evaluated by the doctor. This would also include pain management.

The veterinary technician could assist in establishing protocols by collaborating with all members of the team, including the veterinarians, client care representatives (front desk personnel), and veterinary assistants.

> **TECHNICIAN NOTE** The following is a format that can be used to create a protocol:
> - Create a list of specific conditions and disease processes routinely addressed in emergency receiving.
> - Determine specific point of care (POC) data to collect drugs and/or fluid therapy to receive and initial procedures to begin after owner consent is received.
> - Define follow-up procedures and communication with clients. Post-care handouts for owners can also be developed for specific conditions.

PREPARATION—THE READINESS ASSESSMENT

Take your own pulse rate; then begin. It is important to give yourself a moment to collect yourself before entering a triage situation. Many clients will be visiting the emergency department for the first time and will not be familiar with the staff or operations of the emergency clinic. It is the duty of the hospital to provide an excellent first impression in 5 minutes or less. The time that is spent providing an excellent first impression will decrease the amount of time required to earn the trust of the client.

Hospitals choose to employ people who have different skills sets, to create a team. The veterinarians rely on the support staff to assist in facilitating the care of the patients. Client care representatives (CCRs); veterinary assistants (VAs); and licensed, registered, or certified veterinary technicians (LVTs, RVTs, CVTs) are some common terms used to define specific roles. All personnel should wear badges that clearly indicate who they are and their position. It is important for veterinary

technicians to always identify themselves as veterinary technicians, because owners often assume that they are the veterinarian.

Verbal and written communication with all members of the team throughout the shift provides opportunities for information exchange that will benefit patient care and client service.

Whiteboards can be placed in treatment rooms and updated regularly with information regarding incoming patients. The information listed may include the following: patient name, patient condition, and estimated time of arrival (ETA). Another column can be added to include updates of status for all to view quickly. The use of "virtual whiteboards" is becoming more common, with hospital management systems providing this information, as well as in-hospital information on a TV screen or monitor. Either method acts as a quick reference, and assists with communication as well as maintaining situational awareness.

Huddles are an activity that can be performed periodically through the day to continue to involve all members of the team and maintain situational awareness. A huddle is called to update all in a group of the status of incoming, hospitalized, and any other information pertinent to the flow of care of the patient and client. Assigning duties, determining resources, and expressing concerns are also shared at this time. Anyone on the team can call a huddle and is encouraged to do so when necessary.

EXAMPLE OF A HUDDLE

CCR: Kathy enters treatment area. Dr. Clark and the VT Melissa are preparing to anesthetize a coonhound that encountered a porcupine. The VA, Sheila, and the other VT, Dave, are obtaining blood samples from a cat that presented with a cough.

Kathy: Can we touch base quickly? I have some updates. Can everybody hear me?

All respond: Yes.

Kathy: I have just received a call from the local dog shelter. They have two dogs they are bringing in for an assessment of neglect and abuse. The one dog sounds like it may be critically ill and I'm concerned may be infectious based on the statement that other dogs in the house have died after experiencing vomiting and diarrhea. They will be arriving in the next 15 minutes. We also have a 9-year-old Labrador on his way with respiratory distress. Owners stated wheezing after a walk. They will be arriving in 30 minutes. Would you like me to contact our on-call veterinarian?

Melissa: I will be able to complete the de-quilling in 10 minutes.

Sheila: I will prepare to assist Dave with the initial exam of the shelter dogs in our isolation room.

Dr. Clark: I will prepare to receive the Labrador so I do not think we will need to call in back-up support at this time; however, if you receive any more calls, we may receive another critically ill or injured pet within the next hour; then contact Dr. McCarthy.

Kathy: Ok. I will contact Dr. McCarthy if we are to receive any more critically ill or injured within the next hour.

Most clinics will have hospitalized patients to care for in addition to those they are receiving. A rotation of duties has been a successful way of improving job satisfaction. The duties for the veterinary technician may include laboratory, treatment, phone triage, and admissions. Assigning duties at the beginning of the shift will assist in creating an efficient work flow.

FACILITY

The Veterinary Emergency and Critical Care Society (VECCS) has created three levels of certification for hospitals. This has assisted in the development of better equipped facilities by establishing guidelines for personnel, equipment, medical records, communications, and stock items including fluid and drug therapies, blood products, and catheters. Visiting www.veccs.org will provide all the details necessary to obtain certification.

ENTRANCE

Signage of where clients need to enter with their pet should be clear. A gurney must be quickly accessible to safely transport patients into the hospital. Garbage cans and an area marked for dog walks are advised. A station for disposal of feces is also helpful for infectious disease control.

WAITING ROOM

It is ideal that the waiting room is open and the front desk personnel can visualize activities of clients and their pets. Signage reminding owners that the emergency room is not a place for pets to socialize is recommended. Reading materials can include brochures

explaining the operations of the hospital and understanding the different roles of the personnel. Child friendly materials are appreciated. A pet loss hotline or other local support group information should be made available as indicated. Many facilities have a television, coffee makers, and snack machines for the comfort of their clients.

A place to dispose of trash and a clean-up station for pet accidents is advised. Exam gloves in three sizes are made available to use for this purpose.

Security systems including video monitoring of the outside areas are encouraged. The team should also be trained on how to address difficult or disruptive clients. Emergencies are not planned events and all have different coping mechanisms. Clients may be arriving under the influence of drugs or alcohol, may have mental instabilities and communication barriers, and/or may lack financial resources. This adds to a person's stress and may cause violent behaviors. Local police departments are an excellent resource and direct access using "panic buttons" are an option that can be easily installed.

The team should also create a way to quickly communicate to others in the hospital when a threatening situation with a client in the front greeting area occurs. An established code word can be used to alert the others. For example, if a client becomes irate, the CCR can contact the team members in other areas by stating, "Dr. Green could use you to come to the front." This alerts the entire team that more assistance will be needed. The team should be aware of the individual roles they will need to play, including defusing the client, moving other clients to safe area, addressing needs of the pet, and contacting police reinforcement if deemed necessary.

TREATMENT AREA

Creating an inventory system to avoid running out of key items is ideal. Many systems are available including electronic inventory controls that are web based. A simple, inexpensive method involves the use of tags. A tag system involves the following: colored tags, with the item written on the tag, are placed on the specific stock item when reordering is needed; for example, on the second-to-last box of an oral antibiotic. The person who takes the tagged item then places the tag in an inventory box. The person responsible for ordering will then use this as a tool to establish order lists.

Organization of items is imperative for effective work flow. Creating emergency procedure kits can be a time-saving system. The list of kits to create can include, for example, fluid packs, chest tape kit, and blocked cat kit (Figure 12-1). All items used for these procedures are placed in an easy-to-open zip-lock bag or tray. Creation of kits removes the time required to collect all the items, and leads to a more efficient stabilization of the emergent patient. It is important kits are labeled and all item expiration dates are considered. Lists should be prepared of items to be included in each kit, so they are created consistently, and a system should be in place to replace kits as they are used.

Essential items needed to stabilize a patient should be located in an area where the stabilization will occur. A mayo stand or a rolling cart can be used for initial stabilization items including clippers, scrub materials, IV catheters (22, 20, and 18 gauge) (IO needles [24, 16, and 14 gauge] are also sizes that should be in close proximity), tape and wrap material for stabilization of the IV catheter, syringes for point of care (POC) blood work, and flush solution for the IV catheter. IV fluid lines should be available and ready to spike a bag of fluids (Figure 12-2).

Other essentials to consider for the area (Figure 12-3) where the emergent patient is to be received include the following:

- A cart with necessary drugs, syringes with needles attached, endotracheal tubes, ambu-bag for CPR. A medical cart or simple tool box can be used to keep all drugs and other items well organized. Lists of items needed are included in Chapter 14 (Figure 12-4).
- Clearly labeled drawers and cabinets listing the specific items located in the areas
- Additional towels and bandage materials
- Syringes, needles, other items needed for taking samples for POC data
- Otoscope, ophthalmoscope
- Heating units
- Fluid pumps specific for station
- ECG, BP, pulse oximeter, and defibrillator
- Oxygen and suction
- Variety of muzzles
- Surgical pack for wound closures
- Long towel clamp for removal of oral foreign bodies
- Wire cutters for fishing hooks, traps, chains
- Hemostats, scissors
- Exam gloves

The items located in emergency receiving are not to be removed or borrowed.

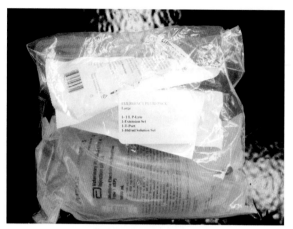

FIGURE 12-1 Fluid pack.

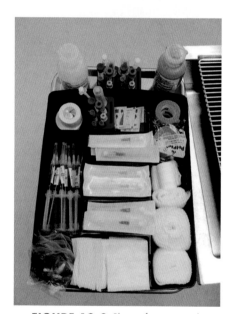

FIGURE 12-2 Photo of mayo stand.

THE CLIENT

Preparing the client for what to expect upon arrival begins with the phone call. Many clients will request treatment information over the phone, or a diagnosis based on the information or observations they share about their pet's condition or behavior. It is not recommended to provide this information over the phone and any suggestions made could worsen the condition or delay necessary treatment.

Canned phone statements can be developed to establish consistency of information delivered. Information

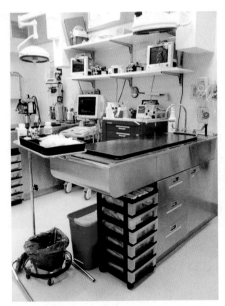

FIGURE 12-3 Photo of emergency area.

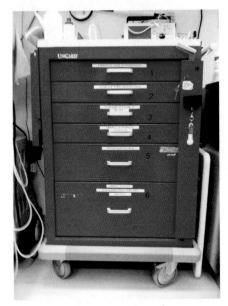

FIGURE 12-4 Photo of cart.

can include the initial greeting, explanation of what to expect when they arrive, and payment policy. Clients who arrive unexpectedly can be handed forms to complete, but also will need a verbal exchange confirming they understand the processes associated with providing care for their pet (Figure 12-5).

A written policy regarding owner visitation and presence in the treatment room during stabilization can be provided at this time as well. There may be situations where having the client present during the initial stabilization will be beneficial to both the pet and the client. This can build trust and eliminate the stress for the client and pet when separation occurs. It is not advisable to allow the client to assist in restraining their own pet, due to potential liability if the client is injured during the process. It is recommended the client sit in a chair provided to avoid injury if dizziness or nausea is experienced (Figure 12-6).

ASSESSMENT OF THE EMERGENT PATIENT

TRIAGE

The word triage is derived from the French term "to sort" or "choose." The process was used by the military to sort large numbers of injured soldiers. The goal was to determine the soldiers who could be saved if treated, those who would benefit from immediate treatment, and those who would not improve, regardless of treatment. This process also allowed for a quick assessment of those who could return to the battlefield.

Veterinary emergency medicine brings many types of emergency receiving scenarios. The location of the practice often determines the number and types of cases that may be seen, and if a triage situation will present itself. More populous areas tend to have more traffic, especially in the evenings and weekends. It is not uncommon to have multiple patients arrive within minutes of each other.

The two primary purposes of triage are assessment of those patients who need immediate care and prioritization of care for incoming patients. Rapid assessment and classification of ill or injured pets is essential to maximize efficiency in the emergency room. Correct prioritization and distribution of resources is often the role of the emergency receiving veterinary technician.

Triage is accomplished by determining a patient's **acuity** level by observing, taking a history, and obtaining vital signs. The goal should be to rapidly gather sufficient information for the assessment. This is also the time to assess the client's emotional well-being and need for further support (Figure 12-7).

Emergency Treatment Consent Form   Case Name/Number: ________________

Your pet has been evaluated and is considered critical ill or injured and requires immediate treatment.

A veterinarian is examining your pet now. A representative from the emergency medical team will provide you with an update and a cost estimate for additional care as soon as possible.

Payment information: There are no payment plans or billing options for service at the ______________ *(Hospital name)*

Payment is required at the time of service.

Estimated Cost of Initial Medical Interventions: ______________________

Radiographs: $ __________

IV Catheter/Fluid Therapy: $ __________

Pain Management : $ __________

Other Diagnostics: $ __________

I Give Consent for immediate treatment and accept payment conditions outlined above. *(Initial)*

I DO NOT Give Consent for immediate treatment and would like to speak to veterinarian. I understand the delay in treatment of my pet may result in an adverse outcome. *(Initial)*

Signature: ____ Date: ______________

Client Care Representative: ____________________________ Date: ______________

FIGURE 12-5 Informed consent.

Visitation Policy

We are dedicated to providing your pet with the best possible care. We understand it is difficult to leave your pet and encourage you to visit if it is determined they will need to stay over a 24-hour period.

The following is our visitation policy in order to maintain excellent patient care:

- Please call to arrange a time for a visit.
- Patients housed in our Environmental Oxygen Therapy Unit will be allowed 5-10 minute visitations and no more than every 12-hours. The oxygen delivery is an important part of your pet's treatment and you may only be able to observe.
- Cage side visitations—limit to 2 people and maximum 15 minutes twice daily.
- Exam room visitation—up to 30 minutes and twice daily.
- No small children allowed in treatment areas.
- To protect privacy of other clients, please limit questions regarding your own pet.
- Do not approach any of the other hospitalized patients.

Visitation may not be possible at times due to case load, emergencies or procedures being performed. We may also advise no visitations if pet becomes distressed after you leave. We appreciate your trust in our ability to provide care for your pet and will be as accommodating as possible. Please do not hesitate to call if any questions or concerns.

FIGURE 12-6 Visitation policy.

GREETING THE CLIENT

> **TECHNICIAN NOTE**   A mirror hanging on the back door of the entrance into the waiting room provides a moment of reflection.
> - Did you remember to wipe off the charcoal that sprayed on your face during the last toxicity treatment or clean the blood from your hands?
> - Just had lunch? Dinner? ...Snacked on onion rings? Mints are ideal (avoid gum) and remove the greenery from between your teeth.
> - Breathe—Be calm. Speak slowly. Both the client and the pet will quickly recognize someone who is experiencing stress or nervousness. Present a confident, professional demeanor.

READINESS

- Pen, stethoscope, thermometer, exam gloves, and watch are necessities.
- A bandage cart should be available to quickly cover open wounds.
- Note patient name and case number on questionnaire.
- Review the form the owner has completed with necessary information including name and sex of the patient.

APPROACH

- Introduce yourself and your role as the emergency receiving technician.
- Greet the pet by stating his/her name and note the response.
- Ask the owners the primary reason they have brought their pet to the clinic and use form to guide questioning and record information provided.
- Quick assessment through observation is performed in the waiting room to determine if you need to proceed to an exam room to complete obtaining vitals (temperature, pulse, respiration [TPR]) or if others in waiting room are more urgent.

Nonurgent (0)

- Client is informed of any wait times, if applicable, and encouraged to notify front desk personnel if pet's condition declines.
- All findings and history are presented to the veterinarian and a plan is created. A more thorough exam with diagnostics is recommended. The cardiopulmonary resuscitation (CPR) code will be discussed with the owner if it is determined that the pet requires hospitalization.
- Clients are updated if wait time exceeds 10 minutes.

Urgent (1)

- Client is informed of concerns and escorted into exam room where a full TPR is completed. Treatment consent form is signed.
- CPR code is discussed with owner and owner determines if he/she wants team to proceed with CPR if indicated.
- All findings and history are presented to the veterinarian and a more thorough exam and discussion with client occur. Plan is determined, with treatment after owner consent is provided.

Emergent (2)

- Client is informed immediate stabilization is necessary; verbal client consent is obtained and the consent form is signed.
- CPR code is discussed with owner and owner determines if he/she wants team to proceed with CPR if indicated.
- Initial stabilization of pet begins. History is obtained while stabilization is occurring.
- Updates to client are provided within 10 minutes.

Life Threatening (3)

- Client is informed immediate stabilization is necessary because of life-threatening condition; verbal client consent is obtained and consent form is signed.
- CPR code is discussed with owner and owner determines if he/she wants team to proceed with CPR if indicated.
- Initial stabilization of pet begins. History is obtained while stabilization is occurring.
- Updates to client are provided within 10 minutes.

The initial assessment and determination of level of acuity of the pet should take an average of 5 minutes. Providing the client with realistic expectations of wait times, if any, can occur at this time as well. Most clients will understand wait time increases when a critically ill or injured pet arrives. Regular updates are always appreciated.

The Emergency Severity Index (ESI) has been developed in human medicine and it includes 2 to 5 acuity systems. The 3-tier (emergent, urgent, and nonurgent) or 5-tier (resuscitation, emergent, urgent, nonurgent, referred) categories tend to be the more popular. The benefits of establishing the ESI have included the following: each person is assessed by an experienced triage nurse, a person in need of immediate care is identified, first aid is provided, and the emotional needs of the patient and family are addressed.

Emergency Receiving Questionnaire

Date:	Arrival time: [　　]	Case number:	Pet name/client name:
Sex/age/species:		Presenting complaint:	

History

Duration of illness or condition?			
Current medications?			
Over-the-counter medication given?			
Exposure to potential toxins?			
How is pet housed?	Indoors	Outdoors	Roams freely	Always supervised
Environmental changes?	Yes	Describe:	No
Diet?			
Appetite?	Normal	Decreased	Absent
Rabies vaccine date: (Proof needed)			
Other vaccine date:			
Vomiting/diarrhea? .	Yes	Describe:	No
Urinating without difficulty?	No	Describe:	Yes
Ambulating normally?	No	Describe:	Yes
Other changes?			

Initial Exam

Respiratory rate/ventilatory nature
Lung sounds
Heart rate/sounds
Pulse rate/quality
CRT/MM color
Temperature
Pain scale rating*
If painful, location
Ambulatory?
Activity level (BAR-bright alert reactive, QAR Quiet alert reactive, Lethargic)
Behavior (Blue-friendly, interactive, Yellow-reserved, Red-caution)

Overall Assessment

Non-urgent	Urgent	Emergent	Life threatening
Time assessment completed: [　　]			

*http://www.vasg.org/pdfs/CSU_Acute_Pain_Scale_Canine.pdf

*http://www.csuanimalcancercenter.org/assets/files/csu_acute_pain_scale_feline.pdf

FIGURE 12-7 Triage questionnaire.

The ESI has also challenged the triage nurse to be able to determine the number of resources that will be needed to address the patient's condition. Resources include diagnostics, IV fluid therapies, other medications, or simple (e.g., urinary catheter) or complex procedures (e.g., chest tube). Establishing a formalized way of identifying acuity levels has proven to increase team effectiveness and customer service.

Veterinary scoring systems are commonly used to assess pain, level of consciousness, and trauma. The following is the modified Glasgow coma scoring scale and trauma patient scoring scale that have been developed and can be used as a reference to establish consistent ways of communicating the status of patents (Figure 12-8).

A cardiopulmonary resuscitation (CPR) code is also discussed with the owner to determine if the owners approve the healthcare team proceeding if the patient experiences a respiratory or cardiac arrest. Color codes are common: red, no CPR; yellow, closed-chest CPR only; green, open-chest CPR included if necessary.

COMMUNICATION

Once the **level of severity** is determined, the plan on how to proceed is developed and communicated to the members of the team. It is important to confirm that communicated information is received appropriately. This can be accomplished by using a check-back or closed-loop communication technique. It involves both the sender (person providing the information or order) and the receiver (person listening and responsible for sharing information or carrying out order) confirming accuracy of communication.

Example of Closed-Loop Communication

Dr. Clark (sender) is the receiving emergency veterinarian who has left the exam room and needs to share the plan for the patient in exam room 2. Melissa (VT receiver) is the emergency receiving technician for the day.

Dr. Clark: Melissa, I have a medium-sized mixed breed dog in exam room 2 that I need you to obtain a blood sample for a Lyme's test. Please use the 4DX. Also draw additional blood in case we want to run any more tests if this is negative. He may bite, so use caution.

Melissa: Ok, Dr. Clark. I will complete the 4DX and hold blood for additional tests on the dog in exam room 2. I understand he may bite and will need a muzzle.

Dr. Clark: This is correct. Thank you.

Emergent situations are notorious for creating poor communication scenarios. The hospital can establish clear expectations and guidelines in how they are going to communicate to eliminate errors.

Use of check back in emergent situation:

Mixed breed dog arrives actively seizing. The owners have consented to immediate stabilization and the triage team carries the dog to the treatment area. An IV catheter is placed.

Dr. Clark: Melissa, Give 5 mg of Valium IV please.

Melissa: Drawing up 5 mg (1 ml) of Valium and administering IV

Dr. Clark: Correct, Thank you.

Implementing this style of communication will help avoid errors, and improve patient safety. The check back also allows others to confirm what they have heard and maintain situational awareness.

Documentation also assists with preventing errors. Check lists and admission forms can be developed to assist in confirming orders are clear and accurate. The form can also act as a record when the request is completed. The admission form is printed on a unique colored paper for quick identification. It contains a brief statement of presentation, initial vitals, recommended therapies, and procedures requested. Boxes are placed by each item listed and marked off once completed. The sheets can be a tool used to prioritize treatments or procedures that need to be completed once the patient is hospitalized (Figure 12-9). Many hospital information management computer systems are available that will maintain all of this information in a paperless environment. Television screens or monitors will display inpatient information, upcoming treatments, and so on, and allow for electronic notes that can be easily accessed by all staff.

All results of diagnostics and continued care are transferred to the treatment form or electronic record. A quick reference card that contains emergency drug calculations and client contact information is also a useful reference.

RE-ENERGIZING

The role of the emergency receiving technician involves providing compassionate care not only for the animal but also for the owner as well. Encounters with death, human, and animal suffering, and the possibility of resuscitation efforts failing, are some of the difficult realities of working in emergency medicine. Veterinary

A Trauma scale

Grade	Perfusion	Cardiac	Respiratory	Eye/Muscle/Integument	Skeletal	Neurological
0	*mm* pink & moist CRT – 2 sec rectal temp ≥ 37.8°C (100°F) femoral pulses strong or bounding	HR: C - 60–140 F - 120–200 Normal sinus rhythm	Regular resp rate with no stridor No abdominal component to resp	Abrasion, laceration: none or partial thickness Eye: no fluorescein uptake	Weight bearing in 3 or 4 limbs, no palpable fracture or joint laxity	Central: conscious, alert →sl dull; interest in surroundings Periph: normal spinal reflexes; purposeful movement and nociception in all limbs
1	*mm* hyperemic or pale pink; mm tacky CRT 0–2 sec Rectal temp ≥ 37.8°C (100°F) Femoral pulses fair	HR: C - 140–180 F - 200–260 Normal sinus rhythm or VPC's < 20/min	Mildly ↑ resp rate & effort, ± some abdominal component Mildly ↑ upper airway sounds	Abrasion, laceration: full thickness, no deep tissue involvement eye: corneal Laceration/ulcer, not perforated	Closed appendicular/rib fx or any mandibular fx Single joint laxity/luxation incl. sacroiliac joint Pelvic fx with unilateral intact SI-ilium-acetab Single limb open/closed fx at or below carpus/tarsus	Central: conscious, but dull, depressed, withdrawn Periph: abnormal spinal reflexes with purposeful movement and nociception intact in all 4 limbs
2	*mm* v pale pink & v tacky CRT 2–3 sec Rectal temp < 37.8°C (100°F) Detectable but poor femoral pulses	HR: C - > 180 F - > 260 Consistent arrhythmia	Moderately ↑ resp effort with abdom component, elbow abduction Moderately ↑ upper airway sounds	Abrasion, laceration: full thickness, deep tissue involvement, and arteries, nerves, muscles intact eye: corneal Perforation, punctured globe or proptosis	Multiple Grade 1 conditions (see above) Single long bone open fx above carpus/tarsus with cortical bone preserved non-mandibular skull fx	Central: unconscious but responds to noxious stimuli Periph: absent purposeful movement with intact nociception in 2 or more limbs or nociception absent only in 1 limb; anal and/or tail tone
3	*mm* gray, blue, or white CRT > 3 sec Rectal temp < 37.8°C (100°F) femoral pulse not detected	HR: C - 60 F - 120 Erratic arrhythmia	Marked respiratory effort or gasping/agonal respiration or irregularly timed effort Little or no detectable air passage	Penetration to thoracic/abdo cavity Abrasion, laceration: full thickness, deep tissue involvement, and artery, nerve, or muscle compromised	Vertebral body fracture/luxation except coccygeal Multiple long bone open fx above tarsus/carpus Single long bone open fx above tarsus/carpus with loss of cortical bone	Central: nonresponsive to all stimuli; refractory seizures Periph: absent nociception in 2 or more limbs; absent tail or perianal nociception

mm, Mucous membranes.

FIGURE 12-8 A, Trauma scale. (**A** From Rockar RA, Drobatz KJ, Shofer FS: Development of a scoring system for veterinary trauma patient, *J Vet Emerg Crit Care* 4(2): 77-84, 1994.)

Continued

B   Modified Glasgow Coma Scale

	Score
Motor activity	
Normal gait, normal spinal reflexes	6
Hemiparesis, tetraparesis, or decerebrate activity	5
Recumbent, intermittent extensor rigidity	4
Recumbent, constant extensor rigidity	3
Recumbent, constant extensor rigidity with opisthotonus	2
Recumbent, hypotonia of muscles, depressed or absent spinal reflexes	1
Brain stem reflexes	
Normal pupillary light reflexes and oculocephalic reflexes	6
Slow pupillary light reflexes and normal to reduced oculocephalic reflexes	5
Bilateral unresponsive miosis with normal to reduced oculocephalic reflexes	4
Pinpoint pupils with reduced to absent oculocephalic reflexes	3
Unilateral, unresponsive mydriasis with reduced to absent oculocephalic reflexes	2
Bilateral, unresponsive mydriasis with reduced to absent oculocephalic reflexes	1
Level of consciousness	
Occasional periods of alertness and responsive to environment	6
Depression or delirium, capable of responding but response may be inappropriate	5
Semicomatose, responsive to visual stimuli	4
Semicomatose, responsive to auditory stimuli	3
Semicomatose, responsive only to repeated noxious stimuli	2
Comatose, unresponsive to repeated noxious stimuli	1

C   Modified Glasgow Coma Scale score category and suggested prognosis

Score Category	Actual MGCS Score	Suggested Prognosis
I	3–8	Grave
II	9–14	Guarded
III	15–18	Good

MGCS, Modified Glasgow Coma Scale.

FIGURE 12-8, cont'd B, Modified Glasgow Coma Scale. **C,** Modified Glasgow Coma Scale score category and suggested prognosis. (**B** and **C** From Platt SR, Radaelli ST, McDonnell JJ: The prognostic value of the modified Glasgow Coma Scale in head trauma in dogs, *J Vet Inter Med* 15(6):581-584, 2001.)

medicine has the additional stressor of having to euthanize even when treatment could save the pet. The client's choice remains the final decision.

It is not uncommon to hear someone involved in emergency medicine state that he/she enjoys the adrenaline rush. This adrenaline rush may have negative effects if not managed. One study showed that emergency medical personnel have a lack of recovery in cortisol values after handling patients in life-threatening situations. The degree of severity of the patient's condition is directly related to the response.

The fight or flight response, associated with the rise in adrenaline and cortisol levels, speeds the heart rate, decreases digestion, shunts blood flow to major muscle groups, and causes changes to other autonomic nervous systems. This provides the burst of energy and strength to react, but a relaxation response should occur after the perceived threat or emergency has resolved. Healthcare professionals involved in emergency and critical care medicine experience this fight or flight response frequently throughout the day when addressing the needs of their patients and clients. Job experience appeared to have a protective effect on the degree of physiologic response.

Many terms have been used to define this condition, including **trauma-induced stress**, helping-induced trauma, and secondary stress disorder. All can lead to burn out and chronic stress syndrome. Stress has been linked to heart disease, depression, and other physical and emotional health problems. Work performance, job satisfaction, and knowledge retention are negatively impacted as well.

Practicing **wellness** and developing coping mechanisms are a vital part of becoming a successful emergency and critical care veterinary technician. Five- to 10-minute breaks after a traumatic event should be considered a mandatory exercise practiced in the hospital. The break includes movement off the floor or away from the area where the event occurred. Each person has his or her own abilities to cope and how the person utilizes the time-out period should be respected. All are encouraged to use known destressing exercises, including breathing techniques, meditation, exercise, and music.

Debriefing is another tool successfully used to open lines of communication, provide support, and review the event, with all who were involved. The debriefing exercise can also include ideas from the team about how to adjust a method or approach for better success in the

Emergency Intake Form

Date:	Time:	Case number:	Pet name/client name:

Sex/age:	Breed:	Weight:

Disposition:	Presenting complaints:

Admission TPR	T- ▭ P- ▭ R- ▭	Level of severity ▭	CPR CODE ▭

Problem List	1.	2.	3.
	4.	5.	6.

IV Catheter Placement

Type	Size	Location	Initial

Other Indwelling Tubes

Type	Size	Location	Initial

Fluid Therapy/Blood Products

Type	Rate	Route	Total recd	Time

Pain Management/ Sedation

Type	Dosage	Route	Dose	Time

Other Medications

Type	Dosage	Route	Dose	Time

Point of Care Diagnostics

Time	Type	Results	Initial

Monitoring

Time/initial				
Temp				
HR				
RR				
PQ				
MM/CRT				
BP				
Pulse ox				
ECG				

Lab Monitoring

Time/initial				
PCV/TS				
BG				
Azo				
Lactate				

FIGURE 12-9 Example of admissions form.

future. Debriefs are most effective when initiated by one of the considered leaders on the team and the culture of the hospital should view mistakes as a learning opportunity.

> **TECHNICIAN NOTE** The following is the format for a debriefing session and should only require 3 to 5 minutes:
> - Debriefing begins with an accurate review and documentation of key events.
> - All staff members analyze why the event occurred and which interventions were successful or unsuccessful.
> - There should be a discussion of what was gained from the experience and what changes could be made if the situation recurs.
> - Plan to implement changes for better success if there is a reoccurrence of the situation.

Grief is another familiar emotion experienced by the emergency veterinary technician. Grieving occurs when interventions have been unsuccessful and the death of a patient occurs or we experience the grief of the client.

Supporting the grieving client includes the following:
- Ask them what they need.
- Help them connect with family or friends, and provide them with additional resources, including pet loss support groups.
- Answer any questions they may have, and offer to find answers you cannot answer.
- Offer an opportunity to say goodbye to their pet and provide a quiet private room.
- Offer a memory option, such as a paw print or a lock of hair.
- Do not judge the grieving client.

Supporting yourself:
- Be aware of how the exposure to pets in an emergent state, and their owner's grief, is an important part of the healing process.
- You must provide yourself with time to grieve and deal with emotions.
- Utilize resources available on how to deal with grief.
- Seek outside assistance if you find you are unable to manage your grief.
- Find a self-care strategy that works for you.
- Recommendations for coping include regular exercise, no smoking, limited alcohol use, weight control, living within one's means, and creating a support network among colleagues, family, and friends.
- The emergency receiving role provides the technician with the opportunity to use a variety of skill sets and perfect his/her technical abilities. It is important for the veterinary technician to invest in himself/herself to maintain health and wellness. This will help to maintain job satisfaction and provide the necessary support for our clients and their pets (Figure 12-10).

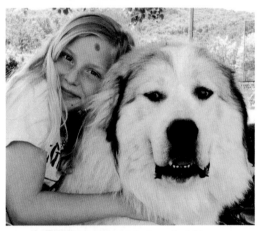

FIGURE 12-10 Pet with child.

SUGGESTED READINGS

Emergency Nurses Association: *Use of protocols in the emergency setting.* Available at www.ena.org.

Escriba-Aguir V, Martin-Baena D, Perez-Hoyos S: Psychosocial work environment and burnout among emergency medical and nursing staff, *Int Arch Occup Environ Health* 80:127–133, 2006.

Flannery RB: Managing stress in today's age: a concise guide for emergency services personnel, *Int J Emerg Mental Health* 6(4):205–209, 2004.

Gilboy N, Tanabe P, Travers D, et al.: *Emergency severity index, version 4: implementation handbook*, Rockville, MD, May 2005, AHRQ Pub No. 05-0046-2. Agency for Healthcare Research & Quality. *J Emerg Trauma Shock* 22(3):147–149, Sept-Dec 2009.

Keene E, Hutton N, Hall B, et al.: Bereavement debriefing sessions: an intervention to support health care professionals after the death of a patient, *Pediatr Nurs* 36(4):185–189, July-Aug 2010.

Mace SE, Mayer TA: Triage. In Baren J, Rothrock SG, Brennan J, et al, editors: *Pediatric emergency medicine*, Philadelphia, 2008, Saunders, pp 1087–1096.

Platt SR, Radaelli ST, McDonnell JJ: The prognostic value of the modified Glasgow Coma Scale in head trauma in dogs, *J Vet Intern Med* 15(6):581–584, 2001.

Rockar RA, Drobatz KJ, Shofer FS: Development of a scoring system for the veterinary trauma patient, *J Vet Emerg Crit Care* 4(2):77–84, 1994.

Santana-Cabrera L: Whats new in emergencies, trauma and shock? Study stress in emergency medicine, *J Emergency Trauma Shock* 2(3):147–149, 2009.

Sluiter JK, vanderBeck AJ, Frings-Dresen MH: Medical staff in emergency situations: severity of patient status predicts hormone reactivity and recovery, *Occup Environ Med* 60(5):373–374, May 2003; discussion p 375.

Stamm BH: Work related secondary traumatic stress, *PTSD Res Q* 8(2), 1997.

Team Strategies and Tools to Enhance Performance and Patient Safety: Available at www.teamstepps.org. Accessed July 2, 2014.

What's Your Grief: *Supporting grieving families: tips for RNs and others on the front line.* Available at www.whatsyourgrief.com /supporting-grieving-families-tips-rns-nurses. Accessed Aug 6, 2014.

Wiler J, Gentle C, Halfpenny J, et al.: Optimizing emergency department front-end operations, *Ann Emerg Med* 55(2):142–160, Feb 2010.

www.ena.org/sitecolection documents/position%20statements/us eofprotocols.pdf. Accessed July 23, 2014.

SCENARIO

Purpose: To provide the veterinary technician with the opportunity to build or strengthen the ability to quickly evaluate a situation faced in a typical emergency clinic.

Stage: Emergency clinic is considered a Level II facility and always has at least four staff members available including one ER clinician, two veterinary technicians, and one receptionist who also assist with animal handling when necessary. There is a back-up clinician on call to assist with surgeries.

Scenario

Sunday morning.

Patient 1: A 7-year-old, male German shepherd walks into the hospital at 11:00 AM. Owner is relaxed and describes dog as not wanting to lie down through the night; dog attempted to vomit once and not eating.

Initial assessment determines tachycardia (HR: 160 beats/min), pulse deficits, respiratory rate—pant, temperature 103.2° F, mucous membranes dark pink, wet with CRT of >1 sec. Dog is pacing and not wanting to sit.

Patient 2: A 4-year-old female miniature pincher is carried in by owner at 11:00 AM. Owner is very distraught, crying with visible blood on hand. Owner described incident that occurred 20 minutes ago that included an attack of the miniature pincher by a large mixed breed dog (stray).

Initial assessment determines normal TPR (T: 101.8° F, HR: 125 beats/min; RR: 36 breaths/min). Dog appears comfortable with no visible bite wounds.

Patient 3: A 2-year-old male cat is carried into the clinic in a carrier at 11:05 AM. Owner is unhappy about having to invest any time or money in this cat. Only reason for visit is because owner believes cat is in pain. Owner describes the cat walking around house howling and not eating. Initial assessment is based on visual only due to cat's aggressive behavior.

Initial assessment reveals cat is tachypneic (RR: 60 breaths/min), growling.

Patient 4: An 8-year-old male Labrador walks into hospital at 11:15 AM. Owner appears under the influence of alcohol and begins to allow his dog to greet others in the waiting area. Owner states that dog has been lame in the right back leg since he jumped off the dock this morning.

Initial assessment determines tachycardia (HR: 134 beats/min); pulses normal; respiratory rate 30 breaths/min; temperature 100.3° F; mucous membranes pink, moist. Dog is wagging tail and very interactive.

Delivery

- Write case ideas on separate cards and place cards on chairs.
- Staff reviews cards and has **3-5 minutes** to review each case.
- Questions following case evaluations are answered.
- Discussion should continue without goal being to find the right answer.

Questions

- Which patient/owner would you decide needs to be evaluated by a clinician first? Explain why.
- How would you approach each patient?
- Which patient would you complete an initial assessment including TPR? Explain why.

Continued

SCENARIO—cont'd

- How would you rate each patient before initial TPR using the nonurgent, urgent, emergency, life-threatening categories?
- Which patient would you decide needs immediate stabilization including IV catheter, IV fluids, pain management, diagnostics? Explain why.
- Which patient/owner would you decide would need to wait?
- How would you explain to owner reasons for the delay in service?
- What are the possible complications if this patient is not evaluated?
- What are the possible complications if medical intervention is delayed?
- What would you do for patient/owner who needs to wait?

Key Teaching Points

- Provides veterinary technicians opportunity to review hospital procedures and guidelines on how to approach a triage situation.
- Provides opportunity to view client as part of the evaluation.
- Veterinary technician can evaluate ability to assess situations and provides opportunity for open discussion.

References

- Triage questionnaire
- Trauma scoring system

CHAPTER OUTLINE

Types of Shock
Oxygen Delivery
Pathophysiology of Shock
  Cardiogenic Shock
  Distributive Shock
  Obstructive Shock
  Hypovolemic Shock
Initial Assessment and Recognition
  Physical Assessment
  Shock Index
  Lactate Concentration

Therapy
  Oxygen Therapy
  Venous Access
  Fluid Resuscitation
  Sympathomimetics
Monitoring
  Physiologic Monitoring Parameters
  Laboratory Parameters
Summary

KEY TERMS

Cardiac output
Lactate
Oxygenation
Resuscitation
Shock

LEARNING OBJECTIVES

After studying this chapter, you will be able to:

- Define and understand the types of shock.
- Understand the different treatment for types of shock.
- Recognize shock.

The veterinary technician plays an integral role in the management of the emergent or critically ill patient. Many of these patients suffer a disease process associated with inadequate tissue perfusion, resulting in poor oxygen delivery. The condition is often assessed as **shock**. Shock is defined as inadequate cellular energy production. Shock most commonly occurs secondary to poor tissue perfusion from low or unevenly distributed blood flow that causes a critical decrease in oxygen delivery in relation to oxygen consumption (de Laforcade and Silverstein, 2014). Shock has been typically classified into several categories (e.g., cardiogenic, septic, hypovolemic), and the causes of shock are numerous. Regardless of the form of shock, the goal is to optimize oxygen delivery. This discussion provides an overview of the determinants of oxygen delivery and a review of the pathophysiology, assessment, and the management of shock.

TYPES OF SHOCK

Many different categorization schemes have been used to define shock. In some instances, overlap between categories exists. For the purposes of this discussion, shock is categorized into four different forms based on the causative pathophysiologic mechanism. Ultimately, the focus of therapy will be to optimize oxygen delivery. *Cardiogenic* shock is a form of shock that results from heart failure but excludes those factors outside the heart (i.e., cardiac tamponade, caval syndrome). Pump failure may be caused by hypertrophic or dilative cardiomyopathy, valvular insufficiency or stenosis, arrhythmias, or fibrosis. *Distributive* shock is often used to describe shock states associated with flow maldistribution. Initiating causes for this form of shock include sepsis, anaphylaxis, trauma, and neurogenic problems. *Obstructive* shock results from a physical obstruction in the circulatory system. Heartworm disease, pericardial effusion, pulmonary embolism, and gastric torsion can all contribute to impaired blood flow. *Hypovolemic* shock is the result of decreased intravascular volume. The decreased volume may be caused by blood loss, third-space loss, or fluid losses because of excessive vomiting, diarrhea, and diuresis. Hypovolemic shock is the most common form of shock seen in small animals.

TECHNICIAN NOTE It is important for the technician to understand the different types of shock, because each type will be treated differently.

OXYGEN DELIVERY

Oxygen delivery (DO_2) represents the amount or volume of oxygen transported to the tissues each minute. DO_2 is the product of cardiac output and the oxygen content in arterial blood (CaO_2). Calculating DO_2 is not possible in most practice situations. However, the concept is important, and several components of DO_2 (Figure 13-1) can be addressed. **Cardiac output** is the product of stroke volume and heart rate. To improve or increase cardiac output, the heart rate or stroke volume has to increase. Stroke volume is the amount of blood pumped out of the heart with each beat, and three primary determinants of stoke volume exist. Stroke volume is increased in proportion to (1) the stretch of the walls of the ventricles during diastole (preload), (2) the strength

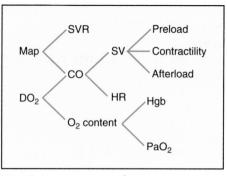

FIGURE 13-1 Determinants of DO_2. *CO,* Cardiac output; *Hgb,* hemoglobin; *HR,* heart rate; *Map,* mean arterial pressure; *PaO_2,* partial pressure of oxygen; *SV,* stroke volume; *SVR,* systemic vascular resistance.

$$CaO_2 = (1.34 \times Hb \times SaO_2) + (PaO_2 \times 0.003)$$

FIGURE 13-2 Oxygen content (CaO_2) equation.

of contraction (contractility), and (3) the decrease in the forces that oppose blood flow from the heart (afterload).

Oxygen content (CaO_2) is the amount of oxygen in arterial blood. Oxygen is either dissolved in plasma or bound to hemoglobin (Hb). CaO_2 is defined by the equation in Figure 13-2.

Hb is the main carrier of oxygen in the blood. Each gram of Hb has the capacity to carry 1.34 ml of oxygen, which is 20.1 ml of oxygen per deciliter of blood when the Hb concentration is 15 g/dl (150 g/L). Only 0.3 ml of oxygen per deciliter blood is dissolved in the plasma when the partial pressure of oxygen in arterial blood (PaO_2) is 100 mm Hg.

PATHOPHYSIOLOGY OF SHOCK

CARDIOGENIC SHOCK

Several factors come into play with regards to cardiogenic shock: they include ineffective forward blood flow, structural problems, arrhythmias, and decreased myocardial perfusion. The end result is poor tissue perfusion and oxygen delivery. Cardiogenic shock results when forward flow failure causes inadequate tissue perfusion despite adequate intravascular volume; in this case cellular energy demands are not met. Cardiogenic shock ensues from alterations in the determinants of stroke volume (preload, contractility, and afterload). Either systolic or diastolic dysfunction may result in decreased stroke volume and cardiogenic shock.

Potential causes of systolic dysfunction include dilated cardiomyopathy (DCM), or structural causes (stenosis, hypertrophic cardiomyopathy, and backflow regurgitation). DCM results in poor contractility leading to decreased stroke volume and forward flow. Reduced forward flow may also result from stenosis (obstructive) or hypertrophic cardiomyopathy (diastolic failure). Valvular insufficiency may result in a backflow regurgitation that can reduce forward flow sufficiently to result in cardiogenic and pulmonary edema.

Diastolic dysfunction may be caused by hypertrophic cardiomyopathy and arrhythmias. Hypertrophic cardiomyopathy results in a decreased end-diastolic volume (preload) because of the inability of the myocardium to relax. The resultant decreased preload leads to a decreased stroke volume and cardiac output.

Arrhythmias can result in poor preload or reduced contractility. Tachyarrhythmias do not allow the heart sufficient time to fill, causing decreased end-diastolic volume and resulting in decreased stroke volume and cardiac output. Poor cardiac output can result in poor myocardial perfusion, which may result in poor contractility and arrhythmias and worsen cardiac dysfunction.

DISTRIBUTIVE SHOCK

A state of distributive shock has occurred in those cases in which the vascular compartment expands (vasodilation), a normal volume of blood is insufficient to fill the compartment, and blood is displaced away from the heart and central circulation. Preload is diminished and ultimately stroke volume and cardiac output are decreased but not a total decrease in blood volume. The expansion of the vascular compartment is due to a loss of vessel tone. Two mechanisms contribute to a loss of vessel tone: a decrease in sympathetic control of vasomotor tone and the presence of vasodilatory mediators.

Sepsis, anaphylaxis, and neurogenic states can lead to distributive shock. Sepsis is the systemic inflammatory response to an infection. In sepsis, various mediators are released that affect capillary permeability and the distribution of blood flow to the tissues and organs. Prostaglandin is one example of a mediator that is released and can cause vasodilation. Anaphylaxis is a result of an immune-mediated response to something, such as an insect venom or drug. The immune mediated

response is the release of a vasodilatory mediator such as histamine. These mediators cause an increase in capillary permeability, and dilation of arterioles and venules. Disruption of the sympathetic nervous system can also result in a loss of vasomotor tone. Output from the vasomotor center of the brainstem can be disrupted by hypoxia, depressant drugs, or hypoglycemia. The end result of this neurogenic response is a decreased preload, decreased stroke volume, decreased cardiac output, and finally decreased DO_2. In summary, distributive shock is inappropriate vasodilation, which leads to a relative hypovolemia or the failure of effective vasoconstriction.

OBSTRUCTIVE SHOCK

In obstructive shock there is a mechanical obstruction of blood flow in the vascular system. The obstruction can occur in the great vessels, heart, or lungs. The location, degree of obstruction, and resulting compromise to systemic perfusion are important determinants of whether flow occlusion will lead to shock. Elevated right heart pressures (central venous pressure [CVP]) and impaired venous return (preload) may be seen.

HYPOVOLEMIC SHOCK

Hypovolemic shock is a complex and dynamic process involving many compensatory mechanisms. An initiating cause results in a decreased intravascular volume. As a result of the decreased intravascular volume, venous return and ventricular filling (i.e., preload) are decreased. With the decreased ventricular filling, decreased stroke volume and cardiac output occur. The end result is inadequate tissue perfusion and oxygen delivery.

Decreased cardiac output and hypotension cause a baroreceptor-mediated sympathoadrenal reflex that activates the patient's compensatory mechanisms to help maintain perfusion. Norepinephrine, epinephrine, and cortisol are released from the adrenal gland. Epinephrine and norepinephrine cause an increase in heart rate and contractility and arteriolar constriction (which increases systemic vascular resistance and redirects blood flow to the heart and brain and away from skin, muscles, kidneys, and gastrointestinal tract). Cortisol enhances the effects of the catecholamines on arterioles. Sodium and water are conserved, because of renin-angiotensin-aldosterone system activation, causing an increased intravascular volume.

INITIAL ASSESSMENT AND RECOGNITION

The initial recognition of shock is based on historical and physical findings. There are other tools available for patient assessment of perfusion; they include shock index and lactate concentration. Historically, the owner may be able to provide information that supports a reason for hypovolemia, such as trauma, excessive urination, diarrhea, or vomiting.

PHYSICAL ASSESSMENT

There are six physical examination perfusion parameters (Table 13-1) that allow a rapid evaluation of the circulatory status. Keep in mind that circulatory shock is a clinical diagnosis. These clinical findings should be evaluated in combination; an abnormality in a single parameter does not have the clinical significance of multiple abnormalities.

1. *Mentation*

    A reduced level of mentation is indicated by a loss of interest in the surrounding environment and diminished or absent responses to stimuli such as noise and touch. This can be described as obtundation or depression. Because depression implies an assessment of the animal's emotional state, obtundation may be a more appropriate term. If there is a loss of consciousness it is considered to be either stupor or coma. Stupor refers to a patient that is unconscious and only responsive to noxious stimuli. Coma refers to a completely unconscious, nonresponsive state. Unconscious animals may require intubation to protect their airway.

    An altered level of mentation can be the result of primary intracranial disease or significant systemic abnormalities such as hypoperfusion or hypoglycemia. Any abnormality in mentation should be considered serious and a complete triage examination is warranted immediately.

2. *Mucous membrane color*

    Pale or white mucous membranes are a consequence of a reduced quantity of red blood cells perfusing the capillary beds of the mucosal tissue. This can be the result of vasoconstriction in compensation to circulatory shock or severe anemia. This abnormality in combination with other evidence of poor perfusion or inadequate tissue **oxygenation** warrants emergency intervention.

    Vasodilation will increase the flow of blood through the mucous membranes, changing the membranes' color to deep pink to red. Vasodilation may be an appropriate response as seen in a hyperthermic animal post exercise or it can be pathologic as seen in vasodilatory shock. Patients with vasodilatory shock commonly present with concurrent hypovolemia and therefore will often have pale mucous membranes; it is only after adequate fluid **resuscitation** that red mucous membranes are noted.

3. *Capillary refill time*

    Capillary refill time (CRT), the time it takes for mucous membranes to regain their color following blanching by digital pressure, is a reflection of local blood flow. When perfusion is normal, CRT is 1 to 2 seconds. Vasoconstriction will reduce the flow of blood through the mucous membranes via arteriolar and precapillary sphincter contraction and it will take longer for the color to return to the tissue after blanching. In severe vasoconstriction when the mucous membranes appear white, it is often impossible to appreciate any CRT. In patients with vasodilation the CRT can be more rapid than normal since there is less resistance to blood flow and the capillary beds rapidly refill with blood after the digital pressure is removed. A slow CRT is always a concern and suggestive of poor perfusion. A rapid CRT in conjunction with other perfusion abnormalities can suggest vasodilatory shock.

4. *Heart rate*

    The normal heart rate of an animal varies with body size. In general, large breed adult dogs have resting heart rates of 60 to 140 beats per minute (beats/min); medium adult dogs have heart rates of 70 to

TABLE 13-1	Perfusion Parameters
PARAMETER	
Mentation	
Mucous membrane color	
Capillary refill time	
Heart rate	
Pulse quality	
Extremity temperature	

160 beats/min; and small dogs, puppies, and cats are in the range of 100 to 220 bpm. When arterial blood pressure is threatened either by a drop in stroke volume or as a result of vasodilation, there will be a baroreceptor-mediated increase in sympathetic tone resulting in a reflex tachycardia. Because tachycardia is a normal response to anxiety, excitement, and exercise, it is a common physical examination finding. The presence of tachycardia in conjunction with other signs of abnormal perfusion (vasoconstriction or vasodilation) is suggestive of hemodynamic compromise.

Tachycardia is the appropriate and expected response to circulatory shock. The presence of normocardia or bradycardia in canine shock patients (i.e., patients with abnormalities of the other five parameters) is of concern because it suggests decompensated shock and is associated with greater severity of illness and a poorer prognosis. Feline shock patients will often present without tachycardia and this is not considered to have prognostic relevance as it does in dogs.

Auscultable arrhythmias may or may not require immediate medical therapy. Femoral pulse evaluation should be performed simultaneously with auscultation for both time efficiency and recognition of pulse deficits. Arrhythmias without any other signs of poor perfusion are far less concerning, but these patients should always be prioritized for a secondary evaluation including an electrocardiogram (ECG) since the clinical evaluation of these abnormalities is considerably limited.

5. *Pulse quality*

Pulse quality is subjectively determined by the digital palpation of the femoral pulse. Obvious abnormalities in pulse quality are concerning and if present in conjunction with other signs of poor perfusion the patient should receive immediate medical attention. Unfortunately, patients can have considerable hemodynamic compromise without palpable changes in pulse quality. As a result, the palpation of an adequate femoral pulse cannot be used to indicate a stable patient.

The pulse quality is determined by the difference between diastolic and systolic arterial blood pressures as well as the duration of the pulse and the size of the vessel. The greater the diastolic-systolic difference the "stronger" the pulse will feel. For example,

a normal arterial blood pressure would be a systolic blood pressure of 120 mm Hg, a mean of 85 mm Hg, and a diastolic of 70 mm Hg. The systolic-diastolic pressure difference (pulse pressure) is 50 mm Hg. If there is a fall in blood pressure such that the patient is hypotensive with a systolic pressure of 90 mm Hg, mean of 55 mm Hg, and diastolic of 40 mm Hg, the pulse pressure would still reflect a systolic-diastolic difference of 50 mm Hg. The examiner may be challenged to detect the change in pulse quality.

Vasoconstriction will tend to diminish palpable pulse quality—the "thready pulse." In contrast, vasodilation will increase vessel size and compliance. In addition, vasodilated patients usually have an elevated stroke volume such that the pulse quality is often appreciated to be normal or exaggerated (bounding) in these patients.

6. *Extremity temperature*

The sympathetic-mediated vasoconstriction that occurs in response to a drop in cardiac output will tend to shunt blood from venous capacitance vessels to the central circulation, preserving blood flow to vital organs at the expense of less vital tissue. This reduction in peripheral circulation will cause a fall in extremity temperature in comparison with core body temperature. If the patient is generally hypothermic, cool extremities that are essentially the same temperature as the rest of the animal do not indicate an abnormality in perfusion. For this reason the temperature of the extremities (evaluated by digital palpation of the paws and distal limbs) should always be interpreted with reference to the measured body temperature. Vasodilation will be associated with warm extremities if the patient is fluid resuscitated.

The clinical signs seen during shock may differ because of changes in vasomotor tone (Table 13-2). Typically, the physical findings are indicative of sympathoadrenal activation (tachycardia and vasoconstriction). In the early stage or compensatory phase of shock, tachycardia, decreased pulse quality, prolonged capillary refill time (CRT), pale mucous membrane (MM) color, and cool extremities are seen. This may be called *stage I, compensated shock.* In *stage II, decompensated shock,* the patient is tachycardic and has decreased pulse quality, variable CRT, "muddy" mucous membrane color,

TABLE 13-2	Changes in Clinical Signs due to Changes in Vasomotor Tone	
CLINICAL SIGNS	**VASOCONSTRICTION**	**VASODILATION**
Mentation	Altered	Altered
MM color	Pale to white	Injected (brick red)
CRT	Slow to absent	Fast
Heart rate	Increased	Increased
Pulse quality	Poor	Bounding
Extremity temp	Cool	Warm

decreasing BP, and obtunded mental status. When the patient is suffering from severe systemic hypoperfusion and therapies cease to be effective, the patient is said to be in *stage III, irreversible shock*. The stages of shock are a continuum. Progression through the stages is based on patient-related factors, as well as the timeliness and effectiveness of therapy.

Patients with vasodilatory shock can have red mucous membranes, rapid CRT, bounding pulses, and warm extremities. Because these animals are likely to present with concurrent hypovolemia these signs of vasodilation may not be evident until after adequate fluid resuscitation.

> **TECHNICIAN NOTE** Remember that each of these clinical signs can be seen independent of the others, and not associated with shock. When all six are present, however, even in varying degrees, an animal can be suspected to be in shock.

SHOCK INDEX

The shock index (SI) is a tool that was developed in human medicine as a simple means to quantify the severity of shock and the response to therapy in the emergency room. The SI is the ratio of heart rate (HR) to systolic blood pressure (SBP). It is calculated by dividing the HR by the SBP (SI = HR/SBP). This tool may be advantageous in that it may identify poor perfusion states in the face of seemingly normal cardiovascular parameters. While the majority of work has looked at the hemorrhagic porcine model and people, work has also been conducted in dogs (Peterson et al, 2013; Porter et al, 2013). In one study, an SI of >1.0 was a highly sensitive

and specific indicator to distinguish emergency room dogs not in shock and healthy dogs from dogs with biochemical evidence of moderate to severe shock (Porter et al, 2013). The other study showed that an SI of 0.9 had high sensitivity but low specificity as a triage tool (Peterson et al, 2013). While there was some overlap and limitations in the studies SI can be used along with physical exam findings as an additional tool for assessment.

LACTATE CONCENTRATION

Hyperlactatemia is an increased **lactate** concentration. Lactic acidosis is the result of hyperlactatemia and a decrease in systemic blood pH. Lactic acidosis may be classified in one of two subclassifications: type A and type B (Pang and Boysen, 2007). Type A lactic acidosis can be subclassified as that resulting from inadequate DO_2 or increased oxygen demand. Shock is a classic example of decreased DO_2. Type B lactic acidosis can be subclassified into inadequate utilization of oxygen and several other subcategories. Systemic inflammatory response and sepsis are potential causes for inadequate oxygen utilization. When perfusion decreases and DO_2 is reduced, the body shifts from aerobic to anaerobic metabolism, resulting in lactate formation. Hyperlactatemia (lactate >2 mmol/L) has been proposed as an indicator of inadequate tissue oxygenation. Although elevated blood lactate levels often signify generalized tissue hypoxia, a normal value does not rule out regional lactate production. Detection of increased lactate concentrations with or without acidosis should raise the index of suspicion for hypoperfusion.

THERAPY

The goal of therapy is to improve oxygen delivery. The veterinary technician's focus should be directed at correcting or improving the components of the oxygen delivery algorithm (see Figure 13-1).

OXYGEN THERAPY

Maintaining oxygen saturation is one of the primary goals in maintaining blood oxygenation. If any question exists concerning a patient's blood oxygenation, then supplemental oxygen should be provided until assessment of arterial blood gases or hemoglobin (Hb) saturation confirms that oxygen supplementation is not necessary. When this equipment is not available, assessment will have to be based on clinical signs of respiratory

TABLE 13-3	Fluid Flow Rates Based on Catheter Gauge and Height of Fluid Bag	
	HEIGHT, 3 FEET	**HEIGHT, 6 FEET**
CATHETER GAUGE	**FLOW RATE (ml/min)**	**FLOW RATE (ml/min)**
16	88	152
18	75	114
20	45	75

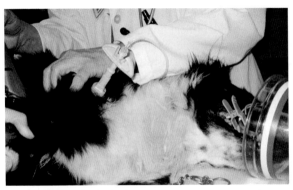

FIGURE 13-3 Fluid administration via intraosseous catheter.

distress or auscultable abnormalities and clinical signs of hypoxemia: cyanosis of the mucous membranes or dark-colored blood, tachypnea, tachycardia, and anxiety. Individually, the clinical signs do not prove hypoxemia, but together they are suggestive of hypoxemia.

VENOUS ACCESS

Selection of a vein to catheterize depends on several factors, such as the size and species of the animal, the skill of the operator placing the catheter, the therapeutic goals, and the animal's problem or disease. Any vessel that is visible or palpable should be considered a candidate for percutaneous catheterization. The cephalic and saphenous veins offer easily accessible routes that can be catheterized quickly. The internal diameter and the length of the catheter and the height of the fluid bag above the patient primarily determine the maximum fluid flow rate of a catheter (Table 13-3) (Fulton and Hauptman, 1991).

A short, large-gauge catheter is needed if fluids are to be rapidly administered. Keeping administration tubing short is also advisable, as well as avoiding excessive use of extension tubing and unnecessary connectors that reduce flow rates.

In the event vascular access cannot be obtained, the establishment of an intraosseous line (Figure 13-3) is a reasonable alternative. Fluid or drugs administered by this route are rapidly absorbed into the circulatory system.

> *TECHNICIAN NOTE* A short, large-gauge catheter is always the best choice for fluid resuscitation, but you can successfully use ANY size that you are able to get into the patient rapidly. Ideally, avoid 24 gauge because the impedance to flow is too large; but, 22- to 18-gauge catheters will often allow sufficient volume to reverse shock until a larger catheter can be obtained.

FLUID RESUSCITATION

The most effective way to improve oxygen delivery is to increase cardiac output by optimizing preload with the administration of fluid.

Crystalloids

Isotonic crystalloids, which have electrolyte concentrations (i.e., sodium, chloride, potassium, and bicarbonate-like anions) similar to those of extracellular fluid, are commonly used in the treatment of hypovolemic shock. These fluids freely and rapidly distribute between the intravascular and interstitial compartments. After 30 minutes, 98% of the volume of fluids infused into the intravascular compartment shifts into the interstitial compartment. Examples of commonly used crystalloids include lactated Ringer's, normal saline, Plasma-Lyte A pH 7.4 (Abbott Laboratories, North Chicago, IL), and Plasma-Lyte 148 (Baxter, Deerfield, IL). A commonly cited "shock" fluid dose of isotonic crystalloids is 80 to 90 ml/kg/hr for the dog and 50 to 55 ml/kg/hr for the cat (equivalent to 1 blood volume). Individual animal requirements are variable; increments of one fourth to one third of the calculated shock dose can be given and the patient reassessed at the end of each bolus. Frequently reassessing the patient's condition (i.e., about every 5 to 10 minutes) is necessary during large- or rapid-volume fluid administration. Many cases may not require the full "shock" dose of fluids for resuscitation whereas other cases may require greater volumes to effectively resuscitate the patient.

Hypertonic crystalloids such as 7.5% saline have been recommended for use in shock therapy in cases in which it is difficult to administer large volumes of fluids rapidly enough to resuscitate the patient. Hypertonic saline causes fluid shifts from the intracellular space to the extracellular (including intravascular) space, resulting in improved venous return and cardiac output. Hypertonic saline also causes microvascular vasodilation and improves tissue perfusion. It is also thought that hypertonic saline may be beneficial in the treatment of traumatic brain injury by reducing brain edema. The recommended dose ranges are 4 to 6 ml/kg and 3 to 4 ml/kg in dogs and cats, respectively, given over 5 minutes. Very rapid administration of hypertonic saline can cause vasodilation and cardiovascular collapse, so it is essential to give the dose slowly over 5 minutes. Hypertonic saline does not replenish the volume deficit of a hypovolemic patient and isotonic fluid resuscitation is still required. Synthetic colloids, such as 6% Hetastarch (Hospira, Lake Forest, IL), have been added to hypertonic saline to potentiate and sustain vascular volume augmentation. There are growing concerns regarding the safety of synthetic colloids and they are no longer recommended for routine resuscitation.

> **TECHNICIAN NOTE**　Hypotonic fluids such as 5% dextrose in water, half-strength saline, and half-strength lactated Ringer's should not be used to treat hypovolemic shock. These fluids contain too much free water and distribute excessively to the intracellular compartment.

Colloids

Colloids are high molecular weight solutions that do not cross capillary membranes readily. Colloids are better blood volume expanders than are isotonic crystalloids, because 50% to 80% of the infused volume remains in the intravascular space. Human studies have been unable to demonstrate that use of synthetic colloids such as Hetastarch or Tetrastarch in shock resuscitation is advantageous compared with isotonic crystalloids. Because synthetic colloids can cause coagulation defects and have been associated with kidney injury, they are not recommended for routine treatment of hypovolemia. It may be necessary to use colloids for the resuscitation of hypoproteinemic patients. When the total protein or albumin levels are decreased to less than 3.5 g/dl (35 g/L) or 1.5 g/dl (15 g/L), respectively, it may be difficult to maintain intravascular volume with isotonic crystalloids alone. Colloids include plasma, and the synthetics— 6% Hetastarch (HES), Hextend, Voluven (Hospira,

Lake Forest, IL), and VetStarch™ (Abbott Laboratories, North Chicago, IL). Plasma provides albumin, immunoglobulins, platelets, and clotting factors. The approximate dose of plasma is 10 to 30 ml/kg; however, it should be administered to effect. Large volumes of plasma are required to affect a change in total protein or albumin concentrations, which is often not economical.

Whole Blood or Packed Red Blood Cells

Red blood cells are the source for Hb. Hb must be available in sufficient concentrations to ensure adequate CaO_2. If Hb concentration decreases from 15 g/dl (150 g/L) to 10 g/dl (100 g/L), then CaO_2 is reduced by one third; cardiac output will need to increase to maintain adequate delivery of oxygen (see Figure 13-1). In the absence of Hb level measurements, Hb concentration can be estimated from the micohematocrit (micro-HCT). The Hb level is usually about one third of the HCT values. Oxygen delivery is limited when the HCT decreases below 20%. When treating hemorrhagic shock, whole blood and packed red blood cells are administered at 10 to 30 ml/kg and 5 to 15 ml/kg, respectively; again, this will need to be administered to effect. These doses will increase the HCT level by approximately 5% to 15%.

SYMPATHOMIMETICS

Sympathomimetics, such as dopamine (American Regent, Shirley, NY) and dobutamine (Hospira, Lake Forest, IL), are indicated when the patient is unresponsive to vigorous fluid therapy and arterial BP, vasomotor tone, and tissue perfusion have not returned to acceptable levels. These drugs support myocardial contractility and BP. BP monitoring is recommended. Dopamine, a precursor of norepinephrine, has dose-dependent effects. At 0.5 to 3.0 mcg/kg/min, dilation of renal, mesenteric, and coronary vascular beds will occur because of the dopaminergic effect. Increase of heart rate or contractility (or both) is seen at a dose range of 3.0 to 7.5 mcg/kg/min (a result of beta$_1$ activity). At doses greater than 7.5 mcg/kg/min, alpha-receptor stimulation and vasoconstriction occur. Dobutamine has primarily beta activity. It increases cardiac contractility and has minimal effect on heart rate and peripheral vascular resistance except at higher doses. The dose range is 2 to 15 mcg/kg/min. Sympathomimetics should not be a substitute for adequate volume restoration. Fluid resuscitation remains the cornerstone of shock therapy.

Dosage (µg/kg/min) × (kg) (body weight) = Drug (mg) to place in 250 ml/fluids

Administer at 15 ml/hr

FIGURE 13-4 Quick formula for calculating microgram per kilogram per minute constant rate infusions.

BOX 13-1 | **Summary of Therapy to Improve Oxygen Delivery (DO$_2$)***

Correct Primary Problem
- Control fluid loss
- Treat infection

Oxygenation
- Provide supplemental oxygen (mask, nasal or transtracheal catheter, cage)

Fluid Resuscitation
- Crystalloids
  Dogs: 80-90 ml/kg (dosed to effect)
  Cats: 50-55 ml/kg (dosed to effect)
- 7.5% hypertonic saline
  Dogs: 4-6 ml/kg
  Cats: 3-4 ml/kg
- Synthetic colloids
  Dogs: 10-20 ml/kg
  Cats: 5 ml/kg increments over 15 to 20 minutes
- 7.5% hypertonic saline and synthetic colloid
  Dogs: 1.5-3 and 3-6 ml/kg
  Cats: 1.5 and 3 ml/kg
- Plasma 10-30 ml/kg
- Whole blood 10-30 ml/kg
- Red blood cells 5-15 ml/kg

*NOTE: All fluids given to effect. Consider sympathomimetics—dopamine 5-10 mcg/kg/min, dobutamine 2-15 mcg/kg/min.

The technician should be able to calculate constant rate infusions using the formula shown in Figure 13-4.

The goal of therapy is to improve perfusion so that oxygen can be delivered to the tissues. Many options are available to achieve this goal (Box 13-1).

MONITORING

Many of the signs associated with shock are related to the compensatory mechanism the body invokes to maintain life. Frequently assessing clinical signs is important because the hemodynamic and metabolic sequelae of shock are continually changing. The monitoring process

begins with the reassessment of the perfusion parameters and is integrated with physiologic monitoring and evaluation of cellular function (acid-base balance and other laboratory values).

PHYSIOLOGIC MONITORING PARAMETERS

Oxygen Saturation

Hb saturation measured by pulse oximetry (SpO$_2$) provides noninvasive and continuous information about the percent of oxygen bound to Hb. Normal SpO$_2$ is greater than 95%. The patient is seriously hypoxemic when the SpO$_2$ is less than or equal to 90%. Caution should be exercised when interpreting SpO$_2$ values with animals breathing 100% oxygen. Animals with a Pao$_2$ of 500 mm Hg still show SpO$_2$ values ranging from 98% to 99%.

Arterial Blood Pressure

Arterial blood pressure (measured by indirect and direct methods) is the product of stroke volume, HR, and systemic vascular resistance (vasomotor tone). Should one of the three become subnormal, the other two determinants should compensate. Normal systolic, diastolic, and mean blood pressure values are approximately 100 to 160, 60 to 100, and 80 to 120 mm Hg, respectively. Systolic and mean BPs less than 90 and 60 mm Hg, respectively, warrant therapy. Causes of hypotension include hypovolemia, peripheral vasodilation, and decreased cardiac output. Hypertension may be caused by chronic renal failure, the presence of an adrenal tumor, pheochromocytoma, or any other factor that causes increased cardiac output.

Electrocardiogram

Tachycardia and bradycardia have several causes, some of which may be related to abnormal rhythms. If arrhythmias are auscultated, then an ECG is indicated.

Central Venous Pressure

Central venous pressure (CVP) is the BP in the intrathoracic anterior vena cava compared with a column of water in a plastic manometer or a pressure transducer and oscilloscope. Changes in pressure in the thorax produce fluctuations in the water manometer or waveforms on the oscilloscope. CVP is a measure of the heart's ability to pump fluids returned to it and is also an estimate of the relationship of blood volume to blood volume capacity. CVP should be measured when heart failure is suspected or as an aid in determining the endpoint to aggressive fluid therapy. Clinicians generally assume that a reasonable preload has been achieved when the CVP approaches 10 cm of water (7.5 mm Hg). If cardiac output, pulse quality, BP, and perfusion parameters are acceptable, the clinician can assume that effective blood volume restoration has been accomplished. If not, then the clinician can assume that the heart is unable to handle the venous return.

Urinary Output

Bladder size can be monitored either by palpation or by ultrasound. In some cases a urinary catheter may be warranted. Normal urine production is 1 to 2 ml/kg/hr; it decreases when perfusion is decreased or when mean arterial blood pressure is less than 60 mm Hg.

LABORATORY PARAMETERS
Hematocrit and Total Protein

HCT and total protein (TP) measurements can be used to gauge fluid therapy, estimate Hb concentration, and, to a certain degree, assess blood loss. The two tests should be interpreted together to minimize errors in interpretation. Increases in both HCT and TP values indicate dehydration; decreases in both HCT and TP levels are suggestive of recent blood loss or clear fluid administration. Increase in TP amount and normal HCT measurements may indicate anemia with dehydration. Both HCT and TP measurements may be normal in peracute blood loss. TP level may decrease with reduced albumin levels; albumin is a contributor to oncotic pressure.

Electrolytes

Electrolytes play a major role in the maintenance of extracellular compartmental water balance and cell function. Baseline electrolyte levels should be obtained and monitoring should be continued as therapy progresses. Fluid therapy can alter various serum electrolyte concentrations, and may require adjustment of the electrolyte composition in the fluids being administered. Commonly measured electrolytes include serum potassium, sodium, chloride, magnesium, and ionized calcium.

Blood Gases and pH

Arterial blood gases are an excellent way to assess ventilation and oxygenation. Testing $PaCO_2$ reveals how well the patient is ventilating the lungs. A $PaCO_2$ value less than 35 mm Hg or greater than 45 mm Hg indicates hyperventilation or hypoventilation, respectively. Testing PaO_2 levels reveals how well the patient is oxygenating. A PaO_2 value less than 80 mm Hg is considered hypoxemia, and a PaO_2 measurement approaching 60 mm Hg is severe hypoxemia. Arterial or venous pH combined with bicarbonate or base balance reveals the metabolic acid-base status of the patient. Normal pH is 7.35 to 7.45; a pH less than 7.35 is termed *acidemia,* and a pH greater than 7.45 is termed *alkalemia.* A patient has metabolic acidosis if the bicarbonate level is less than 18 mmol/L or the base deficit is more negative than −4. Alkalosis is identified by bicarbonate concentrations greater than 27 mmol/L and a base excess greater than +4.

Jugular venous PO_2 samples less than 30 mm Hg or greater than 60 mm Hg may be caused by decreased oxygen delivery to the tissues and reduced oxygen uptake by the tissues, respectively. No correlation exists between venous PO_2 and arterial PO_2 measurements.

Colloid Osmotic Pressure

Colloid osmotic pressure (COP) can be measured and used to guide fluid therapy. COP is a force created by large plasma proteins that do not move freely across capillaries. The presence of colloids in the vascular space keeps fluid in the vascular space and reduces the likelihood of fluid redistributing to the interstitial space. Normal COP is 20 to 25 mm Hg; the goal is to maintain a COP greater than 18 mm Hg.

SUMMARY

Shock is a dynamic and complex syndrome; the focus of therapy and monitoring is oxygen delivery. To improve the CaO_2 component of oxygen delivery, the veterinary technician might administer oxygen or Hb in the form of packed red blood cells or whole blood. To improve the cardiac output component, the technician might administer fluids in the form of crystalloids or colloids that, in turn, improve preload. Drug therapy may also be needed to improve contractility and heart rate and, in some cases, to reduce afterload. By improving cardiac output and systemic vascular resistance the patient's BP is improved. Having a basic understanding of the pathophysiologic and compensatory mechanism of this complex syndrome will aid the veterinary technician in meeting therapeutic and monitoring goals.

REFERENCES

de Laforcade A, Silverstein DC: Shock. In Silverstein DC, Hopper K, editors: *Small animal critical care medicine*, ed 2, St Louis, 2014, Elsevier, pp 26–30.

Fulton RB, Hauptman JG: In vitro and in vivo rates of fluid flow through catheters in peripheral veins of dogs, *J Am Vet Med Assoc* 98(9):1622–1624, 1991.

Pang DS, Boysen S: Lactate in veterinary critical care: pathophysiology and management, *J Am Anim Hosp Assoc* 43:270–279, 2007.

Peterson KL, Hardy BT, Hall K: Assessment of shock index in healthy dogs and dogs in hemorrhagic shock, *J Vet Emerg Crit Care* 23(5):545–550, 2013.

Porter AE, Rozanski EA, Sharp CR, et al.: Evaluation of the shock index in dogs presenting as emergencies, *J Vet Emerg Crit Care* 23(5):538–544, 2013.

SCENARIO

Purpose: To provide the veterinary team with examples of how to simulate patient assessment.

Stage: A small animal practice with a team of five members: one veterinarian, two credentialed veterinary technicians, one veterinary assistant, and one receptionist.

Scenario

Late afternoon walk-in 2 hours before closing—there is no medical supervision after-hours.

A 30-kg mixed breed dog was hit by a car 20 minutes ago. On presentation you find that it has a RR of 60 breaths/min and shallow; absent breath sounds; HR of 180 bpm; poor pulse quality; CRT >2 seconds; cool extremities; mucous membranes are pale; obtunded; pupils are equal and responsive; systolic BP 70 mm Hg; and temperature 100° F (37.7° C).

Questions

Group discussion, using the following discussion points:

1. How should the receptionist respond when presented with an emergency?
2. What is the triage technician's assessment of the patient?
   a. Are there any airway, breathing, circulatory, neurologic, or other life-threatening problems?
3. What should be done immediately for the patient?
   a. The technician should anticipate what the veterinarian will want to do based on the assessment.
   b. Think in terms of the problems that have been identified.
4. How can you tell the therapy is improving the patient's condition?
5. Assuming the patient has been stabilized, what follow-up care should be provided?
   a. Consider if the veterinarian will want to perform further diagnostics.
   b. What type of continued monitoring should be performed? (Think respiratory, cardiovascular, and neurologic.)
   c. What are the patient's comfort needs?
   d. What are the nursing concerns for the patient?
6. What are the options for continued care when the clinic closes?

Key Teaching Points

1. Provides the veterinary healthcare team the opportunity to review procedures for handling the emergency patient.
2. Enhances the triage and assessment skills of veterinary technicians/assistants.
3. Encourages the technician to be proactive and anticipate the needs of the patient and veterinarian.

MEDICAL MATH EXERCISE

What is the shock index of a dog with a heart rate of 200 beats/min and a systolic blood pressure of 60 mm Hg?

    a. 0.033
    b. 0.33
    c. 3.3

KEY TERMS

Agonal breaths
Cardiopulmonary arrest
Compressions
Defibrillation

CHAPTER OUTLINE

Preparation
  Staff
  Facilities
  Equipment
Recognition
Phase One: Basic Life Support
  Mechanism of Blood Flow
  Chest Compressions
  Ventilation

Assessing Effectiveness
Advanced Life Support
Drugs
Defibrillation
Precordial Thump
Cardiac Rhythms
Phase Three: Post–Cardiac Arrest
  Care
Summary

LEARNING OBJECTIVES

After studying this chapter, you will be able to:

- Understand the definition of cardiopulmonary arrest (CPA).
- Understand how to prepare for CPA.
- Identify patients who are at risk for CPA.
- Understand the correct way to administer compressions during CPR.
- Provide an introduction to the RECOVER project.

Cardiopulmonary arrest (CPA) is the sudden cessation of spontaneous and effective ventilation and systemic perfusion (circulation). CPA may be a result of any disease process carried out to its extreme that disrupts cardiac or pulmonary homeostasis (or both). Potential causes of CPA include hypoxia, metabolic disorders, trauma, vagal stimulation, anesthetic or other drugs, and environmental influences (i.e., hypothermia or hyperthermia). In a recent study the most common cause of CPA in dogs and cats was reported to be cardiovascular failure including hypovolemia, hemorrhage, and anemia. Respiratory failure was the second most common cause (McIntyre et al, 2014).

In another study, CPA was associated with anesthesia with or without preexisting diseases in 55% of the animals, cardiovascular collapse in 28% of the animals, and chronic disease with an imposed stress in 17% of the animals (Waldrop et al, 2004). Almost 50 years have elapsed since the combined techniques of positive pressure ventilation, external precordial compression, and defibrillation were introduced in

TABLE 14-1	Cardiopulmonary Resuscitation Responsibilities and Tasks	
RESPONSIBILITY	**TASK**	
Airway management	Establish airway	
	Ventilate	
Cardiovascular management	Compress chest	
Venous access	Place IV or IO access	
	Start IV fluids if indicated	
Monitor	Attach ECG	
	Check pulse	
	Check Doppler flow	
	Measure end-tidal carbon dioxide (ETCO$_2$)	
Drug administration	Administer drugs	
	Document drugs given and response	

human medicine. Today clinicians know these combined techniques as cardiopulmonary resuscitation (CPR) and are fortunate that much of the CPR research conducted has been carried out in animal subjects. In June of 2012 the *Journal of Veterinary Emergency and Critical Care* published a supplement containing the results of the Reassessment Campaign on Veterinary Resuscitation (RECOVER) project. The RECOVER project detailed the science and scientific gap in evidence in 101 clinical resuscitation guidelines for small animals. In short, they published consensus guidelines on veterinary CPR.

Many of the techniques or procedures used in human medicine are also used in veterinary medicine. The goal of CPR is to provide adequate ventilatory and circulatory support until spontaneous function returns. CPR has three phases: (1) basic life support (BLS), (2) advanced life support, and (3) post–cardiac arrest care. This chapter covers preparation for this ultimate emergency, recognition of CPA, and the three phases of CPR.

PREPARATION

STAFF

Like many other aspects of emergency care, the team approach to the management of the CPA patient is essential. The ideal number of participants in a resuscitation attempt is probably three to five; all are required to meet several responsibilities (Table 14-1) of CPR. Each member of the hospital staff (including reception and kennel

help) should be trained to carry out one or more of those responsibilities. The team leader is usually the veterinarian; if the veterinarian is not available, then the person with the most experience in performing CPR should lead the team. Ideally the team leader should not actually participate in performing CPR but oversee and direct the team in the resuscitation endeavor. People will be needed to provide ventilation and chest **compressions,** establish IV lines, administer drugs, attach monitoring equipment, record the resuscitation effort (also inform the team every 2 minutes at the end of a BLS cycle), and monitor the team's effectiveness. Practice drills should be held on a regular basis. The benefits are tremendous when the staff can respond quickly and efficiently. A CPR manikin is ideal for practice but you can use a stuffed animal if a manikin is not available. Each person should understand what his or her responsibilities are during an arrest. After each practice session or true resuscitation, a self-evaluation should be performed.

> **TECHNICIAN NOTE** Three to five people are needed for effective CPR. Ensure that all laystaff in the hospital are trained in some aspect of CPR so they may be incorporated into the CPR effort.

FACILITIES

The area in which the resuscitation endeavor takes place should provide enough space for a CPR team (a minimum of three people) and equipment. An oxygen source should be readily available. Good lighting is required; it facilitates endotracheal intubation and visualization of veins. If open chest massage is attempted, then good lighting will allow visualization of internal structures. If CPR is to be performed on a table, then the height of the table should be adjustable. If a table is too tall for the person performing chest compressions, then he or she will find it difficult to perform effectively. If the height of the table is not adjustable, then a footstool should be made available or CPR should be performed on the floor. Grated surgical preparation tables should be avoided if at all possible; they have too much "give," which can be counterproductive when performing chest compressions. If the team has no choice and must use a preparation table, then a board should be placed on or below the grate to provide extra support. The table must have a solid surface. If some form of crash cart is not used, then the necessary drugs, electrocardiogram (ECG), suction, and defibrillator should

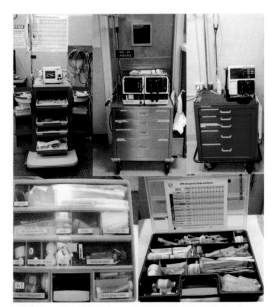

FIGURE 14-1 Examples of an emergency kit and crash cart.

be in close proximity. A shelf and a few drawers may be set aside for the emergency supplies. Visual aids such as drug dosage charts and CPR algorithms posted on the wall are helpful in aiding the CPR endeavor.

> *TECHNICIAN NOTE* The crash area should be well stocked and organized, with everything needed for CPR readily available and within easy reach.

EQUIPMENT

The use of a crash cart or kit makes the resuscitation endeavor more efficient by having the necessary supplies readily available. The crash cart or kit may be as simple as a fishing tackle box or as elaborate as a mobile tool chest (Figure 14-1). If a cart is used, then in addition to the standard emergency supplies (Box 14-1), additional equipment may be stored on the cart (e.g., suction machine, ECG, defibrillator). The crash cart or kit should be checked at the beginning of each shift and restocked immediately after each use.

> *TECHNICIAN NOTE* Every clinic should have an emergency crash kit/cart. All drugs should be assessed frequently for expiry, and a detailed stocking checklist should be prepared to ensure the kit is appropriately stocked at all times.

RECOGNITION

Veterinary technicians are often in a position to recognize impending problems such as CPA. The technician's efforts should be directed toward identifying those patients who are at risk for developing CPA. The technician should observe for decreasing mentation or lack of response; change in respiratory rate, depth, and pattern; change in pulse rate, rhythm, or quality; abnormal rhythms on ECG; or unexplained changes in anesthetic depth. If the patient's condition begins to deteriorate, then medical and nursing interventions will be required. Preventing an arrest is often easier than treating an arrest. CPA should be suspected in patients that are unresponsive with no obvious signs of breathing and no palpable pulse or heartbeat. **Agonal breaths** are not considered adequate breathing and very

BOX 14-2	Basic Life Support

Airway—Endotracheal intubation (or tracheostomy)
  • Intubation in lateral recumbency without interrupting chest compressions is ideal.
Breathing—Once every 6 seconds (10 breaths/min), 10 ml/kg tidal volume, 1-sec inspiration
Circulation—100-120 compressions/min*

*Note: Chest compressions should be initiated immediately.

little time should be spent making this assessment. If any questions arise as to whether the patient is in CPA, then CPR should be initiated until proven otherwise.

> **TECHNICIAN NOTE** Avoiding CPA is the key!

PHASE ONE: BASIC LIFE SUPPORT

The primary objective of BLS is to temporarily support the patient's oxygenation, ventilation, and circulation (Box 14-2). This is accomplished by administering external chest compressions and manual artificial ventilation. The RECOVER project guidelines recommend that chest compressions be started immediately; airway and ventilation management should not delay the start of chest compressions if multiple team members are present. Chest compressions may be performed in either left or right lateral recumbency. Intubation should be carried out in lateral recumbency while chest compressions are being performed. In veterinary medicine, respiratory and vagally mediated arrests are common causes of CPA. In addition, CPA in animals is most often a result of conditions that are not primarily cardiac in origin. Given the causes of CPA in the veterinary patient, early ventilation is more likely to be of benefit.

MECHANISM OF BLOOD FLOW

Two theories explain mechanisms of forward blood flow during CPR. The classic theory is the cardiac pump theory. The heart is compressed between the two thoracic walls, forcing blood out of the heart and into the arterial circulation. This is equivalent to the systolic phase of a normal heartbeat. Atrioventricular valves prevent retrograde blood flow. Chest relaxation creates subatmospheric intrathoracic pressure, allowing venous return and heart filling, similar to the normal diastolic phase.

The thoracic pump mechanism of blood flow is a newer theory that was recognized a little more than 25 years ago. It is hypothesized that chest compressions cause a rise in intrathoracic pressure that is transmitted to the intrathoracic vasculature; intrathoracic structures are compressed. Collapse of venous structures also occurs in the thorax, which prevents retrograde venous blood flow. Intrathoracic pressure falls when chest compressions are relaxed, allowing return of venous blood from the periphery into the thoracic venous system. Determining which mechanism plays the predominant role in blood flow during cardiopulmonary resuscitation (CPR) is difficult; it may depend on several factors. Some of the factors include patient size, chest compliance, the presence or absence of pleural filling defects, and cardiomegaly. Maximizing the effects of both mechanisms is perhaps best.

CHEST COMPRESSIONS

Artificial circulation can be accomplished through external or internal cardiac compression. The effectiveness of cardiac compression depends on the transmission of force to the heart and intrathoracic vessels.

External Cardiac Compression

External cardiac compression can be carried out with the patient in lateral or dorsal recumbency. For most medium to giant breed dogs it is suggested that they be placed in lateral recumbency. The hands are placed one on top of the other over the widest portion of the chest (taking advantage of the thoracic pump mechanism). In keel-chested patients (e.g., greyhounds) or patients weighing less than 10 kg, the patient is placed in lateral recumbency; the hands are placed on the lateral thoracic wall over the area of the heart (fourth to fifth intercostal space at the costochondral junction). With the arms extended and locked, the compressive force is applied by bending at the waist (Figure 14-2). The person delivering the chest compressions should not compress the chest by bending the elbows; it will be difficult to generate an appropriate force to affect perfusion. Alternately in cats and small dogs, a one-handed circumferential chest compression with the hand wrapped around the sternum directly over the heart or the thumb and first two index fingers can be used to compress the chest (taking advantage of the cardiac pump mechanism). Placing barrel-chested (also known as flat-chested) dogs in dorsal recumbency and compressing the sternum may aid in increasing intrathoracic pressure (taking advantage of the thoracic pump

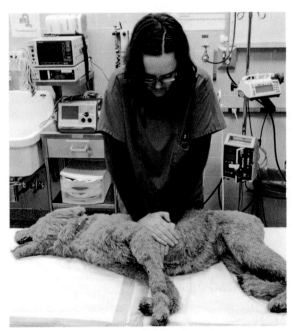

FIGURE 14-2 Proper technique for applying chest compressions. Note that the arms are extended and the technician is bending at the waist.

mechanism) and subsequent forward blood flow. It is recommended that the compressions be delivered with enough force to displace the thorax by 25% to 33% of its diameter. The rate of compressions ranges from 100 to 120 per minute. Chest compressions should be performed for 2 minutes without interruption; this is a BLS cycle. At the end of a cycle the person performing chest compressions should be rotated out with a replacement so that compressor fatigue does not affect the effectiveness of chest compressions (Hopper et al, 2012). This is also the time to *briefly* assess the ECG rhythm.

> **TECHNICIAN NOTE** Using straight arms and bending at the waist are critical to successful compressions. Ensure that no body weight remains on the patient during chest recoil.

Internal Compression

Internal or direct cardiac compression has been shown to be more effective than external chest compression. The advantages over external compression include greater cardiac output and blood pressure; better cerebral, myocardial, and peripheral tissue perfusion; and

higher survival rate with improved neurologic recovery. Other advantages of internal compression include the ability to assess ventricular filling between compressions and to determine what type of cardiac arrest is present in the absence of an ECG monitor. With the chest open, the descending aorta may also be compressed to force blood to the brain and coronary circulation. It has been suggested that a pericardectomy be performed to prevent cardiac tamponade.

Immediate internal compression is indicated if the patient has rib fractures, pleural effusion, pneumothorax, or cardiac tamponade. Otherwise, internal cardiac compression should be considered if return of spontaneous circulation (ROSC) with external compressions is not evident within 5 minutes of cardiac arrest. If external compressions are effective (evident by generation of a palpable pulse) but ROSC is not attained within 10 minutes of CPA, internal compressions may be indicated. Although frequently indicated, internal chest compressions are often not performed for financial or logistical reasons.

The patient is placed in lateral recumbency for an emergency thoracotomy. Time is not wasted performing a surgical preparation; however, the coat is clipped in longhaired dogs enough to see the rib spaces. An incision is made at the fourth or fifth intercostal space from just below dorsal epaxial muscles down to 2 cm short of the sternum but not through the pleura. The person ventilating the patient should stop while the chest cavity is entered with a pair of curved Mayo scissors. The scissors are then opened slightly and slid along the cranial edge of the caudal rib to enlarge the opening. A gloved hand is inserted into the chest and the heart compressed between the fingers and the palm of the hand. Small hearts can also be compressed between two fingers. Internal cardiac compression is performed rhythmically. Care should be taken not to puncture the heart with fingertips or twist the heart. Should spontaneous beating return and the patient stabilize, the chest cavity is irrigated with sterile saline; a sterile surgical skin preparation is performed, and the chest cavity is closed.

> **TECHNICIAN NOTE** Although often indicated, the decision to perform internal compressions must be weighed against the clinic and staff's ability to manage a patient that has had a thoracotomy, should ROSC occur.

Interposed Abdominal Compression

Interposed abdominal compression (IAC), alternating with external chest compression (alternating abdominal and chest compressions), can improve venous return to the chest (this has been reported to improve arterial blood pressure and cerebral and myocardial perfusion). This technique is reasonable when sufficient personnel trained in its use are available (Fletcher et al, 2012).

VENTILATION

An endotracheal tube is inserted to ensure a patent airway. On occasion, a tracheostomy tube may be indicated if an upper airway obstruction exists. If tracheostomy tubes are not available and the patient has an upper airway obstruction, then an endotracheal tube may be used like a tracheostomy tube. A variety of different-sized endotracheal and tracheostomy tubes and the associated airway management supplies (e.g., laryngoscopes, stylets, roll gauze, syringes) should be readily available to the team. In addition, suction should be available to remove blood, mucus, pulmonary edema fluid, and vomitus from the oral cavity and trachea. Properly placing the endotracheal tube is imperative. Proper placement is confirmed by visualization and chest auscultation for breath sounds.

Following intubation the patient is attached to a breathing source that delivers 100% oxygen such as an Ambu bag, or anesthetic machine. The patient's lungs are then ventilated once every 6 seconds (10 breaths per minute) with a tidal volume of 10 ml/kg and an inspiratory time of 1 second. Hyperventilation should be avoided. Higher respiratory rates, longer inspiratory times, and higher tidal volumes lead to impaired venous return because of increased intrathoracic pressure as well as decreased cerebral and coronary perfusion because of vasoconstriction, all of which has led to poor outcomes in people. Expired carbon dioxide with a capnometer in the CPA patient does not reflect the effectiveness of the artificial ventilation and should not be used as a guide.

In the case of a single rescuer, CPR or intubation is not a possible option; therefore, mouth to snout breathing may be attempted. The rescuer holds the mouth closed with one hand; places his or her mouth over the patient's nostrils, creating a seal; and blows into the nostrils to achieve a normal rise in the chest. It is important to keep the neck straight and extended to keep the airway open. The suggested compression to ventilation ratio is 30:2. This means you perform 30 chest compressions, then stop and provide 2 breaths, and then repeat another 30 chest compressions.

> **TECHNICIAN NOTE**   Compressions should not be withheld while intubating. Practice intubating patients of all sizes and breeds in lateral recumbency during routine surgeries.

ASSESSING EFFECTIVENESS

The effectiveness of the team's efforts must be monitored frequently. The presence of a palpable pulse during CPR is commonly used for assessing effectiveness. However, even in the best of circumstances palpation of a pulse can be difficult. The placement of a Doppler flat probe on the cornea has been suggested as a method of assessing blood flow through the common carotid artery and hence the effectiveness of CPR; however, there is no evidence to support the efficacy of this monitoring tool. If it is used, it should be interpreted with caution because of motion artifact or from venous flow and not arterial flow. If a direct arterial line is in place, then arterial pressure waveforms and pressures can be used to assess effectiveness of therapy. In essence, the clinician will have a compression-to-compression assessment of the technique; the goal is to achieve a diastolic pressure of 40 mm Hg or greater. Some investigators have shown that when aortic diastolic pressure was raised above 40 mm Hg, usually with α-adrenergic drugs or other special maneuvers, dogs could be successfully resuscitated from CPA (Kern and Niemann, 1996). Measurement of end-tidal carbon dioxide ($ETCO_2$) has been recommended to noninvasively assess resuscitation efforts (Brainard et al, 2012). Capnometers are used to measure $ETCO_2$ (Figure 14-3). Studies have shown that $ETCO_2$ varies directly with cardiac output (not ventilation) during cardiac arrest. Dramatic decreases in $ETCO_2$ occur during cardiac arrest; with CPR, an increase in $ETCO_2$ is expected. The higher the reading the more effective are the resuscitation efforts. A dramatic increase of $ETCO_2$ suggests ROSC has occurred. In humans the initial $ETCO_2$ measurement obtained at the outset of CPR is very low (11 to 12 mm Hg), compared with normal $ETCO_2$ values of 40 to 45 mm Hg.

If resuscitation efforts are not effective, then the resuscitation techniques must be changed. It may be necessary to increase or decrease the rate, duration, and

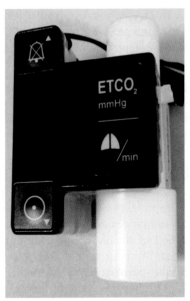

FIGURE 14-3 The Masimo EMMA capnometer used for measuring the level of expired carbon dioxide.

depth of compression; change the hand or patient's position; or change the person performing compressions.

ADVANCED LIFE SUPPORT

Once BLS objectives have been achieved, they must be maintained and a shift is made to advanced life support. During advanced life support, drugs and countershock are administered based on ECG and clinical findings. The type of cardiac arrest present dictates drug therapy during CPA; therefore ECG monitoring is required.

DRUGS
Epinephrine

Epinephrine possesses both α- and β-adrenergic properties. Epinephrine's strong α-adrenergic properties cause arterial vasoconstriction. Diastolic blood pressure is increased, which results in augmented coronary and cerebral blood flow. Aortic diastolic pressure is the critical determinant of success or failure of resuscitative efforts in animals and humans. The drug also causes constriction of large veins that displace blood out of the venous capacitance vessels. It has been reported that higher doses of epinephrine (0.1 mg/kg) may be more effective in establishing ROSC but it is not associated with increased survival to discharge. Initial doses of epinephrine should be low (0.01 mg/kg) and administered every 3 to 5 minutes or every other 2-minute BLS cycle

(Rozanski et al, 2012). After prolonged CPR, high doses of epinephrine may be administered.

Vasopressin

Vasopressin is the naturally occurring antidiuretic hormone. In doses higher than those required for the antidiuretic hormone effect, vasopressin acts as a direct peripheral smooth muscle vasoconstrictor. Vasopressin is a vasoconstrictor and may be used as an alternative to, or in conjunction with, epinephrine in the treatment of cardiac arrest. Evidence of the efficacy of vasopressin compared to epinephrine in dogs and cats is limited. One study suggested that vasopressin in addition to epinephrine is beneficial when administered to dogs undergoing CPR (Hofmeister et al, 2009) while another study found equivalent survival rates (Buckley et al, 2011). The guidelines consider its use in asystole/pulseless electrical activity and ventricular fibrillation/pulseless ventricular tachycardia. A suggested dose for vasopressin is 0.8 unit/kg given intravenously as an alternative or in combination with epinephrine every 3 to 5 minutes or every other 2-minute BLS cycle (Fletcher et al, 2012).

Atropine

Atropine has predominant parasympatholytic effects. Its use in cardiac arrest is based on its vagolytic action. It plays a central role in the prevention and management of CPA associated with intense vagal stimulation. Atropine is not strongly supported by the literature; it is most likely to be of use in dogs and cats with ventricular asystole or pulseless electrical activity (PEA). Because of the lack of detrimental effects, routine use of atropine in CPR may be considered. The recommended dose is 0.04 mg/kg.

Lidocaine 2%

Lidocaine is a class 1 antiarrhythmic agent and is most commonly used to treat ventricular tachycardia. Lidocaine may also be used to supplement treatment of refractory ventricular fibrillation and is used as a background drug to raise the fibrillatory threshold. Studies suggest that lidocaine increases the energy requirements for defibrillation and is not recommended to be given to patients with ventricular fibrillation. The dose is 2 mg/kg in dogs. Amiodarone is the only agent that has shown consistent benefit and is considered in cases of ventricular fibrillation/pulseless ventricular tachycardia resistant to defibrillation, but the drug is not commonly stocked in veterinary practices.

Reversal Agents

Drugs such as naloxone, flumazenil, and atipamezole should be administered if an opioid, benzodiazepine, or α_2-agonist, respectively, has been administered recently before the cardiac arrest.

Sodium Bicarbonate

The use of sodium bicarbonate ($NaHCO_3$) has been deemphasized. It was one of the primary drugs used in the treatment of cardiac arrest. The premise for its use was that it corrected metabolic acidosis, which was generated by anaerobic metabolism in hypoxic tissues. It was felt that the metabolic acidosis was associated with decreased cardiac function and lowered ventricular fibrillation threshold. Intracellular pH, not blood pH, determines cardiac viability and the likelihood of resuscitation. Ideally, $NaHCO_3$ administration should be guided by venous blood gas results; however, in the absence of blood gas measurements, $NaHCO_3$ may be given empirically if the CPA is greater than 10 to 15 minutes at a dose of 1 mEq/kg. Proper ventilation is necessary as a result of CO_2 development when $NaHCO_3$ is administered.

Calcium Therapy

Calcium is not currently recommended in the routine treatment of cardiac arrest. Calcium was used routinely during CPR to augment cardiac contractility. Excessive intracellular calcium concentrations, however, cause sustained muscular contraction ("stone heart") and myocardial and cerebral vasoconstriction. Calcium has also been implicated in reperfusion injury. Reperfusion injury occurs when ischemic tissue is reperfused or reoxygenated, leading to cellular damage. It remains to be seen whether calcium is beneficial in patients with prolonged arrest. Calcium is indicated when the patient is hyperkalemic, or moderate to severely hypocalcemic.

Fluids

Fluids are not used as liberally as they once were during CPR. Studies have shown that if fluids are administered during CPR in the euvolemic patient there is the potential for decreased coronary perfusion. As a result, routine intravenous fluid administration during CPR is not recommended in the euvolemic or hypervolemic dog or

---

BOX 14-3	Methods of Drug Delivery

- Jugular venous
- Peripheral venous (cephalic)
- Intraosseous
- Intratracheal
- Intracardiac

---

cat. Those patients suffering from or suspected to be hypovolemic are likely to benefit from fluid administration during CPR.

Route of Drug Administration

Selecting a site for drug administration during CPR requires the following considerations:

- Speed with which venous access can be obtained
- Technical abilities of the person attempting venous access
- Difficulties encountered in obtaining venous access
- Rate of drug delivery to the central circulation
- Duration of effective drug levels after injection

Several options (Box 14-3) are available for the delivery of drugs during CPA. Although drug circulation time is dependent on the cardiac output generated during CPR, it appears that the central or jugular vein is the most desirable, because drugs will be deposited near the heart. Drugs administered at the central venous site have the advantage of providing higher drug concentrations in a shorter period of time. Aside from patient movement during CPR, placing a jugular catheter in a patient suffering CPA (the jugular vein is usually palpable) is relatively easy. Peripheral venous drug administration tends to deliver the drug to the heart in a lower blood concentration and at a slower rate as compared with the central venous route. Experimental studies in animals demonstrate that drug delivery after peripheral injection is enhanced after the injection with 10- to 30-ml saline flushes (depending on patient size; use caution in cats) and elevation of the extremity. The circulation time was shorter, and the peak concentration was higher. In one study a 0.5 ml/kg flush solution permitted a peripherally administered model drug to reach the central circulation as quickly and in an equivalent concentration as a centrally administered drug during CPR in a canine cardiac arrest model (Gaddis et al, 1995).

BOX 14-4	Drugs That Can Be Administered by the Intratracheal Route

Atropine
Lidocaine
Epinephrine
Vasopressin

TECHNICIAN NOTE Ensure that large-volume flushes are drawn up with emergency drugs during CPR to ensure the drug reaches the heart. (Use 10- to 30-ml saline flushes, depending on the size of the patient, and use caution in cats.)

Few studies have examined the intraosseous (IO) route for the delivery of drugs during CPR; however, it remains an option. The intraosseous route has been used in human medicine for treating pediatric CPA. This route requires the placement of an intramedullary cannula inserted into the femur, humerus, or tibial crest. "Shock" treatment volumes of fluids and drugs can be injected into the medullary canal and rapid uptake is provided by the abundant endosteum medullary blood supply.

The intratracheal route can be used to administer a limited number of drugs (Box 14-4).

The intratracheal route has been advocated for drug administration when venous access is not accessible, but peak concentrations will be lower than those obtained by other routes. Some studies have indicated that drug uptake from the tracheal surface during resuscitation is sporadic, undependable, and delayed. If this route is to be used, the person administering the drugs can use up to 10 times the standard dose (in the case of epinephrine), diluting it with sterile saline or water (if needed) to provide enough volume; there are no data regarding optimal dose. The drug is injected via a long catheter placed through the endotracheal tube to the carina (Rozanski et al, 2012).

Several years ago the American Heart Association deemphasized the use of intracardiac injections. Chest compressions must be stopped while the injection is made. In addition, several potential complications are associated with this procedure: myocardial trauma, lacerated coronary arteries, pericardial effusion, and refractory ventricular fibrillation if the heart muscle is injected with epinephrine. As a result, use of this route is probably best reserved as a last resort after all other methods have failed, if at all.

Regardless of the drug administration route, effective chest compressions must be maintained throughout the CPR endeavor so that the drug can circulate.

DEFIBRILLATION

The purpose of defibrillation is to eliminate the chaotic asynchronous electrical activity of the fibrillating heart. **Defibrillation** is accomplished by passing an electrical current through the heart, causing the cardiac cells to depolarize and (it is hoped) to repolarize in a uniform manner with resumption of organized and coordinated electrical and contractile activity. Defibrillation stands a better chance of being successful if performed early in the CPR endeavor. The defibrillator paddles are placed firmly over the heart on each side of the chest after a contact gel has been applied. The person performing the defibrillation should yell "Clear" and make sure that no personnel (including themselves) is in contact with the patient (or anything associated with the patient) immediately before discharging the defibrillator. An energy level is set, and the defibrillator is discharged. The energy necessary for external defibrillation is 4 to 6 J/kg with a monophasic defibrillator or 2 to 4 J/kg for a biphasic defibrillator. The internal defibrillation energy level is at least 0.5 to 1 J/kg monophasic and 0.2 to 0.4 J/kg biphasic defibrillation. Excessive energy levels and repeated defibrillation can cause myocardial damage; therefore starting at the lower energy levels and increasing as needed is best.

Defibrillation is recommended for the treatment of ventricular fibrillation (VF) or pulseless ventricular tachycardia (PVT). If the duration of VF or PVT is less than 4 minutes or the shockable rhythm is identified between BLS cycles, then defibrillation is performed immediately. If it is suspected that the duration of VF or PVT is greater than 4 minutes the patient will likely benefit from 2 minutes of a BLS cycle before defibrillation. Necessary energy substrates are depleted after 4 minutes of VF/PVT. Alcohol or alcohol-based solutions should not be used on or near the CPA arrest patient in the event defibrillation is likely. There is a risk of igniting a fire.

TECHNICIAN NOTE The person defibrillating must ensure that all other participants are clear before discharging the defibrillator. This can be achieved by yelling "clear" and doing a quick visual check before discharging the paddles.

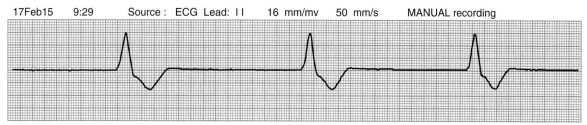

17Feb15   9:29   Source : ECG Lead: II   16 mm/mv   50 mm/s   MANUAL recording

FIGURE 14-4 ECG example of pulseless rhythm; note you would not be able to feel a pulse or hear the heart with this rhythm.

PRECORDIAL THUMP

The precordial thump is a method of mechanical defibrillation where the patient is struck with the heel of the hand directly over the heart in the hopes of converting the patient. Although there is minimal efficacy for this technique, it should be considered when a defibrillator is not available.

CARDIAC RHYTHMS

In a study the three types of ECG rhythms noted during CPA were (1) pulseless electrical activity (23.3%), (2) asystole (22.8%), and (3) ventricular fibrillation (19.8%) (Rush and Wingfield, 1992). Additional rhythms that may be encountered during a CPR event include sinus bradycardia (19%), sinus tachycardia, and ventricular tachycardia. Early recognition of the cardiac rhythm will dictate the type of therapy needed. A focused and directed approach is needed to treat CPA. An algorithm or flowchart aids the CPR team in making therapeutic decisions.

Pulseless Electrical Activity

The electrical pattern in pulseless rhythms may be near normal in appearance or wide and bizarre QRS complexes (Figure 14-4). In addition, pulse and heartbeat will not be detectable. Because pulseless electrical activity is common in the arrest patient, it is essential to always evaluate the pulse or heartbeat when assessing the ECG. Therapy (Box 14-5) should be aimed at determining the underlying cause such as hypoxia, acidosis, hyperkalemia, hypovolemia, cardiac tamponade, and tension pneumothorax. Epinephrine and atropine administration is indicated, and a fluid bolus should be considered.

Asystole

Asystole is characterized by no electrical (a flat line on the ECG) or mechanical activity (Figure 14-5). Pulse

BOX 14-5	Asystole and Pulseless Electrical Activity Therapy

Continue Effective BLS
- Epinephrine 0.01 mg/kg given every 3 to 5 min or every other BLS cycle
- Vasopressin 0.8 unit/kg in conjunction with or as an alternative to epinephrine, given every 3 to 5 min or every other BLS cycle
- Atropine 0.04 mg/kg

Consider the Following:
- High-dose epinephrine (if CPA >10 min)
- Sodium bicarbonate 1 mEq/kg (if CPA >10 min)

PEA Search for Treatable Causes
- Hypoxia
- Acidosis
- Hyperkalemia
- Hypovolemia
- Cardiac tamponade
- Tension pneumothorax

and heartbeat will not be detectable, and heart movement will not be visible (if the heart was viewed). Epinephrine, vasopressin, and atropine are the primary drugs used to treat this rhythm (see Box 14-5).

Ventricular Fibrillation

Ventricular fibrillation is characterized by chaotic electrical activity (Figure 14-6) and no mechanical activity. The ECG display will show no definable pattern and marked irregularity in rhythm; P waves and QRS complexes are unidentifiable. Pulse and heartbeat are undetectable. The heart would look like a quivering bag of worms if viewed. Defibrillation is the treatment of choice (Box 14-6).

17Feb15   9:28   Source : ECG Lead: I I 16 mm/mv 50 mm/s MANUAL recording

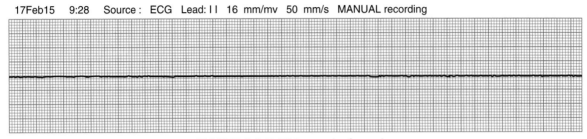

FIGURE 14-5 ECG example of asystole.

17Feb15   9:27   Source : ECG Lead: I I   16 mm/mv   50 mm/s   MANUAL recording

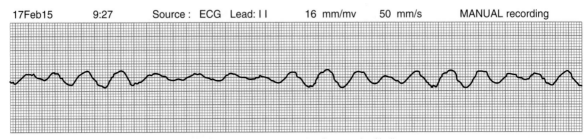

FIGURE 14-6 ECG example of ventricular fibrillation.

BOX 14-6	Ventricular Fibrillation Therapy/ Pulseless Ventricular Tachycardia

Continue Effective BLS
- Defibrillation (or precordial thump if no defibrillator)
- If suspect the duration of VF is >4 min, then perform 2 min of BLS cycle

	MONOPHASIC (J/KG)	BIPHASIC (J/KG)
External	4-6	2-4
Internal	0.5-1	0.2-0.4

With Prolonged Ventricular Fibrillation or Pulseless Ventricular Tachycardia Consider
- Lidocaine
- Epinephrine or vasopressin
- Defibrillate—increase dose by 50%

PHASE THREE: POST–CARDIAC ARREST CARE

Once the heart is beating spontaneously, the patient should be monitored closely. Special attention should be paid to the cardiovascular, pulmonary, and central nervous systems. Monitoring as many parameters as possible for each system is helpful. Asking the following questions gives the team a clear overview of the patient's status:

- What is the heart rate and rhythm? (If arrhythmias are present, then administration of antiarrhythmic drugs, correction of electrolyte abnormalities, or provision of oxygen therapy may be indicated.)
- What is the state of the patient's blood pressure, central venous pressure, and pulse pressure? (All are indications of the heart's mechanical activity.)
- What is condition of the patient's mucous membrane color, capillary refill time, pulse quality, urine output, and extremity temperature? (These are indications of the peripheral perfusion.)
- What is the patient's respiratory rate and character of breathing?
- Does the patient seem to be taking adequate breaths?
- Can airway sounds be auscultated? (If airway sounds cannot be heard, pleural filling defects must be ruled out.)
- What is the patient's mental status?
- Is the patient's neurologic condition improving or deteriorating? (Mannitol or diuretics may be indicated.)

TECHNICIAN NOTE There is a very high likelihood of re-arrest after CPR. Effective and continuous monitoring must be performed.

SUMMARY

Ideally the team will have an idea of the owner's wishes with regard to CPR. Knowing how far owners want to go should their animals arrest is important. Do the owners want an emergency thoracotomy performed, closed chest CPR, or no resuscitation? Many factors come into play when deciding whether CPR is to be attempted: the patient's current condition, the prognosis for recovery, the age, and the owner's financial limitations. The number of animals with CPA that attain ROSC is relatively high but only a very small number of animals survive to leave the hospital. The animals that survive CPR are often those that were young and healthy before the arrest or those that had a drug reaction or drug overdose.

A recent study from the University of California-Davis reported the rate of ROSC in dogs and cats to be 58%; 10% were alive at 24 hours, and 6% of dogs and 3% of cats were discharged alive from the hospital (McIntyre et al, 2014). Even with the dismal survival rates, if resuscitation is to be undertaken, then it needs to be managed aggressively. The veterinary team needs to have a plan regarding how the CPA will be managed; cases in which resuscitation is successful often are due, at least in part, to an informed, prepared, and efficient CPR team.

REFERENCES

Brainard BM, Boller M, Fletcher DJ: RECOVER evidence and knowledge gap analysis on veterinary CPR. Part 5: Monitoring, *J Vet Emerg Crit Care* 22(S1):65–84, 2012.

Buckley GJ, Rozanski EA, Rush JE: Randomized, blinded comparison of epinephrine and vasopressin for treatment of naturally occurring cardiopulmonary arrest in dogs, *J Vet Intern Med* 25(6):1334–1340, 2011.

Fletcher DJ, Boller M, Brainard BM, et al.: RECOVER evidence and knowledge gap analysis on veterinary CPR. Part 7: Clinical guidelines, *J Vet Emerg Crit Care* 22(S1):102–131, 2012.

Gaddis GM, Dolister M, Gassis ML: Mock drug delivery to the proximal aorta during cardiopulmonary resuscitation: central vs. peripheral intravenous infusion with varying flush volumes, *Acad Emerg Med* 2(12):1027–1033, 1995.

Hofmeister EH, Brainard BM, Egger CM, et al.: Prognostic indicators for dogs and cats with cardiopulmonary arrest treated by cardiopulmonary cerebral resuscitation at a university teaching hospital, *J Am Vet Assoc* 235(1):50–57, 2009.

Hopper K, Epstein SE, Fletcher DJ: RECOVER evidence and knowledge gap analysis on veterinary CPR. Part 3: Basic life support, *J Vet Emerg Crit Care* 22(S1):26–43, 2012.

Kern KB, Niemann JT: Perfusion pressure. In Paradise NA, Halperin HR, Nowak RM, editors: *Cardiac arrest: the science and practice of resuscitation medicine*, Baltimore, 1996, Williams & Wilkins, pp 270–285.

McIntyre R, Hopper K, Epstein SE: Assessment of cardiopulmonary resuscitation in 121 dogs and 30 cats (2009-2012) in a university teaching hospital, *J Vet Emerg Crit Care* 24(6):693–704, 2014.

Rozanski EA, Rush JE, Buckley GJ, et al.: RECOVER evidence and knowledge gap analysis on veterinary CPR. Part 4: Advanced life support, *J Vet Emerg Crit Care* 22(S1):65–84, 2012.

Rush JE, Wingfield WE: Recognition and frequency of dysrhythmias during cardiopulmonary arrest, *J Am Vet Med Assoc* 200:1932–1937, 1992.

Waldrop JE, Rozanski EA, Swanke ED, et al.: Causes of pulmonary arrest, resuscitation management, and functional outcome in dogs and cats surviving cardiopulmonary arrest, *J Vet Emerg Crit Care* 14:22–29, 2004.

SCENARIO

Purpose: To provide the veterinary team with scenarios with which to practice CPR in the clinic.

Stage: A general veterinary practice offering routine care to veterinary patients.

Scenario

Afternoon appointments.

A client is scheduled to bring her 5-year-old Labrador retriever, Bentley, in for vaccinations. She gets out of the car, and Bentley, excited as usual, jumps out of the car without his leash and runs out onto the road where he is struck by a car. In the clinic, you are alerted to the incident by the sounds of squealing brakes, and run to the front to see what has happened. Seeing the dog prone in the middle of the road, you grab a stretcher and an assistant and run out to help.

Arriving at the scene, Bentley is not responsive and has obvious trauma to the head and back right leg. You quickly place him on the stretcher and run into the clinic with the owner.

Questions

1. What are the two best indicators that the patient is in CPA?

Continued

SCENARIO—cont'd

2. You identify that Bentley has suffered a cardiopulmonary arrest, and quickly ask the owner about CPR. She insists you "do everything."
   a. Bentley is quickly taken to the back treatment room, and what is the first intervention?
   b. What is the second intervention?
3. Given Bentley's breed and typical body type, what type of compressions will be performed?
4. Where will the compressions be performed on the chest?
5. How long should one compressor work before changing compressors?
6. What rate should IPPV be delivered?
7. What rate should compressions be delivered?

Discussion

1. Unresponsive and apneic
2.
   (a) Start compressions.
   (b) Intubate and start IPPV.
3. Thoracic pump compressions because Labradors are typically barrel-chested breeds.

4. In lateral recumbency, the compressions should be performed at the widest part of the chest, approximately the seventh intercostal space.
5. 2-minute cycles
6. 10 breaths per minute
7. 100-120 compressions per minute

Other Considerations

This is a true emergency arrest, with very little information being provided to the owner regarding costs for CPR and post-CPR care. It is important for the team to discuss a policy with regards to CPR, such as an emergency release waiver and quote, which will provide the owner with a small estimate for the CPR itself. If the patient gains ROSC, an additional quote must be provided to ensure that the owner is prepared for post–resuscitative care, which may require referral to a 24-hr hospital.

MEDICAL MATH EXERCISE

Epinephrine is available in two concentrations: 1:1000 (1 mg/ml) and 1:10,000 (0.1 mg/ml).

1. The doctor has ordered 0.01 mg/kg for a 3-kg cat in asystole. What volume of 1:10,000 epinephrine will you draw up?

a. 0.003 ml
b. 0.03 ml
c. 0.3 ml
d. 3.0 ml

15 Traumatic Emergencies

Jennifer J. Devey

CHAPTER OUTLINE

Introduction
Readiness
  Ready Area and Crash Cart
  Suction
  Fluids
  Autotransfusion
  Radiology and Ultrasound
  Laboratory
  Surgery
  Warming Devices
  Veterinary Team
  Protocols
  First Aid and Safety
Patient Assessment
  Triage
  Primary and Secondary Survey
  Initial Database
  History
  Additional Diagnostic Tests
  Scoring Systems
Trauma Triad of Death
Resuscitation
  Goals

  Oxygenation and Ventilation
  Fluids
  Hemorrhage Control
  Resuscitating the Patient with Severe
    Intraabdominal Hemorrhage
Analgesia
Wounds, Bandages, and Splints
Surgical Resuscitation
Basic Monitoring
Advanced Monitoring
Postresuscitation Care: the First 24
  Hours
Nutrition
Communication
Assessment and Management of
  Specific Injuries
  Head and Facial Trauma
  Cervical Soft Tissue Injury
  Chest Injury
  Abdomen
  Musculoskeletal System
Conclusion

KEY TERMS

Analgesia
Autotransfusion
Hemorrhage
Readiness
Resuscitation
Trauma management

LEARNING OBJECTIVES

After studying this chapter, you will be able to:

- Understand how to be ready for a patient arriving with an injury.
- Understand the types of trauma and how to approach assessment of trauma emergencies in a systematic way.
- Understand the importance of the team approach to the trauma patient and the importance of including owners.

INTRODUCTION

A well-equipped hospital with a well-trained team of doctors, veterinary technicians, and receptionists is essential for treating the seriously injured patient. The team must be prepared to address both the medical needs of the patient and the emotional needs of the owners. Medical skills go hand in hand with caring and compassion.

> **TECHNICIAN NOTE** Although the information in this chapter deals primarily with the medical management of trauma, taking care of the distraught owner can be as important as taking care of the medical needs of the animal.

Survival of the injured patient depends on many factors, including the type and severity of the injury and the medical treatment provided. Recognition, assessment, action, and reassessment are the four essential components of effective **trauma management.** Technicians and doctors must be able to recognize critical injuries quickly, because the outcome of a very severe injury often is determined within the first few minutes. Technicians usually have the first contact with patients in the hospital; therefore, they must be able to assess the patient rapidly and determine whether potentially life-threatening problems are present. The veterinary team must be able to act immediately and treat the problems in order of priority. **Resuscitation** may entail invasive procedures, laboratory tests, advanced diagnostic tests (including contrast radiographic studies and ultrasound), and potentially emergency surgery, often during the first or so-called golden hour after the injury. The hospital must be equipped, and the team trained to deal with all these components.

> **TECHNICIAN NOTE** It should always be assumed that the patient has a serious injury until proven otherwise. By anticipating the worst, the team is more likely to recognize injuries and their secondary effects.

All patients should be evaluated in the same stepwise fashion, starting with the *ABCs* of *airway, breathing,* and *circulation.* A patient with a distal forelimb fracture

BOX 15-1	Responsibilities of Veterinary Technician Related to Trauma Patient

Ensuring readiness (including emergency department and operating room)
Receiving phone calls
Providing first aid instructions
Securing airway on arrival of patient (oxygen [O_2], intubation if indicated)
Managing positive pressure ventilation with positive end-expiratory pressure (if needed)
Establishing IV access
Setting up and interpreting monitoring devices
Managing pain
Recording in charts
Communicating

sustained during a fall may also have pneumothorax, which can be overlooked easily if a complete assessment is not performed.

Intensive monitoring is vital.

> **TECHNICIAN NOTE** Tracking changes in vital signs and other physiologic parameters allows technicians and doctors to determine if the patient's status is improving or deteriorating.

Detailed flowsheets and treatment sheets must be used. Because injured patients are at serious risk for secondary complications such as pneumonia, delayed healing, and the systemic inflammatory response syndrome, intensive monitoring and treatment may help to prevent some of these complications (Box 15-1).

READINESS

READY AREA AND CRASH CART

Each hospital should have a ready area where all emergency patients requiring immediate care are brought for examination and treatment. The ready area should also be where in-hospital emergencies are treated. It is usually centrally located, such as in a main treatment room. It should be near the operating room, because seriously injured trauma patients may require surgery as part of their resuscitation. The ready area must have all the

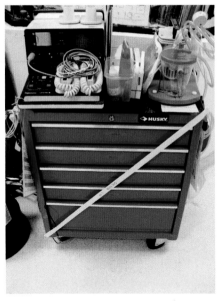

FIGURE 15-1 Tape across crash cart.

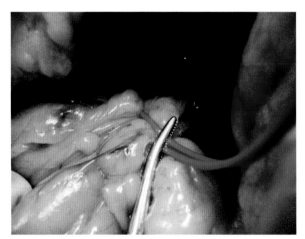

FIGURE 15-2 Modified Rumel tourniquet using a red rubber tube to perform a modified Pringle maneuver (temporary occlusion of the hepatic artery, portal vein, and common bile duct).

necessary equipment for all types of resuscitation, including open-chest cardiopulmonary resuscitation. Oxygen (O_2), airway and vascular access devices, fluids (e.g., crystalloids, colloids), suction, monitoring equipment, and basic bandaging supplies must be available. A crash cart with multiple drawers should be outfitted with all the necessary supplies. The crash cart should be checked once or twice daily to ensure all the necessary supplies are present and equipment is connected and in good working condition. A piece of tape placed diagonally across the cart can be used as an indicator of whether or not materials have been removed (Figure 15-1). When the cart is used, the tape is taken down and not replaced until the missing supplies have been replaced. The tape also can be dated and initialed after each check so that other members of the team can be certain that the cart has all the necessary equipment.

Monitoring equipment should be kept on the top of the crash cart and should include suction and equipment to continuously monitor an electrocardiogram (ECG), blood pressure (BP), capnography, and pulse oximetry. Several sizes of BP cuffs should be available (1 to 5 cm widths). Good overhead lighting is essential. Both a wide-beam dish light and a focusing high-intensity cool-beam light should be available. Direct light sources that can be worn, such as a head loupe or inexpensive hiking headlamps or snake lights (available

from hardware stores), allow the airway, oral cavity, and wounds to be closely assessed while freeing both hands.

A limited number of sterile surgical supplies should be kept with the crash cart, including scalpel blades, curved Mayo scissors, curved hemostats, and various sizes of polypropylene suture material (sizes from 2 to 5-0) for vascular suturing, tracheotomy, or resuscitative thoracotomy. Satinsky forceps, although expensive, are invaluable as vascular forceps for controlling **hemorrhage** from large vessels such as the vena cava or the aorta. Ideally, a pair of Balfour retractors or Finochietto rib retractors should be available. Sterile laparotomy pads and towels, which can be used to cover and protect open wounds from infection, and to apply pressure to bleeding wounds, should be available. Red rubber tubes are effective vascular occlusive devices. When wrapped around a vessel and pulled tightly with hemostats, a red rubber tube acts as an atraumatic modified Rumel tourniquet (Figure 15-2).

SUCTION

Suction equipment should be capable of generating pressures of up to 760 mm Hg. Electronic suction devices are ideal; however, hand-held suction devices (Mityvac, Neward Enterprises, Cucamonga, CA) are an inexpensive but effective alternative. A suction trap placed between the suction tip and the tubing will help prevent clogging of the tubing. Several different types of suction tips should be available. A Yankauer suction tip is useful for oral and pharyngeal secretions. A dental suction tip can be used to remove vomitus and clots from the rima glottidis and trachea. Tracheal whistle-tip catheters can be used for removing frothy secretions, vomit, and blood from the trachea. Suction also can be attached directly to the end of the endotracheal tube if the patient is intubated and fluid or exudate is obstructing the tube. The suction device should always be ready for immediate use. This means that the suction tip should be attached to the tubing and the tubing should be attached to the suction unit. If an electric unit is being used, then the machine should be plugged into an outlet.

FLUIDS

Trauma patients often need large volumes of intravenous (IV) fluids. Balanced isotonic solutions that are buffered are the preferred crystalloid solutions, for example, lactated Ringer's solution (Lactated Ringer's Injection USP, Abbott Animal Health, Abbott Park, IL), Normosol-R (Normosol®-R, Hospira, Lake Forest, IL), and Plasma-Lyte A (Plasma-Lyte A® Injection pH 7.4, Abbott Animal Health, Abbott Park, IL). Both synthetic colloids (hydroxyethyl starch, Vetstarch®, Abbott Animal Health, Abbott Park, IL) and biologic colloids (blood products) should be readily available. Because trauma patients are at risk for developing coagulopathies secondary to loss of clotting factors and platelets, fresh whole blood and fresh frozen plasma are frequently indicated in the severely hemorrhaging patient.

AUTOTRANSFUSION

Autotransfusion can be lifesaving. If large volumes of blood are present in the thoracic or abdominal cavity, then the blood can be collected into sterile containers and reinfused as an autotransfusion (Crowe, 1981). Alternatively, a multi-holed catheter placed into the abdominal cavity can be connected to the patient's IV catheter via a three-way stopcock and extension sets. The blood can then be aspirated from the abdomen and infused directly back into the bloodstream using a closed system. Anticoagulant is not required because this blood is deficient in fibrin and platelets (Broadie et al, 1981); however, a blood filter should be used. When using a suction unit to collect the blood, care should be taken to prevent suctioning air simultaneously since this can cause red blood cell lysis. Commercial autotransfusion systems are available, but the cost may be prohibitive for most veterinary hospitals. A simple but effective way to

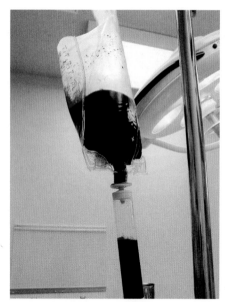

FIGURE 15-3 Autotransfusion using a sterile IV fluid bag.

administer an autotransfusion is to use a bag designed for delivering liquid enteral nutrition as the transfusion bag. These bags have a large opening at the top with a cap. The cap is removed and the blood is poured into the bag. Blood administration sets can be attached to the food bags and gas-sterilized as a unit. A simpler method is to use a sterile 1-L IV fluid bag (Figure 15-3). The top is cut along approximately 30% of the front panel. In this way the bag can still be hung and blood poured into the bag through this hole. Blood is collected from the patient and placed into the transfusion bag. Ideally, this blood should be administered through a filter; however, in an emergency a filter is not essential. It often is more important that the patient receives the blood rapidly, and filters significantly decrease the infusion rate. If large volumes of autotransfused blood are administered, then fresh frozen plasma will also be needed as a source of fibrin.

RADIOLOGY AND ULTRASOUND

An x-ray machine capable of producing high-quality radiographs is a necessary part of evaluating injured patients. If digital radiography is not available then a 300- to 500-mA machine and an automatic processor that can develop films within minutes are needed. Accurate technique charts should be available for taking the standard lateral and ventrodorsal views. The technician should be trained to perform contrast radiographic studies such as IV urography, double-contrast cystography, and barium series. Contrast dyes, tubes, and catheters should be stocked in the radiology department for these studies. Both positioning charts and protocols for contrast studies should be posted or be readily available.

Injured patients who are nonambulatory or unconscious should be secured to Plexiglas or wood spinal boards and radiographed through the boards. Trauma films or survey radiographs of the animal from nose to tail can be effectively taken through both materials to look for obvious injuries. A variety of positioning devices should be available to help decrease the exposure of the staff to radiation. This includes items such as V trays, foam pads, sand bags, and cushions filled with beads.

An ultrasound machine should be available for immediate scanning of trauma patients since ultrasound is one of the diagnostic tests of choice for rapid evaluation of the internally hemorrhaging trauma patient. A portable unit that can easily be brought to the patient is ideal.

LABORATORY

Laboratory equipment ideally includes a centrifuge for spinning packed cell volumes (PCVs) as well as for separating serum; a refractometer for blood, urine, and fluid analysis; and the capability for analyzing blood gases, basic chemistries, complete blood cell counts, and coagulation parameters. Point-of-care devices allow for rapid (i.e., 1 to 2 minutes) assessment of blood gases; acid-base status; electrolyte, glucose, and lactate levels; and coagulation parameters using very small volumes of whole blood (0.05 ml). A good microscope is essential for performing manual differentials and evaluating urine and fluid cytology.

SURGERY

Many seriously injured trauma patients require surgery as part of their resuscitation. Because time is of the essence for many of these patients, the anesthetic machine must be ready and the operating room must be kept prepared. A major surgical pack and gowns should be laid out and ready to be opened at a moment's notice. The suction unit must be functional and ready to receive suction tubing from the surgeon. Electrocauterization devices should be connected, and the ground plate should be in place. The use of a surgical headlight will greatly enhance visualization of bleeding and traumatized tissues and vessels; it should be a standard part of

---

BOX 15-2 Surgical Trauma Pack

Saline bowls (small and large)
Scalpel handle and no. 10 and no. 11 blades
Towel clamps (minimum of eight)
Mayo scissors (curved)
Metzenbaum scissors (curved)
Sharp blunt scissors
Kelly hemostatic forceps (eight curved)
Halsted mosquito forceps (eight curved)
Rochester-Carmalt hemostatic forceps (six curved)
Sponge forceps (curved)
Allis tissue forceps (four)
Right-angle forceps (small and large)
DeBakey or Cooley tissue forceps (short and long)
Russian thumb forceps
Brown-Adson tissue forceps
Serrefine forceps (two bulldog clamps)
Balfour retractors (small and large)
Mayo-Hegar needle holders (small and large)
Yankauer, Poole, and Frazier suction tips
Silastic tubing
Bulb syringe
Laparotomy pads (eight)
Rumel tourniquet (umbilical tape, silastic or red rubber tubing)
Cotton towels (four small and four large)

---

the operating room equipment. Trauma surgical packs should contain the basic equipment for an exploratory laparotomy or thoracotomy (Box 15-2). In addition, towels and laparotomy pads (for packing large bleeding wounds) and red rubber tubes for use as vascular occlusion devices should be sterilized and ready for use. Many trauma patients are hypothermic or develop hypothermia during resuscitation and surgery; therefore a means of warming the patient should be available.

WARMING DEVICES

Keeping a patient normothermic is very important because hypothermia interferes with normal metabolic functions, leading to problems such as altered perfusion, cardiac dysfunction, and interference with coagulation. Ideally the core should be warmed since warming the periphery leads to vasodilation and can worsen both core hypothermia and shock. The immobile patient should always be monitored closely, because almost any warming device has the potential to cause burns.

Warm-air circulating blankets are an extremely effective means of keeping patients warm. Artificial warming devices and hot-water bottles should not come in direct contact with the patient's skin. Instead, they should be wrapped or covered in a towel before being applied to the patient. A blanket warmer is handy for keeping towels and blankets warm. Warm-water bottles can be kept in an incubator or heated in a microwave. If IV fluid bags are being used as warm-water bottles, then food coloring should be added to the bags so that they can be easily identified for reuse. This also prevents inadvertently using them for parenteral fluids. Homemade warming bags can be made from fabric sacks filled with rolled oats. These can be heated in a microwave and are reusable. Bubble wrap can be warmed in the microwave in a bowl of water and wrapped around the patient; the air cells will retain heat well. Bubble wrap or plastic food wrap can be sterilized and used in the operating room to help prevent hypothermia. IV fluids should be kept warm in an incubator or warmed in a microwave. Fluids administered rapidly at room temperature can significantly lower a patient's temperature and ideally fluids should be administered through fluid warmers. Commercially available infant isolettes and tables can be purchased at reasonable cost through used hospital equipment suppliers. Heat lamps that either are commercially available or are even made from an exposed light bulb can provide additional external heat. These always have the potential to overheat the patient, and close monitoring is required. Temperatures should never exceed 106° to 110° F (41° to 43° C).

VETERINARY TEAM

The veterinary team (i.e., technicians, doctors, receptionists) must be mentally and physically ready to perform the necessary tasks. All team members must be dedicated and trained to do their jobs. Technicians must be familiar with the location and operation of all the equipment needed for diagnostics and treatment. They must be trained to place IV catheters, bandage wounds, and provide anesthesia. Team members must also understand the various procedures involved in preparing instruments and equipment and assist when asked to do so. Familiarity with the techniques, tests, procedures, and treatments means the nurse is able to help monitor for complications and for efficacy.

Drills are the most effective way to prepare the team for emergencies. These drills can be performed on stuffed animals or cadavers (assuming appropriate permission has been obtained). This encourages teamwork and the chance to practice psychomotor skills. It allows each individual to know exactly what his or her responsibility is during an emergency situation. Through practice sessions, recognition, assessment, and treatment become more automatic during a true emergency.

PROTOCOLS

It has been shown in human hospitals that the implementation of protocols for treating patients significantly decreases morbidity and mortality. These protocols should be readily available for everyone to use. Resuscitation algorithms should be posted so that under the stress of the emergency situation, resuscitation is undertaken in an orderly fashion and important treatments are not overlooked.

FIRST AID AND SAFETY

Initial treatment often begins at the scene of the accident, and prehospital care may significantly influence outcome. Safety and first aid information can be provided to owners during the initial telephone contact to help both at the scene of the accident and en route to the hospital. Most owners will be stressed and frightened because their pet has just been hurt. Calming the owner is important in order to gain accurate information so that appropriate first aid instructions can be given. A calm owner is also much more capable of following instructions. The tone of voice that the technician uses may be as important as the information dispensed. If the owner has not had any previous first aid experience, then it may be best to advise him or her to confine the injured pet to a box, strap it to a board (or otherwise limit the animal's movement), and transport it to the clinic as rapidly as possible.

All team members should follow several basic rules:
1. Ensure that the scene is safe. This means watching for other vehicles, broken glass, spilled chemicals, and other hazards.
2. Ensure that the owner and staff are safe while working directly with the animal. Blood on the patient may be human blood. To prevent contact with contagious diseases such as hepatitis and human immunodeficiency virus, direct contact with blood should be prevented until the source of the blood is determined. At the scene, towels or clothing should be

used to apply direct pressure on wounds. In the hospital, gloves should always be worn before handling animals with blood on their fur. Injured animals often are frightened and in pain. Appropriate precautions for restraint should be used. Muzzles should be placed when available. Plastic muzzles that cover the entire nose and mouth and contain multiple holes to enable breathing and drainage of oral secretions are often easier to place, less painful, and more comfortable for the trauma patient than the standard muzzles that fit tightly over the bridge of the nose. If a muzzle is not available, a tie or belt can be wrapped around a dog's muzzle. If facial hemorrhage or making a muzzle is not possible, then a blanket or large jacket can be used to cover the patient's head.

3. Minimize movement of the patient until the full extent of the injuries is known. The pet should be transported on a board or in a box if it is nonambulatory. If ambulatory, then the animal should not be allowed to jump in and out of the vehicle and walking should be kept to a minimum. This will help to prevent making any potentially minor problem into a major problem. For example, a partial body wall hernia may become a complete hernia if the animal jumps out of the car.

4. Apply direct pressure to wounds with a clean cloth whenever possible. Alternatively, with bleeding from extremities, hands can encircle and squeeze the limb or tail proximal to the wound to help control hemorrhage. Newspaper, large sticks, or pieces of wood can be used as splints for lower limb fractures.

PATIENT ASSESSMENT

TRIAGE

Triage is the sorting of patients according to the severity of injury or illness to ensure that the most critical patients are treated first. The technician usually performs the triage, which involves quickly evaluating each patient on arrival in order to determine how rapidly each needs to be seen by the doctor.

TECHNICIAN NOTE Patients who have been involved in any serious accident should be triaged immediately to the ready area of the hospital for evaluation by the doctor.

PRIMARY AND SECONDARY SURVEY

The animal should be approached from the rostral direction and quickly surveyed for level of consciousness, breathing and respiratory pattern, abnormal body or limb posture, the presence of blood or other materials in or around the patient, and any other gross abnormalities. A primary survey, which assesses level of consciousness and the ABCs, should be completed within 30 to 60 seconds. Resuscitation is started as the primary survey is being completed. If the primary survey indicates severe abnormalities such as an inadequate airway, then the airway is immediately established before the physical examination is completed and diagnostics or other treatments are performed.

The airway is checked for patency by looking, listening, and feeling. If visual examination of the oral cavity and oropharynx is required, appropriate precautions should be taken to ensure no one is bitten. If the patient shows signs of an exaggerated inspiratory effort, the airway may not be patent. The presence of increased respiratory effort, paradoxic chest wall movement, abdominal wall movement with respiration, nasal flare, open mouth, extended head and neck, abducted elbows, and cyanosis are all indicators of respiratory distress that require immediate treatment. Airway assessment is followed immediately by breathing assessment done by watching chest wall motion and auscultating the trachea as well as lung sounds bilaterally. Lung sounds should be auscultated before the heart, because the ear is much less discerning of softer sounds once it has adjusted to louder sounds. Percussion of the thorax may be indicated to help rule out a pneumothorax or hemothorax (Box 15-3). Circulation is assessed by checking mucous membrane color and capillary refill time and auscultating for heart tones at the same time as central (femoral) and peripheral (dorsal metatarsal) pulses are palpated. Finally, a very rapid assessment and palpation of the abdomen, flank, pelvis, spine, and limbs is carried out.

Once the primary survey is completed and resuscitation has been initiated then a secondary survey including measurement of vital signs is completed. Vital signs are taken *after* the primary survey is completed. The secondary survey entails a complete examination of the patient in a systematic fashion from nose to tail. The five vital signs are respiratory rate, heart rate, temperature, blood pressure, and pain. The temperature should be checked after a respiratory rate and heart rate have been taken. Patients with extremely

Method

Lay the hand on the chest wall or body surface being examined.

Tap firmly (using the top of the middle finger of the hand) on the patient, with the middle and ring finger of the opposite hand.

Strike or tap several times until consistency is reached (interpreting the strength of the tap, the sound, and the vibration generated).

Interpretation

A very low-pitched resonant sound (hollow sound) indicates an air-filled structure under the body wall.

A moderate-pitched sound with slight resonance (solid sound) indicates a fluid- or tissue-filled structure under the body wall.

A high-pitched sound with significant resonance indicates a solid structure (possibly under pressure) or a fluid-filled structure under pressure under the body wall.

slow heart rates can have a vagally induced arrest with stimulation of the rectum. In these patients an axillary or ear temperature should be taken. In addition, respiratory and heart rates will usually increase once a cold thermometer is inserted.

BP measurement is very important and should be monitored in all trauma patients. For example, the combination of a high heart rate and a high BP is consistent with pain, whereas the presence of a high heart rate and low BP indicates hypovolemic shock. A jugular vein should be clipped and assessed for distention when the vein is clamped at the thoracic inlet as an estimate of central venous pressure (CVP) (Crowe, 2006). A mildly distended jugular vein will normally be noted when the animal is in lateral recumbency. A highly distended jugular vein or one that is distended with the animal standing or in sternal recumbency is consistent with an elevated CVP, which is usually associated with a severe pneumothorax or pericardial effusion in the patient in shock. A flat jugular vein is consistent with hypovolemia. Peripheral vein distention can be assessed in some breeds of dogs. When the patient is in lateral recumbency, mild distention of the lateral saphenous vein should be evident if the vein is below the level of the right atrium. Raising the limb should cause the vein to flatten. The difference in the height of the leg from when the vein is distended to when it becomes flat can be measured. During resuscitation this can be remeasured as a crude assessment of a change in venous volume during resuscitation.

Cyanosis may be difficult to detect in patients with severe hemorrhage because 5 g/dl of hemoglobin (Hb) (equivalent to a hematocrit of 15%) is required for the eye to be able to discern cyanosis. Fluorescent lights also interfere with accurate evaluation of mucous membrane color in the face of pallor; therefore, a direct light source such as a penlight or transilluminator should be used.

INITIAL DATABASE

Once vital signs have been measured and resuscitation has been started, baseline data can be collected. This will usually include lab work, a lead II ECG, and abdominal focused assessment with sonography for trauma (AFAST)/thoracic focused assessment with sonography for trauma (ATFAST). A minimum laboratory database should include measurement of a PCV and total solids (TS), and blood glucose level. If point-of-care testing is available, then the blood urea nitrogen value, or preferably creatinine level, along with electrolyte and blood gas measurements can often be assessed simultaneously as part of an extended database. Although point-of-care machines may provide a hematocrit, assessment of a PCV and TS is always recommended because the hematocrit can be significantly different from a spun PCV. The technician can collect the blood sample by inserting hematocrit tubes into the hub of the catheter stylet. A more extended database should include measurements of serum albumin, prothrombin time, and activated partial thromboplastin time or activated clotting time and a platelet estimate. A complete database includes a complete blood count with evaluation of a blood smear for the white blood cell differential, red cell morphology and platelet estimate, chemistry panel, urinalysis, and arterial blood gas. Usually the minimum or extended database is collected initially, and further tests are considered once the patient has been fully examined and preliminary resuscitation has been completed. Treatment for arrhythmias or laboratory abnormalities should be instituted as indicated.

HISTORY

Once the secondary survey is completed, the history is taken. If the patient is stable, then a capsule history can be taken at the time the patient arrives at the hospital. A useful mnemonic is AMPLE:

A—Allergies—Does the animal have any known allergies?

M—Medications—Is the animal taking any medications? If so, then what drugs and what doses?

P—Past history—Has the animal had any past medical problems?

L—Lasts—When was the pet's last meal, defecation, urination, medication?

E—Events—What is the problem now? Details should be given.

Important historic facts relating to the injury include the time elapsed since the injury, the cause of the injury (e.g., fall, hit by car, gunshot), the speed of the car if the animal was hit, evidence of loss of consciousness at the scene, approximate amount of blood lost at the scene, and deterioration or improvement in the patient since the time of injury. The technician should also determine if the patient has other underlying medical diseases or is currently being treated with any medication. Having the owner complete a history sheet helps provide comprehensive information on the pet, as well as giving the owner something to do while the preliminary evaluation and resuscitation is being completed.

ADDITIONAL DIAGNOSTIC TESTS

Once the patient has been completely examined, a history has been taken, and resuscitation has been initiated, further tests may be instituted. Ultrasonographic assessment of both the abdomen and the thorax provides a rapid means of ruling out significant injuries. AFAST has been validated in the dog as an effective means of determining the presence of free fluid in the abdomen (Boysen et al, 2004). The scan, which is ideally performed with the dog in left lateral recumbency, interrogates the subxiphoid region, the region around the apex of the urinary bladder and the left and right flanks (Figure 15-4). TFAST, which has been shown to be a very sensitive test for detecting abnormalities consistent with pneumothorax and pulmonary contusions, can normally be completed in less than 5 minutes (Lisciandro et al, 2008). Trauma radiographs are survey radiographs taken of the entire body. If the patient is on a wooden or Plexiglas board, then radiographs should be taken through the board, and the patient should not be

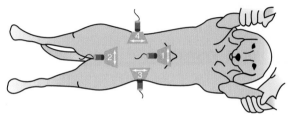

FIGURE 15-4 Illustration of the probe placements and movements used to obtain ultrasonographic views of the abdomen via focused assessment of sonography for trauma (FAST) in a dog. The FAST examination involves transverse and longitudinal views at the subxiphoid region (1), the midline position over the bladder (2), and the right (3) and left (4) flanks (respectively gravity-dependent and gravity-independent locations in dogs in lateral recumbency). (From Boysen SR, Rozanski EA, Tidwell AS et al: Evaluation of focused assessment with sonography for trauma protocol to detect free abdominal fluid in dogs involved in motor vehicle accidents, J Am Vet Med Assoc 225:1198-1204, 2004. Reprinted with permission.)

moved into dorsal recumbency until spinal injury and significant thoracic injury have been ruled out. If the patient is stable, then lateral and ventrodorsal views should be taken. Survey radiographs should be taken and assessed before radiographing extremities or other more localized injury. Once again, treatment should be instituted as abnormalities are detected.

If abdominal hemorrhage or rupture of an abdominal viscus (i.e., urinary bladder, gallbladder, bowel) is a possibility, then ultrasound and ultrasound-guided abdominocentesis should be performed. Four-quadrant abdominocentesis can be performed, but a high incidence of false-negative results are possible if only small amounts of abdominal fluid are present (Crowe, 1986). If ultrasound is not available, then diagnostic peritoneal lavage should be performed. Diagnostic peritoneal lavage requires a multiholed catheter, warm 0.9% saline, and a collection bag. The patient is placed in left lateral recumbency, and the ventral midline of the abdomen is surgically prepared. Local anesthetic is infused, and the catheter is inserted approximately 2 cm caudal to the umbilicus on the midline or just lateral to the midline. Fluids are infused into the abdomen (20 ml/kg), the abdomen is gently massaged to mix the fluid, and a sample is collected. If the patient's respiration becomes compromised during infusion of the fluids, then infusion should be discontinued. Fluid is analyzed for PCV, TS, and creatinine (if a ruptured urinary bladder is a possibility), bilirubin (if a ruptured gallbladder is a possibility), and cytology. The catheter can be left in the animal and the

PCV can be reassessed at 5- to 10-minute intervals for signs of ongoing hemorrhage.

SCORING SYSTEMS

A number of different scoring systems—such as the animal trauma triage score (Rockar et al, 1994), the small animal coma scale (Shores, 1983) (Table 15-1), and the

TABLE 15-1	Small Animal Coma Scale*	
PARAMETER		**SCORE**
Motor Activity (choose one)		
Normal gait, normal spinal reflexes		6
Hemiparesis, tetraparesis, decerebrate rigidity		5
Recumbent, intermittent extensor rigidity		4
Recumbent, constant extensor rigidity		3
Recumbent, constant extensor rigidity with opisthotonos		2
Recumbent, hypotonia of muscles, depressed or absent spinal reflexes		1
Brainstem Reflexes (choose one)		
Normal pupillary light reflexes and oculocephalic reflexes		6
Slow pupillary light reflexes and normal to reduced oculocephalic reflexes		5
Bilateral unresponsive miosis with normal to reduced oculocephalic reflexes		4
Pinpoint pupils with reduced to absent oculocephalic reflexes		3
Unilateral unresponsive mydriasis with reduced to absent oculocephalic reflexes		2
Bilateral unresponsive mydriasis with reduced to absent oculocephalic reflexes		1
Level of Consciousness (choose one)		
Occasional periods of alertness and responsive to the environment		6
Depression or delirium, capable of responding but response may be inappropriate		5
Semicomatose, responsive to visual stimuli		4
Semicomatose, responsive to auditory stimuli		3
Semicomatose, responsive only to repeated noxious stimuli		2
Comatose, unresponsive only to repeated noxious stimuli		1

*Each of the categories is given a score and the score is totaled. A score of 3 to 8 likely indicates a grave prognosis, 9 to 14 guarded, and 15 to 18 good.

abdominal fluid scoring system (Lisciandro et al, 2009), which may be useful in determining prognosis—have been developed in veterinary medicine.

TRAUMA TRIAD OF DEATH

The trauma "triad of death" is acidosis, hypothermia, and coagulopathy (Rotundo et al, 1993). The acidosis can have a respiratory component secondary to pulmonary contusions, pneumothorax, diaphragmatic hernia, or pain from blunt or penetrating trauma to the chest wall. Metabolic acidosis develops secondary to poor tissue perfusion and the ensuing hypoxia. Significant acidity causes dysfunction of all enzyme-driven functions in the body. These enzymatic reactions drive everything from muscle contraction to coagulation. Hypothermia can develop secondary to environmental conditions, from alterations in perfusion, and from treatment with cold intravenous fluids. Hypothermia may lead to further complications by decreasing the metabolic rate, causing a decrease in sinoatrial node automaticity, an increase in ventricular irritability, a decrease in enzymatic reactions, an increase in membrane permeability, and a failure of ion pumps. Mild hypothermia can be protective during shock but significant hypothermia is associated with higher morbidity and mortality. Coagulopathy results from loss of clotting factors; alterations in the coagulation cascade secondary to inflammatory mediators, acidemia, and hypothermia; and also dilution from fluid therapy. All efforts should be made clinically to avoid this triad.

RESUSCITATION

GOALS

To be able to resuscitate the patient in shock, the signs of shock must be recognized. Signs include increased respiratory rate and effort; tachycardia with weak or bounding pulses; pale or muddy mucous membranes; delayed capillary refill time; and low body temperature, cool extremities, or both.

The goal of resuscitation is to reverse the signs of shock and provide effective O_2 delivery to the cells. This means that O_2 must be delivered to the alveoli; once there, the pulmonary circulation must take it up. Adequate hemoglobin (Hb) to transport the O_2 must be present, because the content of O_2 in the arterial blood

(CaO_2) is far more dependent on Hb concentration than the dissolved O_2 level:

$$CaO_2 = 1.34 \times Hb \times \text{saturation of Hb } [SaO_2] + 0.003 \times \text{partial pressure of } O_2 \text{ } [PaO_2]$$

Once the O_2 is taken into the blood it must be transported to the peripheral tissues. This requires adequate circulating volume and a heart that can pump effectively. Preload, or the amount of venous volume that returns to fill the heart, should be maximized. Treatment is aimed at restoring O_2 levels and blood flow to all tissues.

OXYGENATION AND VENTILATION

O_2 should be provided immediately at high flow rates, either by flow-by, mask, baggie, or O_2 collar to all seriously injured trauma patients. An unconscious patient without a good gag reflex should be intubated immediately, and O_2 should be provided via the endotracheal tube. Nasal O_2 provides an inspired fraction of O_2 of 0.4 to 0.6 (Mann et al, 1992), whereas O_2 collars and baggies provide an inspired fraction of O_2 closer to 0.7 to 0.95 (Engelhardt et al, 2004); therefore, nasal O_2 may not be the ideal initial means of providing O_2. O_2 cages are not ideal because patients cannot be monitored adequately. Every time the door to the O_2 cage is opened, significant fluctuations occur in inspired O_2 concentration. In addition, most O_2 cages do not allow the inspired fraction of O_2 to exceed 0.4.

If the respiratory rate and effort and mucous membrane color are not improving with O_2 supplementation, then the patient either has an injury that is interfering with ventilation or has inadequate pulmonary circulation. Injuries leading to impaired ventilation include pneumothorax, hemothorax, fractured ribs (causing pain that leads to hypoventilation), diaphragmatic hernia, or severe pulmonary contusions. Thoracentesis is indicated if lung sounds are dull and hemothorax or pneumothorax is a possibility. Thoracentesis should always be performed in the patient with possible pneumothorax before taking radiographs, because the distress caused by positioning for radiographs may cause the patient to arrest. If negative suction is not obtained during thoracentesis, then a chest tube must be placed immediately. If the patient might have significant intrapulmonic hemorrhage and the site of the hemorrhage is known, then the patient should be placed in lateral recumbency with the affected side down. If the patient has severe pulmonary contusions and is decompensating despite O_2 supplementation, then the patient may need to be rapidly anesthetized, intubated, and started on positive pressure ventilation. Some of these patients require ventilatory support for up to several days until the contusions resolve.

Critical patients should be intubated in lateral recumbency. Technicians should be able to intubate patients in both lateral and dorsal recumbent positions and to use a laryngoscope proficiently. If a patient is significantly hypotensive, then raising the head may cause a sufficient decrease in cerebral blood flow to lead to cardiac arrest. Laryngeal stimulation that can occur with blind intubation can cause a vagal response potentially leading to cardiac arrest in the severely hypotensive or bradycardic patient. Once the patient is intubated, the lungs should be auscultated bilaterally to ensure the trachea has been intubated and that the tube is not in a bronchus. If lung sounds cannot be auscultated, then the esophagus may have been intubated (or the patient may have either an airway obstruction or an airway disruption). If the patient cannot be orotracheally intubated because of oral, pharyngeal, or laryngeal injuries, then a tracheotomy is indicated.

FLUIDS

IV fluids must be provided to the patient in shock at the same time as O_2 is being supplemented. One or more large-bore IV catheters must be placed (14 to 16 gauge in medium and large dogs; 18 to 20 gauge in small dogs and cats). A vascular cutdown may be required for those patients in severe shock. Because flow is directly proportional to the radius to the fourth power and inversely proportional to the length of the catheter, a short large-bore catheter will be more effective for rapid fluid administration than a long small-bore catheter. Peripheral catheters are suitable in most cases. Ideally, a jugular catheter should be placed if large volumes of fluids are to be administered; this allows for measurement of CVP, which is the only way of estimating preload.

A combination of crystalloids and colloids should be delivered at an appropriate rate to improve the patient's hemodynamic status. The patient that is dying from hypovolemic shock requires fluids at a much faster rate than the patient showing mild signs of shock. Patients in shock require intravascular volume resuscitation, not interstitial resuscitation; therefore, large volumes of crystalloid should be infused with caution. Crystalloids are administered in 20 to 30 ml/kg increments.

To maintain adequate intravascular volume, colloids should be infused if response to the initial bolus of crystalloids is limited or not seen. Synthetic colloids such as hydroxyethyl starch should be administered in 5 ml/kg increments to a maximum volume of 20 ml/kg with pentastarch and 50 ml/kg with tetrastarch. Synthetic colloids can be bolused to dogs but should be infused over 10 to 20 minutes in cats. Because many of these patients are in shock from blood loss, the most effective colloid for resuscitation is whole blood. Blood products should be infused as indicated to maintain PCVs of approximately 30% in dogs and 27% in cats and an albumin concentration greater than 2.0 g/dl.

The goal of IV fluid therapy is to restore an effective circulating volume, and therefore, fluids should be administered incrementally until hemodynamic parameters have normalized. In dogs this can be most effectively monitored clinically by ensuring the elevated heart rate decreases to a more normal level and that BP is a minimum of 100 mm Hg systolic. Cats often develop a significant bradycardia in response to shock, unlike the tachycardic response seen in dogs. The goal in bradycardic cats is to have the heart rate increase to a more normal rate.

Patients that are not responding to fluid therapy may have ongoing serious internal abdominal hemorrhage. Serious intraabdominal hemorrhage can come from blunt liver trauma, which leads to liver fractures, splenic lacerations, and renal avulsion. Hypotensive resuscitation, placement of limited external counterpressure, or both may be needed in these patients. Alternatively, surgery may be required as part of the resuscitation.

HEMORRHAGE CONTROL

Hemorrhage is controlled as resuscitation is being initiated. Sterile gauze, sterile laparotomy pads, and sterile towels can all be used as pressure bandages. If strikethrough occurs, then the initial dressing should not be removed; a second dressing should be placed over the top of the first one. In some cases, applying digital pressure to superficial major arteries supplying the hemorrhaging area can control bleeding (Crowe and Devey, 1994). Pressure to the deep area adjacent to and ventral to the mandible controls maxillary artery flow and will help control hemorrhage to the head. Pressure to the axillary area will help control brachial artery blood flow, and pressure applied to the inguinal and femoral canal region controls femoral artery blood flow. In smaller animals, pressure can be placed on the caudal abdomen, thus occluding external iliac blood flow. If significant bleeding occurs from a distal extremity, BP cuffs can be placed proximal to the wound and inflated to 20 to 40 mm Hg greater than systolic pressure. This will effectively control most serious hemorrhage while more definitive treatment is being instituted. Narrow band tourniquets should ideally never be used because they can cause permanent neurologic and vascular damage within minutes.

In cases of severe hemorrhagic shock or ongoing significant abdominal or pelvic hemorrhage, limited external abdominal counterpressure using a wrap incorporating the pelvic limbs, pelvis, and abdomen may be needed (Figure 15-5). Pressure is applied indirectly to blood vessels under the bandage. Because flow is directly proportional to the radius of the vessel to the fourth power, any decrease in the radius of the vessel will significantly decrease flow (and hemorrhage) through that vessel (Niemann et al, 1983). If the pelvic limbs are not included in the bandage, then blood may pool in the pelvic limbs and a risk exists of occluding the caudal abdominal vena cava. The wrap can be made either of towels and duct tape or of rolled cotton and a full bandage, with the former being much quicker to place. A towel is placed between the pelvic limbs. A second large towel is used to wrap the patient in a spiral fashion, starting at the tip of the toes of the pelvic limbs and extending to the diaphragm. The towels are held in place with duct tape. Respiration must be monitored closely, because incorporation of the cranial abdomen in the wrap will

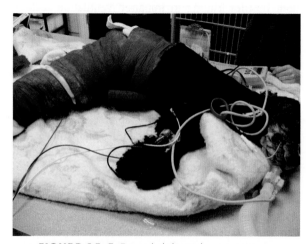

FIGURE 15-5 External abdominal counterpressure.

compromise movement of the diaphragm. If this occurs, then a decision will need to be made either to loosen the bandage, which may lead to further hemorrhage, or to place the patient on a ventilator. Two fingers should be able to be placed easily under the wrap when it is completed. If desired, a BP cuff can be partially inflated and incorporated into the bandage. The wrap then is secured, placing approximately 30 mm Hg pressure on the abdomen. The goal is to ensure intraabdominal pressures remain less than 20 mm Hg. Higher pressures can lead to abdominal compartment syndrome and serious circulatory compromise to the gastrointestinal tract and the kidneys, which can lead to irreversible damage. A urinary catheter should be inserted rapidly in male dogs before placement of the wrap to prevent soiling and to allow urine output to be monitored. The wrap is left in place until the patient is hemodynamically stable, usually from 6 to 24 hours. BP is monitored constantly during removal. The wrap is removed slowly from the cranial extent proceeding caudally. If systolic BP drops by more than 5 mm Hg, then removal is stopped and fluids are infused. If pressure continues to drop, then the wrap is replaced.

RESUSCITATING THE PATIENT WITH SEVERE INTRAABDOMINAL HEMORRHAGE

Hypotensive resuscitation is reserved for those patients in whom hemorrhage will worsen if the BP is restored to normal. It may be appropriate in these patients to restrict fluid resuscitation until the source of the hemorrhage is controlled (Herold et al, 2008). In hypotensive resuscitation fluids are infused to reach a systolic BP of 85 to 100 mm Hg. Elevations in BP are controlled in an effort to prevent disrupting soft clots that are starting to form. In addition, decreasing the amount of fluids administered reduces the chance that the patient will develop a dilutional coagulopathy and minimizes the risk of iatrogenic hypothermia. External abdominal counterpressure is usually needed in these patients.

ANALGESIA

Analgesics are always indicated once the patient has been evaluated and resuscitation has been started. Pain not only is detrimental to the overall well-being of the patient but also is detrimental to the healing process. Catecholamine release can lead to vasoconstriction and poor flow to injured areas.

TECHNICIAN NOTE It is important to realize that pain kills and no patient is too critical to receive analgesics.

Doses may need to be decreased to 25% to 50% of normal in critical patients, but all patients should receive appropriate **analgesia.** Patients with chest trauma should always have their pain aggressively controlled, since thoracic pain can interfere significantly with ventilation, potentially leading to hypercarbia and hypoxia. Opioids are the primary class of drug used for pain control; they can be given intravenously, intramuscularly, or subcutaneously. Pure *mu* agonists are preferred. The intravenous route is preferred over the intramuscular route (painful over time) and subcutaneous route (absorption is unpredictable). If the intramuscular route is used, the injection should be given in the epaxial muscles since blood flow to this muscle bed is more consistent even in the face of alterations in tissue perfusion. Constant rate infusions of fentanyl or morphine are indicated in patients with significant pain and are very useful in patients that will require surgery. Local anesthetics (lidocaine, bupivacaine) can be injected as local or regional blocks. Intercostal blocks will help substantially to improve ventilation in dogs with fractured ribs. Pain related to the acidic nature of the local anesthetic can be modified by warming the drug to body temperature (Mader et al, 1994) or by adding 10% of the volume of lidocaine as sodium bicarbonate.

WOUNDS, BANDAGES, AND SPLINTS

Most wound infections in acute trauma patients occur after the patient enters the hospital. Hospital bacteria and bacteria from human hands often are the cause. Whenever possible, sterile dressings (e.g., sterile bandage material, laparotomy pads, towels) should be placed in direct contact with the wound to help prevent secondary complications. Ideally, wounds should be clipped and cleaned before dressings are placed. The wound must be kept moist and protected from further injury, contamination, and infection. When time permits, the wounds can be cleaned and treated properly.

All wounds should be clipped and cleaned once resuscitation is complete. Placing sterile water-soluble lubricant in wounds before clipping helps prevent hair from getting lodged in the wound and prevents wound desiccation. Tap water can be safely used to wash large wounds (Bansal et al, 2002). Wounds should be cleaned with a surgical disinfecting solution and should not be irrigated in the conscious patient that has not received analgesia because this is a painful procedure. Wounds should be irrigated using a bag of saline pressurized to 300 mm Hg attached to any size needle (Gall and Monnet, 2010). Irrigation using the previously recommended 35-ml syringe attached to an 18-gauge needle often exceeds safe pressure and may lead to tissue trauma. Puncture-type wounds should not be flushed under pressure, because this may force dirt and debris deeper into the wound.

Once the wound has been cleaned, a sterile dressing is placed. Wet-to-dry dressings are used if residual contamination is present or necrotic tissue is seen that requires debridement. In some cases, sterile water-soluble lubricant is placed in the wound, and the wound is covered with a nonadherent dressing such as a Telfa pad. The wound dressing is then covered with a padded layer followed by roll gauze and a water-repellent outer wrap. Bandages must be kept clean and dry; if they become wet or soiled, they must be changed immediately. This is especially important if urine gets into the bandage, because urine is very caustic to tissues. Bandages must be changed as soon as strike-through occurs to prevent wicking of external contaminants and bacteria into the wound through the wet bandage. To prevent infection, gloves should be worn whenever dressings on an open wound are changed.

Effective temporary splints can be placed on distal extremity injuries before radiographs are taken. Splinting can prevent a closed fracture from becoming an open fracture; help stabilize fractures and prevent further injury, from bone fragments that may create shearing injury to the soft tissue; and promote patient comfort by immobilizing the injury. Temporary splints can be placed using newspaper and white porous tape or duct tape. Bubble wrap secured with duct tape also makes a very effective lightweight splint (Figure 15-6).

A properly placed splint stabilizes the joint above as well as below the fracture. Limb bandages should always be placed from the digits proximally and should incorporate the lateral two digits. Toes must be monitored to ensure they stay warm and do not start to swell. If either problem is noticed, then circulation to the foot is compromised and the splint or bandage should be removed immediately.

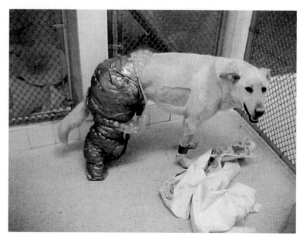

FIGURE 15-6 Splint made of bubble wrap and duct tape stabilizing a femoral fracture.

SURGICAL RESUSCITATION

Surgery may be required to resuscitate and stabilize some trauma patients (Devey, 2013). Examples of patients to whom this applies include those with severe external hemorrhage (e.g., lacerated artery), severe ongoing internal hemorrhage, penetrating gut injuries, and diaphragmatic hernias. Anesthesia in these patients can be challenging, and a dedicated anesthetist is essential for these patients. The severely hemorrhaging patient will need large volumes of warmed fluids and blood products intraoperatively.

BASIC MONITORING

The trauma patient should be monitored closely during resuscitation, during any intraoperative period, and in the intensive care unit after resuscitation. The frequency of monitoring depends on the severity of the patient's condition and should range from as frequently as every 15 minutes in the more critical animal to as infrequently as every 4 to 8 hours in the more stable one. Trends of change often are more important than the exact numbers. Basic monitoring includes measuring level of consciousness, respiratory rate and effort, heart rate, pulse rate and strength, jugular venous distention, BP, and temperature. Monitoring the difference between rectal and toe web temperature can help assess peripheral perfusion. The temperature difference under normal circumstances should be no more than 7° F (4° C).

The lungs should be auscultated frequently (every 1 to 2 hours) to check for the presence of signs consistent with pneumothorax, hemothorax, or pulmonary contusions. Variation in pulse quality or detection of pulse deficits is consistent with ventricular premature contractions (VPCs) or rarely pericardial effusion.

Urine output of a minimum of 0.5 ml/kg/hr helps ensure that renal perfusion is adequate. Fluid intake and output should be monitored and fluids adjusted every 4 to 6 hours as indicated.

Analgesics should be administered regularly and supplemented based on whether the animal appears to be in pain (rather than based on a set schedule). Pain has detrimental effects both physiologically and psychologically and should be controlled as much as possible.

Basic laboratory monitoring should include serial assessment of the PCV and TS. In cases of possible active hemorrhage, the PCV may need to be monitored every 30 minutes; in the more stable patient the PCV can be checked at 2 hours and then every 4 to 8 hours (Table 15-2).

ADVANCED MONITORING

More advanced monitoring includes the use of electrocardiography, CVP, and pulse oximetry. VPCs and ventricular tachycardia are the most common arrhythmias seen in trauma patients. The VPCs should be treated if they are multifocal or affecting perfusion (significant pulse deficits), if the heart rate is elevated (usually above 160 beats per minute), or if evidence of R on T phenomenon is seen. Treatment includes administering supplemental O_2, ensuring tissue perfusion is being maximized, providing analgesia, and ensuring a constant rate infusion of antiarrhythmic drugs (e.g., lidocaine, procainamide).

Pulse oximetry can be monitored on the awake patient; however, measurements are often subject to significant technical errors. If perfusion is poor, then the pulse may not be strong enough for the oximeter to provide an accurate measurement. Strong ambient light and motion can also cause artifacts; percent O_2 saturation should normally read about 97% on room air. If the patient has O_2 saturation readings of 90% to 92% on supplemental O_2, then an arterial blood gas should be checked because the patient may require mechanical ventilation.

Adequate CVP does not necessarily mean venous volume is adequate, but it is a test that can be performed in the conscious patient to help estimate preload. CVP monitoring should ideally be performed in all patients in which fluid overload is a potential complication. Monitoring trends may be more important than exact numbers. Ideally, the CVP should be kept between 5 and 8 cm of water in critical patients where maintaining adequate perfusion is proving to be difficult. CVP does not reflect circulating venous volume if the patient has a pneumothorax, an abdominal counterpressure wrap, or right ventricular heart failure. If CVP is normal and none of the previously mentioned conditions exists but BP is still low, then cardiac function likely is inadequate and positive inotropic support may be indicated.

Advanced laboratory monitoring includes regular assessment of electrolytes and blood gas parameters. A venous blood gas can be used to assess acid-base status and carbon dioxide tension as long as perfusion is not significantly altered to the site of the venipuncture, but an arterial blood gas measurement is required to monitor oxygenation. Albumin levels, coagulation parameters, and platelet numbers should be assessed in more

TABLE 15-2	Goals for Measured Parameters for Trauma Patients	
PARAMETER	**GOAL**
Respiratory rate	>18 and <36 breaths/min
Heart rate	>60 and <130 beats/min
Heart rhythm	*Sinus:* If ventricular premature contractions (VPCs)—unifocal, no significant pulse deficits, heart rate <160 beats/min, no R on T phenomenon
Temperature	Normal; ΔT^* <7° F
Blood pressure (BP)	Systolic >90 and <130 mm Hg Diastolic >60 and <100 mm Hg
Blood flow	Doppler sounds good
Central venous pressure (CVP)	>5 and <10 cm water
Urine output	>0.5 ml/kg/hr
Pulse oximetry	>94%
Packed cell volume (PCV)	>25% and <50%
Total solids (TS)	>4.5 and <7.5 g/dl
Albumin	>2.0 g/dl
Platelet estimate	>5-8/hpf (high-powered field)

*ΔT, Difference between rectal and axillary or rectal and toe web temperatures.

critical patients. If the patient has an indwelling urinary catheter, then daily urine sediments should be evaluated to monitor for possible urinary tract infection. The frequency of laboratory monitoring depends on how critical the patient's condition is; typically parameters are assessed every 8 to 24 hours.

POSTRESUSCITATION CARE: THE FIRST 24 HOURS

The severely traumatized patient is at risk for developing the systemic inflammatory response syndrome (SIRS). Respiratory and cardiovascular parameters must be maintained as close to normal as possible. In addition, laboratory parameters should be monitored and values kept as close to normal as possible.

Patients with significant blood loss have lost a substantial amount of endogenous clotting factors. In addition, tissue trauma is a trigger for activating the coagulation cascade and, if left uncontrolled, may lead to disseminated intravascular coagulation (DIC). Patients in shock frequently are hypothermic and acidotic, which can cause dysfunction of the coagulation system. Infusion of large volumes of crystalloids or synthetic colloids can dilute the remaining coagulation factors, thus leading to a dilutional coagulopathy.

Many of these patients will have multiple tubes in place. All tubes should be carefully labeled to ensure that O_2 is not delivered into a nasogastric tube and enteral feedings are not infused intravenously. If nasal tubes are in place, then the patient should be monitored for signs of skin irritation at the suture site (at the naris) and signs of rhinitis. If adhesive tape is used to secure the tube and it gets wet, it can lead to a moist dermatitis. Complications are usually mild and self-limiting; however, if the patient is experiencing discomfort, then the tube may need to be moved to the other nostril or removed. Feeding tubes, such as esophagostomy, gastrostomy, and jejunostomy tubes, should have daily to twice-daily bandage changes during the initial healing period (3 to 5 days). Ostomy sites should be examined visually for signs of inflammation or discharge and should be palpated for signs of pain. Any abnormalities should be reported because infection may be present.

Bandages on chest tubes should be changed daily to twice daily, and the ostomy site should be inspected by observation and by palpation. The site should be cleaned with an antibacterial solution, and a sterile dressing should be placed. Broad-spectrum antibiotic ointment should be used in generous quantities at the exit site to help form a seal. Patients should wear Elizabethan collars as needed to prevent them from chewing or removing the tubes. Urinary catheter care includes cleaning of the vulva or prepuce with an antibacterial solution and application of a broad-spectrum antibiotic ointment around the tube entry site. Closed collection systems, like IV fluid administration systems, should be replaced every 48 to 72 hours.

Many of these patients will be inactive or have trouble ambulating. Patient comfort is very important; therefore analgesics should be administered as frequently and at as high a dose as necessary to keep the patient comfortable. Uncontrolled pain can cause harmful physiologic effects such as tachycardia, vasoconstriction, and compromised ventilation. Pain should never be used as a means of restricting an animal's movement. For instance, if a patient has a possible soft tissue injury to a limb, then controlling the pain and supporting the limb in a padded bandage or splint are better than keeping the animal immobile through pain. Analgesics ideally should be administered parenterally (locally or regionally). Epidural catheters provide an alternative route that is very effective. Topical fentanyl and fentanyl patches are effective; however, in some severely injured patients, the sedation and cardiovascular depression caused by these formulations can be excessive.

Recumbent patients should be kept on padded bedding and turned every 2 to 4 hours. Larger patients should be monitored closely for the development of decubitus ulcers. Gentle physiotherapy should be performed on all possible limbs when the patient is recumbent. This not only will improve patient comfort but also will stimulate circulation; once the patient is able to ambulate, it will be able to do so more rapidly. This becomes especially important in more geriatric animals or animals with arthritis.

NUTRITION

Nutritional support is vital to trauma patients because they are in a hypermetabolic state. Patient morbidity can be altered significantly if enteral nutritional support is provided within the first 12 to 24 hours (Moore et al, 1992). Enteral nutrition is preferred over parenteral nutrition; enteral nutrition helps preserve the gastrointestinal barrier, thus decreasing the likelihood of bacterial translocation, as well as helping to preserve immune function and normal intestinal, pancreatic, and biliary secretions. Enteral nutritional support can be provided most easily by tube feeding if the patient will not eat. Nasoesophageal or nasogastric tubes can be placed. If longer-term nutritional support is anticipated, then an esophagostomy or gastrostomy tube may be indicated. Feeding tubes can be placed easily at the time of any exploratory celiotomy for use postoperatively. Microenteral nutrition (i.e., the provision of small amounts of glucose and a balanced electrolyte solution) may be beneficial (Devey and Crowe, 2009). Rates start at 0.1 to 0.5 ml/kg of body weight per hour. If the patient cannot tolerate full enteral nutrition, then this can be slowly increased and liquid enteral diets can be added to the infusion. It can be delivered by a constant rate infusion or as intermittent boluses. Caloric intake initially should be estimated based on resting energy requirements. Overfeeding the respiratory compromised patient should be prevented, because excess carbon dioxide will be produced, which requires a compensatory increase in respiratory rate.

COMMUNICATION

Communication with the owner is one of the technician's most important responsibilities. When the critically injured patient arrives and the doctor cannot leave the patient, the technician often can relay basic information on the status of the pet, reassure the owner, and gain permission for procedures or treatment. Because technicians work with patients more closely than do doctors, they are often much more informed about the nuances of the pet's condition and can provide information about the patient's comfort, urination and defecation habits, appetite, and water intake. Owners need to feel that their pets are being taken care of—not only from a medical perspective but also from a psychologic and emotional perspective.

> *TECHNICIAN NOTE* The veterinary technician is the patient's and the owner's advocate. If any part of the patient's care is not being addressed adequately, then the technician's responsibility is to inform the veterinarian and make recommendations to resolve the issues.

ASSESSMENT AND MANAGEMENT OF SPECIFIC INJURIES

The degree of tissue trauma varies with the type of trauma and the velocity and mass of the impact. Force is equal to the mass multiplied by the velocity squared ($F = MV^2$). The greater the force, the more significant the tissue trauma. For instance, a dog hit in the head with a baseball bat will suffer a significantly different injury than one shot in the head; a dog hit by a bicycle will suffer much less force of injury than one hit by a car.

Trauma is generally divided into two types: (1) blunt and (2) penetrating. Blunt trauma, which involves crushing forces, usually occurs from collision with an object. This can occur if the animal falls, is stepped on, or is hit by an object such as a car or baseball bat. Penetrating injuries generally are those inflicted by knives, arrows, bullets, and larger objects that cause impalement (e.g., sticks, metal rods). Bite wounds can cause both penetrating and blunt trauma. Significant shearing forces can be applied after penetration, especially with bite wounds. The seriousness of the injury often will depend on the body part that is penetrated. A better understanding of the mechanism of injury allows for greater appreciation of possible internal injuries, which can enable the team to minimize patient morbidity and mortality.

Several types of traumatic injury can lead to death rapidly if the injury is not assessed accurately and treated immediately. These include airway disruptions or obstructions, tension pneumothorax, severe pulmonary contusions, and massive internal thoracic or abdominal hemorrhage. A high index of suspicion should be maintained for these injuries.

In the following sections, injuries are grouped by anatomic location. A brief overview of how to assess, manage, and monitor these patients during the resuscitation period is provided. The reader is referred to more detailed descriptions of individual injuries for more information. In all cases it is assumed that O_2 will be provided, as well as IV fluid support and analgesics. It is also assumed that basic diagnostics and monitoring as outlined previously are being performed. The list is not all-inclusive, but it is designed to provide an overview of the more common injuries that will arrive at the emergency department. A word of caution: No impaled object should be removed until the wound tract is explored. The object may have passed through or may be lodged in a major vessel such as the heart or the abdominal aorta. Premature removal may lead to rapid exsanguination. The only exception to this rule is any object that is thought to be compromising respiration to the point of impending arrest.

HEAD AND FACIAL TRAUMA

Assessment

Patients with head trauma have varying levels of consciousness from normal mentation to coma. Head trauma can lead to traumatic brain injury (TBI). Trauma to the brainstem is life threatening and can lead to alterations in respiratory pattern and cardiovascular derangement. Facial fractures may lead to intraoral and intranasal hemorrhage and subsequent respiratory difficulty. Blood can pool in the oropharynx, leading to an effective airway obstruction. Use of the small animal coma scale (see Table 15-1) provides an objective evaluation and may help with prognosis.

Management

A clear airway is the first priority. The airway should be cleared of as much of the blood, vomitus, or other secretions as possible using instrument sweeps with gauze in between the jaws of the instrument or using suction; however, extreme care should be taken to ensure no one is bitten. A gagging response should be avoided in the patient with traumatic brain injury (TBI), because this will elevate intracranial pressure and decrease cerebral blood flow. If patients are unconscious with no gag reflex, then they must be intubated rapidly, without lifting the head because the decrease in blood flow to the brain caused by this maneuver may lead to cardiac arrest. A laryngoscope should be used to assist with intubation to avoid excessive manipulation of the larynx. Nasal tubes should not be used, because sneezing may elevate intracranial pressure.

The second priority is to ensure adequate cerebral blood flow. The intracranial volume is comprised of the brain tissue, the cerebrospinal fluid, and the blood vessels. Because the skull contains the brain, any change in one of the compartments will affect the other two. Pressure on the jugular veins during venipuncture or placement of catheters should be avoided, because this may raise intracranial pressure (ICP) and decrease perfusion to the brain. Fluids should be administered to maintain normal BP. These patients must not be volume overloaded or allowed to become hypertensive, because this may exacerbate intracranial hemorrhage; however,

hypotension is even more detrimental. Hypertonic saline (5% to 7.5%) is useful in patients with systemic hypotension and elevated ICP. Corticosteroids do not improve and may even worsen outcome and should not be used (Edwards et al, 2005). Although mannitol has the potential to worsen active intracranial hemorrhage, its benefits generally outweigh its potential disadvantages. Sedatives may be needed if the patient is severely disoriented or hypertensive. The $PaCO_2$ should not be allowed to rise because this causes cerebral vasodilation. Mild hyperventilation to a $PaCO_2$ of 30 to 35 mm Hg may be indicated to help lower ICP. If a compressed skull fracture is seen or the patient's neurologic status is worsening, then emergency surgery for a decompressive craniotomy may be required.

Hyperbaric O_2 therapy delivered within 2 to 6 hours of the head injury has been shown to be effective in ameliorating ongoing secondary neuronal ischemia caused by edema and swelling, as well as to decrease ongoing hypoxic injury to the brain (Niklas et al, 2004). Recumbent patients should be kept in a horizontal position with mild elevation of the head up to 30 degrees and turned every 2 to 4 hours. When placing the patient in a cage, care must be taken to ensure the neck is not flexed, which may potentially lead to a compromised airway and compromised venous outflow via the jugular veins.

Severe epistaxis may necessitate the use of intranasal epinephrine or nasal packing. Surgery is rarely required. Sneezing and hypertension will worsen the epistaxis and should be controlled. These animals must be kept very quiet and often require sedation.

Monitoring

Small animal coma scale score, pupil size and symmetry, respiratory pattern, heart rate, mucous membrane color, BP, CVP, PCV, and TS should be monitored. Blood gases and an ECG should be evaluated as indicated. Platelet numbers, a buccal mucosal bleeding time to check for platelet dysfunction, and a coagulation screen are indicated if epistaxis persists or the clinician is concerned about an underlying coagulopathy.

CERVICAL SOFT TISSUE INJURY

Assessment

Cervical trauma can lead to airway avulsion or disruption, airway obstruction from hemorrhage or swelling, esophageal laceration, and laceration of major vessels.

These animals can experience varying degrees of respiratory distress. Blood loss is highly variable, as is injury to other soft tissues including muscle, subcutaneous tissue, and skin.

Management

The animal's respiratory rate and pattern must be closely observed. Any animal that has noisy breathing has a compromised airway, which may progress to an obstruction. Exaggerated chest movement without airway sounds is a hallmark for an airway obstruction. The animal that is struggling to breathe and has pronounced respiratory efforts may have an avulsed larynx or trachea. These patients require immediate anesthesia and intubation or an awake tracheostomy; transtracheal or nasotracheal O_2 administration may help in the interim. The trachea should be auscultated and the entire area carefully palpated and thoroughly clipped of hair to evaluate the wounds, extent of hemorrhage, and swelling. Any wound should be cleaned and a sterile bandage placed unless a tracheal injury is possible. Bandaging a tracheal laceration should be avoided because this may cause subcutaneous emphysema and a pneumomediastinum. Extreme care should be taken when placing a cervical bandage, because patient movement often tightens these bandages. If there is a concern for an associated spinal injury, then the patient must not be moved before stabilizing the injury. Cervical spinal injuries at or above the level of C4-C6 can lead to loss of diaphragm function and subsequent respiratory compromise.

Monitoring

Mucous membrane color, respiratory rate and effort, heart rate, BP, and pulse oximetry should be monitored. The PCV, TS, blood gases, and ECG should be evaluated as indicated. Neck bandages should be checked every 4 to 6 hours and loosened as needed.

CHEST INJURY

Assessment

Chest trauma can lead to musculoskeletal injuries such as fractured ribs, lacerated muscles, and bruising. Intrathoracic trauma most commonly leads to pneumothorax, hemothorax, pulmonary contusions, and cardiac contusions. These patients will have varying degrees of respiratory distress. Hypoventilation caused by pain from fractured ribs is a significant concern.

Management

The technician should provide O_2 immediately if he or she believes the animal has a chest injury. Rapid, shallow ventilation often indicates pain from fractured ribs and a pleural space abnormality (pneumothorax or pneumohemothorax). Tension pneumothorax should be considered if the patient has shallow, rapid respiration, an expanded thorax, limited movement of the chest wall with ventilation, and distended jugular veins. Deep, gasping breaths often indicate severe pulmonary contusions. Auscultation and percussion of the thorax should be performed. Dull lung sounds are consistent with pulmonary contusions or pleural space disease, and dull or hyperresonant areas on percussion are consistent with pleural space abnormalities. In either situation, thoracentesis is indicated. Thoracentesis always should be done bilaterally and should always precede radiographs. Analgesia should be provided early using intrapleural analgesia, intercostal nerve blocks, or frequent parenteral injections of opioids. All wounds should be clipped and cleaned, and sterile dressings should be placed. The exception may be a large wound into the pleural space. If this is sealed, then a tension pneumothorax may result. A chest tube may need to be placed through this hole first followed by placement of an occlusive dressing. Alternatively, an occlusive patch dressing that is sealed on three sides only is placed over the hole, with the fourth side acting as a pop-off valve. When the patient inhales, the dressing will be pulled inward, creating a seal against the thorax; when the patient exhales, the unsealed dressing will act as a relief valve and allow excess air to be expelled. If the patient has a flail chest and is in lateral recumbency, then the flail side should be placed downward. A flail chest is a segment of chest wall that moves paradoxically with each breath (*in* when the patient inhales and *out* when the patient exhales). The cause of this condition is three or more adjacent ribs that are fractured in more than one location, which create a free-floating segment of chest wall. Many of these patients can be managed medically but a severe flail chest may require surgical stabilization.

Monitoring

Patients with chest injuries must be monitored on a continuous basis until they are stable. Vital signs, including respiratory rate and effort, mucous membrane color, heart rate, and BP, should be assessed frequently. Measurement of arterial blood gases is ideal but positioning to enable collection of an arterial sample may stress the patient excessively. In this case, pulse oximetry should be performed. Patients with chest trauma may develop ventricular premature contractions (VPCs) and ventricular tachycardia secondary to traumatic myocarditis. These patients should have continuous ECG monitoring, and pulses should be palpated routinely for deficits. Chest tube connections should be checked frequently for signs of loosening or dislodgment. If continuous underwater suctioning is being applied then the tubing should be stripped every 4 to 6 hours and intermittent hand aspiration should be performed.

ABDOMEN
Assessment

Intraabdominal injury can lead to significant hemorrhage from solid visci (e.g., liver, spleen), vascular injury to major vessels, and lacerations to the bowel leading to peritonitis. Persistent vomiting, increasing abdominal pain, and abdominal distention are all indicators of a significant intraabdominal injury. Percussion may indicate areas of dullness, fluid waves, or areas of resonance, suggesting intraabdominal air accumulations. Splenic injuries frequently are associated with VPCs. Retroperitoneal injuries can be more difficult to diagnose; however, if the patient is becoming more anemic and no other known source for the blood loss is found, then the bleeding may be coming from the retroperitoneal space.

Management

Patients with abdominal injuries often have multiple injuries; airway and breathing should always be assessed and managed before addressing abdominal injuries. Nasogastric decompression is important to decrease vomiting from gastric distention (either from aerophagia or from fluid) and to encourage the stomach to return to normal motility (Moss, 1984). This is especially important if the patient has had surgery for abdominal injuries or has an open abdomen. Pharmacologic control of vomiting may be required. Urine should be assessed for the presence of hemorrhage grossly (using a dipstick test) and microscopically. If the patient is not producing urine within the first 4 hours of hospitalization, then the possibility of a ruptured urinary bladder should be considered. The stool should be monitored for signs of hemorrhage and melena. The hair covering the ventral and lateral aspects of the abdomen and caudal rib cage should be clipped and the area examined for the presence of a wound and bruising.

Monitoring

Physical parameters including mucous membrane color, respiratory rate and effort, heart rate, and BP should be closely monitored. Ongoing hemorrhage is always a concern; therefore, serial PCV and TS measurements should be assessed. The abdomen should be monitored for signs of distention or excessive bruising. Urine output should be monitored hourly during initial resuscitation, and then every 4 hours.

MUSCULOSKELETAL SYSTEM
Assessment

Animals with suspected musculoskeletal injury should not be allowed to be too mobile in case they injure themselves further; they should be restrained in lateral recumbency or confined to a small space until they are examined. Some musculoskeletal injuries are readily apparent because of the soft tissue trauma surrounding the injury. Non–weight-bearing lameness usually indicates luxation, fracture, or severe ligament injury, whereas partial weight bearing usually indicates a less severe injury. Severe hemorrhage into muscle compartments can lead to compartment syndrome. This occurs when the pressure rises within the muscle belly to the point that circulation to the affected area is obstructed. Because compartment syndrome rapidly leads to tissue necrosis, the condition must be recognized early. Clinical signs can include severe swelling, signs that the affected area is becoming more painful than would be expected, decreased temperature of the toes of the affected limb in comparison to a normal limb, and increasing loss of movement or loss of sensation. Fractures can lead to laceration of underlying soft tissue. For instance, rib fractures can be associated with a lacerated lung and pneumothorax, femoral fractures can lead to laceration of major femoral vessels, and pubic fractures can lacerate the urethra. Patients with possible spinal fractures should be immobilized (taped to a board with duct tape or similar material). These patients must be radiographed before they are allowed to move, because movement may cause a significant worsening of the injury.

Management

All distal limb fractures should be splinted before radiographs are taken or the patient is moved. Pain should not be used as a way of immobilizing patients, and analgesics should always be administered. As discussed previously, wounds should be protected with sterile dressings or covered with sterile towels. If it is suspected that compartment syndrome is present, then pressure must be released immediately. The clinician does this by performing a fasciotomy in the operating room under aseptic conditions.

Monitoring

The patient should be monitored closely for evidence of soft tissue injury under fracture sites (i.e., monitored for urination with pubic fractures, pneumothorax with rib fractures, and compartment syndrome with long bone fractures).

CONCLUSION

The severely injured patient's survival depends on a well-equipped facility and an educated and trained staff. The technician plays a vital role in ensuring the ready area is properly prepared to receive any emergency, in triage (which ensures the seriously injured patient is recognized immediately), and in being able to assist with resuscitation. The technician must be able to use a wide variety of monitors and monitoring techniques. An understanding of the pathology that can occur with different injuries helps ensure the patient is monitored and treated appropriately. Good communication between team members is essential to minimize patient morbidity and mortality.

REFERENCES

Bansal BC, Wiebe RA, Perkins SD, et al.: Tap water for irrigation of lacerations, *Am J Emerg Med* 20:469–472, 2002.

Boysen SR, Rozanski EA, Tidwell AS, et al.: Evaluation of focused assessment with sonography for trauma protocol to detect free abdominal fluid in dogs involved in motor vehicle accidents, *J Am Vet Med Assoc* 225:1198–1204, 2004.

Broadie TA, Glover JL, Bang N, et al.: Clotting competence of intracavitary blood in trauma victims, *Ann Emerg Med* 10:121–130, 1981.

Crowe DT: Autotransfusion in the critically injured patient: a historic review and current recommendations, *J Vet Crit Care* 4:14–39, 1981.

Crowe DT: Assessment and management of the severely polytraumatized small animal patient, *J Vet Emerg Crit Care* 16:264–275, 2006.

Crowe DT, Crane SW: Diagnostic abdominal paracentesis and lavage in evaluations of abdominal injuries in dogs and cats: clinical and experimental investigations, *J Am Vet Med Assoc* 168:700–705, 1986.

Crowe DT, Devey JJ: Assessment and management of the hemorrhaging patient, *Vet Clin North Am Small Anim Pract* 24:1095–1122, 1994.

Devey JJ: Surgical considerations in the emergent patient, *Vet Clin North Am Small Anim Pract* 43:899–914, 2013.

Devey JJ, Crowe DT: Microenteral nutrition. In Bonagura JD, editor: *Current veterinary therapy XIV*, Philadelphia, 2009, Elsevier. (Electronic chapter: evolve.Elsevier.com/Bonagura/Kirks/.)

Edwards P, Arango M, Balica L, et al.: Final results of MRC CRASH, a randomised placebo-controlled trial of intravenous corticosteroid in adults with head injury—outcomes at 6 months, *Lancet* 365:1957–1959, 2005.

Engelhardt MH, Crowe DT: Comparison of six non-invasive supplemental oxygen techniques in dogs and cats, *J Vet Emerg Crit Care* 14:S1–S17, 2004.

Gall TT, Monnet E: Evaluation of fluid pressures of common wound-flushing techniques, *Am J Vet Res* 71:1384–1386, 2010.

Herold LV, Devey JJ, Kirby R, et al.: Clinical evaluation and management of hemoperitoneum in dogs, *J Vet Emerg Crit Care* 18:40–53, 2008.

Lisciandro GR, Lagutchik MS, Mann KA, et al.: Evaluation of a thoracic focused assessment with sonography for trauma (TFAST) protocol to detect pneumothorax and concurrent thoracic injury in 145 traumatized dogs, *J Vet Emerg Crit Care* 18:258–269, 2008.

Lisciandro GR, Lagutchik MS, Mann KA, et al.: Evaluation of an abdominal fluid scoring system determined using abdominal focused assessment with sonography for trauma in 101 dogs with motor vehicle trauma, *J Vet Emerg Crit Care* 19:426–437, 2009.

Mader TJ, Playe SJ, Garb JL: Reducing the pain of local anesthetic infiltration: warming and buffering have a synergistic effect, *Ann Emerg Med* 23:550–554, 1994.

Mann FA, Wagner-Mann C, Allert JA, et al.: Comparison of intranasal and intratracheal oxygen administration in healthy awake dogs, *Am J Vet Res* 53:856–860, 1992.

Moore FA, Feliciano DV, Andrassy RJ, et al.: Early enteral feeding, compared with parenteral, reduces postoperative septic complications, The results of a meta-analysis, *Ann Surg* 216:172–183, 1992.

Moss G: Efficient gastroduodenal decompression with simultaneous full enteral nutrition: a new gastrostomy catheter technique, *J Parenter Enteral Nutr* 8:203–207, 1984.

Niemann JT, Stapczynski JS, Rosborough JP, et al.: Hemodynamic effects of pneumatic external counterpressure in canine hemorrhagic shock, *Ann Emerg Med* 12:661–667, 1983.

Niklas A, Brock D, Schober R, et al.: Continuous measurements of cerebral tissue oxygen pressure during hyperbaric oxygenation—HBO effects on brain edema and necrosis after severe brain trauma in rabbits, *J Neurol Sci* 219:77–82, 2004.

Rockar RA, Drobatz KJ, Shofer FS: Development of a scoring system for the veterinary trauma patient, *J Vet Emerg Crit Care* 4:77–84, 1994.

Rotondo MF, Schwab CW, McGonigal MD, et al.: Damage control: an approach for improved survival in exsanguinating penetrating abdominal injury, *J Trauma* 35:375–382, 1993.

Shores A: Craniocerebral trauma. In Kirk RW, editor: *Current veterinary therapy X*, Philadelphia, 1983, Saunders, pp 847–854.

SCENARIO

Scenario

A 20-kg male neutered mixed breed is presented 20 minutes after being hit by a car. The dog has evidence of head trauma and is stuporous. Chest radiographs reveal signs of pulmonary contusions with no signs of a pneumothorax or hemothorax. There are no other injuries.

Questions

1. The systolic blood pressure is 100 mm Hg. Is this an adequate blood pressure for this patient? Why or why not?
2. What does stuporous mean?
3. A decision is made to give more crystalloid fluids to the dog. What are two potentially major complications of this necessary treatment? Discuss how the patient can be monitored for these complications.
4. What nursing care should be instituted to try and help prevent the intracranial pressure from becoming higher than it already is?

Discussion

1. No; it is not adequate. Discussion should focus on the pathophysiology of increased intracranial pressure, how cerebral perfusion pressure is defined, and how hypotension impacts cerebral perfusion pressure.
2. Stuporous is an altered level of consciousness where the patient is recumbent and appears unaware of its surroundings and is only responsive to painful stimuli.
3. Primary complications of extravasation into the brain causing worsening of the brain injury and extravasation into the lungs causing worsening of lung function should be discussed.
4. Discussion of monitoring should focus on how to determine that brain injury and respiration have worsened using a combination of parameters such as physical exam findings, scoring systems, and lab work, for example.
   - Elevate the head and neck approximately 30 degrees.
   - Avoid pressure on the jugular veins.
   - Avoid any treatment that may lead to sneezing (e.g., intranasal medications, insertion of a nasal tube).

MEDICAL MATH EXERCISE

Patient order states: *Give 20 mg/kg cefazolin.* The patient weighs 40 kg. The concentration of the cefazolin is 100 mg/ml.
   a. What dose in mg should be given?
   b. What dose in ml should be given?

16 Hematologic Emergencies

Kenichiro Yagi

CHAPTER OUTLINE

Hemostasis
Disorders of Primary Hemostasis
Disorders of Secondary Hemostasis
Disorders in Anticoagulation
Clinical Assessment
History
Physical Examination
Laboratory Tests
Primary Hemostatic Tests
Platelet Estimation

Bleeding Time Test
Secondary Hemostatic Tests
Anemia
RBC Loss
RBC Destruction
Reduced or Ineffective Erythropoiesis
Dysfunctional Hemoglobin Species
Clinical Assessment
Treatment and Management

KEY TERMS

Anemia
Coagulation
Coagulopathy
Disseminated intravascular coagulation
Erythropoiesis
Heinz body
Hemolysis
Hemophilia
Hemostasis
Hypoxemic shock
Thrombocytopenia
Thrombopathia
Vitamin K antagonism
von Willebrand's disease

LEARNING OBJECTIVES

After studying this chapter, you will be able to:

- Understand the consequences, causes, and treatment of anemia.
- Understand basic hemostasis and common hemostatic disorders and their treatment.
- Recognize clinical signs and a working knowledge of diagnostics involved in hematologic emergencies.

HEMOSTASIS

The hemostatic system is a complex protective mechanism sealing off avenues of blood loss through the vascular system upon damage. Although cessation of blood loss is vital in preventing subsequent **anemia** and eventual death, **coagulation** of the blood is normally controlled, limiting it within the intravascular space to maintain normal blood flow and minimizing chances of thrombosis. This delicate balance and interaction of procoagulant and anticoagulant mechanisms is essential to the proper function of the hemostatic system. It occurs through a complex series of events involving the vessels, platelets, plasma coagulation factors, and the fibrinolytic system. The role that each component plays in **hemostasis** is dependent on the size of the vessel and the amount of damage that has occurred. Bleeding in smaller vessels may be controlled by a simple response involving the vasculature and platelets, known as primary hemostasis. With larger vessel injury, plasma coagulation factors are needed to form a stable clot, a process known as secondary hemostasis. Dysfunctions of the hemostatic system lead to life-threatening conditions through a variety of mechanisms.

When a patient has abnormal bleeding, its cause must be determined. Animals may bleed after injury or trauma, but they may also suffer from either an inherited or an acquired hemostatic defect. Although the veterinarian is responsible for diagnosing and choosing an appropriate therapy for each patient, the veterinary technician should be knowledgeable and anticipate the needs of the veterinarian and, most importantly, the patient. This requires a basic understanding of the physiology of hemostasis.

The first response to blood vessel injury is vasoconstriction, temporarily diverting blood flow around the injured area. Once the endothelial lining of the vessel is disrupted, the subendothelial connective tissue (collagen) is exposed. Circulating platelets pool to the area of injury and adhere to the endothelial lining (platelet adhesion) through binding of surface glycoprotein complexes with collagen-bound von Willebrand's factor (vWF). Platelets are activated upon adhesion (platelet activation), experiencing a cascade of events starting with increased cytosolic calcium concentration, leading to production of procoagulants (thromboxane A_2 and platelet activating factor). The membrane skeleton changes in shape and exposes receptors for collagen, fibronectin, and other components, furthering adhesion and activation. The procoagulants are secreted, enhancing platelet layering in the injured area (platelet aggregation, resulting in the formation of a temporary hemostatic plug). This portion of the hemostatic process is referred to as *primary hemostasis*.

Coagulation factors are involved in forming a stable hemostatic plug *(secondary hemostasis)*. Plasma coagulation factors (denoted by Roman numerals) are produced in the liver, many with the help of vitamin K (II, VII, IX, and X), and are enzymes or cofactors to enzymatic processes. They circulate in the blood in the inactive form and, when exposed to certain substances, become activated (denoted by the letter "*a*") in a cascade-like effect (Table 16-1). Blood coagulation involves a complex process by which the multiple coagulation factors contained in blood interact. A classic model divides the process into three major pathways: tissue factor (extrinsic), contact activation (intrinsic), and common pathways (Figure 16-1).

TABLE 16-1	Coagulation Factors	
COAGULATION FACTOR	NAME	VITAMIN K DEPENDENT
I	Fibrinogen	
II	Prothrombin	X
III	Tissue factor	
IV	Calcium	
V	Proaccelerin	
VI	No factor VI	
VII	Proconvertin	X
VIII	Antihemophilic	
IX	Christmas factor	X
X	Stuart factor	X
XI	Plasma thromboplastin antecedent	
XII	Hageman factor	
XIII	Fibrin-stabilizing factor	

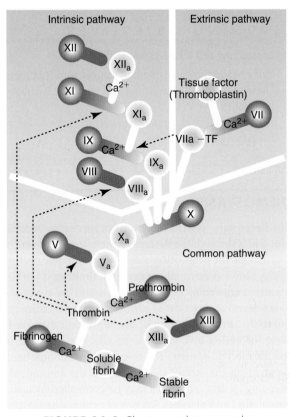

FIGURE 16-1 Classic coagulation cascade.

A new understanding of hemostasis involving the role of platelets and tissue factor (TF) bearing cells (cell-based model) describes the process in overlapping phases of initiation, amplification, and propagation (Figure 16-2) (Weiss and Wardrop, 2010).

TF expressed by cells located outside of the vasculature serves as the initiator for coagulation. The localization of TF in the extravascular compartment prevents the activation of coagulation in normal circumstances where the endothelium is intact. TF is also expressed by some cells in circulation but is kept in an inactivated form. During the *initiation* phase, injury of the endothelium exposes TF, leading to the binding of factor VIIa (FVIIa), which in turn activates more TF-FVII complexes. The complex activation leads to generation of FIXa, FXa, and FVa. FXa and FVa form the prothrombinase complex, leading to small amounts of thrombin generation through cleavage of prothrombin.

The *amplification* phase amplifies the small signaling for coagulation through thrombin generation in the initiation phase. Platelets are activated by the generated thrombin as they leave the intravascular space through the injured endothelium. Through changes in membrane surfaces incited by thrombin binding to receptors, platelets degranulate to release fibronectin, platelet factor, von Willebrand's factor (vWF), calcium, and other procoagulants. These factors further activate platelets and promote binding of coagulation factors to the membrane surface. Thrombin then activates FXIa and FVa on the platelet surface, and cleaves vWF from FVIII, releasing vWF and activating FVIII to FVIIIa.

Propagation occurs through the effect of platelet degranulation, including the expression of platelet surface ligands resulting in platelet aggregation. FIXa (generated during initiation and amplification) and FVIIIa (generated during amplification) form the tenase complex on the platelet surface. Tenase then rapidly generates FXa on the platelet surface, binds to FVa (generated in the amplification phase), and cleaves prothrombin into thrombin. Thrombin is the protease responsible for fibrin formation. When there is a significant amount of thrombin generated, conversion of fibrinogen to fibrin occurs, allowing for clotting. Thrombin further promotes coagulation by activating FVII, FXI, FVIII, and FV; activating platelets; and activating FXIII (a transglutaminase responsible for crosslinking fibrin fibrils).

The final step in the hemostatic process is fibrinolysis. Once the damage is repaired through healing mechanisms, removal of the clot is required to reestablish unimpeded blood flow. Fibrinolysis is the process of dissolution of the fibrin clot, performed by an enzyme called plasmin created from plasminogen by the action

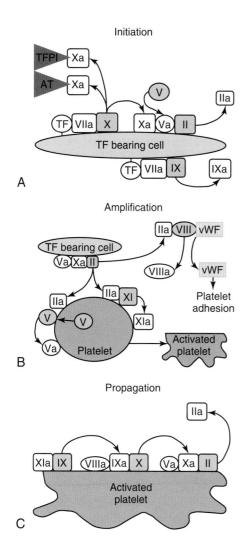

FIGURE 16-2 Cell-based model of coagulation. **(A)** Initiation phase triggered by TF-bearing cells resulting in a small amount of thrombin (IIa) formation. **(B)** Amplification phase: Thrombin signal is amplified through platelet-mediated activation of FV, FVIII, and FXI. **(C)** Propagation phase: Factors activated in previous phases form intrinsic tenase, eventually leading to a burst of thrombin generation. (From Weiss DJ, Wardrop KJ, editors: *Schalm's veterinary hematology*, ed 6, Ames, Iowa, 2010, Wiley-Blackwell.)

of plasminogen activators. Clot dissolution produces small pieces of fibrin, referred to as *fibrin split products (FSPs)* or *fibrin degradation products (FDPs),* which are cleared from the circulation by the liver. After clot digestion, vessel wall endothelium is reestablished and returned to its original state. Small levels of FSPs always appear in the circulation as a result of bleeding and clotting secondary to normal wear-and-tear on vessels. FSP levels may increase during episodes of excessive bleeding with diffuse coagulation (i.e., **disseminated intravascular coagulation** [DIC]) and in patients with compromised liver function.

DISORDERS OF PRIMARY HEMOSTASIS
Thrombocytopenia

Patients with a low platelet count, known as ***thrombocytopenia,*** experience bleeding when inadequate numbers of platelets are available to form a platelet plug (spontaneous bleeding typically does not occur unless platelet concentration is less than 20,000 to 30,000/µL). Platelet production in both dogs and cats is affected by various means (e.g., drugs, bone marrow neoplasia, and infection). Massive transfusion may cause thrombocytopenia from a combination of the rapid consumption of platelets and the dilution of platelet concentration by fluid solutions and blood components. Thrombocytopenia can also result from an increased consumption of platelets attributable to DIC, infection, neoplasia, inflammation, immune-mediated disorders, and drug interactions.

Immune-mediated thrombocytopenia (IMT) is a common cause of increased platelet sequestration and destruction with subsequent thrombocytopenia. IMT occurs when immunoglobulin G (IgG) antibodies against platelet membrane elements are produced and bound, resulting in premature removal by the reticuloendothelial system. IMT can be classified as a *primary disorder,* referred to as *idiopathic thrombocytopenic purpura (ITP),* if the production of antiplatelet antibodies is truly autoimmune and has no apparent cause. Classification as a secondary disorder is warranted if antibodies are produced in response to antigenic stimuli (e.g., drugs, vaccines, infections, and neoplasia). A complete medical history, including recent vaccinations, medications, and tick exposure, as well as recent or concurrent illness, is important in identifying a potential antigenic stimulus. IMT may be acute, chronic, or recurrent, and can range from mild to severe in presentation.

Thrombopathia

A platelet function defect, or thrombopathia, is considered in patients with a history of bleeding (especially surface bleeding) and a normal platelet count. When the platelet quality is compromised, platelet adhesion or aggregation (or both) at the site of endothelial damage may be abnormal. Thrombopathia may be classified as an *inherited* or an *acquired* defect.

Congenital disorders of platelet function have been recognized in small animals but are rare. Some of the more common inherited thrombopathia are listed in Table 16-2. Certain drugs may have a pronounced adverse effect on platelets by inhibiting platelet function (e.g., aspirin, ibuprofen, naproxen, aminophylline, diltiazem, and nonsteroidal antiinflammatory drugs [NSAIDs]). Drug-induced hemostatic abnormalities usually resolve when the drug is discontinued. However, aspirin causes irreversible platelet inactivation persisting throughout the life span of the platelet. Bleeding abnormalities may also be a clinical manifestation of

TABLE 16-2	Common Hereditary Bleeding Disorders
PLATELET DYSFUNCTION	
DISORDER	**BREED**
Delta storage pool disease	Cocker spaniel
Glanzmann thrombasthenia	Otterhound, Great Pyrenees
Chédiak-Higashi syndrome	Persian cat
Other thrombopathias	Basset hound, boxer, spitz, domestic shorthair
COAGULOPATHIES	
Factor I (fibrinogen) deficiency	Bichon frisé, borzoi, collie, cats
Factor II (prothrombin) deficiency	Boxer
Factor VII deficiency	Beagle, malamute, schnauzer, cats
Factor VIII deficiency (hemophilia A)	Many canine breeds, cats
Factor IX deficiency (hemophilia B)	Many canine breeds, cats
Factor X deficiency (Stuart-Power trait)	Cocker spaniels, Jack Russell terrier, cats
Factor XI deficiency (hemophilia C)	English springer spaniel, Kerry blue terrier, cats
Factor XII deficiency	Miniature poodle, Shar Pei, cats

patients with acute or chronic renal failure from platelet dysfunction induced by uremia.

Clinically significant bleeding from thrombocytopenia or thrombopathia is an indication for platelet transfusions. Preparation of platelets in a volume needed to measurably increase platelet numbers, especially in larger breed dogs, is difficult (1 unit/10-kg body weight for 35,000/μL increase). In some patients, however, cessation of bleeding after platelet transfusion has been achieved without a measurable increase in platelet number. In situations of platelet destruction, such as IMT, the survival of transfused platelets is transient and not recommended except in cases of severe, life-threatening hemorrhage. In patients with IMT, the veterinarian must treat the underlying disease (e.g., ehrlichiosis) or remove the triggering agent (e.g., drugs) and source of immunosuppression (glucocorticoids, azathioprine, cyclosporine, mycophenolate, vincristine, human immunoglobulins) in primary IMT.

Platelet transfusion may be warranted if the patient is acutely bleeding into a vital structure (e.g., brain, myocardium, pleural cavity) or in severe, uncontrolled bleeding. In veterinary medicine, treatment of thrombocytopenia and thrombopathia with active bleeding is more practical using fresh whole blood, from which the patient will receive both platelets and oxygen-carrying support. In most instances, however, medical management is the treatment of choice.

von Willebrand's Disease

The most common hereditary bleeding defect in dogs (recognized in more than 60 breeds) is **von Willebrand's disease** (vWD), a deficiency of von Willebrand's factor (vWF) (a large plasma protein produced by and stored in endothelial cells). vWF facilitates platelet adhesion and aggregation, and acts as a carrier for factor VIII. The size of vWF multimers varies, with the larger multimers being more hemostatically active. Assays are available to quantify vWF in circulation, to determine vWF-dependent platelet activity, and to establish its multimeric distribution (Ettinger and Feldman, 2010).

The three major types of vWD are differentiated by the vWF concentration and multimer pattern: type 1 (mild to moderate disease with low vWF and normal multimer distribution), type 2 (moderate to severe disease with a lack of higher molecular weight multimers), and type 3 (complete absence of vWF).

Mucosal surface bleeding and hemorrhage after surgery or trauma characterize the bleeding tendency in vWD. Severity of bleeding is variable in dogs with type 1 vWD and may not correlate with plasma vWF concentration in each dog. Dogs with types 2 and 3 vWD generally experience the most severe bleeding episodes (Table 16-3).

Blood component therapy is generally indicated preoperatively in dogs with clinically severe forms of vWD and a history of bleeding. Cryoprecipitate, a concentrate of specific coagulation factors (vWF, FVIII, fibrinogen, fibronectin) derived from fresh-frozen plasma (FFP), is ideal in managing bleeding as a result of vWD. FFP or fresh whole blood (FWB) contains viable vWF, but carries higher risks of transfusion complications.

Desmopressin (DDAVP), a synthetic analog of vasopressin, may be sufficient to control minor bleeding in some (but not all) dogs with type 1 vWD. In humans, DDAVP causes a significant increase in plasma vWF

TABLE 16-3	Canine von Willebrand's Disease*	
TYPE	**PLASMA VON WILLEBRAND'S FACTOR (vWF)**	**EXAMPLES OF BREEDS WITH KNOWN MUTATION**
1	Variably reduced vWF levels; all multimer sizes proportionately reduced; most common—recognized in >70 breeds; hemorrhage tendency variable, often with surgery or trauma	Doberman pinscher, German shepherd, golden retriever, rottweiler, Manchester terrier, Cairn terrier, Pembroke Welsh corgi, Bernese mountain dog, Kerry blue terrier, poodle, papillon
2	Disproportionately low vWF activity; deficiency of high molecular weight multimers; larger, more effective multimers absent; bleeding can be severe	German shorthair pointer, German wirehair pointer
3	Complete vWF deficiency (<1% plasma vWF); most severe in that all multimers are absent	Scottish terrier, Shetland sheepdog, Chesapeake Bay retriever, Kooikerhondje

*Enzyme-linked immunosorbent assay results: normal = >70%, borderline = 50% to 69%, affected = 0% to 49%.

concentration; however, the plasma vWF concentration increases only marginally in dogs, despite improvement in hemostasis. The beneficial hemostatic effects of DDAVP are evident within 30 minutes after administration and may last for up to 4 hours.

DISORDERS OF SECONDARY HEMOSTASIS

When coagulation factor deficiencies are present, fibrin stabilization of the platelet plug cannot occur and hemostasis is impaired. Clotting defects may result from decreased factor synthesis, factor loss or consumption, factor molecular defects interfering with function, and factor inactivation by inhibitors (e.g., warfarin), overactive fibrinolysis, or antibodies resulting from certain drugs. Coagulation factor deficiencies may be inherited or acquired.

Hereditary Coagulopathies

A hereditary disorder should always be considered when a bleeding patient arrives at the emergency service given the variety of coagulation factor deficiencies described in small animals.

Hemophilias are the most common severe hereditary coagulopathies in the dog. Hemophilia A is caused by a factor VIII deficiency, whereas hemophilia B is due to a factor IX deficiency. They are sex-linked, autosomal recessive disorders carried on the X chromosome; therefore, both hemophilia A and hemophilia B are expressed only in males (although females may be asymptomatic carriers). Hemophilias A and B have also been identified in cats.

Affected animals usually hemorrhage into cavities (e.g., hematoma, hemarthrosis, hemoperitoneum) after trauma or surgery or exhibit prolonged bleeding from minor wounds. These animals often experience recurrent bleeding episodes that require transfusion support. Treatment with cryoprecipitate for hemophilia A (FVIII) and cryosupernatant for hemophilia B (FIX) is ideal. Based on component availability, FFP or FWB may be used. FWB is especially useful if the patient is concurrently anemic.

Many other hereditary coagulopathies have been identified in the dog and cat but occur less frequently (see Table 16-2).

Acquired Coagulopathies
Factor Activation Defect

The activation of coagulation factors II, VII, IX, and X is accomplished through the addition of gamma-carboxyglutamic acid, allowing the factors to interact with calcium, bind to membrane surfaces, and form active enzyme complexes. Vitamin K is essential in the activation of these factors in the liver, aiding the carboxylation through oxidation from vitamin K hydroquinone (KH_2) to vitamin K epoxide (KO). Vitamin K epoxide reductase converts KO back to KH_2, recycling a limited supply of vitamin K in the body.

A commonly seen **coagulopathy** in emergency and critical care is anticoagulant rodenticide toxicity, caused by the toxic component (coumarins) inhibiting the activity of vitamin K epoxide reductase. The inhibition of this enzyme results in the depletion of KH_2 and the subsequent depletion of functional vitamin K–dependent coagulation factors. The body does not contain an excessive store of vitamin K, so vitamin K1 must be administered to allow activation of vitamin K–dependent factors. First-generation rodenticides (e.g., warfarin, indanedione) have a relatively low toxicity and generally require repeated ingestion. Second-generation rodenticides (e.g., bromadiolone, brodifacoum) are more potent and have longer half-lives (weeks); therefore, the type of anticoagulant rodenticide ingested determines the duration of vitamin K therapy. Removing the toxic substance and supplementing vitamin K is the key treatment, but patients may need coagulation factor support in the form of FFP, frozen plasma, cryosupernatant, or fresh whole blood transfusion to stop hemorrhage more immediately.

In small animals, a dietary deficiency of vitamin K is not likely to be encountered, but intestinal malabsorption and biliary obstruction may lead to a deficiency state. In vitamin K deficiency, the liver produces inactive factors known as *proteins induced by* **vitamin K antagonism** (PIVKA).

Dysfunctional Synthesis

The liver is the site of synthesis of all coagulation factors. Although liver dysfunction affects the production of procoagulant and anticoagulant factors, patients with severe liver disease frequently develop coagulopathies because of impaired coagulation factor synthesis and vitamin K malabsorption. Bleeding tendencies will vary from mild to severe hemorrhage. Coagulation factors with the shortest plasma half-lives (FVII, with a half-life of 6 hours, for example) will be depleted first. Liver dysfunction may also lead to defective fibrin formation from production of dysfunctional fibrinogen.

Coagulation factor replacement is achieved by administering plasma products. Whole blood–derived components include FFP, frozen plasma, cryoprecipitate, and cryosupernatant. Before receiving transfusion support, patients must be evaluated to determine whether multiple or specific coagulation factor replacement is needed.

Factor Consumption and Dilutional Coagulopathies

A significant demand on coagulation factors as seen in disseminated intravascular coagulopathy (DIC, discussed later) will lead to a consumptive coagulopathy, with liver synthesis unable to meet the demands. Snake envenomation can cause coagulation factor depletion and defibrination through proteases contained within the venom activating clotting factors or directly degrading available fibrinogen. In cases of high-volume fluid resuscitation or massive transfusions, a dilutional coagulopathy can manifest. The coagulopathy arises from diluted concentration of the procoagulants as the intravascular space is filled with fluid without coagulation factors. Dilution results from fluid shift from the intracellular and interstitial spaces into the intravascular space in response to a change in hydrostatic pressure during hypovolemia, and additional intravenous administration of crystalloids, synthetic colloids, or red blood cell (RBC) products. In the case of breach in endothelial integrity (e.g., trauma), activation of coagulation and consumption of coagulation factors and platelets contribute to a reduction in available procoagulants. If blood products are used, hypocalcemia from citrate and hypothermia can lead to further exacerbation. Simultaneous administration of FFP and platelets along with RBCs in massive transfusions have been observed to increase survival in humans, presumably due to replacement of coagulation factors and platelets leading to a less severe dilutional effect.

DISORDERS IN ANTICOAGULATION

Thrombosis—or the formation of matrices of platelets, fibrin, and cellular debris—occurs within the intravascular space, potentially leading to thromboembolism attributable to three factors (described by Virchow's triad): hypercoagulability, blood stasis, and endothelial injury. Thrombosis can be further divided into macrovascular thrombosis (leading to clinical manifestations of aortic thromboembolism and pulmonary thromboembolism [PTE]) and microvascular thrombosis (leading to microvascular ischemia and coagulation factor depletion, which may result in DIC).

Hypercoagulability can result from platelet hyperreactivity, excessive coagulation factor activation, natural anticoagulant deficiency, hypofibrinolysis, or a combination of any of these causes. Platelet hyperreactivity can result from increases in platelet activators. This includes direct stimulation by inflammatory cytokines, release of other platelet agonists, and hypoalbuminemia-mediated increase in thromboxane A_2 (a prothrombotic). Endothelial damage leading to decreased availability of platelet inhibitors (prostacyclin, nitrous oxide, and adenosinediphosphatase [ADPase]) or administration of antiplatelet drugs can lead to reduced platelet inhibition. Excessive coagulation factor activation occurs when there is increased expression of TF by endothelial cells, macrophages, and cell-derived microparticles, induced by endotoxins or inflammatory mediators. An increased exposure of already existing TF can also occur as a result of endothelial damage. Deficiencies in natural anticoagulants may be genetic or acquired in origin (we will focus on acquired origins because they are more prevalent in animals). Deficiency in antithrombin (AT), a protein that inactivates certain coagulation factors, can arise from hepatic failure, protein-losing nephropathies, consumption attributable to a pathologic increase in thrombin (DIC or massive thromboembolism), or suppression from drugs. Deficiency in protein C, an enzyme that inactivates FVa and FVIIIa, can result from sepsis, malignancy, pancreatitis, DIC, and hepatic or cardiac failure. Tissue factor pathway inhibitor (TFPI) deficiencies are seen in hypercholesterolemia, and are a risk factor for thromboembolism. Hypofibrinolysis has not been very well-defined in veterinary medicine, but is thought to occur with an increased level of plasminogen activator inhibitor 1 (PAI-1) and/or α_2-antiplasmin. Hypoplasminogenemia has been reported in traumatized dogs and horses with strangulating obstructions. Areas of impaired blood flow can lead to varying degrees of blood stasis. Changes in cardiovascular anatomy and cardiovascular function can cause abnormal or reduced flow, risk factors of thrombosis. Left atrial dilation causing an aberrant blood flow is a well-known cause of feline aortic thromboembolism. Other conditions associated with altered blood flow include hypovolemia, hyperviscosity disorders, neoplasia, and vascular and cardiac abnormalities.

Thrombotic disorders in canine patients typically involve multiple causes, and are most often reported in patients with protein-losing nephropathy, neoplasia, immune-mediated hemolytic anemia (IMHA), necrotizing pancreatitis, hyperadrenocorticism, and corticosteroid therapy. Both venous and arterial thromboembolism is seen, with more than one organ involvement. Patients with IMHA have a predisposition to PTE. Aortic thromboembolism secondary to cardiomyopathy is the most common form of thromboembolism in feline patients, and although other forms do occur, they are rare.

Disseminated Intravascular Coagulation

In certain pathologic situations, the coagulation response may become accelerated and the fibrinolytic system overwhelmed. This imbalance between bleeding, coagulation, and fibrinolysis is called disseminated intravascular coagulation *(DIC)*. Diffuse thrombosis within the vasculature without localization occurs, leading to microvascular thrombosis.

DIC is not a primary disorder, and always has an underlying cause. Many stimuli may trigger the coagulation cascade in this way, with neoplasia and systemic inflammation (e.g., sepsis, pancreatitis, IMHA) being the most common causes. DIC is initiated with a supraphysiologic expression of TF through severe endothelial injury or TF expression on intravascular cells (monocytes, tumor cells) stimulated by proinflammatory cytokines. TF-independent triggers exist, such as snake venoms and neoplastic cells activating coagulation. Thrombosis in the initial phase of DIC is controlled by antithrombotic and fibrinolytic mechanisms (non–overt DIC), but as they become overwhelmed with the degree of coagulation, control of thrombosis is lost. Uncontrolled thrombosis leads to microvascular thromboembolism and ischemia. Additional compromise to perfusion occurs through hemodynamic instability from release of vasoactive peptides (e.g., bradykinin, endothelin), combined, leading to tissue hypoxia and multiple organ dysfunction. Consumptive depletion of coagulation factors as well as platelet and coagulation factor dysfunction attributable to acidosis leads to the development of the hemorrhagic stage of DIC (overt DIC).

No pathognomonic test for DIC exists; however, the presence of schistocytes, thrombocytopenia, and hypofibrinogenemia; elevated levels of fibrin degradation products and D-dimer; decreased amount of antithrombin; and prolonged prothrombin time (PT), partial thromboplastin time (PTT), and activated clotting time (ACT) are evaluated in conjunction with clinical signs. Thromboelastography gives insight into the patient's coagulation status, although it does not necessarily diagnose DIC. Interpretation of laboratory values is difficult since they vary depending on the stage of progression of DIC.

Therapy for DIC is treatment of the underlying disease process. In the non–overt phase of DIC, administration of unfractionated or low molecular weight heparin is thought to slow or stop the coagulation process by partnering with antithrombin, thereby inhibiting critical substances of hemostasis. The efficacy of this treatment modality remains unknown, and a wide range of doses has been suggested. Regardless of the dose, patients receiving heparin require careful monitoring for the duration of therapy.

In overt DIC, administration of blood components directed at coagulation factor and platelet replacement (FFP, platelet concentrate, FWB) may be necessary to maintain hemostatic function in actively bleeding patients. Cryoprecipitate may be useful if the patient primarily lacks fibrinogen. PRBCs may be necessary if clinical anemia exists from coagulopathic bleeding. Fluid replacement with crystalloids and colloids may be warranted for volume replacement as well (Ralph and Brainard, 2012).

CLINICAL ASSESSMENT

An accurate history, thorough physical examination, and certain laboratory tests must be performed to evaluate a bleeding patient, reach a diagnosis, determine a prognosis, and define an appropriate therapeutic plan.

HISTORY

A complete history is critical in beginning a workup for a hemostatic defect. Obtaining and assessing a complete and detailed history will help define the nature, severity, and duration of bleeding and other clinical signs, as well as aid in making a correct diagnosis. Attention to detail will help in establishing probability for each possible differential early in the diagnostic process.

Questions should be clear, nonleading, and thought provoking. Devising a list of questions for owners to review should help to stimulate them to think of some very important (most likely, not obvious) facts. For example, does the animal have any previously diagnosed diseases? Is the animal currently taking any medication?

A list of any prescription or over-the-counter medications should be included, because many drugs have potentially harmful or complicating side effects (resulting in a toxic effect on RBCs, white blood cells [WBCs], and platelets, as well as the vasculature and coagulation factors). Complete vaccination history should not be overlooked. The animal's environmental history may suggest potential exposure to toxic or organic substances such as anticoagulant rodenticide, poisons, or zinc. Ectoparasite exposure should also be investigated.

Evaluation of the current bleeding episode is vital, and the bleed should be characterized as localized or multifocal. Is this the animal's first bleeding episode, or is there a history of bleeding tendency? Did the bleeding start spontaneously, or was it caused by initial trauma? The answers to these questions may help to differentiate between an acquired and a hereditary bleeding disorder. Although hereditary coagulopathies may occur in any breed, each coagulopathy has thus far only been reported in certain breeds. Because specific breeds may suggest a specific coagulopathy, any information the owner may have regarding breed history could provide helpful clues.

PHYSICAL EXAMINATION

A complete physical examination and multiple monitoring procedures may be required to properly assess the patient in a bleeding crisis. Optimal assessment cannot be based on the result of a single parameter, and should be based on the results of several physical examinations and monitored parameters that are always evaluated in relation to one another.

Certain clinical signs found on physical examination may help determine the origin of the bleeding episode. Small surface bleeds (e.g., petechiation, ecchymosis, epistaxis, hematuria) (Figure 16-3) are usually suggestive of platelet or vascular abnormalities. Larger bleeds or bleeding into body cavities (e.g., hematoma formation, hemarthroses, deep muscle hemorrhage, hemothorax, hemoabdomen) are suggestive of clotting factor deficiencies. A combination of these clinical signs is not uncommon. The presence of blood in more than one general location is suggestive of a bleeding disorder.

Mucous membrane color, capillary refill time, pulse rate and quality, and respiratory rate and effort should also be evaluated to determine bleed severity and the presence of possible life-threatening complications and shock.

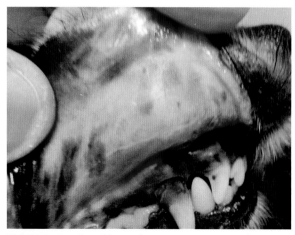

FIGURE 16-3 Mild petechiation on a patient with immune-mediated thrombocytopenia.

LABORATORY TESTS

Hemostatic tests are indicated whenever an animal is bleeding excessively, before surgery when an increased bleeding tendency is possible, to monitor therapeutic interventions, and for genetic screening in certain breeds with a known bleeding disorder.

To summarize the status of the hemostatic mechanism, the difference between primary and secondary hemostasis must be understood. Information obtained from the history and specific clinical signs may suggest a diagnosis, and laboratory tests interpreted in the clinical context are necessary for a definitive diagnosis. All laboratory tests should be performed as soon as possible, and therapy should be instituted promptly after test samples are obtained.

PRIMARY HEMOSTATIC TESTS

A platelet count should be performed on any patient that arrives at the clinic in a bleeding crisis. A normal platelet count in dogs is 200,000 to 500,000/µL, and 200,000 to 600,000/µL in cats. Abnormal bleeding may occur in animals with platelet counts below 20,000 to 30,000/µL; however, each patient varies and some animals may not exhibit clinical signs associated with bleeding with a platelet count of 2000/µL. In an animal exhibiting signs of surface bleeding with a normal platelet count, platelet function should be evaluated.

Because vWD is such a common mild primary hemostatic defect in dogs, plasma vWF measurements (most often by enzyme-linked immunosorbent assay) are indicated. The reference range depends on the assay method and laboratory used (see Table 16-3).

The following are simple, in-house tests requiring no specialized equipment. They are quick, inexpensive, practical tests that allow recognition of primary hemostatic defects.

PLATELET ESTIMATION

A quick, reasonably accurate estimation of platelet number can be made from a stained blood smear and is much faster than an actual platelet count. After routine preparation and staining, the blood smear is scanned to ensure even platelet distribution with no evidence of platelet clumping. The average number of platelets in approximately 5 to 10 oil immersion fields is counted to estimate platelet numbers. One platelet per oil immersion field represents approximately 15,000 to 20,000 platelets/μL. Approximately 8 to 15 platelets per oil immersion field are considered normal.

Although platelet estimation helps determine the presence of thrombocytopenia in an emergency situation, a true platelet count is necessary to classify the severity of depletion. After obtaining baseline values, ongoing platelet quantitation can be helpful in monitoring the course of a disease or the patient's response to certain therapies.

BLEEDING TIME TEST

Bleeding time is the time it takes for bleeding to stop after severing a vessel. The most commonly used bleeding time test in veterinary medicine is the buccal mucosal bleeding time (BMBT). The buccal mucosal bleeding time assesses platelet and vascular contribution to hemostasis, thereby evaluating primary hemostasis. A disposable template with two spring-loaded blades is used to produce standardized incisions in the buccal mucosal surface of the upper lip. The blades create 5 mm long × 1 mm deep incisions. The duration of bleeding from these incisions is monitored (Figure 16-4 and Box 16-1). Normal bleeding time is less than 4 minutes in dogs, and 3 minutes in cats (Harvey, 2012).

The buccal mucosal bleeding time is a screening test. As with any screening test, sensitivity is not 100%. Therefore not all primary hemostatic defects will be discovered. This test also will not differentiate between vascular defects or platelet function defects. The buccal mucosal bleeding time is prolonged in cases of

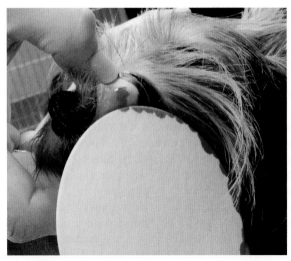

FIGURE 16-4 Buccal mucosal bleeding time test.

BOX 16-1	Buccal Mucosal Bleeding Time Supplies

The materials needed for this test are as follows:
- Bleeding time device
- Gauze strip
- Filter paper or gauze sponges
- Timing device

Buccal Mucosal Bleeding Time Procedure
1. Place animal in lateral recumbency position.
2. Expose the mucosal surface of the upper lip. Position a gauze strip around the maxilla to fold up the upper lip. Tie the strip gently, just tightly enough to partially block venous return.
3. The incision site should be void of surface vessels and slightly inclined so that shed blood from the incision can flow freely toward the mouth. Place the bleeding time device flush against the mucosal surface, applying as little pressure as possible; press the tab to release scalpels.
4. Let the stab incisions bleed freely, undisturbed; time the bleeding until it stops. Excessive blood should be blotted as often as necessary to prevent blood flow into the patient's mouth. Place either filter paper or gauze sponge approximately 3 to 4 mm below the incision, taking care not to disturb the incision site and any clot that may be forming.
5. The end point is recorded when the edge of the filter paper or sponge does not soak up free-flowing blood. The bleeding time is the mean bleeding time for the two incisions. Normal bleeding time is less than 4 minutes in dogs, and 3 minutes in cats (Harvey, 2012).

thrombocytopenia and thrombopathia, vWD, uremia, and aspirin therapy. The BMBT does not yield any additional information for patients with thrombocytopenia since bleeding time is expected to be prolonged. Patients with anemia will often have a prolonged BMBT from a lower viscosity of blood.

Patients seem to tolerate the procedure well, eliminating the need for chemical restraint. The incisions produced are well above the concentrated pain fibers in the lip. Sometimes the animal will reflex on hearing the noise the scalpels make when released from the device, but the procedure itself is not painful. Although the BMBT does have limitations, several advantages to the test exist:

- Commercial bleeding time devices are readily available.
- The templates are standardized and therefore results are reproducible.
- The test is simple and quick to perform, and the results are almost immediately available.

SECONDARY HEMOSTATIC TESTS

Several standardized coagulation screening tests are useful to define coagulopathies in clinical practice. Blood samples for hematologic testing are ideally collected directly into a plastic syringe containing 3.2% or 3.8% trisodium citrate at a ratio of 1:9 with blood to be collected. Atraumatic venipuncture and smooth blood flow into collection tubes are necessary to prevent extraneous clotting mechanism activation. Samples should be processed immediately after collection and testing performed without delay. If samples are to be sent to an outside laboratory, the plasma should be frozen before shipment. Extra plasma should be saved in case further individual factor analysis becomes necessary.

Prothrombin Time

The clinician may assess the extrinsic and common pathways by the prothrombin time (PT) (Figure 16-5). A prolongation in PT can be caused by liver failure, vitamin K antagonism, malabsorption, hereditary factor deficiencies, or consumptive factor deficiencies. A normal PT does not necessarily rule out factor deficiencies, because it is not affected until there is severe depletion of extrinsic pathway factors. A shortening of PT does not consistently correlate with a hypercoagulable state.

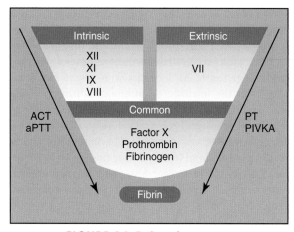

FIGURE 16-5 Coagulation testing.

Proteins Induced by Vitamin K Antagonism

The PIVKA test is a modified PT test developed and used to detect anticoagulant toxicity. PIVKA tests detect any coagulation factor deficiency of the extrinsic and common pathways and are not specific for the detection of anticoagulant rodenticide poisoning. There is no advantage in using the PIVKA test over the PT aside from possibly having higher sensitivity in certain species.

Activated Partial Thromboplastin Time

The intrinsic and common pathways are assessed by activated partial thromboplastin time (aPTT). Prolongation of aPTT indicates deficiencies in coagulation factors in the intrinsic or common pathway. Some causes are liver failure, vitamin K antagonism, malabsorption, hereditary factor deficiencies, consumptive deficiencies, and vWD.

Prolongation of PT and aPTT will be seen when clotting factors are depleted below 30% of normal. Each test should be interpreted in terms of the pathway or pathways it specifically evaluates. Although hereditary coagulopathies can be suggested based on the pattern of coagulation test abnormalities, specific factor analyses are needed to confirm a diagnosis.

Activated Clotting Time

The activated clotting time (ACT) test is a simple, inexpensive screening test for severe abnormalities in the intrinsic and common pathways of the clotting cascade. It evaluates the same pathways as aPTT, but is less sensitive at detecting factor deficiencies (because factors must be decreased to less than 5% of normal to prolong ACT). The ACT is a useful diagnostic test because results are available within minutes.

Prolongation of ACT occurs with severe factor deficiency in the intrinsic or common clotting pathway (e.g., hemophilia) in the presence of inhibitors (e.g., heparin, warfarin). Prolongation may also occur in cases of severe thrombocytopenia because of the lack of platelet phospholipid (mild prolongation of 10 to 20 seconds). The ACT is inexpensive, easily learned, quickly performed, and reproducible, and provides immediate results. In addition, it provides a useful measurement of coagulation in emergency situations. When compared with the PTT, the role that technical and laboratory error can have on the test results must be taken into consideration. This is not to suggest that one should rely solely on the ACT. In most situations, the ACT should be followed with an aPTT.

Thrombin Clotting Time

Thrombin clotting time (TCT) or thrombin time (TT) is used to assess an animal's ability to produce fibrin and the fibrin meshwork to form a clot. Prolonged TCT can result from decreased fibrinogen, heparin administration, dysfibrinogenemia, and elevated FDPs.

Thromboelastography

Thromboelastography (TEG), while not commonly available in private practice, is a method of visualizing the viscoelastic properties of whole blood as clotting occurs. Measurements and tracings made include initiation time, clot strength and stability, clot formation, and clot breakdown. The tracing provides information of whether the patient is in a hypercoagulable or hypocoagulable state, giving supplemental information that better guides treatment of patients with hemostatic disorders (Figure 16-6).

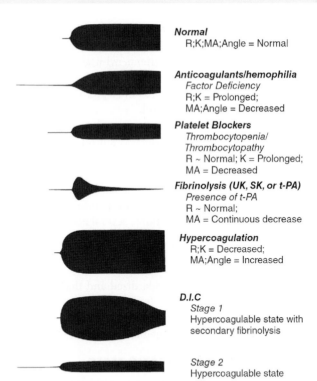

Normal
R;K;MA;Angle = Normal

Anticoagulants/hemophilia
Factor Deficiency
R;K = Prolonged;
MA;Angle = Decreased

Platelet Blockers
*Thrombocytopenia/
Thrombocytopathy*
R ~ Normal; K = Prolonged;
MA = Decreased

Fibrinolysis (UK, SK, or t-PA)
Presence of t-PA
R ~ Normal;
MA = Continuous decrease

Hypercoagulation
R;K = Decreased;
MA;Angle = Increased

D.I.C
Stage 1
Hypercoagulable state with secondary fibrinolysis

Stage 2
Hypercoagulable state

FIGURE 16-6 Example of thromboelastographic tracings. *DIC,* Disseminated intravascular coagulation; *K,* clotting time; *MA,* maximum amplitude; *R,* reaction time; *t-PA,* tissue plasminogen activator. (From Weiss DJ, Wardrop KJ, editors: *Schalm's veterinary hematology,* ed 6, Ames, Iowa, 2010, Wiley-Blackwell.)

ANEMIA

Anemia, most accurately described, is a deficiency in the blood's oxygen-carrying capacity attributable to a reduction in the circulating red cell mass. Measurement of total red cell mass requires specialized testing and is difficult to accomplish in clinical practice. Measurements of PCV, HCT, hemoglobin (Hb), and RBC count are more common methods in the assessment of the erythrocyte content of blood. Thus, anemia is commonly defined as a reduction in these values, and occurs when the rate of red blood cell loss or destruction exceeds the rate of production. Anemia is caused by various diseases, many of them resulting in the patient requiring immediate attention.

PCV, HCT, and RBC count all translate into the amount of Hg available, representing the patient's oxygen-carrying capacity and the ability for the cardiovascular system to provide oxygen delivery (DO_2) to body systems. The importance of maintaining adequate DO_2 lies in the difference in the amount of adenosine triphosphate (ATP) produced in the presence and absence of oxygen. ATP is considered the "currency of cellular energy," providing energy for cellular processes required to maintain life when phosphate groups are cleaved, resulting in energy release and formation of adenosine diphosphate (ADP) or adenosine monophosphate (AMP). ATP is involved in cellular signaling, DNA and RNA synthesis, muscle contraction, cytoskeletal maintenance, active transporting, and many other cellular functions.

There is a finite amount of ATP available within a body, and a constant recycling of ADP and AMP into ATP is required to keep up with energy demands. In the presence of oxygen, 38 ATP molecules are generated from metabolism of a single glucose molecule undergoing oxidative phosphorylation in the mitochondria. In contrast, a single glucose molecule yields two ATP molecules through anaerobic metabolism. The presence of oxygen is imperative in efficient energy generation.

> **TECHNICIAN NOTE** Provided there is adequate intravascular volume and tissue perfusion, DO_2 is dependent on the oxygen level contained in the blood (arterial oxygen content, CaO_2) and how quickly the body can circulate the blood to the tissues (cardiac output, CO). The resulting mathematical expression of DO_2 is: $DO_2 = CaO_2 \times CO$.

Oxygen contained within blood exists in two forms: dissolved in the plasma or bound to hemoglobin. The amount of oxygen dissolved in arterial plasma is expressed as the partial pressure of oxygen (PaO_2), with 1 mm Hg creating enough tension to result in 0.0031 ml of dissolved O_2 per deciliter (dl) of plasma. Each gram of hemoglobin is able to theoretically carry 1.39 ml of O_2 when fully bound with oxygen, comprising a significant portion of oxygen content of blood. In reality, there are portions of dysfunctional hemoglobin lowering this to approximately 1.34 ml. In addition, not every hemoglobin molecule will be fully bound to oxygen in every situation (SaO_2, or arterial oxyhemoglobin saturation), adding some variability. The resultant formula to quantify DO_2 is the following, expressing the impact lowered hemoglobin concentration and saturation of the hemoglobin will have on overall delivery of oxygen:

$$DO_2 = [(1.34 \times Hb \times SaO_2) + (0.0031 \times PaO_2)] \times CO$$

In animals without disease, DO_2 is significantly higher than oxygen consumption (VO_2), supplying a very comfortable buffer of available oxygen for energy production. This buffer allows for sudden changes in oxygen demand through changes in cellular metabolic rate or reduction in CaO_2. When DO_2 is significantly compromised (termed critical oxygen delivery, DO_{2Crit}), tissue hypoxia results and increased lactate levels and lowered pH are seen. The oxygen extraction ratio (OER or O_2ER) can also be used to express the level of oxygen consumed in relation to DO_2 ($O_2ER = VO_2/DO_2$). Higher oxygen consumption or lower DO_2 leads to a higher ratio. The normal O_2ER value is approximately 0.2, although different organ systems have varying O_2ER values (normal O_2ER of the heart is 0.6, making it more sensitive to hypoxemia). Normal values for DO_2, VO_2, and O_2ER in dogs were observed to be 790 ml/min/m^2, 164 ml/min/m^2, and 0.205 (Haskins et al, 2005), respectively, in one study. A couple of other studies observed a normal DO_2 of 20 to 25 ml/kg/min and critical oxygen delivery levels of 8 to 11 ml/kg/min (Van der Linden et al, 2006) regardless of the cause (anemia, hypoxemia, and cardiac tamponade). A patient is said to be in **hypoxemic shock** when Hb, SaO_2, or PaO_2 levels are low enough for DO_2 to be below DO_{2Crit}. In clinical settings, measurements of specific values such as CO and VO_2, although they can be estimated, are rather difficult. It is important, however, to have an understanding of these concepts in patients suspected to be in hypoxemic shock.

Anemia is a clinical sign or laboratory test abnormality, not a diagnosis for a specific disease. Clinical signs and a patient's history indicate the possibility of anemia. The severity of signs depends on the rapidity of onset, the degree and cause of the anemia, and the extent of the animal's physical activity. Once anemia is confirmed, its cause should be thoroughly investigated to determine proper therapeutic management of the patient.

Anemia may result from increased loss (acute or chronic) (i.e., hemorrhage), increased destruction (i.e., intravascular or extravascular **hemolysis**), or decreased production (i.e., hypoplasia or aplasia of the bone marrow) of red blood cells. The red cell life span is usually normal in blood loss anemias and hypoproliferative anemias but is characteristically reduced in hemolytic anemias. Based on the erythropoietic response seen in peripheral blood, anemias may also be classified as *regenerative* or *nonregenerative*. Classification is helpful in differentiating blood-loss and hemolytic anemias (which are generally responsive) from bone marrow depression anemias (which are generally nonresponsive).

RBC LOSS

Normal blood volume is 8% to 9% of body weight (80 to 90 ml/kg) in dogs and 6% to 7% (60 to 70 ml/kg) in cats. The relative blood volume is determined by the animal's age, splenic reserve, and hydration status.

A significant loss of blood over minutes to hours results in hypovolemia and potential cardiovascular collapse. Healthy animals can tolerate as much as a 20%

reduction in blood volume, but signs of shock generally develop when blood volume is reduced to 60% to 70% of normal. The therapeutic goal in the treatment of acute hemorrhagic hypovolemia is to stop the hemorrhage and support the cardiovascular system. Aggressive, rapid restoration of vascular volume must be instituted while preventing further blood loss if possible. In cases of external hemorrhage, direct pressure can be applied to the bleeding site or sites; however, the veterinary technician should watch for continued blood loss from uncontrolled sites after intravascular volume resuscitation. Although internal hemorrhage may not be evident on presentation, it should be considered if shock occurs following trauma.

When choosing resuscitation fluid for vascular space replacement, volume and composition are critical in determining the effectiveness of volume expansion and the duration of its effect. Following blood loss, the intravascular space is depleted; and only later does interstitial fluid shift from the extravascular into the intravascular space, providing much needed volume. In the early stages of hemorrhage, replenishing intravascular space losses is a priority and can be accomplished easily using crystalloid fluid solutions. Crystalloid solutions also enter the extravascular space; consequently, administering two to three times the amount of crystalloid as volume lost is necessary. Risk of fluid overload is of concern when a large volume of crystalloids is administered, especially in older patients or patients with some degree of cardiovascular compromise. Colloid solutions should be considered when a need exists to maintain intravascular oncotic pressure without administering large volumes of fluid, as well as when blood loss continues and a substantial portion of the blood volume is depleted.

The symptoms that occur immediately following hemorrhage are a result of blood volume depletion, not a decrease in RBC mass. Although fluid administration will improve tissue perfusion, patient assessment is necessary to help determine whether enough Hb is present to provide oxygen to vital organs. The need for transfusion should be based on clinical assessment of the signs of anemia, because no laboratory value exists as a definitive transfusion trigger. Red cell replacement may not be necessary during initial therapy of acute blood loss. The aggressiveness of therapy will depend on the volume of blood lost, the rate at which it was lost, and the patient's condition.

Patients may also present with a chronic blood loss anemia resulting from gastrointestinal bleeding, ectoparasites, endoparasites, neoplasia, and chronic thrombocytopenia. Clinical signs of chronic blood loss anemia may not be obvious because of the body's compensatory mechanisms and ability to adapt to this compromised state.

RBC DESTRUCTION

Various types of defects in RBCs can cause an increased rate of destruction, leading to a reduced hemoglobin level. Hemolytic anemia results in lowered red cell mass and subsequent reduction in oxygen-carrying capacity without significant changes in plasma volume. Hemolysis can be intravascular (destruction of RBC within the bloodstream), extravascular (phagocytosis by macrophages in the spleen, liver, bone marrow, and lymph nodes), or both. Intravascular hemolysis will result in the presence of free hemoglobin in the plasma, leading to hemoglobinemia and hemoglobinuria (when renal threshold is exceeded). Hemoglobinuria leads to tubular necrosis resulting in acute kidney injury in humans, posing similar concerns in veterinary medicine. Icterus may be seen in patients with extravascular hemolysis and bilirubin production at rates exceeding the liver's processing ability. Hemolytic anemias can be classified as *immune-mediated hemolytic anemia (IMHA),* inherited RBC defects, hemolysis associated with chemical ingestion, and hemolysis associated with infection.

IMHA may be a primary disease, also known as *idiopathic* or *autoimmune hemolytic anemia,* in which autoantibodies are produced against the unaltered RBC membrane. Hemolysis may be caused by an immunoglobulin G (IgG) or immunoglobulin M (IgM) mediated type II hypersensitivity (cytotoxic) reaction involving antibody or complement response to the surface antigens of RBCs (intravascular hemolysis). Phagocytic loss of RBC membranes reduces the surface area of the RBC, leading to formation of spherocytes (RBCs that have lost the biconcave structure) or destruction (extravascular hemolysis). Gross agglutination of red cells may also be seen (Figure 16-7, *A*). The specific stimulus provoking an individual to develop antibodies to its own tissue remains unidentified. Researchers hypothesize that a change in antigenicity of the red cells or in an individual's immune status may cause the immune system to recognize and attack its own RBCs.

usually more severe, with myelofibrosis, osteosclerosis, and death occurring before the age of 4. Phosphofructokinase deficiency tends to be associated with mild-to-moderate, intermittent intravascular hemolysis, often exacerbated by exercise. Both disorders exhibit marked reticulocytosis associated with chronic hemolytic disease. Hereditary RBC disorders should be included as a differential for any dog belonging to an affected breed that arrives with regenerative anemia and even mild signs of hemolytic disease. Special laboratory tests are required to definitively diagnose an inherited erythrocyte defect. Additionally, carrier detection can be used in breeding programs to limit the frequency of these genetic disorders in the affected breeds.

Many compounds have been reported to cause damage to the RBC. For example, an oxidizing agent found in onions, *n*-propyl disulfide, may cause hemolysis. Oxidation results in structural changes to the RBC (i.e., Heinz bodies), leading to hemolysis that may range from subclinical to severe. A single ingestion of large quantities of onion or repeated meals containing small amounts of onion can produce marked hemolysis and anemia in both dogs and cats. Heinz bodies, as well as eccentrocytes (RBC with Hb shifted to one side), appear within 24 hours after onion ingestion. When stained with new methylene blue, Heinz bodies appear as blue to purple refractile bodies on the periphery of the RBC. The key to diagnosing onion-induced hemolytic disease in dogs rests on patient history of onion ingestion and specific laboratory tests. Other causes for **Heinz body** anemia include toxins contained in food (garlic, propylene glycol), drugs (acetaminophen, vitamins K_1 and K_3, benzocaine), and chemicals (copper, naphthalene, skunk musk, zinc). Cats are more prone to Heinz body formation, but are also more forgiving towards red cells containing Heinz bodies, allowing for a longer survival time. Because of this, feline RBCs may show Heinz bodies without anemia. Cats can develop Heinz bodies when exposed to propylene glycol, and are more prone if inflicted with diabetes mellitus, lymphoma, or hyperthyroidism.

Zinc toxicosis in dogs is often associated with a hemolytic crisis of rapid onset. Zinc-induced hemolytic disease in dogs occurs most commonly after ingestion of zinc-containing materials (e.g., coins, nuts and bolts, skin ointments). All pennies minted in the United States after 1983 contain 96% zinc and represent the most common source of zinc intoxication in

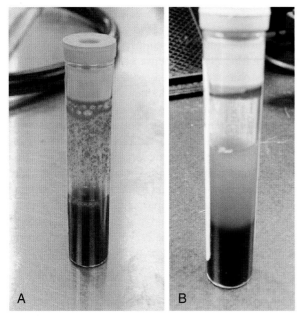

FIGURE 16-7 (A) Severe macroscopic agglutination of blood obtained from a patient with IMHA. **(B)** Severe hyperbilirubinemia seen in the plasma of settled whole blood.

IMHA can also be a secondary immune response directed toward a foreign antigen, ultimately leading to inadvertent damage to normal patient cells. Causes of secondary IMHA include neoplasia, infectious disease (i.e., parasitic, viral, bacterial, rickettsial), toxin exposure, and drug therapy. Neoplasia is reported to be the most frequent cause of secondary IMHA. Passive acquirement of anti–red cell antibodies through blood transfusions and colostrum can cause an IMHA. The latter results in a phenomenon called neonatal isoerythrolysis.

Although IMHA is the most common cause of hemolytic disease in dogs, other important causes of hemolysis exist. Differentiation of the cause of hemolysis is important, given the wide variability between therapy and prognosis. Additionally, immunosuppressive drugs used in the treatment of IMHA may be associated with significant side effects that are far from benign.

Several inherited defects in erythrocyte metabolism that cause hemolysis have been described in a number of canine breeds. The most common are phosphofructokinase deficiency in the English springer spaniel and pyruvate kinase deficiency in the basenji, beagle, and West Highland white terrier. Pyruvate kinase deficiency is dogs. Signalment and history help establish an index of suspicion of zinc intoxication; many of these dogs are young and may have a history of repeated foreign body ingestion. Although Heinz bodies are associated with zinc toxicosis, the exact mechanism of zinc-induced hemolysis is unknown (Clancey and Murphy, 2012). Intravascular hemolysis often occurs, thereby causing hemoglobinemia and hemoglobinuria.

Various forms of microangiopathic diseases, including DIC, hemangiosarcoma or metastatic tumors, snake bites, and heartworm infestation, may result in direct red cell damage occurring in the microvasculature, causing clinical signs of hemolysis. In microangiopathic hemolytic anemias, fragmented schistocytes and keratocytes are seen on blood smears as an indication of mechanical damage. RBCs are mechanically fragmented because of fibrin deposition in small blood vessels. DIC can be a cause of fragmentation, and at the same time precipitate DIC. Cats with diabetes mellitus or hepatic lipidosis can develop hypophosphatemia resulting in fragile membranes and hemolysis; phosphate supplementation is recommended if a phosphate level less than 0.5 mmol/L is seen.

REDUCED OR INEFFECTIVE ERYTHROPOIESIS

All blood cells develop from early stage cells in one of the largest organs in the body—the bone marrow. The bone marrow is stimulated to differentiate cells into RBCs, platelets, and specific types of WBCs according to the requirements of the body. As the cells mature, they proceed through developmental stages before being released from the bone marrow into the circulation where they become fully functional. The development of mature red blood cells is referred to as **erythropoiesis.**

Anemia caused by reduced or ineffective erythropoiesis may result from nutritional deficiencies (e.g., iron, vitamin B_{12}, gastrointestinal malabsorption), drugs, infection (e.g., feline leukemia virus, feline immunodeficiency virus), chronic disease, bone marrow infiltration (e.g., leukemia, multiple myeloma), and organ disorders (e.g., renal, liver, and endocrine disease). These anemias are chronic and usually nonregenerative or poorly regenerative.

Anemia of chronic disease is probably the most common form of nonregenerative anemia and is associated with a variety of chronic diseases (e.g., chronic infections, inflammation, neoplasia). The most common

example is chronic kidney disease of dogs and cats. Decreased levels of erythropoietin (EPO), a hormone produced by the kidney that stimulates the bone marrow to produce RBCs, lead to reduced erythropoiesis. Patients with chronic kidney disease often become anemic as EPO production by the kidneys is diminished. Other factors such as uremic toxins leading to a lowered red cell half-life, hemorrhagic loss attributable to gastrointestinal (GI) ulcers, increased bleeding tendencies resulting from platelet dysfunction, inhibition of iron store release, suppression of erythropoiesis by the parathyroid gland, and reduced nutrient intake may also contribute. The degree of anemia is approximately proportional to the degree of uremia and may be more severe in young animals; however, decreased erythropoietin production is the main cause.

Suppression of response to EPO is another cause for reduced production. In the presence of chronic inflammatory disease (such as chronic infections, chronic immune conditions, malignant cancers) or acute inflammatory diseases, red cell production is reduced. This is attributed to an increased production of hepcidin by hepatocytes during inflammatory disease, which inhibit the iron exporting action of ferroportin in macrophages and enterocytes. This reduces the iron available for erythropoiesis. In addition, inflammatory mediators (tumor necrosis factor alpha and interleukin-1) released from leukocytes reduce surface EPO receptors on erythroid stem cells, leading to a suppression of erythropoiesis.

Dysfunction of the bone marrow may be another cause for reduced RBC production. Irradiation, toxicities, viral or bacterial infections, and administration of certain drugs can result in marrow aplasia, leading to a lack of marrow stem cells. Myelophthisis, or marrow suppression secondary to marrow infiltration by tumors, can displace or inhibit production of hematopoietic cells. Both of these situations result in pancytopenia. In FeLV infections in cats or immune-mediated erythroid stem cell destruction in dogs, erythrocyte precursor cells are specifically reduced in number, leading to red cell aplasia.

When nutrients required for producing the signaling system for erythropoiesis and functional erythrocytes are deficient, anemia will occur. Folic acid, vitamin B_{12}, cobalt, and intrinsic factor (a glycoprotein aiding in the absorption of vitamin B_{12}) deficiency can result in a dysfunction of DNA and RNA synthesis, leading to the production of erythrocytes of abnormal shape and size. These abnormal cells are destroyed in the bone marrow, thus never making it into circulation. Potential causes include administration of drugs that antagonize folate (methotrexate for malignant tumors), inhibit folate metabolism (sulfonamides), and deplete folate concentrations (phenobarbital). A genetic disorder in giant schnauzers, beagles, and border collies involving selective malabsorption of vitamin B_{12} has been reported and leads to a nonregenerative anemia. A deficiency in iron results in the production of erythrocytes with a reduced concentration of Hb, or may lead to a delay in red cell production causing anemia.

Nonregenerative anemia can be clinically classified according to the number of cell types involved. When only erythrocytes are decreased, this is considered a *refractory anemia,* which may be the result of chronic disease, iron deficiency, or other organ disorders (i.e., external effects that influence bone marrow). When other cell types are involved (pancytopenia), the anemia is called *aplastic anemia,* which can be caused by disease within the marrow, exposure to radiation or chemicals, infection, leukemia, or other tumors; or it can be idiopathic. A bone marrow examination is usually necessary to distinguish these two classifications.

DYSFUNCTIONAL HEMOGLOBIN SPECIES

Although not necessarily resulting from a reduction in RBC mass or hemoglobin number, dysfunctional hemoglobin species (or hemoglobin molecules structurally altered in their ability to carry and deliver oxygen) contribute to a reduction of DO_2.

Methemoglobinemia

When ferrous iron (Fe^{2+}) in the heme groups of hemoglobin undergoes oxidation to ferric iron (Fe^{3+}), it is called methemoglobin (metHb). MetHb is unable to bind oxygen and does not contribute to oxygen-carrying capacity. In addition, the oxidation of iron in one heme group increases the oxygen affinity of the remaining heme groups on the hemoglobin, reducing oxygen unloading. The proportion of total hemoglobin existing as metHb from natural oxidation is kept at approximately 1% at any given time, since the change is reversed by cytochrome-b_5 reductase (Cb5R, also known as methemoglobin reductase). Methemoglobinemia occurs when the animal is exposed to high levels of oxidative compounds (acetaminophen ingestion, phenazopyridine

therapy, skunk musk exposure, vitamin K_3 administration, benzocaine administration) or has reduced levels of Cb5R (inherited conditions), such that the reversal mechanism is overwhelmed. Significant methemoglobinemia manifests in chocolate-brown colored blood and can be measured via co-oximetry. Treatment lies in eliminating the oxidative factor through diuresis and administration of medication enhancing elimination (e.g., *N*-acetylcysteine for acetaminophen).

Carboxyhemoglobin

Smoke inhalation and exposure to car exhaust, heating systems, gasoline-powered generators, and other forms of smoke and fume inhalation can lead to carbon monoxide toxicity. Carbon monoxide binds to hemoglobin at greater than 200 times higher affinity than oxygen, leading to formation of carboxyhemoglobin (COHb). Carbon monoxide binds to two of the four heme groups resulting in a 50% reduction of oxygen-carrying capacity, and reduces the functional heme groups' ability to unload oxygen. The presence of a significant amount of COHb manifests in cherry red–colored mucous membranes, and is treated with 100% oxygen therapy to compete with CO binding and decrease the half-life of carbon monoxide through displacement.

Sulfhemoglobin

A toxic ingestion of sulfur containing chemicals can lead to sulfhemoglobinemia through sulfide bonding with hemoglobin, inducing the inability of carrying oxygen. The condition is rare and is most commonly associated with toxic ingestions of sulfur compounds (sulfonamides, sulfasalazine). Treatment is supportive.

CLINICAL ASSESSMENT

An accurate history, thorough physical examination, and appropriate laboratory tests must be performed to properly evaluate an anemic patient, determine a diagnosis, and define a therapeutic plan.

History

All pertinent information regarding patient history must be gathered from the owners. Obtaining and assessing a complete and detailed history will help define the nature, severity, and duration of clinical signs and aid in making a correct diagnosis. Attention to detail allows the clinician to establish probability for each possible differential early in the diagnostic process. For example, an anemic English springer spaniel with pigmenturia, especially after physical exertion, should alert the clinician to the possibility of phosphofructokinase deficiency. When a puppy has signs of hemolytic disease, the owner should be questioned about the possibility of foreign body ingestion of certain zinc-containing metallic objects.

> TECHNICIAN NOTE   Complete vaccination history should not be overlooked, because a relationship between recent vaccination and onset of IMHA has been demonstrated. One study showed that 25% of all IMHA cases were vaccinated within 1 month of presentation and that this complication occurred independent of the type of vaccine used.

The animal's environmental history may suggest possible exposure to toxic and organic substances that will create hemolytic conditions (e.g., onions, zinc). Tick exposure should also be investigated because various infectious agents may cause a hemolytic anemia (e.g., hemobartonellosis, babesiosis, ehrlichiosis, leptospirosis).

Information regarding previously diagnosed diseases and any recently or currently administered medication is very important. Many drugs have potentially harmful or complicating side effects, resulting in a toxic effect (i.e., drug-induced IMHA) on RBCs, WBCs, and platelets.

Physical Examination

As always, a complete physical examination and multiple monitoring procedures may be required to properly assess the patient in an anemic crisis. Optimal assessment cannot be based on the result of a single parameter; instead, it should be based on the results of several physical examinations and monitored parameters should always be evaluated in relation to one another.

In anemic patients, the development and progression of clinical signs depend on the rapidity of onset of the anemia, the degree and cause of the anemia, and the animal's physical activity. Common physical findings are those associated with a decrease in red cell mass: lethargy, weakness, pale mucous membranes, tachycardia, tachypnea, and bounding pulses. Anorexia,

exercise intolerance, and collapse may also be seen. The cardiovascular and respiratory systems should be carefully evaluated. Assessment of perfusion is based on mentation, core to extremity temperature gradient, mucous membrane color, capillary refill time, and heart rate as well as pulse rate, strength, and character. In a severe anemic state, a low-grade systolic flow murmur may occur secondary to decreased blood viscosity. Assessment of respiratory rate and effort, as well as careful auscultation, may help differentiate between decreased oxygen-carrying capability and possible pulmonary thromboembolism. Tachypnea and dyspnea may be evident as a result of increased respiratory drive from hypoxemia or compensatory respiratory alkalosis, but are not typical signs unless the anemia is severe. Fever is sometimes observed and may be caused by red cell destruction, or secondary or underlying inflammation and infection. Monitoring and considering all parameters will lend information regarding bleed severity and potentially life-threatening complications.

Patients should be evaluated for signs of underlying or concurrent disease. For example, dogs with IMHA should be carefully examined for signs of other immune-mediated disease, such as concurrent IMT (i.e., Evans syndrome). If petechiation is present, then IMT or other coagulopathies, such as liver disease or DIC, should be investigated.

Other common physical findings in dogs with hemolytic disease are those relating to an accumulation of bilirubin or Hb (or both), in blood, urine, and soft tissue. As a result of extravascular RBC destruction, increased quantities of bilirubin are presented to the liver for conjugation and excretion. Bilirubin begins to accumulate in blood, urine, and soft tissue when the quantity of bilirubin present exceeds the liver's capacity to excrete it in the bile. Consequently, dogs with severe extravascular hemolysis have icterus and pigmenturia, caused by the presence of bilirubin or Hb in the urine. Given the low threshold for urinary excretion of conjugated bilirubin in dogs, bilirubinuria develops early in the disease process and precedes hyperbilirubinemia (see Figure 16-7, *B*) and icterus. Icterus is easily recognized on all skin surfaces when severe. When more subtle, icterus is best recognized on the gingiva, sclera, conjunctiva, and inner pinna. Hemoglobinemia with or without hemoglobinuria may be present if intravascular hemolysis occurs.

Splenomegaly, hepatomegaly, or both may be discovered on abdominal palpation. This occurs as a result of increased RBC clearance by the mononuclear phagocytic system in these organs, by extramedullary hematopoiesis, and by hemosiderosis (accumulation of iron in the liver). Dogs with IMHA may also develop hepatopathy, particularly after glucocorticosteroid therapy.

Laboratory Tests

Although information obtained from the history and specific clinical signs can suggest a diagnosis, certain laboratory tests are necessary for a definitive diagnosis. Laboratory tests will help define the severity of the anemia, classify the anemia, and identify the underlying disease process.

Anemia is suggested when one or more of the red cell parameters (i.e., RBC count, PCV, hematocrit) are less than normal for the age, sex, and breed of the species concerned. Of these three parameters, PCV provides a simple, quick, and accurate means of detecting anemia, and it allows for classification of the anemia as *mild, moderate,* or *severe.*

> **TECHNICIAN NOTE** Dehydration and splenic contraction may mask anemia, whereas hemodilution may cause a temporary reduction in red cell parameters; therefore, determination of both PCV and total plasma protein (TP) level may help in differentiating these variables.

Dehydration is associated with increases in PCV and TP, but splenic contraction only elevates PCV. Hemodilution after acute blood loss or fluid therapy is associated with decreases in both PCV and TP, whereas hemolytic anemias are usually associated only with a reduction in PCV. TP is usually normal in anemia secondary to decreased production or increased destruction of erythrocytes, compared with blood loss, in which PCV and TP may be decreased because of loss of erythrocytes and plasma proteins and a compensatory shift of fluid from the interstitial space to the intravascular compartment.

Reticulocyte Count

The reticulocyte count is the best indicator of the effectiveness of bone marrow activity. The reticulocyte count during regenerative anemia generally varies with the degree of anemia; the greater the stimulation of marrow erythropoiesis, the greater the reticulocytosis. This is not the case with nonregenerative anemias; therefore the degree of reticulocytosis must be viewed in concert with the degree of anemia. The technician can do this by calculating a corrected reticulocyte count (percent [%]) or an absolute reticulocyte count (numbers/microliter [μL] of blood). The absolute reticulocyte count is calculated by multiplying the percentage of reticulocytes by the RBC count. Alternatively, the percentage of reticulocytes can be corrected for the degree of anemia by the following formula:

$$\text{Corrected reticulocyte } \% = \\ (\text{Observed reticulocyte count in percent}) \times \\ (\text{PCV of patient/mean normal PCV for species})$$

The mean normal PCV is 45% and 37% for dogs and cats, respectively. A corrected reticulocyte count greater than 1% in the dog and cat indicates a regenerative anemia. An absolute reticulocyte count of greater than 60,000/μL of blood in the dog is evidence of a regenerative response.

The degree of reticulocytosis is generally greater in hemolytic anemia and is evident earlier than in blood loss anemia; 3 or 4 days are typically needed for a significant reticulocytosis to be found in blood after an acute hemolytic or hemorrhagic episode, and a maximal response may take 1 to 2 weeks or longer. Thus reticulocytosis in an anemic patient indicates increased red cell destruction or blood loss. Conversely, the absence of reticulocytosis in an anemic patient suggests reduced erythropoietin production, marrow depression or failure, defective iron use, or ineffective erythropoiesis. Bone marrow evaluation is necessary to assess the production of RBCs in these patients.

Hemogram and Blood Smear

Much information can be gathered from a complete blood count (e.g., Hb concentration, cell counts, RBC indices). On careful microscopic examination of a stained blood film, RBC indices and morphology can help characterize an anemia. The mean cell volume (MCV), which represents the average size of the RBC, classifies erythrocytes as *normocytic* (normal), *macrocytic* (larger than normal), and *microcytic* (smaller than normal). For example, an increased MCV may result from cells being released from the bone marrow before they reach full maturity. This is called a *macrocytic anemia*. The mean corpuscular Hb concentration (MCHC) is represented by the terms *normochromic* (normal Hb content) and *hypochromic* (less than normal Hb content). For example, a decreased MCHC may result from increased numbers of circulating immature red cells. This is called a *hypochromic anemia*.

The blood smear can also show appropriate morphologic features, such as spherocytosis, polychromasia, and anisocytosis. Marked spherocytosis is indicative of IMHA in dogs. During the IMHA episode, macrophages bind to the RBC membrane and remove a piece. The RBC escapes complete phagocytosis, but its membrane is tightened, creating a small, swollen, densely stained erythrocyte. A small number of spherocytes may also be observed in microangiopathic hemolytic anemia, DIC, zinc intoxication, and heartworm disease.

Platelet Count

IMHA and IMT may occur concurrently. If thrombocytopenia is present, then a diagnostic workup for IMT should be performed and appropriate treatment instituted. With any clinical evidence of bleeding, other coagulation studies should be performed to rule out concurrent thrombocytopenia, DIC, or other coagulopathies (see discussion in section on hemostatic testing).

Saline Agglutination Test

RBC autoagglutination indicates anti–RBC antibodies are present and therefore strongly suggests IMHA. Agglutination appears as grapelike clustering of erythrocytes in the blood smear and can be distinguished from rouleaux formation by examining a wet-mount preparation of a blood sample. The veterinary technician should mix one drop of blood with one drop of isotonic saline on a clean microscope slide, cover it with a coverslip, and examine it under the microscope. Rouleaux, unlike agglutination, should be dispersed by the addition of the saline. This test is not infallible, because weak agglutinins may cause false-negative results. Blood should also be evaluated for macroagglutination (seen grossly on the slide). Persistent agglutination precludes any further blood typing, crossmatching, or Coombs' test.

Coombs' Test

Serologic diagnosis of IMHA is based on the demonstration of immune-mediated antibody or complement on the surface of red cells or in the patient's serum via Coombs' antiglobulin tests. The direct Coombs' test demonstrates the presence of antierythrocyte antibody or activated complement components on the surface of the patient's red cells. The indirect Coombs' test reveals the presence of antierythrocyte antibody in patient serum. A suspension of washed cells of the patient (direct Coombs' test) or of normal washed red cells exposed to the patient's serum (indirect Coombs' test) is allowed to react with species-specific antiglobulin to induce visible agglutination of red cells. In cases of drug-induced IMHA, the offending drug must be incorporated into the test system, or the test may yield negative results. The diagnosis of IMHA is supported by demonstrating the presence of these antibodies or complement (evidenced by the appearance of agglutination).

Chemistry Profile and Urinalysis

A serum biochemistry profile and urinalysis is important in detecting and assessing concurrent metabolic disease (e.g., renal, hepatic). Electrolyte disturbances should be monitored closely. Decreased bilirubin and albumin or globulin levels may indicate blood loss. Elevated bilirubin levels suggests hemolysis. Bilirubinuria and bilirubinemia are observed with active hemolysis, but bilirubinemia may be very modest.

Blood sample collection technique is critical, because hemolysis associated with traumatic venipuncture can cause serum bilirubin measurements to be falsely elevated.

Tick Titers

Various infectious agents may cause a hemolytic anemia; therefore serologic testing for tick-borne diseases should be performed if tick exposure is a possibility.

Miscellaneous Information

With IMHA, the leukocyte count is often elevated with a slight to marked neutrophilia and left shift as a result of maximal bone marrow stimulation. A patient in hemolytic crisis may exhibit a marked neutrophilia (60,000 to 70,000/μL with increase in banded neutrophils) in the absence of infection; therefore one must evaluate the clinical presentation of each patient and look for other signs that might support infection along with the WBC count.

TREATMENT AND MANAGEMENT

Anemic animals often arrive at the emergency service in advanced stages of disease, on the verge of cardiovascular collapse, and in need of immediate therapeutic intervention. Although a definitive diagnosis is important in the ultimate treatment of these patients, stabilizing the patient's emergent clinical problem is critical. This stabilization may include controlling hemorrhage and replacing lost blood volume with the appropriate intravenous fluid solutions, blood components, or both, as well as improving DO_2 with oxygen support and taking all necessary measures to combat shock. Once the patient is stabilized, the clinician should classify the anemia, proceed with diagnostic evaluation, determine the underlying cause, and begin appropriate therapy. Clinical laboratory tests should be performed immediately and therapy instituted promptly after test samples are obtained. The goal is to correct the condition responsible for the blood loss (e.g., provide surgery, withdraw offending drug, administer anthelmintics).

Animals do not tolerate an acute onset of anemia secondary to hemolysis or hemorrhage as well as they tolerate chronic anemia caused by hemolysis or decreased RBC production.

> **TECHNICIAN NOTE** With chronic anemia, a much lower hematocrit can be tolerated as a result of the body's compensatory mechanisms (e.g., increase in heart rate, stroke volume, and plasma volume). The rapidity and severity of an acute anemic crisis necessitate allocating these patients a priority status. The animal should be kept quiet and provided with oxygen if needed. Intensive care consisting of warmth, oxygen, intravenous fluid support, and blood transfusion may be required, keeping in mind that the benefit of transfusion therapy must be weighed against its inherent risks.

In IMHA, transfusion support has been viewed as a controversial treatment because even more RBCs will be destroyed—those of the patient and of the donor. However, transfused RBCs are not preferentially attacked by the patient's immune system. Blood typing and crossmatching is essential when treating these patients.

When a bleeding problem is identified in a patient, nursing care should be directed toward minimizing further loss of blood. Special attention should be given to minimizing trauma to decrease the chance of hemorrhage. A small-gauge needle (e.g., 25 gauge) should be used for venipuncture, and extended application of pressure to venipuncture sites will be necessary. Avoidance of central vessels for blood collection is very important. Patient activity should be restricted and extra padding used during cage confinement. Invasive and surgical procedures may need to be postponed until the patient is hemostatically stable. Ultimately the extent of nursing support for the bleeding patient will vary based on the severity of the condition.

The veterinary technician plays a critical role in supporting the patient with hemostatic disorders and anemia. Involvement with patient triage and with blood component procurement and administration as well as consistent and careful monitoring is crucial in ensuring a successful patient outcome.

SUGGESTED READINGS

Brooks MB: Section VII: Hemostasis. In Weiss DJ, Wardrop KJ, editors: *Schalm's veterinary hematology*, ed 6, Ames, Iowa, 2010, Wiley-Blackwell, pp 633–707.

Brooks MB, Catalfamo JL: Immune-mediated thrombocytopenia, von Willebrand disease, and platelet disorders. In Ettinger SJ, Feldman EC, editors: *Textbook of veterinary internal medicine*, ed 7, St Louis, 2010, Saunders, pp 772–783.

Callan MB: Section VIII: Transfusion medicine. In Weiss DJ, Wardrop KJ, editors: *Schalm's veterinary hematology*, ed 6, Ames, Iowa, 2010, Wiley-Blackwell, pp 709–795.

Clancey NP, Murphy MC: Zinc-induced hemolytic anemia in a dog caused by ingestion of a game-playing die, *Can Vet J* 53:383–386, 2012.

Day MJ, Kohn B: *BSAVA manual of canine and feline haematology and transfusion medicine*, ed 2, Gloucester, 2012, British Small Animal Veterinary Association.

Harvey JW: Evaluation of hemostasis. In Harvey JW, editor: *Veterinary hematology: a diagnostic guide and color atlas*, St Louis, 2012, Saunders, pp 191–233.

Haskins S, Pascoe PJ, Ilkiw JE, et al.: Reference cardiopulmonary values in normal dogs, *Comp Med* 255:156–161, 2005.

Ralph AG, Brainard BM: Update on disseminated intravascular coagulation: when to consider it, when to expect it, when to treat it, *Top Compan Anim Med* 27:65–72, 2012.

Van der Linden PJ, De Hert SG, Belisle S, et al.: Critical oxygen delivery during cardiopulmonary bypass in dogs: pulsatile vs. non-pulsatile blood flow, *Eur J Anaesthesiol* 23:10–16, 2006.

SCENARIO

Purpose: To provide the veterinary technician with the opportunity to build or strengthen his/her knowledge about different causes of hemostatic disorders.

Stage: Emergency clinic is considered a level I facility with access to PRBCs, FFP, cryoprecipitate, fresh platelet concentrate (most of the time), synthetic colloids, and isotonic crystalloids, as well as most drugs.

Scenario

Consider the following patients:

Patient 1: A 4-year-old male cocker spaniel weighing 13.1 kg presents for lethargy. Upon examination he is found to have the following: HR 140 beats/min, RR 28 breaths/min with no obvious effort, lungs auscult clear, mucous membrane (MM) pink with a capillary refill time (CRT) of 1 sec. Pulse quality is normal. Small, diffuse, round bruising is seen on the mucous membranes and abdominal skin. Initial blood work shows PCV 32%, TP 6.5 g/dl, platelet count 45,000/μL, and BMBT 5 min, but a normal PT/PTT value. The patient was recently seen and given a vaccine booster.

Patient 2: A 6-month-old intact female Bassett hound weighing 20.1 kg is brought to the hospital because she has had occasional bleeding from the gums after shedding deciduous teeth. Upon examination she is found to have normal heart rate and sounds, as well as normal respiratory rate, character, and sound. Her MMs are pink, and CRT is 1-2 sec. Pulses feel normal. Initial blood work shows her PCV is 38%, her TP is 5.8 g/dl, and her platelet count is 250,000/μL.

Patient 3: A 2-year-old female mix breed dog weighing 29.2 kg walks into the hospital having difficulty breathing and also coughing some blood; bruising is seen on the abdomen. Upon examination she is found to be tachycardic (HR 150 beats/min) and tachypneic (RR 56 breaths/min) with increased effort, lungs auscult harsh with some crackles, and mucous membranes (MMs) are pink with a capillary refill time (CRT) of less than 1 sec. Pulse quality is normal. Initial blood work shows packed cell volume (PCV) of 39%, platelet count of 214,000/μL, and PT/PTT is prolonged. Thoracic radiographs show signs of pulmonary edema. The patient is hospitalized for respiratory support, and the owner calls later informing you that his/her neighbors have placed some rat bait in their yard.

Patient 4: An 11-year-old female DSH is brought in after suddenly not being able to use her hind limbs. She weighs 5.2 kg. The owner reports her suddenly seeming very painful, crying in a room. The owner thinks she may have fallen off the nearby dresser. Upon examination she seems to have paresis in both hind legs; peripheral pulses in the hind limbs cannot be felt. HR is 160 beats/min with a gallop rhythm, RR is 28 breaths/min when not panting. PCV is 33%, and TP is 6.0 g/dl.

Delivery

- Present all cases to the staff.
- Initial discussion: Allow *10-20 minutes* for staff to review the cases and determine the type of hemostatic disorder.
- Have staff explain their rationale.
- Follow-up discussion: Discuss potential causes and treatment options for each case.

Questions

- Initial question
  - Which findings indicate a hemostatic disorder, if any?
  - What type of hemostatic disorder is this?
  - Which aspect of hemostasis is impaired to cause these symptoms?
  - Is there any additional testing or examination needed?
- Follow-up questions
  - What are potential causes of this hemostatic disorder?
  - What questions regarding history may help delineate the causes?
  - What treatments do you anticipate will be asked by the veterinarian?

Key Teaching Points

- Provides veterinary technicians the opportunity to review presentation signs of hemostatic disorders
- Provides opportunity to consider diagnostics for confirmation of the disorder
- Veterinary technicians can consider all potential causes in relation to history and physical examination findings.

Discussion

Patient 1

Initial discussion:

- The patient is showing small, diffuse, round shaped bruising indicating possible bleeding disorder.
- Hypocoagulation (hemorrhaging coagulopathy)

SCENARIO—cont'd

- Thrombocytopenia (note: 45,000/μL is often sufficient to prevent spontaneous bleeding, but in this case it is not)
- The cause of the thrombocytopenia should be pursued.

Follow-up discussion:
- Bone marrow dysfunction, infectious, immune-mediated
- Any medication, travel history, and medical history
- The treatment is dependent on the potential cause. If it is due to medications, it should be stopped. If the cause is infectious, the correct antibiotics should be used. If the cause is immune-mediated, immunosuppressive agents are used.

Patient 2

Initial discussion:
- The patient is showing occasional bleeding, especially after sources of trauma.
- Hypocoagulation (hemorrhaging coagulopathy)
- Thrombopathia or a coagulation factor deficiency is possible.
- BMBT prolongation would point towards thrombopathia.

Follow-up discussion:
- Thrombopathia may be drug induced. Coagulation factor deficits can be inherited.
- History on tendencies to bleed from young age would indicate possible inherited disease. Obtain information on any current medications.
- Transfusion of plasma products may be needed if coagulation factor deficiency.

Patient 3

Initial discussion:
- Dyspnea, coughing up blood, bruising on the abdomen, all are signs of coagulopathy.
- Hypocoagulation (hemorrhaging coagulopathy)
- PT/PTT is prolonged, indicating coagulation factor-related problems
- No additional testing is needed.

Follow-up discussion:
- Vitamin K antagonism is very likely, given ingestion of rat bait (anticoagulant).
- The product name or package of the rat bait will allow us to be sure of the cause.
- Plasma product transfusion to stop the bleeding, and vitamin K administration

Patient 4

Initial discussion:
- Acute onset of pain and loss of control of the hind limbs
- Thromboembolism (hypercoagulation)
- Increase in thrombosis, outweighing antithrombosis
- Comparison of pulses, blood pressure, and temperature of front vs hind limbs can further confirm thromboembolism.

Follow-up discussion:
- In cats, hypertrophic cardiomyopathy is often the cause of thrombus formation.
- There are no specific questions.
- Medical interventions with supportive care, thromboprophylactics and thrombolytics (unproven therapy) may allow a patient to recover, though recurrence is likely.

MEDICAL MATH EXERCISE

A patient with refractory immune-mediated thrombocytopenia is being prepared for treatment with vincristine. The veterinarian asks you to prepare *0.02 mg/kg of vincristine for IV injection.* The concentration of vincristine is 1 mg/ml. The patient weighs 18 kg.

  a. How many milligrams of vincristine do you need?
  b. How many milliliters of stock vincristine do you need?

17 Cardiovascular Emergencies*

Deborah Ann Kingston

KEY TERMS

Cardiac arrhythmias
Cardiomyopathy
Electrocardiogram
Endocarditis
Murmur
Rhythm

CHAPTER OUTLINE

Diagnosis of Heart Disease
  Troponin
  Signalment
  History
  Physical Examination
  Electrocardiogram
  Thoracic Radiographs
  Echocardiography
Overview of Cardiac Physiology and Pathophysiology
  Systolic Function
  Preload
  Afterload
  Contractility
  Heart Rate and Rhythm
  Diastolic Function
Heart Failure
  Low-Output or Forward Failure
  Congestive or Backward Failure
  Relationship between Hemodynamic Measurements and Clinical Signs of Heart Failure
Identifying Patients Who May Have Heart Failure
  Client Complaints
  Physical Findings
  Diagnostic Imaging and the Electrocardiogram
  Emergency Treatment of Congestive Heart Failure
  Diuretic Therapy
  Oxygen Therapy
  Vasodilator Therapy
  Positive Inotropic Therapy

Monitoring Therapy for Heart Failure
  Monitoring Vasodilator Therapy
  Monitoring Positive Inotropic Therapy
  Monitoring Diuretic Therapy
Cardiac Arrhythmias
  Client Complaints
  Physical Findings
  Diagnostic Imaging and the Electrocardiogram
  Medical Treatment of Cardiac Arrhythmias
  Role of Electrolytes and Drug Interactions in Antiarrhythmic Therapy
  Treatment of Ventricular Tachycardia
  Treatment of Atrial Fibrillation
  Treatment of Supraventricular Tachycardia
  Treatment of Bradyarrhythmias
  Treatment of Hyperkalemia
  Monitoring Treatment of Cardiac Arrhythmias
  Pacemaker Therapy
  Precordial Thumps in the Treatment of Arrhythmias
Heartworm Disease
  Caval Syndrome
  Client Complaints
  Physical Findings
  Diagnostic Imaging and the Electrocardiogram

*The authors and publisher wish to acknowledge Craig C. Cornell for previous contributions to this chapter. The authors would also like to acknowledge Dr. Lynne O'Sullivan, DVM, DVSC, DACVIM (cardiology), for her assistance with this chapter.

Surgical Treatment of Caval
    Syndrome
Monitoring
Complications of Adulticide
    Therapy
**Cardiac Tamponade and
    Pericardial Effusion**
    Client Complaints
    Clinical Signs
    Diagnostic Imaging and the
        Electrocardiogram

Treatment of Cardiac Tamponade
    and Pericardial Effusion
Monitoring
Feline Aortic Thromboembolism
    Client Complaints
    Diagnostic Imaging and the
        Electrocardiogram
    Clinical Signs
    Treatment

LEARNING OBJECTIVES

After studying this chapter, you will be able to:

- Describe common cardiac emergencies.
- Introduce treatment options for cardiac disease.
- Discuss the role of the veterinary technician during a cardiac emergency.

Heart disease is one of the most common health problems seen in small animal practice. The technician plays a very important role in the treatment and management of the cardiac patient. The technician also contributes to the diagnosis by obtaining an accurate history from the client, whether during the initial emergency phone call or during the physical examination upon admission to hospital. Once the status of the patient is gauged, there are initial diagnostic tests that may be performed by the technician, including electrocardiography, blood work, radiography, and blood pressure measurement. Effective treatment is likely to be provided when veterinary technicians have a solid understanding of common cardiac emergencies and the ways in which heart disease is diagnosed as well as the pathophysiology of heart failure. Cardiac emergencies may be divided into three categories: congestive heart failure, thromboembolic disease, and **rhythm** disorders.

DIAGNOSIS OF HEART DISEASE

Although the veterinarian is responsible for making the diagnosis, technicians assist the veterinarian in the initial stabilization of the patient, and by gathering information from clients, examining the patient, performing clinical laboratory tests, measuring noninvasive blood pressure, taking radiographs, and recording and measuring the electrocardiogram (ECG). In some cases a technician may be responsible for performing a diagnostic quality echocardiogram or cardiac ultrasound.

Cardiac ultrasound gives important information about cardiac structure, function, and blood flow. Radiographs may confirm congestive heart failure by allowing the veterinarian to evaluate the cardiac silhouette, pulmonary vessels, pulmonary parenchyma, and pleural space. The level of pulmonary edema and/or effusion will determine the nature and degree of heart failure and will assist with therapeutic decisions. Laboratory tests may include measurement of electrolyte, urea, and creatinine levels. These are especially important to document a pretreatment baseline. The ECG is important for determining initial arrhythmias that may need immediate attention such as atrial fibrillation, other tachyarrhythmias, or bradyarrhythmias. A quick lead II ECG is often adequate in diagnosing most cardiac rhythm abnormalities.

TROPONIN

Measurement of troponin level is an additional test that is becoming readily available. It is not a useful screening tool for heart disease, since it can be elevated with both cardiac and extracardiac disease, but may give supportive information about the myocardium in conjunction with other diagnostic testing, such as echocardiography and ECG.

Troponin's specific biomarkers are I and T, which are thin filament–associated, regulatory proteins of heart muscle. They are crucial to the interaction between actin and myosin, specific to myocyte injury, ischemia, and necrosis. Troponin "I" inhibition measurement is the most sensitive, and is the one most commonly used in small animals. It may be used in cases where myocardial infarction, toxic myocardial disease, myocarditis, or blunt myocardial trauma is suspected.

Blood should be collected in a heparinized tube (green top), and the sample should be separated within 30 minutes of collection. If testing cannot be done within 4 hours, the plasma should be frozen. A total of 0.5 ml of plasma is required. Some laboratories accept whole blood (iStat) or serum depending on their equipment; check with your local lab. The normal reference ranges may vary depending on the assay the lab uses. Results are usually measured in micrograms per liter (mcg/L) or nanograms per milliliter (ng/ml). The two commercial veterinary assays used in the United States are Idexx and Abaxis (iStat).

SIGNALMENT

The age, breed, and gender of an animal provide important information that can aid in the diagnosis of heart disease. Heart murmurs in young animals are sometimes benign but are often a sign of congenital heart disease. Innocent murmurs tend to diminish after 6 months of age, while murmurs related to congenital diseases tend to increase in their intensity as the animal further matures, such as a patent ductus arteriosus (PDA) , subaortic stenosis (SAS), or pulmonic stenosis (PS). Degenerative changes in the heart valves occur in many dogs as they age, with mitral valve disease being a very common cause of heart failure in small breed geriatric dogs. Pericardial disease, aortic stenosis, dilated **cardiomyopathy,** and **endocarditis** are more common in larger breeds.

HISTORY

Clients seek emergency treatment because they have observed something that they perceive to be so serious that it requires immediate attention; this is the presenting complaint. Most patients will present with weakness, lethargy, collapse or syncope, cough, tachypnea, or respiratory distress. Other concerns may be anorexia, vomiting, and/or diarrhea, because cardiac disease may have effects on other major organs in the body. Those working in emergency care do not always have access to

the medical record and need to begin treatment of a life-threatening condition without the benefit of a complete history. In a life-threatening emergency, the veterinarian may need to begin treatment immediately and have a technician gather the history while the patient is being treated. The presenting signs may lead the veterinarian to consider the possibility of heart disease, which may influence the sort of information he or she seeks in the history. A veterinarian treating a patient suspected of having heart disease might look to the client or medical record for information related to the presenting complaint, the patient's history of heart disease, procedures and medications used to treat preexistent heart disease, previous diagnostic procedures and tests, or aspects of history that may be related to heart disease (e.g., activity level, exercise intolerance, difficulty breathing, cough, syncope or collapse, changes in weight, and diet). Box 17-1 lists common signs in cardiac emergencies. Tables 17-1 and 17-2 list various heart diseases and the emergencies associated with them.

PHYSICAL EXAMINATION

The physical examination is the process of gathering information that can be detected with the senses. The veterinarian should be notified if a new sign is observed or if a previously observed sign changes. The following list contains signs that are associated with heart disease and grouped by the sense used to detect them.
Sight:

- Cyanotic or pale mucous membranes
- Cachexia
- Dyspnea
- Tachypnea

BOX 17-1	Common Signs in Cardiac Emergencies

Sudden death
Cyanosis
Dyspnea
Collapse ,
Hind limb paresis
Syncope
Tachypnea
Exercise intolerance
Cough
Abdominal distention (ascites)

TABLE 17-1	Emergencies Associated with Various Forms of Canine Heart Disease
HEART DISEASE	**ASSOCIATED EMERGENCIES**
Heartworm disease	Caval syndrome, right heart failure, pulmonary hypertension
Chronic valvular disease	Pulmonary edema, ruptured chordae tendineae, left atrial tear, cardiac arrhythmias, right heart failure
Dilated cardiomyopathy	Pulmonary edema, right heart failure, cardiac arrhythmias, cardiac arrest (sudden death)
Pericardial disease	Right heart failure, cardiac tamponade
Patent ductus arteriosus (PDA)	Pulmonary edema, cardiac arrhythmias, pulmonary hypertension, cyanosis
Subaortic stenosis	Cardiac arrest (sudden death), cardiac arrhythmias, pulmonary edema (most common with concomitant mitral dysplasia)
Pulmonic stenosis	Right heart failure (most common with concomitant tricuspid dysplasia)
Infective endocarditis	Pulmonary edema, embolism, cardiac arrhythmias
Ventricular septal defect	Left heart failure, pulmonary hypertension, cyanosis, right heart failure
Tetralogy of Fallot	Cyanosis, polycythemia
Tricuspid dysplasia	Right heart failure
Atrial septal defect	Right heart failure, pulmonary hypertension, cyanosis

TABLE 17-2	Emergencies Associated with Various Forms of Feline Heart Disease
HEART DISEASE	**ASSOCIATED EMERGENCIES**
Hypertrophic cardiomyopathy	Thromboembolism, pulmonary edema, pleural effusion, cardiac arrhythmias, sudden death
Restrictive cardiomyopathy	Thromboembolism, pulmonary edema, pleural effusion, cardiac arrhythmias, sudden death
Dilated cardiomyopathy	Thromboembolism, pulmonary edema, pleural effusion, cardiac arrhythmias, sudden death
Cardiomyopathy secondary to hyperthyroidism	Thromboembolism, pulmonary edema, pleural effusion, cardiac arrhythmias, sudden death
Atrioventricular valve dysplasia	Pulmonary edema, pleural effusion
Ventricular septal defect	Pulmonary edema, pleural effusion, cyanosis
Patent ductus arteriosus (PDA)	Pulmonary edema, pleural effusion
Aortic stenosis	Pulmonary edema, pleural effusion, sudden death
Tetralogy of Fallot	Cyanosis, polycythemia

- Ascites
- Jugular distention
- Subcutaneous edema
- Hind limb paresis
- Syncope
- Posture
- Response to environment, level of consciousness

Sound:
- Murmurs
- Cough
- Gallop sounds
- Irregular heart rhythm
- Bradycardia or tachycardia
- Crackles or other abnormal lung sounds
- Muffled heart or lung sounds

Touch:
- Body temperature
- Temperature of extremities
- Abnormal pulses, pulse deficits
- Precordial thrills
- Fluid in abdomen
- Enlarged liver

Auscultation of the heart is one part of the physical examination that deserves particular attention. Heart **murmurs** and gallops are some of the most important signs of heart disease. The ability to detect and characterize these sounds is a skill that can only be mastered by careful practice.

> **TECHNICIAN NOTE** Auscultation skills can be improved by taking the opportunity to examine any animal that is known to have a murmur or gallop sound, while also spending time auscultating normal, healthy patients for comparison.

Murmurs and gallops are sometimes missed because they are soft, intermittent, or very focal. The person examining the patient should be systematic when listening—murmurs are sometimes missed because the examiner failed to listen to the entire chest. Once a murmur is located, its intensity should be noted. Intensity is most often graded on a scale from 1 to 6. A murmur with an intensity of 1 is barely audible in a quiet room, and murmurs with an intensity of 6 are loud enough to be heard without the stethoscope touching the chest wall. Murmurs graded 5 or more will have a precordial thrill present on palpation of the chest wall on either side of the heart. The loudest location of the murmur, referred to as the point of maximum intensity (PMI), may be described as apical or base, right or left sided. Localizing the PMI can assist in determining the etiology or source of the murmur. Murmurs are also described with respect to the time at which they occur in the cardiac cycle. Normally only the first and second heart sounds can be heard in dogs and cats. These *lub dub* sounds mark the beginning and end of systole. Murmurs that occur during this time are systolic murmurs; murmurs that follow the *lub dub* are diastolic murmurs. Diastolic murmurs are less common and generally softer than systolic murmurs. Continuous murmurs occur throughout systole and diastole, with patent ductus arteriosus (PDA) being the most common condition producing a continuous murmur. Diastolic gallop sounds occur when the normally inaudible third and fourth heart sounds can be heard. The third heart sound occurs just after systole, and the fourth heart sound occurs just before systole.

ELECTROCARDIOGRAM

The ECG is the most accurate technique available for the diagnosis of arrhythmias. The ECG may also aid in the diagnosis of chamber dilation or hypertrophy (Table 17-3), electrolyte abnormalities, and pericardial effusion. The presence or absence of conditions other than arrhythmias should be confirmed with other tests. This is particularly true for enlargement of the heart chambers, where the ECG will frequently produce false-positive or false-negative results. Technicians can play a key role in answering the most important initial diagnostic question in relation to the ECG: Is the patient in sinus rhythm? The following are criteria for a sinus rhythm: (1) P wave for every QRS, (2) consistent P-R interval, and (3) positive P waves in lead II. If a sinus rhythm is

not present, then a rhythm algorithm may be useful in determining rhythm diagnosis (Table 17-4).

THORACIC RADIOGRAPHS

The value of thoracic radiography in diagnosing heart disease is in the assessment of heart size and pulmonary vasculature and in the diagnosis of the presence of congestive heart failure. Heart disease usually changes the size and shape of the cardiac silhouette; however, in some cases the changes are subtle. Relying solely on radiographs to diagnose heart disease will frequently lead to misdiagnosis. One factor that limits the ability of radiographs to detect heart disease is that only the external borders of the heart are visible unless contrast medium is used. Some forms of heart disease do not significantly increase the size of the cardiac silhouette. Concentric hypertrophy causes the walls of the ventricles to thicken without increasing the external diameter of the heart. Eccentric hypertrophy and dilation are easier to detect using radiographs, because they increase the external diameter of the heart. As the heart fails, increases in the diameter of the pulmonary veins or vena cava become apparent in thoracic radiographs. Increased opacity of the lungs in dogs with heart disease is a sign of pulmonary edema when accompanied by left atrial dilation and pulmonary venous distention, which indicates left ventricular failure. Radiographic signs of pleural effusion and enlargement of the vena cava in a patient with heart disease may indicate right or biventricular heart failure. The ability to examine the lungs and pulmonary vessels makes thoracic radiographs one the most sensitive techniques for detecting congestive left ventricular heart failure.

Cardiomegaly is a very reliable sign of heart disease when observed, although it will not be seen in every patient with heart disease. Cardiomegaly can be measured objectively by using the length of the thoracic vertebrae as a reference for determining heart size. This technique, known as the *vertebral heart scale* (VHS), was first used in dogs and was published by Buchanan in 1995. Since then, the VHS has been used in cats and other species, and its use as an aid in the diagnosis of heart disease has been studied extensively. Technicians can assist the veterinarian in diagnosing cardiomegaly by measuring VHS.

To use the VHS technique to measure heart size in dogs, a lateral thoracic radiograph is examined and the distance between the lower margin of the left mainstem

TABLE 17-3	Normal Electrocardiographic Parameters in the Dog and Cat	
PARAMETER	**CANINE**	**FELINE**
Heart rate (beats/min)	Adults: 70-160 Toy breeds: up to 180 Puppies: up to 220	160-240
Rhythm	Normal sinus rhythm Sinus arrhythmia Wandering atrial pacemaker	Normal sinus rhythm Sinus tachycardia
Intervals (sec) P	<0.04	<0.04
P-R	0.06-0.13	0.05-0.09
QRS	<20 kg: <0.05 >20 kg: <0.06 Giant breeds: <0.065	<0.04
Q-T	0.15-0.25	0.12-0.18
Amplitudes (mV) in Lead II P	<0.4	<0.2
R	<20 kg: <2.5 >20 kg: <3.0	<0.9
MEA	+40° to +100°	−5° to +160°

Criteria for Chamber Enlargement: Summary

CHAMBERS	ECG PARAMETER	BODY WEIGHT	CANINE	FELINE
Left atrium	PII duration		>0.04 sec	>0.04 sec
Right atrium	PII amplitude		>0.4 mV	>0.2 mV
Left ventricle	RII amplitude	<20 kg	>2.5 mV	>0.9 mV
		>20 kg	>3.0 mV	
Right ventricle	Pattern of SI, SII, and SIII		Present	
	MEA points to Rt vent		Present	Present
	S in V_3		>0.7 mV	
	S in V_3 > R in V_3		Present	

bronchus and the cardiac apex is marked on a piece of paper. The paper is then rotated 90 degrees, and the maximal short axis width is also marked on the paper. Then, beginning with the cranial border of the fourth thoracic vertebra (T4), the length and width of the heart is measured in vertebrae (estimating to one tenth of a vertebra). The sum of the length and width is used to determine overall heart size. Buchanan assumed that VHS was relatively unaffected by breed and that VHS values greater than 10.7 were abnormal. Since then, other studies have shown that some normal dogs have higher VHS values than those reported by Buchanan. Dogs with degenerative valvular disease begin to show signs of congestive heart failure when VHS exceeds

approximately 12 to 13. Figure 17-1 shows the landmarks and technique used to measure VHS in dogs. Table 17-5 shows the normal range for VHS in specific breeds.

The technique for measuring VHS in cats is similar to that used in dogs. The vertebrae beginning at the fourth thoracic vertebra in the left lateral view are still used as a measuring scale. The anatomic landmarks used to measure the heart are slightly different from those used in dogs. In cats the long axis of the heart is measured in a lateral radiograph, beginning at the point where the most ventral cranial lobar vein meets the trachea and ending at the apex of the heart. The maximal short axis is measured just as it was in the dog. In cats the short axis width of the heart in ventrodorsal or dorsoventral

TABLE 17-4		Algorithm to Determine Cardiac Rhythm Disorders by ECG		
RHYTHM	**HEART RATE**	**P WAVES PRESENT?**	**DO QRS COMPLEXES HAVE ASSOCIATED P WAVES?**	**DISORDERS**
Regular	Slow	Yes	Yes	Sinus bradycardia Second-degree heart block
			No	Third-degree heart block
		No		Hyperkalemia Persistent atrial standstill
	Normal	Yes	Yes	Normal sinus rhythm Second-degree heart block Atrial flutter
			No	Ventricular tachycardia
		No		Hyperkalemia Persistent atrial standstill
	Fast	Yes	Yes	Sinus tachycardia Supraventricular tachycardia Atrial flutter
			No	Ventricular tachycardia Nonparoxysmal junctional tachycardia
		No		Supraventricular tachycardia (P waves present but buried in QRS or T)
Irregular	Slow	Yes	Yes	Sinus bradycardia Sinus arrhythmia Sick sinus syndrome Second-degree heart block
			No	
		No		Slow atrial fibrillation
	Normal	Yes	Yes	Sinus arrhythmia Second-degree heart block Atrial flutter
			No	Ventricular tachycardia (rhythm is usually regular)
		No		Atrial fibrillation
	Fast	Yes	Yes	Sinus tachycardia Atrial flutter Supraventricular tachycardia
			No	Ventricular tachycardia (rhythm is usually regular) Nonparoxysmal junctional tachycardia
		No		Atrial fibrillation

radiographs may be just as useful a diagnostic sign as the sum of the long and short axis measurements in the lateral view. The measurement is made by examining the dorsoventral or ventrodorsal radiograph and drawing a line from the apex to the base of the heart. Next the maximal width of the heart perpendicular to that line is marked on a piece of paper. Then, starting at the fourth thoracic vertebra on the lateral radiograph as a ruler, the distance between the marks on the paper is measured to determine the width of the heart. The combined long and short axis lengths in the lateral view should be less than eight vertebrae, and the short axis width in dorsoventral or ventrodorsal radiograph should be less than four vertebrae in the cat. It may be difficult to measure heart size in obese cats, because fat surrounding the heart may obscure the true cardiac border. Figure 17-2 shows the landmarks and technique used to measure VHS in cats (Table 17-6).

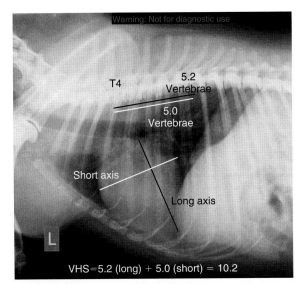

FIGURE 17-1 Landmarks for measuring vertebral heart scale (VHS) in dogs. Lateral radiograph illustrating the VHS measurement method. The long axis *(L)* and short axis *(S)* heart dimensions are transposed onto the vertebral column and recorded as the number of vertebrae beginning with the cranial edge of the fourth thoracic vertebra. These values are then added to obtain the VHS. *T*, Trachea.

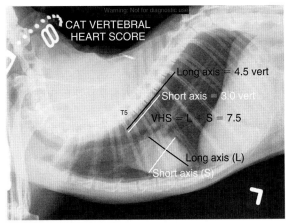

FIGURE 17-2 Landmarks for measuring VHS in lateral radiographs in the cat. Radiograph of lateral view of the thorax of a cat illustrating the VHS method. The long axis *(L)* and short axis *(S)* dimensions of the heart are transposed onto the vertebral column and recorded as the number of vertebrae beginning with the cranial edge of the fourth thoracic vertebra. These values are then added to obtain the VHS. The depth of the thorax *(D)* is measured from the dorsocaudal border of the seventh vertebra to the closest edge of the vertebral column. Precordial distance *(P)* is the minimum distance from the heart to the sternum. Falciform fat *(F)* is the minimum distance from the dorsocaudal border of the xiphoid cartilage to the liver. *T*, Trachea.

TABLE 17-5	Normal Range for Vertebral Heart Scale (VHS) in Specific Breeds
BREED	**NORMAL RANGE**
Boxer	10.3-12.6
Cavalier King Charles spaniel	9.9-11.7
Doberman pinscher	9.0-10.8
German shepherd	8.7-11.2
Labrador retriever	9.7-11.7
Whippet (includes dogs trained for racing)	10.3-12.3
Yorkshire terrier	9.0-10.5
Generic (Buchanan)	8.7-10.7

Data from Lamb CR, Boswood A: Role of survey radiography in diagnosing canine cardiac disease, *Compend Contin Educ Pract Vet* 24(4):316-326, 2002; Buchanan JW, Bücheler J: Vertebral scale system to measure canine heart size in radiographs, *J Am Vet Med Assoc* 206(2):194-199, 1995; Bavagems V, Van Caelenberg A, Duchateau L, et al: Vertebral heart size ranges specific for whippets, *Vet Radiol Ultrasound* 46(5):400-403, 2005.

TABLE 17-6	Ranges of Severity of Vertebral Heart Scale (VHS) in Dogs and Cats		
SEVERITY IN DOGS	**VHS**	**SEVERITY IN CATS**	**VHS**
Normal	8.5-10.7	Normal	6.7-8.1
Normal to mild	11-12	Mild	8.2-8.5
Mild to moderate	12-13	Moderate	8.6-8.9
Moderate to severe	13-14	Severe	9-10
Very severe	>14	Very severe	>10

ECHOCARDIOGRAPHY

Echocardiography has become a very important tool for the diagnosis of canine and feline heart disease. It allows the production of a moving two-dimensional image of the heart and the interpretation of cardiac morphology, wall movement, valve function, and blood flow within the heart. Patients with heart disease are often referred to veterinary cardiologists for an echocardiographic examination. The following discussion is designed to explain how echocardiography is used to diagnose heart disease.

Each echocardiographic mode provides a unique glimpse at the structure and function of the heart. M-mode echocardiography is used primarily to measure the size of structures in the heart. It can also be used to measure certain systolic time intervals. Two-dimensional echocardiography allows the size and relationship of structures that lie in the same plane to be examined; it can also be used to measure the length and area of structures in the heart. Doppler echocardiography is used to detect turbulence and measure the velocity of blood flow. A relationship exists between the increase in velocity and the pressure gradient across an area of stenosis or leaking heart valve. Doppler echocardiography can be used to estimate the pressure in a particular region of the heart by using this relationship. These pressure estimates are useful in determining the severity of pulmonic and aortic stenosis, as well as pulmonary hypertension. The pressure gradient (PG) across the stenotic region or leaking valve can be calculated using the following equation:

$$PG = 4V^2$$

The pressure gradient (PG) (in millimeters of mercury) is equal to four times the velocity (V) (in meters per second) squared. The normal velocity across the pulmonic or aortic valves should be less than about 1.5 to 2 m/sec. Values greater than this indicate stenosis of the valve or increased volume of flow across the valve. If tricuspid or pulmonic insufficiency occurs without stenosis, then the peak velocity can be used to estimate pulmonary artery pressure. A peak velocity equal to or greater than 2.8 m/sec across the tricuspid valve or a peak velocity equal to or greater than 2.2 m/sec across the pulmonic valve is considered abnormal. Tables 17-7 and 17-8 show how the pressure gradient is used to determine the severity of semilunar valve stenosis and pulmonary hypertension.

The diameter of the left ventricular chamber measured during diastole (LVIDd) and systole (LVIDs), the thickness (measured during diastole) of the left ventricular septum and free wall, the diameter of the left atrium and aortic root, and the E point to septal separation (EPSS) are some of the most useful measurements that can be made using two-dimensional or M-mode echocardiography. The right ventricle is more difficult to image and measure. Because heart size is related to

TABLE 17-7	How Echocardiographic Flow Velocity and Pressure Gradient Are Used to Determine the Severity of Semilunar Valve Stenosis	
SEVERITY OF STENOSIS	**PRESSURE GRADIENT**	**FORWARD VELOCITY**
Mild stenosis	20-49 mm Hg	2.25-3.5 m/sec
Moderate stenosis	50-80 mm Hg	3.5-4.5 m/sec
Severe stenosis	>80 mm Hg	>4.5 m/sec

TABLE 17-8	How the Pressure Gradient Is Used to Determine the Severity of Pulmonary Hypertension	
SEVERITY OF PULMONARY HYPERTENSION	**PRESSURE GRADIENT (RV TO RA)**	**VELOCITY OF TR BY ECHOCARDIOGRAPHY (RV TO RA)**
Mild	30-50 mm Hg	2.8-3.5 m/sec
Moderate	50-74 mm Hg	3.5-4.3 m/sec
Severe	≥75 mm Hg	≥4.3 m/sec

RA, Right atrium; *RV,* right ventricle; *TR,* tricuspid regurgitation.

body size, these measurements must be compared with values for dogs of the same weight or breed to determine whether or not the measurement is abnormal. Table 17-9 lists normal M-mode values for dogs and cats. Unlike the individual dimensions mentioned previously, the normal ranges of ratios of cardiac dimensions are the same for all dogs regardless of their size, with examples being fractional shortening and the ratio of left atrial diameter to the diameter of the aortic root.

Fractional shortening represents the change in diameter that occurs between diastole and systole: (LVIDd − LVIDs)/LVIDd. Fractional shortening is decreased in diseases characterized by reduced contractility, such as dilated cardiomyopathy. The average value for fractional shortening (FS) is 33%, but the normal range is quite expansive. This is because FS changes significantly with small changes in left ventricular (LV) dimensions. In addition, it is heavily influenced not only by contractility but also by preload and afterload. It must be interpreted cautiously and not used as the sole means of assessing contractility. Values less than 20% generally indicate myocardial failure and animals with values less than 15% have severe heart disease and often show signs of heart failure.

The left atrium/aortic root ratio is useful in determining the likelihood of congestive heart failure. Several echocardiographic techniques are used to measure left atrial size. Each technique has slightly different normal ranges. When the M-mode technique is used, the upper limit of normal in dogs is 1.3 and about 1.6 for cats. Animals begin to develop signs of left heart failure when the left atrial diameter is about one and a half to two times the size of the aorta, though this may not be the case for an acute process

TABLE 17-9	Normal M-Mode Measurements						
BODY WEIGHT (kg)	**LVIDd**	**LVIDs**	**LVWd**	**IVSd**	**Ao**	**LA**	**EPSS**
Dogs							
3	2.1	1.3	0.5	0.5	1.1	1.1	0.1
	1.8-2.6	1.0-1.8	0.4-0.8	0.4-0.8	0.9-1.4	0.9-1.4	
4	2.3	1.5	0.6	0.6	1.3	1.2	0.1
	1.9-2.8	1.1-1.9	0.4-0.8	0.4-0.8	1.0-1.5	1.0-1.6	
6	2.6	1.7	0.6	0.6	1.4	1.4	0.1
	3.1-2.2	1.2-2.2	0.4-0.9	0.4-0.9	1.2-1.8	1.1-1.8	
9	2.9	1.9	0.7	0.7	1.7	1.6	0.2
	2.4-3.5	1.4-2.5	0.5-1.0	0.5-1.0	1.3-2.0	1.3-2.1	
11	3.1	2.0	0.7	0.7	1.8	1.7	0.2
	2.6-3.7	1.5-2.7	0.5-1.0	0.5-1.1	1.4-2.2	1.3-2.2	
15	3.4	2.2	0.8	0.8	2	1.9	0.2
	2.8-4.1	1.7-3.0	0.5-1.1	0.6-1.1	1.6-2.4	1.6-2.5	
20	3.7	2.4	0.8	0.8	2.2	2.1	0.3
	3.1-4.5	1.8-3.2	0.6-1.2	0.6-1.2	1.7-2.7	1.7-2.7	
25	3.9	2.6	0.9	0.9	2.3	2.3	0.3
	3.3-4.8	2.0-3.5	0.6-1.3	0.6-1.3	1.9-2.9	1.8-2.9	
30	4.2	2.8	0.9	0.9	2.5	2.5	0.4
	3.5-5.0	2.1-3.7	0.6-1.3	0.7-1.3	2.0-3.1	1.9-3.1	
35	4.4	2.9	1.0	1.0	2.6	2.6	0.4
	3.6-5.3	2.2-3.9	0.7-1.4	0.7-1.4	2.1-3.2	2.0-3.3	
40	4.5	3.0	1.0	1.0	2.7	2.7	0.5
	3.8-5.5	2.3-4.0	0.7-1.4	0.7-1.4	2.2-3.4	2.1-3.5	
50	4.8	3.3	1.0	1.1	3.0	2.9	0.6
	4.0-5.8	2.4-4.8	0.7-1.5	0.7-1.5	2.4-3.6	2.3-3.7	
60	5.1	3.5	1.1	1.1	3.2	3.1	0.7
	4.2-6.2	2.6-4.6	0.7-1.6	0.8-1.6	2.5-3.9	2.4-4.0	
Cats							
	1.5	0.72	0.41	0.42	0.90	1.17	0.06
	1.1-1.9	0.42-1.02	0.27-0.55	0.28-0.56	0.62-1.18	0.83-1.51	

Data from Cornell CC, Kittleson MD, Della Torre P, et al: Allometric scaling of M-mode cardiac measurements in normal adult dogs, *J Vet Intern Med* 18(3):311-321, 2004; Kittleson MD, Kienle RD: *Small animal cardiovascular medicine*, St Louis, 1999, Mosby, p 104; Sisson DD et al: Plasma taurine concentrations and M-mode echocardiographic measures in healthy cats and in cats with dilated cardiomyopathy, *J Vet Intern Med* 5(4):232-238, 1991.

Ao, Aortic root; *EPSS*, E point septal separation; *IVSd*, thickness (measured during diastole) of the left ventricular septum; *LA*, left atrium; *LVIDd*, diameter of the left ventricular chamber measured during diastole; *LVIDs*, diameter of the left ventricular chamber measured during diastole and systole; *LVWd*, thickness (measured during diastole) of the left ventricular free wall.

where the atrium has not had the time to dilate (e.g., chordal rupture, infectious endocarditis). It should be emphasized that echocardiography alone cannot diagnose left-sided congestive heart failure, which is a radiographic diagnosis.

Despite its usefulness as a diagnostic technique, the results of an echocardiographic examination should be interpreted in conjunction with other diagnostic findings. Just as with most other diagnostic tests, an overlap is often seen between echocardiographic measurements of healthy animals and animals with heart disease.

> *TECHNICIAN NOTE*   The technician should remember that a measurement that falls within the normal range does not always eliminate the diagnosis of heart disease, and a value outside the normal range does not always confirm the diagnosis of heart disease.

The following are some examples of diseases causing LVIDd to increase:

- PDA
- Mitral regurgitation
- Dilated cardiomyopathy
- Aortic insufficiency

Examples of diseases causing the diameter of the right ventricle measured in diastole to increase include the following:

- Tricuspid regurgitation
- Heartworm disease

The following are some examples of diseases causing the left ventricular free wall or left ventricular septum to increase:

- Subaortic stenosis
- Hypertrophic cardiomyopathy
- Systemic hypertension and hyperthyroidism (primarily in cats)
- Hypovolemia (LVIDd should also be decreased)

Examples of diseases causing LVIDs to increase include the following:

- Dilated cardiomyopathy and other diseases that cause myocardial failure

Examples of diseases causing EPSS to increase include:

- Dilated cardiomyopathy and other diseases that cause myocardial failure

OVERVIEW OF CARDIAC PHYSIOLOGY AND PATHOPHYSIOLOGY

SYSTOLIC FUNCTION

The heart is a complex organ that contributes in many ways to maintaining homeostasis. Despite this complexity, the heart's main function, pumping blood, can be explained by looking at four determinants of systolic function. Three of the factors—preload, afterload, and contractility—determine how much blood is pumped with each beat of the heart (i.e., stroke volume). Multiplying stroke volume by the heart rate, the fourth factor, determines the volume of blood pumped in 1 minute (i.e., cardiac output).

PRELOAD

Preload is a measure of how much the ventricle is stretched at the end of diastole. Central venous pressure (CVP), pulmonary capillary wedge pressure, or the left ventricular end-diastolic diameter is commonly used to evaluate preload. Increasing preload is a mechanism by which the body responds to reduced cardiac output caused by heart disease. Initially small increases in ventricular filling pressure, caused by fluid retention and venoconstriction, can increase preload and return cardiac output to near normal levels. If the heart disease continues to progress, then increasing preload to improve cardiac output causes congestive failure.

AFTERLOAD

Afterload is the force against which the heart ejects. Increases in afterload make it harder for blood to leave the heart, causing a decrease in stroke volume. Systemic vascular resistance is an index sometimes used to evaluate afterload. The body is intolerant of hypotension; when blood pressure (BP) drops below normal, the body responds by vasoconstricting. Vasoconstriction improves BP, but it also tends to increase afterload and reduce cardiac output. Animals with poor myocardial function are very sensitive to changes in afterload; a small change in afterload can lead to a much greater change in cardiac output.

CONTRACTILITY

Contractility may refer to the contracting properties of individual cells or to the pump function of the heart as a whole, but in both cases independent of preload or afterload. Increases in contractility may occur when the amount of calcium in heart muscle cells is increased by chemicals produced by the body (such as epinephrine) or by drugs (such as digoxin or dobutamine). Contractility is more difficult to evaluate than the other determinants of systolic function; however, if preload and afterload remain constant, then changes in cardiac output and fractional shortening can be used to assess changes in contractility.

HEART RATE AND RHYTHM

Preload, afterload, and contractility determine stroke volume. The last determinant of systolic function is heart rate. Abnormal heart rhythms can alter the normal sequence and duration of atrial and ventricular contraction (dyssynergy). Changes in heart rate have much more of an effect on the duration of diastole than on the duration of systole. Increases in heart rate usually increase cardiac output. Very fast heart rates can reduce cardiac output by not allowing the ventricles to fill adequately during diastole. Bradycardia also reduces cardiac output. The heart normally maintains adequate cardiac output as the heart rate slows by taking advantage of the increase in preload caused by the extra time spent in diastole. At some point, however, the heart is unable to accept more blood, and cardiac output decreases.

DIASTOLIC FUNCTION

During diastole the ventricle relaxes and fills with blood. Diseases that cause systolic dysfunction often interfere with relaxation and filling, but heart failure caused by diastolic dysfunction can occur even when systolic function is normal. Diastolic dysfunction probably leads to heart failure in many of the cardiac diseases that affect cats, such as hypertrophic cardiomyopathy, hyperthyroidism, and restrictive cardiomyopathy. These diseases can cause the ventricle to become so noncompliant that the filling pressure required to produce a normal end-diastolic volume may be high enough to cause signs of congestive heart failure.

HEART FAILURE

Most forms of heart disease cause heart failure. Heart failure can be defined as the inability of the heart to supply adequate blood flow to meet the metabolic needs of the body or to provide adequate blood flow only by excessive increases in ventricular filling pressure. This definition allows heart failure to exist in three forms: (1) forward or low-output failure, when perfusion is inadequate; (2) congestive failure, when filling pressures are excessive; or (3) a combination of forward and congestive failure. Heart failure takes different forms and varies in severity. One commonly used scale for classifying the severity of heart disease in animals is presented in Box 17-2. Animals with mild failure can tolerate some exercise without showing signs of failure, and severely affected animals show signs of failure while at rest. Because most pets are not required to exercise vigorously, many owners do not recognize heart failure until it affects everyday activities.

LOW-OUTPUT OR FORWARD FAILURE

Low-output failure occurs when the heart cannot pump enough oxygenated blood to the tissues. Severe low-output failure, especially when accompanied by hypotension, is called *cardiogenic shock*. A healthy dog that weighs 30 kg has a cardiac output of about 4 L/min at rest, with each liter of blood containing 200 ml of oxygen (O_2). The dog's tissues consume 25% of the O_2 in the blood. If heart disease forces the dog's cardiac output to drop, then the volume of O_2 delivered to the tissues will also drop. Because O_2 consumption has not changed, the body must somehow compensate if normal function is to be maintained. If the change in cardiac output is not too severe, then the body can compensate by extracting more O_2 from the blood. The limit to this form of compensation is usually reached when cardiac output drops to 2 L/min. Delivery of O_2 has now been cut in half, and the tissues consume 50% of the O_2 in the blood. When blood flow drops below this limit, cardiac

BOX 17-2	ISACHC (International Small Animal Cardiac Health Council) System of Heart Failure Classification

Class I—Asymptomatic patient. Signs of heart disease (e.g., murmur, arrhythmia, cardiomegaly) but no signs of failure (free of clinical signs). Subdivided into Ia (no cardiomegaly) and Ib (cardiomegaly present).

Class II—Mild to moderate heart failure. Signs of heart failure at rest or with mild exercise.

Class III—Advanced heart failure. Signs of heart failure immediately obvious. Subdivided into IIIa (home care possible) and IIIb (hospitalization necessary).

output may not be adequate to meet the metabolic needs of the body, resulting in inadequate O_2 delivery and low-output failure. Exercise increases the body's demand for O_2. If the heart cannot pump enough blood to supply the increased demand, then the animal's ability to exercise will be reduced.

CONGESTIVE OR BACKWARD FAILURE

Congestive heart failure (CHF) occurs when increased pulmonary or systemic venous pressure causes fluid to leak from the capillary beds and accumulate in tissue (edema) or in body cavities (effusions). CHF is generally categorized as right or left heart failure, according to whether systemic or pulmonary venous pressure, respectively, is increased. Normally the pressure in the venous system is low, about 0 to 3 mm Hg in the right atrium and 2 to 5 mm Hg in the left atrium. Right heart failure is usually evident when right atrial pressure reaches 10 to 12 mm Hg, resulting in pleural effusion or ascites. Left heart failure generally occurs when left atrial pressure exceeds 20 to 25 mm Hg, resulting in pulmonary edema. When a disease increases venous pressure equally on both sides of the heart, as in pericardial effusion, right heart failure develops first. This is because signs of congestive failure occur at lower pressure on the right side.

RELATIONSHIP BETWEEN HEMODYNAMIC MEASUREMENTS AND CLINICAL SIGNS OF HEART FAILURE

Cardiac output and right atrial or left atrial pressure indicate whether heart function is adequate or whether heart failure exists. Patients who are not in failure should have a cardiac output that is greater than 2 L/min/m^2 and right and left atrial pressures less than 5 and 12 mm Hg, respectively. Forward failure occurs if the patient's cardiac output is less than 2 L/min/m^2 at rest. Congestive failure should be present if the right atrial pressure exceeds 10 mm Hg or the left atrial pressure exceeds about 20 mm Hg. A patient suffering from both forward and congestive failure would be expected to have a cardiac output of less than 2 L/min/m^2 at rest and a left or right atrial pressure greater than 10 or 20 mm Hg, respectively. Patients with arteriovenous fistulae or hyperthyroidism may have CHF and higher than normal cardiac output at rest. This type of heart failure is known as *high-output failure*. Measuring cardiac output or left atrial pressure rarely is necessary (or possible in most practices) to diagnose heart failure. The physical examination, chest radiographs, and echocardiography generally provide enough information to make an accurate diagnosis of the type of heart failure and its cause.

IDENTIFYING PATIENTS WHO MAY HAVE HEART FAILURE

CLIENT COMPLAINTS

In emergency practice, coughing, dyspnea, tachypnea, abdominal distention, syncope, weakness, and collapse are the most common client complaints associated with heart failure. Coughing is much more common in dogs with heart disease than in cats. Cats typically present with tachypnea in the presence or absence of dyspnea, often manifesting as open-mouth breathing.

PHYSICAL FINDINGS

Systolic murmurs greater than 3 on a scale of 1 to 6, precordial thrills, diastolic murmurs, and diastolic gallop sounds are generally reliable signs of heart disease. The arterial pulse tends to be weak or normal in most types of heart disease, but animals with PDA or aortic insufficiency may have a prominent or bounding pulse. Irregular pulses, pulse deficits, and changes in the quality of the heart sounds may be present in animals with cardiac arrhythmias. Animals in left heart failure may show signs of coughing, dyspnea, tachypnea, exercise intolerance, cyanosis, and weakness. Animals with right heart failure may show signs of venous distention, hepatomegaly, ascites, tachypnea or dyspnea (if pleural effusion is present), exercise intolerance, or weakness. Box 17-3 lists diseases that can cause heart failure.

DIAGNOSTIC IMAGING AND THE ELECTROCARDIOGRAM

Thoracic radiographs are critical to the diagnosis of left-sided heart failure. They show an increase in the size of the pulmonary veins and increased opacity of the lungs in patients with left heart failure. In most cases, signs of left atrial enlargement are seen. Echocardiography is useful both to support the diagnosis and to identify the underlying cause of heart failure. Left atrial enlargement is the most reliable supporting feature on echocardiography for the diagnosis of left heart failure. An enlarged vena cava, right heart enlargement, and a globoid heart suggestive of pericardial effusion are radiographic signs associated with right heart failure. The appearance of the pulmonary arteries (dilated and tortuous) may suggest heartworm disease in some dogs with right heart failure. Echocardiography can again support a diagnosis of right heart failure and provide an underlying cause.

BOX 17-3	Common Causes of Heart Failure

Left Heart Failure in Dogs
Chronic degenerative mitral valvular disease (mitral regurgitation)
Dilated cardiomyopathy
Patent ductus arteriosus (PDA)
Infective endocarditis
Subaortic stenosis (usually with concomitant mitral dysplasia)

Right Heart Failure in Dogs
Pericardial disease
Tricuspid regurgitation (degenerative or dysplasia)
Pulmonic stenosis
Heartworm disease (may be the most common cause of right heart failure in areas with high infection rates)

Generalized (Biventricular) Heart Failure in Dogs
Dilated cardiomyopathy
Some dogs with severe left heart failure

Heart Failure in Cats
Hypertrophic cardiomyopathy
Restrictive cardiomyopathy
Dilated cardiomyopathy
Feline unclassified cardiomyopathy
Cardiomyopathy secondary to hyperthyroidism

The ECG may provide evidence of enlargement of the atria or ventricles; however, these criteria are neither sensitive nor specific, particularly the atrial enlargement criteria. **Cardiac arrhythmias** are often seen in conjunction with the severe heart diseases that cause heart failure. Electrical alternans (alternating R-wave amplitude) and low-amplitude ECG complexes are often seen in patients with large-volume pericardial effusions. Techniques used for routine measurements of the ECG are shown in Figure 17-3, *A-B*.

EMERGENCY TREATMENT OF CONGESTIVE HEART FAILURE

Pulmonary edema, pleural effusion, and severe ascites are the most common emergencies caused by congestive heart failure (CHF). Patients with pleural effusion or ascites can be treated very effectively for the short term by simply removing fluid from the thorax or the abdomen by centesis. Care should be taken to prevent stress in patients that are hypoxic or dyspneic because of their effusions. These effusions will return unless proper medical treatment is started to reduce venous pressure.

Treatment of pulmonary edema consists of the use of several different therapies that reduce pulmonary venous pressure while providing adequate O_2 delivery. O_2 therapy maximizes the O_2 content of arterial blood, which provides some increase in O_2 delivery. Avoiding the use of physical restraint, providing a calm quiet environment, and using sedatives minimizes O_2 consumption and reduces the work of the heart. Furosemide and venodilating drugs decrease pulmonary venous pressure by eliminating fluid from the body and by dilating capacitance

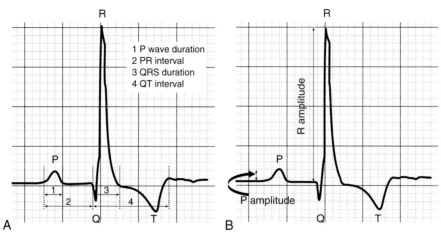

FIGURE 17-3, A-B Methods for measuring ECG.

vessels (large veins). Arterial dilators reduce the regurgitant fraction in patients with mitral regurgitation and improve cardiac output by decreasing afterload. Positive inotropic drugs improve contractility and cardiac output in patients who have low-output failure in addition to congestive failure attributable to systolic dysfunction. For cases of severe CHF complicated by ongoing hypoxemia and increased work of breathing despite the above-mentioned therapies, positive pressure ventilation can be used to eliminate the work of breathing and improve oxygenation. Table 17-10 lists the goals of therapy for pulmonary edema and Table 17-11 lists the therapies used to achieve them.

DIURETIC THERAPY

Water and salt retention is an important compensatory mechanism in heart failure. Diuretics are drugs that act on the kidneys to promote the elimination of water and salt. Furosemide is a potent diuretic that can be used to eliminate fluid from the body quickly. Furosemide's ability to decrease pulmonary venous pressure rapidly makes it one of the most effective emergency treatments for life-threatening pulmonary edema caused by CHF. Overzealous administration of furosemide can cause decreased cardiac output and azotemia, as well as electrolyte abnormalities. It becomes a delicate balance between the lung function and kidney function when determining continued treatment with a diuretic.

OXYGEN THERAPY

CHF often causes hypoxia and hypoventilation because of hydrothorax and pulmonary edema. O_2 therapy can improve oxygenation and reduce the work of breathing. However, the technician should remember that O_2 therapy may only cause a small increase in the O_2 content of the blood.

TECHNICIAN NOTE O_2 therapy can lead to death if the method of administering O_2 increases patient stress or causes the patient to struggle.

Many methods of O_2 administration are available; if one method does not work, then the technician should try another. The success of therapy is measured by improved patient comfort and oxygenation, not by whether the patient has been forced to breathe increased concentrations of O_2.

Almost every practice has the equipment needed to administer O_2 by face mask. A tight-fitting face mask

TABLE 17-10	Goals in Emergency Heart Failure Treatment
GOAL	**SOLUTION**
Reduce oxygen (O_2) consumption, minimize stress	No physical restraint, calm quiet environment, sedatives
Increase O_2 content of blood	O_2 therapy
Decrease venous pressure	Diuretics, venodilators
Decrease regurgitant fraction, decrease afterload	Arterial dilators
Improve contractility and cardiac output	Positive inotropic drugs
Eliminate the work of breathing, improve oxygenation	Positive pressure ventilation
Improve the ability to identify problems and target therapy	Hemodynamic, arterial, and central venous blood gas monitoring

TABLE 17-11	Drugs Used to Treat Heart Failure
Drugs Used to Minimize Stress	
Butorphanol	0.2 mg/kg SQ, IM in dogs 0.2-0.4 mg/kg SQ, IM in cats
Oxymorphone	0.05 mg/kg SQ, IM in dogs and cats
Acepromazine	0.01-0.02 mg/kg SQ, IM in dogs or cats
Drugs Used to Decrease Venous Pressure or Preload	
Furosemide	2-5 mg/kg IM, IV, SQ in dogs 1-2 mg/kg IM, IV, SQ in cats
Nitroglycerin	4-15 mg topically in dogs 2-4 mg topically in cats
Drugs Used to Decrease Afterload	
Amlodipine	0.05-0.2 mg/kg PO, SID in dogs
Hydralazine	0.5-3 mg/kg PO, bid in dogs
Sodium nitroprusside	0.5-10 mcg/kg/min IV
Drugs Used to Increase Contractility	
Dobutamine	2-10 mcg/kg/min IV
Dopamine	2-10 mcg/kg/min IV
Pimobendan	0.25 mg/kg PO bid

bid, Twice daily; *IM*, intramuscularly; *PO*, orally; *SID*, once daily; *SQ*, subcutaneously.

with adequate O_2 flow can deliver 100% O_2. Unfortunately, face masks are poorly accepted by most patients and cannot be used for long periods of time.

Nasal insufflation can be used to deliver high concentrations of O_2 for long periods of time. The placement of nasal catheters has been discussed thoroughly in Chapter 7: Oxygen Therapy Techniques.

Most patients tolerate O_2 cages well, but they require high O_2 flow rates and do not allow hands-on monitoring of the patient. A well-designed oxygen cage should remove exhaled carbon dioxide and lower the temperature in the cage when necessary.

VASODILATOR THERAPY

Vasodilating drugs are effective in treating both congestive and low-output heart failure. Venodilating drugs (e.g., nitroglycerin) expand the capacity of the circulatory system by dilating veins, thereby reducing preload and venous pressure. Venodilation can reduce congestion but will not improve cardiac output. Arterial vasodilators (e.g., amlodipine, hydralazine) decrease systemic vascular resistance, which reduces afterload, improves cardiac output, reduces the regurgitant fraction in animals with valvular disease, and decreases the work of the heart. The main disadvantage of arterial vasodilators is that they may lower BP. Selecting a vasodilator that acts on veins, aterioles, or a combination of the two is possible. Drugs that block the enzyme that converts angiotensin I to angiotensin II (angiotensin-converting enzyme inhibitors) are the most commonly used vasodilators. They also benefit the patient by decreasing the sodium and water retention seen in heart failure by decreasing the plasma concentration of aldosterone. However, these drugs do not take effect quickly enough to be useful in emergency heart failure treatment. Nitroprusside is a potent intravenous arterial and venous dilator that may be used in emergent CHF cases requiring rapid and aggressive preload and afterload reduction.

POSITIVE INOTROPIC THERAPY

Positive inotropic drugs increase stroke volume by increasing contractility, thereby improving cardiac output and BP. Some intravenous positive inotropes are intended for use for only short periods of time. Sympathomimetic drugs such as dopamine and dobutamine lose their effectiveness over time, because their use causes a decrease in the number of available beta receptors. In addition, some positive inotropes can cause tachycardia and arrhythmias, or increase afterload (e.g., dopamine at higher doses).

Sympathomimetic drugs mimic the effect of stimulating the sympathetic nervous system and work by stimulating adrenergic receptors on the cells of the heart and blood vessels. Dopamine and dobutamine are the sympathomimetic drugs used most often in the treatment of heart failure. Dobutamine increases contractility without causing a significant increase in heart rate or vascular resistance. This combination of properties makes dobutamine a good choice for treating heart failure in patients with myocardial failure or mitral regurgitation. Dopamine is useful in situations in which poor contractility is associated with hypotension.

An orally administered positive inotrope that is commonly used in CHF due to mitral valve disease or dilated cardiomyopathy (DCM) is pimobendan. It also has arterial vasodilating properties.

MONITORING THERAPY FOR HEART FAILURE

Animals suffering from dyspnea caused by heart failure appear anxious and are often unwilling to sit or lay down.

> **TECHNICIAN NOTE** Affected animals often assume a characteristic posture, referred to as "orthopnea," with the feet spread apart, the elbows abducted, and the head and neck extended.

Tachypnea is usually evident with respiratory rates often greater than 40 breaths per minute. If therapy has been effective in treating pleural effusion or pulmonary edema, then the patient's attitude should improve, the respiratory rate should decrease, mucous membrane color should improve, and the animal may be able to lie down or sleep. Improvement of pulmonary edema on chest radiographs usually takes longer than improvement of clinical signs.

MONITORING VASODILATOR THERAPY

Vasodilator therapy should improve cardiac output or improve pulmonary edema. Improved cardiac output may be monitored by looking for signs of increased perfusion such as warming of the extremities, increased venous O_2 tension, and a decreased blood lactate concentration. Whenever arteriolar vasodilating drugs are used, BP should be monitored to maintain mean BP around 70 mm Hg. Venodilating drugs reduce venous pressure and should therefore decrease central venous and pulmonary capillary wedge pressures.

MONITORING POSITIVE INOTROPIC THERAPY

Positive inotropic therapy should produce signs of improved cardiac output. Decreases in blood lactate concentration, increased venous O_2 tension, or improvements in measured cardiac output provide more objective assessments of therapy. In addition to increasing contractility, positive inotropic agents can cause vasoconstriction, vasodilation, increased heart rate, or cardiac arrhythmias. Vasoconstriction generally causes an increase in CVP, pulmonary capillary wedge pressure, and arterial blood pressure. Vasodilation may cause a decrease in CVP, pulmonary capillary wedge pressure, or arterial blood pressure depending on the increase in cardiac output. The ECG is helpful in detecting cardiac arrhythmias or sinus tachycardia. Safe, effective use of sympathomimetic drugs requires monitoring of at least the ECG and BP and assessment of perfusion.

MONITORING DIURETIC THERAPY

Diuretic therapy should quickly produce an increase in urine production, particularly with intravenous furosemide. This elimination of fluid should result in a decreased respiratory rate and improved oxygenation and ventilation. Weighing the patient and palpating the urinary bladder to determine its size may be useful for establishing a baseline before diuretic therapy is started. The loss of volume can be estimated by measuring the volume of urine, by measuring the increase in weight caused by urine absorbed in a disposable diaper, or by noting the patient's weight loss during treatment. In some cases, a urinary catheter may be indicated and provide more exact urine output values. Electrolyte and acid-base disturbances can be caused by diuretic therapy, so these values should be monitored. The loss of preload may cause a decrease in cardiac output. This may result in prerenal azotemia or signs of low-output failure.

CARDIAC ARRHYTHMIAS

CLIENT COMPLAINTS

Cardiac arrhythmias should be considered whenever an animal experiences syncope, weakness, or collapse.

BOX 17-4	Emergencies in Which Cardiac Arrhythmias Are Common

Trauma
Splenic tumors
Gastric dilatation volvulus
Canine dilated cardiomyopathy
Urethral obstruction in cats
Heat-induced illness
Feline cardiomyopathies

Some clients may detect tachycardia, bradycardia, or an irregular heart rhythm. Cardiac arrhythmias may be a primary cardiac abnormality or secondary to structural cardiac disease or extracardiac disease. Box 17-4 lists several diseases that are common in emergency medicine and have a high incidence of cardiac arrhythmias.

PHYSICAL FINDINGS

An ECG should be recorded to determine if a cardiac arrhythmia is present whenever changes in the character of heart sounds, tachycardia, bradycardia, irregular heart rhythm, pulse deficits, or changes in arterial or jugular pulses are present.

DIAGNOSTIC IMAGING AND THE ELECTROCARDIOGRAM

The ECG is the gold standard for the diagnosis of cardiac arrhythmias. The main use of radiographs and echocardiography is to provide evidence of a disease that may be the underlying cause of the arrhythmia. The technician may be responsible for applying an ambulatory ECG, known as a Holter system (Figure 17-4), to the patient in order to allow continuous ECG recording over a 24 (or more) hour period. This provides a better representation of the patient's electrical activity over a longer period of time, rather than a snapshot.

MEDICAL TREATMENT OF CARDIAC ARRHYTHMIAS

The efficacy of antiarrhythmic therapy has not been determined in most forms of heart disease found in dogs and cats. In humans the use of certain antiarrhythmic drugs was found to decrease survival in patients with certain forms of heart disease. The following five principles

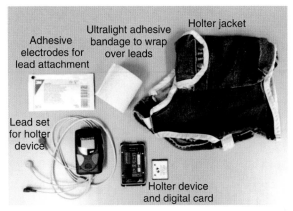

Adhesive electrodes for lead attachment

Ultralight adhesive bandage to wrap over leads

Holter jacket

Lead set for holter device

Holter device and digital card

FIGURE 17-4 Holter system.

should be considered before deciding whether to use antiarrhythmic drugs to treat an arrhythmia:

1. Treating the primary disease or predisposing factors (e.g., hypovolemia, electrolyte disturbances, pain) may eliminate the arrhythmia.
2. Generally, arrhythmias that cause hypotension should be treated.
3. Prolonged tachycardia can damage the heart, even when BP and cardiac output are adequate.
4. The arrhythmia should be treated if it has the risk of progressing to a more severe arrhythmia or cardiac arrest. Multiform ventricular premature contractions, R-on-T phenomenon, more than 20 to 30 ventricular premature contractions per minute, ventricular flutter, and ventricular tachycardia greater than 160 beats per minute are generally considered to be rhythms that have the potential to become more dangerous.
5. When the decision is made to treat an arrhythmia, the veterinarian will select an antiarrhythmic drug based on its ability to eliminate the arrhythmia balanced against the risk of proarrhythmic effects, hypotension, decreased contractility, altered atrioventricular conduction, and interactions with other drugs.

ROLE OF ELECTROLYTES AND DRUG INTERACTIONS IN ANTIARRHYTHMIC THERAPY

Electrolyte and acid-base abnormalities can cause arrhythmias, increase their severity, and influence the effect of antiarrhythmic drugs. Hyperkalemia is one of the more common and easily recognized electrolyte abnormalities

that cause arrhythmias. Hyperkalemia may cause characteristic changes on the ECG: low-amplitude or absent P waves, prolongation of the QRS complexes, increased amplitude of the T wave, and most commonly bradycardia.

Hypomagnesemia has been associated with ventricular arrhythmias, and magnesium administration may be useful as a treatment for some forms of ventricular tachycardia. Hypokalemia, hypomagnesemia, and hypercalcemia can increase the risk of toxicity in patients on digoxin therapy. Restoration of these electrolytes to appropriate levels plays an important role in treating digoxin toxicity. Lidocaine is most effective in regions of the heart in which the pH is decreased and potassium levels are increased. A lack of efficacy of lidocaine therapy may be a result of hypokalemia. Some of the toxic effect of the accidental ingestion or overdose of calcium-blocking drugs (e.g., diltiazem) can be treated by administration of calcium chloride or calcium gluconate.

Interaction between antiarrhythmic drugs is common. In some cases the interaction is additive or synergistic; in others it may be antagonistic. Synergistic or additive interaction is usually beneficial when it applies to antiarrhythmic effects, but adverse effects may also be synergistic. Both calcium-blocking drugs and beta-blocking drugs are effective in the treatment of supraventricular arrhythmias; however, when they are combined the risk of adverse effects such as hypotension, worsening CHF, and bradycardia is increased.

TREATMENT OF VENTRICULAR TACHYCARDIA

Lidocaine and procainamide are the drugs most often used in the emergency treatment of ventricular arrhythmias in the dog. Lidocaine and beta-blockers such as propranolol or esmolol are the drugs used most often in treating cats. Lidocaine is considered the drug of choice for treating ventricular tachycardia in the dog. Lidocaine has little effect on myocardial function, resulting in minimal effect on BP and cardiac output. Adverse reactions such as depression, twitching, or seizures are treated by discontinuation of the drug and administration of diazepam for the latter. Rapid IV administration of procainamide can cause hypotension and decreased cardiac output. Beta-blocking drugs can exacerbate heart failure (because they are negatively inotropic in the short term) and cause bradycardia and bronchospasm. Esmolol has an extremely short duration of action, and any

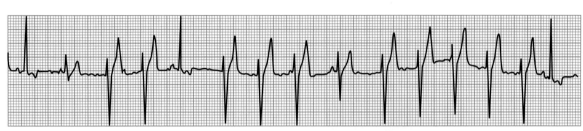

FIGURE 17-5 Accelerated idioventricular rhythm.

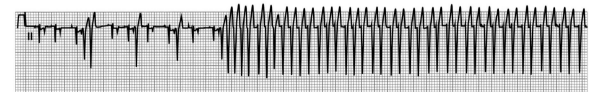

FIGURE 17-6 Ventricular tachycardia, canine. 12.5 mm/sec; 5 mm/mV.

adverse reaction caused by the drug should stop soon after the drug is discontinued. Ventricular tachycardia that causes cardiac arrest should be treated like ventricular fibrillation.

Accelerated idioventricular rhythm is a unifocal ventricular rhythm with a rate that falls within the range of normal sinus rhythm and is sometimes mistaken for ventricular tachycardia. Accelerated idioventricular rhythm rarely causes any hemodynamic dysfunction, is usually benign, and is commonly associated with many diseases. This rhythm probably has a different cause than ventricular tachycardia and usually does not respond to lidocaine treatment. Usually the rhythm disappears when the underlying disease is controlled (Figures 17-5 and 17-6, Table 17-12).

TREATMENT OF ATRIAL FIBRILLATION

Reestablishing normal sinus rhythm in patients with long-standing atrial fibrillation, particularly atrial fibrillation coexisting with structural heart disease, may be unsuccessful or at the very least short-lived. Most often, therapy consists of using a calcium channel blocker such as diltiazem to slow the ventricular rate and improve cardiac function. A constant rate infusion may be used initially to slow the heart rate, followed by oral therapy after weaning from intravenous treatment. Animals that have recently developed atrial fibrillation and do not have significant structural heart disease are the best candidates for conversion to normal sinus rhythm, which is most successfully done by electrical

TABLE 17-12	Drugs Used to Treat Ventricular Arrhythmias
Lidocaine	2-4 mg/kg IV over 1-3 min (max 4 boluses) followed by 40-100 mcg/kg/min IV for dogs or 0.5 mg/kg IV *slowly* for cats
Procainamide	5-15 mg/kg IV *slowly* followed by 25-50 mcg/kg/min IV for dogs
Esmolol	0.05-0.5 mg/kg IV, 50-200 mcg/kg/min IV CRI for dogs and cats
Propranolol	0.01-0.1 mg/kg IV slowly titrated to effect for dogs and cats

cardioversion under general anesthesia. Defibrillators using monophasic waveforms may achieve cardioversion using shocks in the 1 to 5 J/kg range. Biphasic defibrillators are potentially more effective and use less energy (Figure 17-7).

TREATMENT OF SUPRAVENTRICULAR TACHYCARDIA

Beta-blocking drugs, such as esmolol or propranolol, or calcium channel–blocking drugs, such as diltiazem, are the most frequently used therapies for supraventricular tachyarrhythmias (Figure 17-8). If drug therapy is not effective, then nonpharmacologic therapies may be tried. Electrical cardioversion and mechanical methods (e.g., precordial thump) may be effective, and vagal maneuvers (e.g., ocular pressure, carotid sinus massage) are sometimes effective (Table 17-13).

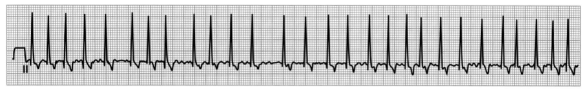

FIGURE 17-7 Atrial fibrillation, canine. 25 mm/sec; 5 mm/mV.

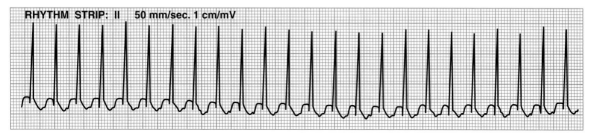

FIGURE 17-8 Supraventricular tachycardia, canine. 50 mm/sec; 10 mm/mV.

TREATMENT OF BRADYARRHYTHMIAS

Sinus bradycardia, sinus arrest, and second-degree atrioventricular block often respond to treatment with anticholinergic drugs like atropine or glycopyrrolate. Anticholinergic drugs are usually ineffective in treating third-degree atrioventricular block, but sympathomimetic drugs like isoproterenol, epinephrine, or dopamine may be tried to increase the ventricular rate to an acceptable level. Drug therapy may be ineffective or only temporarily effective in treating the bradycardia associated with sick sinus syndrome (Figure 17-9). Anticholinergic and sympathomimetic drugs may worsen the tachyarrhythmias in patients with bradycardia-tachycardia syndrome. Pacemaker implantation is the best long-term therapy for most patients with bradyarrhythmias (Table 17-14).

TREATMENT OF HYPERKALEMIA

Hyperkalemia can be treated by giving drugs that cause potassium to move from the vascular space to the intracellular space, such as bicarbonate or insulin, or by giving calcium, which antagonizes the effect of potassium on the heart. Definitive treatment for hyperkalemia should be started as soon as possible, because the effect of calcium, bicarbonate, or insulin therapy is short-lived. To prevent hypoglycemia, glucose must always be given when insulin is used to treat hyperkalemia (Figure 17-10, Table 17-15).

MONITORING TREATMENT OF CARDIAC ARRHYTHMIAS

Continuous ECG monitoring increases the safety and effectiveness of antiarrhythmic therapy. Arterial BP

TABLE 17-13	Drugs Used to Treat Supraventricular Arrhythmias
Propranolol	0.01-0.1 mg/kg IV slowly titrated to effect for dogs and cats
Esmolol	0.05-0.5 mg/kg IV, 50-200 mcg/kg/min IV CRI for dogs
Diltiazem	0.05-0.2 mg/kg IV slow, titrated to effect, followed by 1-5 mcg/kg/min IV CRI for dogs and cats

and clinical signs of perfusion should be monitored to determine whether antiarrhythmic therapy has improved cardiac function. Changes in the P-R interval, QRS duration, and Q-T interval on the ECG may be important signs of toxicity for some antiarrhythmic drugs. Vomiting, twitching, seizures, and syncope are a few of the physical signs that can be associated with toxicity from antiarrhythmic drugs. Levels of electrolytes and glucose should be monitored in patients being treated for hyperkalemia.

PACEMAKER THERAPY

A permanent implantable pacemaker can be used to treat a variety of bradyarrhythmias and restore near-normal quality of life to patients. Temporary pacing is used to treat bradyarrhythmias before or during permanent pacemaker implantation. Several modes of temporary pacing are available. Specific types of equipment are required for each mode of pacing, and each technique has advantages and disadvantages. Transvenous

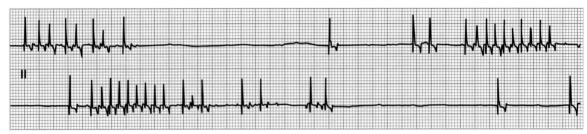

FIGURE 17-9 Sick sinus syndrome. 25 mm/sec; 10 mm/mV.

TABLE 17-14	Drugs Used to Treat Bradyarrhythmias
Atropine	0.01-0.04 mg/kg IV, IM, SQ for dogs and cats
Glycopyrrolate	0.005-0.01 mg/kg IV, IM, SQ for dogs and cats
Dopamine	2-10 mcg/kg/min IV for dogs and cats
Epinephrine	0.03-0.15 mcg/kg/min IV for dogs and cats

IM, Intramuscularly; *IV,* intravenously; *SQ,* subcutaneously.

and transcutaneous techniques are the most safe, most commonly used, and most reliable methods (although transesophageal and transmyocardial techniques are possible). One advantage of transvenous pacing is the ability to insert the lead and use the pacemaker in a conscious animal. A transvenous pacing lead (Figure 17-11) can be inserted into the right ventricle via a percutaneous introducer placed in the jugular vein or the lateral saphenous vein. Transcutaneous pacing has advantages when a patient requires immediate treatment for a life-threatening bradyarrhythmia, because pacing can be started quickly, without the need for vascular access. Adhesive pacing electrodes are attached to the left and right sides of the chest over the heart (Figure 17-12). A disadvantage of transcutaneous pacing is the need to use more energy, which increases discomfort and muscle stimulation, rendering it difficult or impossible to use in a conscious animal. The electrical stimulus applied to the muscles of the chest causes movement, which can interfere with surgery. Esophageal pacing is not commonly used in dogs or cats, but it has potential advantages that could be useful in certain situations. Inserting a transesophageal pacing electrode in the esophagus is simple, and because the electrode is close to the heart, pacing can be achieved with less energy than a transcutaneous electrode. However, only atrial pacing is likely to be achieved via this method, rendering it unsuitable

for arteriovenous (AV) block. The clinician performs transmyocardial pacing by inserting a special pacing lead through the thoracic wall, and then the ventricular wall using an introducing needle. Although the technique is reliable and can be performed quickly, the risk of injury to the heart makes its use rare.

PRECORDIAL THUMPS IN THE TREATMENT OF ARRHYTHMIAS

The precordial thump is a controversial technique. Some studies have shown that the precordial thump can produce a perfusing rhythm in some patients, whereas other studies show deterioration in the rhythm. When synchronized electrical cardioversion, defibrillation, and temporary pacing are available, they should be used; they are consistent, reliable, and controllable. Situations occur in which drugs are not effective, electrical pacing or a defibrillator is not available, and a precordial thump may be life-saving. A precordial thump is administered by striking the chest wall over the heart with the side of the fist. However, precordial thumps can injure a patient from the force of the blow or cause ventricular fibrillation if the thump occurs during the vulnerable period on the ECG (i.e., R-on-T phenomenon). Precordial thumps are often effective in converting supraventricular tachycardia into sinus rhythm and are also effective in treating certain bradyarrhythmias.

HEARTWORM DISEASE

CAVAL SYNDROME

Caval syndrome is a complication of heartworm disease that can occur in both dogs and cats. Caval syndrome occurs when large numbers of heartworms enter the right atrium and entwine themselves in the tricuspid valve apparatus, causing acute and severe tricuspid regurgitation. The heart is not the only organ affected.

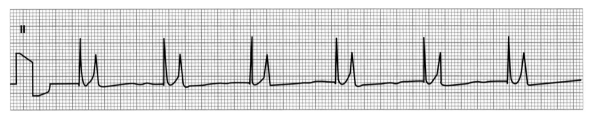

FIGURE 17-10 Hyperkalemia. 12.5 mm/sec; 5 mm/mV

TABLE 17-15	Drugs Used to Treat Hyperkalemia
Calcium gluconate 10%	0.5-1 ml/kg given over 15 min for dogs and cats
Sodium bicarbonate	0.5-2 mEq/kg IV given over 20 min for dogs and cats
Regular insulin	0.1-0.25 U/kg IV followed by 1-2 g/U glucose to prevent hypoglycemia for dogs and cats

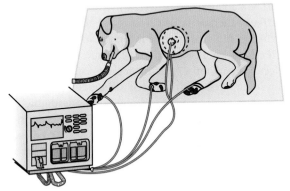

FIGURE 17-12 Transcutaneous pacing.

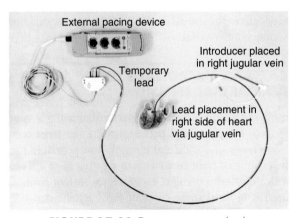

FIGURE 17-11 Transvenous pacing lead.

Hemolysis occurs when red blood cells shear as they are forced through the entangled worms. This also causes hemoglobinuria.

Analysis of the complete blood count and serum chemistry in dogs with caval syndrome may indicate liver and renal dysfunction and signs of disseminated intravascular coagulation.

CLIENT COMPLAINTS

Owners of dogs with caval syndrome typically notice anorexia, weakness, and depression. Some owners may complain that the animal has dark brown urine (hemoglobinuria), dyspnea, or cough. Many animals with caval syndrome will arrive at the clinic in a state of shock.

PHYSICAL FINDINGS

Pale mucous membranes, prolonged capillary refill time, weak pulses, distended jugular veins, ascites, icterus, and dyspnea may be identified on a physical examination. Auscultation of the chest may reveal a systolic murmur, split second heart sound, or a gallop sound.

DIAGNOSTIC IMAGING AND THE ELECTROCARDIOGRAM

Thoracic radiographs will often show right heart enlargement and enlargement of the main pulmonary artery. Peripheral pulmonary arteries are often enlarged relative to the corresponding pulmonary veins. The pulmonary arteries may show other changes characteristic of heartworm disease, such as tortuosity, blunting, or uneven diameter. These radiographic signs are seen in both dogs and cats with heartworm disease, but they tend to be more subtle and difficult to interpret in cats. Using echocardiography, heartworms can be seen as parallel lines about 2 mm apart that look like "equal signs" or "railroad tracks" if heartworms are present in the right heart or main pulmonary artery. Doppler echocardiography may show evidence of pulmonary hypertension. The ECG may show cardiac arrhythmias or signs of right heart enlargement.

SURGICAL TREATMENT OF CAVAL SYNDROME

The presence of heartworms in the right atrium and vena cava is associated with high mortality. Patients with caval syndrome often arrive at the clinic in shock and must be stabilized before heartworm removal is attempted. Fluid therapy is usually needed to improve poor perfusion, but care must be taken to avoid exacerbating preexisting right heart failure. The anesthetic protocol selected should minimize further depression of the cardiovascular system. In severely debilitated patients the procedure can be performed with local anesthesia. For general anesthesia, the lowest possible concentration of inhalational anesthetic and 100% O_2 should be used, and positive pressure ventilation can be used to improve oxygenation and eliminate hypercapnia. The procedure is usually performed with the patient in lateral or dorsal recumbency. After the surgical site is prepared, an incision is made over the jugular vein and the vein is then isolated and tourniquets applied. An incision is made in the jugular vein and alligator forceps are inserted to remove worms, taking great care not to macerate worms or perforate the atrium or vena cava. This technique allows one or more worms to be removed from the right atrium and vena cava (Figure 17-13). Two-dimensional echocardiography can be used to visualize the heartworms and direct the forceps.

MONITORING

Even with treatment, mortality is high in caval syndrome. CVP monitoring is useful for managing fluid therapy and as a prognostic sign. CVP of 20 cm of water or greater is associated with a poor prognosis. Arterial BP, mucous membrane color, capillary refill time, extremity temperature, and urine production should be monitored to evaluate perfusion. Doppler echocardiography or a catheter can be used to determine pulmonary arterial pressure.

COMPLICATIONS OF ADULTICIDE THERAPY

Embolization of dead or dying worms after adulticide therapy is another emergency that can occur as a consequence of heartworm disease. Lethargy, cough, right heart failure, dyspnea, shock, and sudden death may

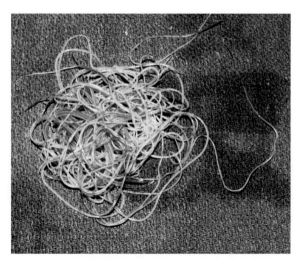

FIGURE 17-13 Heartworms.

occur 7 to 10 days after treatment to kill adult heartworms. Therapy with O_2 and prednisone (as well as cage rest and careful fluid therapy) is generally considered to be effective. The use of heparin, aspirin, and vasodilators is more controversial.

CARDIAC TAMPONADE AND PERICARDIAL EFFUSION

Fluid can accumulate in the pericardial sac for many reasons. Neoplasia and pericarditis are the most common causes of pericardial effusion and generally produce signs of right heart failure as a result of chronic pericardial effusion that accumulates slowly. Trauma, atrial tears, and some cases of right atrial hemangiosarcoma are the most common causes of acute cardiac tamponade. When fluid accumulates slowly in the heart, the pericardium stretches and the heart has time to compensate for the increased pressure on the heart. Effusions that develop slowly tend to produce large volumes of pericardial fluid and cause signs of right heart failure. When fluid accumulates quickly, no time exists for compensation (even a small volume of fluid in the pericardial sac can cause signs of shock). This condition is referred to as cardiac tamponade.

CLIENT COMPLAINTS

Lethargy, dyspnea, anorexia, and collapse are the most common reasons for owners to seek help for dogs with acute signs of pericardial effusion. Abdominal distention, lethargy, anorexia, and cough are common client complaints for dogs with chronic signs of pericardial effusion. Sudden death, collapse, or a history of trauma may be the presenting complaint for animals with cardiac tamponade.

CLINICAL SIGNS

Ascites, jugular venous distention, cachexia, tachycardia, and weak pulses are common findings. An exaggerated weakening of the arterial pulse during inspiration is often associated with pericardial effusion. Auscultation may reveal muffled heart sounds, murmurs, or friction rubs. Signs of shock accompanied by signs of increased systemic venous pressure should raise the possibility of cardiac tamponade.

DIAGNOSTIC IMAGING AND THE ELECTROCARDIOGRAM

When fluid accumulates slowly, thoracic radiographs will usually show a large globoid heart. Acute traumatic cardiac tamponade is unlikely to be detected with radiographs because of the small amount of fluid in the pericardium. Echocardiographic examination of the heart is very sensitive in detecting even small amounts of pericardial fluid. Diastolic collapse of the right atrium and right ventricular free wall are signs associated with tamponade. Echocardiography may also detect a mass, which is frequently the cause of the effusion. Tachycardia, low-amplitude ECG complexes, and electrical alternans are almost pathognomonic signs of pericardial effusion.

TREATMENT OF CARDIAC TAMPONADE AND PERICARDIAL EFFUSION

Pericardiocentesis will rapidly relieve the signs caused by increased pressure in the pericardium. The patient should be prepared by shaving the hair on the right side of the chest over the region of the heart (usually centered on the fifth intercostal space). After aseptically preparing the shaved area, local anesthetic is infiltrated into the tissues between the fourth and fifth intercostal spaces at the level of the costochondral junction. Ultrasound imaging can be used to determine the best location. A 14- to 16-gauge over-the-needle catheter is recommended for the typical patient, which is usually a large breed dog. Many clinicians will cut several side holes near the end of the catheter before insertion; however, if this is done, care must be taken not to weaken the catheter so much that the tip can break off in the pericardium. The catheter is inserted through the right chest wall and into the thoracic cavity. If the patient has concurrent pleural effusion, a flash of clear fluid may appear in the stylet before entering the pericardium. The catheter may be felt to contact the pericardium as it is advanced. Once the catheter has entered the pericardium, fluid flashes into the stylet and the catheter can be advanced over the stylet. The ECG should be monitored during the procedure to help determine if the needle has contacted the myocardium. Contact with the myocardium is indicated by ventricular premature beats. A small sample of the fluid can be saved in a serum vacuum tube or other container, to see if it will clot and to check the hematocrit level. Clotting of the fluid sample after collection indicates active bleeding or entry into a cardiac chamber. As the pericardial fluid is removed, the heart rate may decrease and the ECG may show increased amplitude.

MONITORING

Most animals improve rapidly after the fluid is removed from the pericardium. If the patient does not improve or worsens, then it may be because of active bleeding (in the case of cardiac tamponade) or because of a complication of pericardiocentesis (e.g., laceration of a coronary artery). Monitoring the CVP may help with the initial diagnosis of cardiac tamponade or pericardial effusion. BP should be monitored if cardiac tamponade is a possibility.

FELINE AORTIC THROMBOEMBOLISM

Feline aortic thromboembolism (FATE) is a devastating complication of myocardial disease. Thrombi develop in the heart and then break free and travel into the systemic arteries. These thromboemboli most frequently lodge in the distal aorta where they often cause posterior paresis, paralysis, and pain. Mortality is very high in aortic thromboembolism, with about two thirds of the patients being euthanized or dying during the initial episode. Animals that survive sometimes lose skin, toes, or even a leg to ischemic necrosis. Survivors of the initial episode will require treatment of their underlying heart disease, which is often severe. Survivors are also at increased risk for recurrence.

CLIENT COMPLAINTS

Clients are motivated to seek help quickly because many of the signs seen in patients with FATE (e.g., vocalizing, apparent pain, inability to walk, dyspnea, urinary and fecal incontinence) are very distressing. The majority of clients will be unaware of any problem with the patient's health before embolism occurs.

DIAGNOSTIC IMAGING AND THE ELECTROCARDIOGRAM

Thoracic radiographs often show signs of heart enlargement, pleural effusion, or pulmonary edema. Echocardiography usually shows signs of heart disease, most commonly hypertrophic cardiomyopathy. Left atrial enlargement and spontaneous contrast (smoke) are frequently seen in cats with FATE. In some cases a thrombus may be seen in the left atrium. The majority of cats with FATE will have some abnormality in the ECG.

CLINICAL SIGNS

In about 70% of patients the embolus will affect blood flow to both hind limbs. In 15% a single front limb will be affected (most commonly right), and in 15% a single hind limb is affected. In addition to paralysis and pain, the affected limbs will be cold and pale or cyanotic. Pulses in the affected area will be nonexistent or very weak. A heart murmur, gallop sound, or irregular heart rhythm may be heard. Some cats may show signs of dyspnea or tachypnea. It is very important to measure the patient's rectal temperature (an important prognostic sign). The odds favor survival when the temperature is greater than 37.2° C (98.9° F).

TREATMENT

The long-term prognosis for patients with aortic thromboembolism is poor, but many animals can regain an acceptable quality of life after treatment for some time. To make an informed decision regarding treatment, clients should be educated about what to expect and the role they must play in the patient's care should they decide to proceed. About one third of clients decide to euthanize the patient after the diagnosis is made. Although many of the patients that are euthanized are moribund, some of those euthanized would probably have survived, at least for the short term. Clients should be advised that about one half of the patients that receive treatment survive. Patients with higher rectal temperatures and only one affected limb appear to have the best chance of survival. Patients with taurine deficiency or hyperthyroidism may show significant improvement in their heart disease when these conditions are treated. Clients that elect to treat their cat should be aware that the patient will need some level of nursing care for weeks or months during recovery from nerve damage or ischemic necrosis. Survivors usually need to receive medication for the rest of their lives to treat their heart disease and prevent another episode of thromboembolism.

Patients should be handled carefully, because many have severe underlying heart disease. In one study, 66% of the animals had radiographic signs of CHF. The treatment of pleural effusion and pulmonary edema may be as urgent as the treatment of the aortic embolus.

Three forms of immediate treatment for FATE are available: (1) supportive, (2) extraction of the clot using catheter techniques or surgery, and (3) elimination of the clot with thrombolytic agents. In supportive treatment the patient is treated for its heart disease and pain. Drugs such as heparin and clopidogrel are used to prevent the growth of the clot. Some clinicians also advocate the use of vasodilating drugs to improve circulation, although the benefit of this therapy is unproven. The FATE cat is often in excruciating pain and will usually benefit from CRI and/or multimodal analgesia. See Chapter 9 for various therapies.

Clots have been successfully removed by using one of several different catheter techniques, as well as surgery. Anesthesia for aortic embolectomy in a cat with severe heart disease is particularly challenging and should be performed in an environment in which the patient can be intensively monitored and supported during the procedure. Thrombolytic therapy is expensive, requires careful patient monitoring, and may be contraindicated in patients known to have thrombi in the heart; however, it does not require anesthesia. Importantly, however, the evidence does not show that therapies that eliminate the clot are better at reducing mortality than supportive therapy or that recurrence can be substantially reduced. Therapy to remove the clot appears to improve circulation in the majority of patients, but complications resulting from the use of this type of therapy also appear to have contributed to the deaths of some patients. Box 17-5 lists the goals of therapy for FATE.

BOX 17-5 | Goals of Therapy in Feline Aortic Thromboembolism (FATE)

Stabilize preexisting heart disease.
Administer analgesics for pain.
Administer heparin to prevent the growth of the clot.
Consider using tissue plasminogen activator, streptokinase, surgery, or catheter techniques to remove the clot, recognizing the risks of these therapies.
Prevent and treat the injuries caused by ischemic necrosis.
Use clopidogrel to prevent the formation of clots in the future.

SUGGESTED READINGS

Abbott JA: Traumatic myocarditis. In Bonagura JD, editor: *Kirk's current veterinary therapy XII small animal practice*, Philadelphia, 1995, Saunders, pp 846–850.

Boon JA: *Veterinary echocardiography*, ed 2, Hoboken, NJ, 2011, Wiley Blackwell, pp 632.

Bright JM, Martin JM, Mama K: A retrospective evaluation of transthoracic biphasic electrical cardioversion for atrial fibrillation in dogs, *J Vet Cardiol* 7(2):85–96, 2005.

Buchanan JW, Bücheler J: Vertebral scale system to measure canine heart size in radiographs, *J Am Vet Med Assoc* 206(2):194–199, 1995.

Cornell CC et al.: Allometric scaling of M-mode cardiac measurements in normal adult dogs, *J Vet Intern Med* 18(3):311–321, 2004.

DeFrancesco TC, Hansen BD, Atkins CE: Noninvasive transthoracic temporary cardiac pacing in dogs, *J Vet Intern Med* 17(5):663–667, 2003.

Fletcher DJ, Boller M: Updates in small animal cardiopulmonary resuscitation, *Vet Clin North Am Small Anim Pract* 43:971–987, 2013.

Fox PR, Sisson D, Moïse NS: *Textbook of canine and feline cardiology: principles and clinical practice*, ed 2, St Louis, 1999, Saunders Co.

Gelzer ARM, Kraus MS: Management of atrial fibrillation, *Vet Clin North Am Small Anim Pract* 34(5):1127–1144, 2004.

Gidlewski J, Petrie JP: Therapeutic pericardiocentesis in the dog and cat, *Clin Tech Small Anim Pract* 20:151–155, 2005.

Goutal CM, Keir I, Kenney S, et al.: Evaluation of acute congestive heart failure in dogs and cats: 145 cases (2007-2008), *J Vet Emerg Crit Care* 20(3):330–337, 2010.

Johnson L, Boon J, Orton EC: Clinical characteristics of 53 dogs with Doppler-derived evidence of pulmonary hypertension: 1992-1996, *J Vet Intern Med* 13(5):440–447, 1999.

Kienle RD, Thomas WP: Echocardiography. In Nyland TG, Mattoon JS, editors: *Small animal diagnostic ultrasound*, ed 2, Philadelphia, 2002, Saunders, pp 354–423.

Kittleson MD, Kienle RD: *Small animal cardiovascular medicine*, St Louis, 1998, Mosby.

Knight DH: Reason must supersede dogma in the management of ventricular arrhythmias. In Bonagura JD, editor: *Kirk's current veterinary therapy XIII small animal practice*, Philadelphia, 2000, WB Saunders, pp 730–733.

Lamb CR, Boswood A: Role of survey radiography in diagnosing canine cardiac disease, *Compend Contin Educ Pract Vet* 24(4):316–326, 2002.

Litster AL, Buchanan JW: Vertebral scale system to measure heart size in radiographs of cats, *J Am Vet Med Assoc* 216(2):210–214, 2000.

Lynne O'Sullivan DVM: DVSc, Diplomate ACVIM(cardiology), Dr. Michael O'Grady, DVM, MS, Diplomate ACVIM(cardiology), *Clin Cardiol Notes*, 2011. Vetgo.com.

Reimer SB, Kittleson MD, Kyles AE: Use of rheolytic thrombectomy for the treatment of feline distal aortic thromboembolism, *J Vet Intern Med* 19(3):424, 2005 (abstract).

Rishniw M, Thomas WP: Bradyarrhythmias. In Bonagura JD, editor: *Kirk's current veterinary therapy XIII small animal practice*, Philadelphia, 2000, Saunders, pp 719–725.

Scansen BA: Interventional cardiology for the criticalist, *J Vet Emerg Crit Care* 21(2):123–136, 2011.

Scherf D, Bornemann C: Thumping of the precordium in ventricular standstill, *Am J Cardiol* 5:30–40, 1960.

Sisson DD et al.: Plasma taurine concentrations and M-mode echocardiographic measures in healthy cats and in cats with dilated cardiomyopathy, *J Vet Intern Med* 5(4):232–238, 1991.

Sleeper MM, Clifford CA, Laster LL: Cardiac troponin I in the normal dog and cat, *J Vet Intern Med* 15(5):501–503, Sep-Oct 2001.

Smith SA, Tobias AH: Feline arterial thromboembolism: an update, *Vet Clin North Am Small Anim Pract* 34(5):1245–1271, 2004.

Tilley LP, Smith FWK Jr, Oyama MA, et al.: *Manual of canine and feline cardiology*, ed 4, St Louis, 2007, Elsevier.

Wright KN: Assessment and treatment of supraventricular arrhythmias. In Bonagura JD, editor: *Kirk's current veterinary therapy XIII small animal practice*, Philadelphia, 2000, Saunders, pp 726–733.

SCENARIO

A 7-year-old Doberman, MC, presents at the clinic with a cough, increased respiratory rate, lethargy, and weakness, and has not been eating since yesterday morning. The dog is reluctant to lie down and is leaning against the wall in the waiting room, with his head extended outward, an obvious increase in his respiratory effort.

On physical, his heart rate is 135 bpm, respiratory rate is 45/min, auscultation of the lungs reveal crackles and wheezes, there is a murmur present, pulses are weak and irregular. Mucous membranes are pale. A lead II ECG revealed some ventricular premature beats. No abdominal findings, and no ascites. Body condition is mildly dehydrated. Owner reports the dog has been less active over the past week and more restless at night, and has been coughing 8 to 10 times per day over the past few days.

Questions

- What is the most important clinical sign in this case and what triage score would you give this dog?
- Should this case go back to the treatment area immediately or to an exam room?
- What are your initial interventions, and in what order should they occur?

Treatment/Diagnostic Options

- Radiographic analysis of lungs to determine heart score, and lung status
- Catheter placement
- Furosemide (diuretic) treatment
- Blood pressure
- Fluid therapy
- ECG
- Echocardiography
- Blood work

Discussion

This patient is in the acute stages of heart failure. This particular breed is generally very stoic, and for him to show signs of respiratory effort says he is in imminent trouble.

A catheter should be placed and the administration of diuretic should be given as directed (2-4 mg/kg IV), along with lidocaine 2 mg/kg. As his breathing stabilizes, radiographs and an ECG may be the next best step in determining the cause of his cough, and arrhythmia. Once his heart condition is determined, we can treat the other signs such as dehydration and arrhythmia. Blood can now be collected to look at electrolytes and other organ functions.

- How could we further determine structural heart disease for this dog once he is stable?
- How would this help us with the treatment of this dog in the future?

MEDICAL MATH EXERCISE

LIDOCAINE

Bolus: 2 mg/kg
CRI: 30-50 mcg/kg/min
Supplied as: 2% (20 mg/ml)
Syringe pump administration: Dilute 50-ml bottle in 500 ml of D_5W or 0.9% NaCl, giving a concentration of 2 mg/ml

A Labrador retriever weighing 35 kg presents on emergency; a continuous ECG is placed and he is having VPCs secondary to myocardial trauma; he suddenly goes into ventricular tachycardia at a rate of 220 bpm. The doctor has given you orders on the flowsheet to give a bolus of lidocaine 2%.

1. How much lidocaine bolus do you give (using the information provided above)?

18 Respiratory Emergencies

Andrea M. Steele

CHAPTER OUTLINE

Patient Presentation
Be Prepared
Obtaining Vascular Access
Rapid Intubation Sequence
Primary Survey and Minimum
  Database
Secondary Survey
Continued Management
Common Respiratory Emergencies
Traumatic Conditions
  Laryngeal or Tracheal Trauma
  Pleural Space Conditions
  Chest Wall Deformities

Pulmonary Contusions
Smoke Inhalation
Airway Disorders
  Airway Obstruction
  Laryngeal Paralysis
  Brachycephalic Airway Syndrome
  Feline Asthma
Pulmonary Edema
Pneumonia
  Bacterial Pneumonia
  Fungal Pneumonia
  Viral Pneumonia
  Aspiration Pneumonia

KEY TERMS

Cyanosis
Dyspnea
Orthopnea
Respiration
Respiratory failure

LEARNING OBJECTIVES

After studying this chapter, you will be able to:

- Recognize a respiratory emergency quickly and efficiently.
- Explain how to prepare for a respiratory emergency and how to intervene.
- Demonstrate a solid understanding of common respiratory emergencies.

Emergency respiratory patients can be a challenge for any veterinary technician. Technicians must not only minimize further distress to the patient but also obtain the required diagnostic tests in order to help determine the problem. Sometimes there are subtle signs of respiratory compromise, which often progresses quickly to profound respiratory distress. All technicians must be able to recognize mild, moderate, or severe **dyspnea** as well as **respiratory failure,** and know various techniques that will give the best chance of a positive outcome.

PATIENT PRESENTATION

Normal **respiration** is passive: Our respiratory cycle often remains completely unnoticed, and we only tend to pay attention to our breathing with a respiratory ailment or heavy exertion. Dyspnea has been described as an abnormal breathing effort characterized by changes in respiratory rate, rhythm, and character as well as altered behavior.

319

Common respiratory emergencies include pulmonary edema, pleural effusion, pneumonia, airway obstruction, trauma, and respiratory paralysis. Although each of these presentations requires a different treatment, there are commonalities among them. On a typical triage scale of I to IV, respiratory emergencies must be classified as high (class I or II) and intervention instituted very quickly since respiratory compromise can quickly evolve into respiratory failure.

When triaging a respiratory emergency, a great deal of information can be obtained from a distance evaluation of a patient, before approach. Watch the patient in the waiting room with the owner, or if already in hospital, assess the patient before opening the cage door. Once the patient notices and reacts to your presence, often the patient's demeanor will change, hiding some of the obvious clinical signs. For a more visual approach to the respiratory emergency, see Figure 18-1 (respiratory emergency algorithm).

A patient that is in need of oxygen may display a multitude of different vital signs and abnormalities. Perform the "distance" assessment first, and then approach the patient for a more hands-on assessment. There may be an "Air Hungry" posture, restlessness, anxiety, and other behavioral changes. These patients are frequently oblivious to their surroundings, will focus their gaze on a fixed point, and seem not to notice your presence. Other common presenting signs include tachypnea, increased or paradoxical abdominal movement, open-mouth breathing, reluctance to lie down (dogs) or sternal recumbency (cats), and an abnormal posture characterized by extension of the head and neck and abduction of the elbows, called **orthopnea** (Figure 18-2 and Figure 18-3). Signs of dyspnea with lateral recumbency in a dog or cat usually indicate serious respiratory compromise.

Other signs of increased respiratory effort include abdominal and other accessory muscle involvement, flaring of the nostrils, sucking in at the thoracic inlet

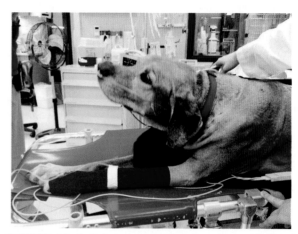

FIGURE 18-2 Orthopnea in the dog. Note the extended head and neck, and adducted elbows. Often dogs are reluctant to lie down, until seriously compromised or weakened.

FIGURE 18-1 Respiratory emergency algorithm.

- Respiratory emergency arrives
- Immediate attention required?
  - Yes
    - Bring to treatment area
    - Administer oxygen
    - Consider sedation
    - Obtain IV access and minimum database
    - Perform palliative procedures
  - No
    - Make triage plan, reassess frequently
- Prepare for emergency intubation and/or procedures

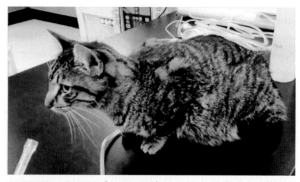

FIGURE 18-3 Orthopnea in the cat. Note the extended head and neck, resting on the sternum with bent elbows. Most cats present in open-mouth respiratory distress.

on inspiration, and pulling back at the commissures of the mouth. As you approach the patient, you may hear noises associated with breathing. Note if the sounds are on inspiration, or expiration. There may or may not be clear evidence of **cyanosis** in the mucous membranes. Cyanosis is usually not readily apparent until the patient has an oxygen saturation of 50% to 60%, suggesting severe hypoxemia. It is important to note slight changes in mucous membrane color, however, because the patient may look "less pink" without appearing blue. This usually starts to make the color of the tongue and mucous membranes dusky pink, rather than a bright pink. Vital signs may be abnormal, with a high heart rate (and often arrhythmias), increased respiratory rate with or without effort, and change in respiratory pattern. Patients may have an elevated temperature, although the converse can also be true, especially in cardiogenic shock. Respiratory distress is not the only clear sign that a patient requires oxygen. There are many conditions that can increase a patient's oxygen demand, or alter the patient's ability to extract oxygen from the blood. Each of these conditions may require supplemental oxygen to reverse the negative effects of having insufficient oxygen available to meet demand.

> **TECHNICIAN NOTE** The initial evaluation of the respiratory patient is of the utmost importance, and noticing audible sounds, posture, respiratory patterns, and behavior will provide the technician with as much information as the physical exam. Do not skip this step!

When a patient presents in respiratory distress, the ultimate goal is to improve the quality of its respirations and relieve the cause of dyspnea. Because dyspnea can be a sign of many different problems requiring many different treatments, an accurate, rapid, primary survey should be performed in order to determine why the patient is dyspneic. In most cases, palliative treatment is performed before a complete physical examination (secondary survey) and many diagnostic tests.

Respiratory patients, arguably more than any other type of emergent patient, are susceptible to the stress of handling, examination, and diagnostics, including obtaining vascular access. The goal in caring for these patients must be to minimize stress. Staff should work in a calm, quiet, and efficient manner, with minimal persons handling the patient. Restraint techniques must be minimal, and technicians should avoid forcibly restraining, scruffing, and muzzling patients in respiratory distress. Often these patients have been removed from their owner for emergency treatment, possibly compounding anxiety. Light sedation will often allow the patient to be managed more easily, and with minimal restraint. Many veterinarians will choose butorphanol, which rarely causes vomiting or panting, but provides some sedation and mild analgesia. This low-dose sedation may relieve some of the anxiety related to dyspnea, and the patient may be better able to deal with handling and diagnostic tests.

BE PREPARED

It is very important that every veterinary practice be prepared to provide emergency oxygen supplementation. This includes having readily available all equipment required for rapid intubation, tracheostomy, and thoracentesis in the emergency area.

Equipment list:
- Devices for oxygen (O_2) administration
- Endotracheal tubes (multiple sizes)
- Tracheostomy tubes (multiple sizes)
- Thoracic drainage tubes (multiple sizes)
- Grasping forceps (long sponge forceps) for foreign body retrieval
- Laryngoscopes with small, medium, and large blades
- Thoracic drainage unit
- Wall or portable suction for airway or thoracic drainage unit
- Suction catheters (small 8 French [Fr] and larger 14 Fr are ideal)
- Three-way stopcocks
- Butterfly catheters, and/or over-the-needle catheters in 20 to 16 gauge
- Bronchoscopes
- Small surgical pack and scalpel blades

In the emergent phase, oxygen supplementation is very important. Oxygen should be provided to respiratory patients in as simple and stress-free a manner as possible. Placing a nasal catheter in this high-anxiety, dyspneic state is often too stressful, even though this is considered one of the most efficient methods of oxygen supplementation. Flow-by oxygen is useful upon presentation, or occasionally with a loose-fitting mask, although even a loose-fitting mask can be stressful. Flow-by oxygen provides the most oxygen enrichment at flow rates of 100 to 150 ml/kg/min, but many patients will resent this high a rate being "blasted" into their face. Human nasal cannulas (prongs), available in adult, pediatric, and infant size, can be a very effective, low-stress method in many dogs and are often very well accepted and quickly placed. An oxygen cage or oxygen hood can be a stress-free method of oxygen supplementation for smaller patients. For more information on oxygen supplementation, please see Chapter 7: Oxygen Therapy Techniques.

TECHNICIAN NOTE Choosing the most appropriate and tolerated oxygen supplementation method will increase your success! Try to have as many choices available to you as possible at your clinic, and be creative.

OBTAINING VASCULAR ACCESS

Obtaining vascular access is critical when presented with a dyspneic patient. That being said, the condition of the patient will dictate if the catheter needs to be placed immediately, since the patient may die at any moment, or if the patient may benefit from some sedation before attempting placement. Sedation will have the benefit of reducing the stress of the placement and restraint, as well as give the patient time to relax with some oxygen, which may relieve some of the clinical signs associated with dyspnea. Sedation may also have undesired effects, such as removing some of the drive to breathe, worsening the patient's condition. The risks must always be weighed against the benefits, but it is rare that the risk of a struggling dyspneic patient being restrained would outweigh the benefit of the patient being sedated. As always when sedating a patient, the technician and team should be prepared for possible undesired outcomes.

Whether the choice has been made to sedate, or not to sedate, vascular access should be obtained quickly and on the first attempt. Intravenous (IV) catheter placement should be performed by a skilled technician, not only to reduce stress but also because hypoxia causes vasoconstriction and shock, leading to a difficult cannulation. Dyspneic dogs are often reluctant to lie down (especially without sedation), because this may further impair respirations. Therefore, being able to place the

IV catheter with the dog standing is a useful skill that will minimize further stress. Minimal restraint is best for these patients, because they often do not like having their heads restrained, and muzzling is highly contraindicated. Technicians who work in teaching institutions must make it clear that dyspneic animals are not suitable practice catheter cases.

Cats are particularly susceptible to sudden death when they are dyspneic and must be handled very carefully. Forcibly restraining a cat for intravenous catheter insertion, oxygen administration, or performance of diagnostic or palliative procedures is contraindicated, and will probably cause the condition of the cat to deteriorate. A common strategy for dyspneic cats is to administer intramuscular or subcutaneous sedation and then place the patient in an oxygen cage or oxygen hood in a cage for 10 to 15 minutes to allow the sedation to take effect, before handling the patient. This also provides an opportunity to perform some "distance evaluations," including respiratory rate, effort, and pattern, while the cat is relaxing in an oxygen-rich environment. Once the sedative has taken effect, the patient can be moved to the treatment area with flow-by oxygen, or the oxygen hood can be moved onto the table with the patient. Oftentimes in dyspneic cats, a hind limb catheter will be the least stressful, allowing the front end to remain sternal under the oxygen hood, or with flow-by oxygen, while the hind end is placed laterally for catheter placement.

TECHNICIAN NOTE Although the choice to sedate or not sedate will always be at the discretion of your veterinarian, do not be afraid to speak up and ask for sedation when it is obvious that the patient is too stressed to handle.

RAPID INTUBATION SEQUENCE

Patients that are at risk of respiratory failure often require emergency interventions beyond oxygen supplementation. These patients may require rapid sequence intubation (RSI) with or without ventilation. RSI is the process of very quickly inducing anesthesia and intubating the patient. It is not the same as intubation during a cardiopulmonary arrest; rather, in this case, the animal is still breathing and will fight intubation without induction. Induction agents chosen must be quick acting, with minimal cardiovascular effects, and are preferably

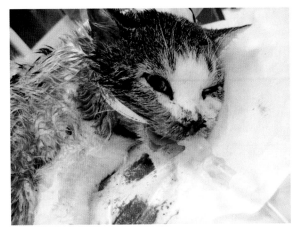

FIGURE 18-4 Rapid sequence intubation is necessary to protect the airway following trauma, or with imminent respiratory failure.

fully or partially reversible. Most veterinarians will have their "go to" induction agents for RSI, and the technician can prepare the required dose in advance when the patient presents. Preparation of appropriately sized endotracheal tubes, laryngoscope, Ambu bag, or anesthetic machine with rebreathing bag, oxygen, and tube ties is essential for success. RSI is a necessity when a patient presents with a profound work of breathing, cyanosis, or severe upper airway disease with obstruction that does not rapidly improve with oxygen, sedation, and emergency therapies such as thoracentesis, or diuretics. The goal of RSI is to intervene before a respiratory or cardiac arrest (Figure 18-4).

In general, endotracheal intubation is preferred in the emergent phase, unless it is physically impossible because of an obstruction, thus requiring a tracheostomy. Preparation of tracheostomy supplies such as a cut-down or small surgical pack, sterile gloves, scalpel, suture material, and a commercial or homemade tracheostomy tube is something the technician can have ready in advance.

PRIMARY SURVEY AND MINIMUM DATABASE

The primary survey should include assessment of temperature, pulse rate, respiratory rate, mentation, mucous membrane color, capillary refill time, and pulse strength. A thorough auscultation of heart and lung fields and the trachea, as well as assessment of the respiratory pattern, is necessary to localize the cause

of the dyspnea. It is important for technicians to auscultate their patients in order to identify worsening or improvement of the patient's condition. Assessing respiration in the emergent patient provides valuable clues to the cause of breathing difficulty. Assessment of the respiratory system involves paying close attention to inspiratory and/or expiratory effort, audible noise during respiration (inspiratory, expiratory, or biphasic), and the character and quality of chest excursion. The primary survey can be performed at any veterinary clinic, without specialized equipment.

The minimum database for a respiratory patient is going to be dependent on what is available at your clinic. In a full-service facility, it will usually include packed cell volume (PCV)/total solids (TSs), blood gases (usually a venous blood gas is obtained first, because an arterial blood gas causes additional stress), electrolytes, glucose, blood urea nitrogen, electrocardiogram, a bedside clotting profile (activated clotting time [ACT] or prothrombin time [PT]/partial thromboplastin time [aPTT]), arterial blood pressure, and pulse oximetry, as long as these measurements can be easily obtained. Blood collection in most cases will have to wait until the patient is calm and somewhat stabilized; this is often done at the time of IV catheter placement. The ACT or PT/PTT is important for rapidly identifying any potential clotting issues, which may contraindicate thoracentesis. If possible, pulling the blood to run a complete blood count/biochemical profile from the catheter at the time of placement will again reduce the stress of multiple blood draws.

SECONDARY SURVEY

Attempting the secondary survey when the patient is suffering from severe dyspnea may cause undue stress. Instead, treating the patient on the basis of the primary survey and history to relieve the dyspnea is often the more prudent course of action. For example, a patient with suspected pleural space disease, based on respiratory pattern, auscultation and history, may benefit more from immediate thoracentesis than from a radiograph (Box 18-1). In this case, thoracentesis is both diagnostic and palliative. Unless it is absolutely necessary, and the veterinarian is not able to pinpoint the cause of the dyspnea, it is generally more appropriate to wait until the patient is more stable before attempting to obtain a radiograph.

BOX 18-1 | Performing a Thoracentesis and Placement of a Chest Tube

Thoracentesis

Placing a needle or catheter into the thoracic cavity is necessary for removing air or fluid from the chest cavity for diagnostic or therapeutic reasons.

Procedure

- The area over the seventh to ninth intercostal space in the midsection of the chest should be clipped and surgically prepared.
- If ultrasound is available, a TFAST (thoracic-focused assessment for trauma) may be performed to identify fluid or air, and location of the largest pocket (of fluid).
- **Air:** Middle to dorsal third of the chest when standing or sternal, highest point of chest when laterally recumbent.
- **Fluid:** Ventral third of the fourth to seventh intercostal space (with caution more cranial than the sixth intercostal, ultrasound guidance preferred to avoid the heart) in an animal that is standing or in sternal recumbency.
- An 18- or 20-gauge butterfly or an over-the-needle catheter can be used. The needle is advanced slowly into the pleural space, in front of the rib (caudal margin of rib is the location of intercostal artery) and at a 45-degree angle.
- Confirmation of placement in the pleural space can be obtained in several ways. (1) Obtain fluid or air on aspiration. (2) Place a drop of sterile saline on hub of catheter, which will be sucked into chest because of negative pressure (generally for fluid only). (3) Catheter can be advanced with a 3-ml syringe attached and gentle negative pressure during advancement; fluid or air will be obtained as soon as in the pleural space.
- At this point, advancement of the needle should stop and the angle of the needle made level with the chest wall.
- A three-way stopcock is attached and aspiration is initiated.

Complications

- Lung laceration
- Iatrogenic pneumothorax

Thoracostomy Tube Placement

Placing a tube in the thoracic cavity is necessary if large amounts of air or fluid are present. A chest tube should be placed if more than two thoracoceteses are needed in the first few hours of presentation. Chest tubes are commercially available both in large-bore rigid tubes and as Seldinger-placed, flexible, fenestrated catheters. Red rubber feeding tubes can be used as an alternative. Three or four holes must be made large enough for fluid to flow through easily.

Procedure

- Sedation and local intercostal nerve blocks are used for the critically ill animal.
- A large section of the lateral thorax is surgically prepared.
- The tube chosen should be approximately the same size as the mainstem bronchus (as estimated from a thoracic radiograph).
- The skin is grabbed at the level of shoulder blade and pulled cranially or caudally. (Use the mnemonic fluid-forward, air-back to determine the direction of pull.)
- A stab incision is made (slightly larger than the tube) into the seventh or eighth intercostal space.
- The clinician bluntly dissects through the incision into the thorax with hemostats. The hemostats are held so that the dominant hand is grasping the instrument near the tip of the hemostats to prevent overpenetration.
- Air is allowed to enter the thoracic cavity (to allow some lung deflation).
- The chest tube is placed in a cranioventral direction for fluid and craniodorsally for air (a stylet will help guide the tube).
- The skin is released to create a subcutaneous tunnel.
- The tube is twisted 180 degrees in each direction to confirm that it is not kinked. Radiographs can be used to confirm proper placement.
- The tube is secured to the periosteum of ribs (using additional local anesthetic).
- A purse-string suture is tied around the tube as it exits the skin to seal the chest.
- The tube is anchored by placing a suture through the skin and around the tube at about the level of the eighth or ninth rib. A Chinese fingertip is placed around the tube to prevent it from slipping out of the chest.
- Triple-antibiotic ointment is placed at the insertion site to create a better seal.
- A wrap is placed around the chest to provide better stability.
- The tube can be connected to a thoracic drain pump for continual suction, or a three-way stopcock can be stabilized to the tube for intermittent suction.
- Lidocaine is infused into the chest tube (1.5 mg/kg). The chest tube is then flushed with saline (1-3 ml depending on the size of the chest tube). The patient is gently rocked and rolled for a complete coating of the area. Bupivacaine is then infused into the chest tube (1.5 mg/kg) and the chest tube is again flushed with saline. The patient is once more gently rocked and rolled for a complete coating of the area. This treatment can be repeated every 6 hours for pain management. The dose may need to be adjusted in cats if the animal becomes too sedate.
- Heimlich valves can be used for animals with pneumothorax that weigh more than 15 kg.

TECHNICIAN NOTE Try to be methodical when dealing with a respiratory patient. Do the least stressful, but most important things first—you do not always need a radiograph before a thoracentesis for a suspected pneumothorax! A diagnostic tap can be performed, the presence of air confirming the pneumothorax.

CONTINUED MANAGEMENT

Once the emergent phase of respiratory distress is successfully addressed, the patient requires continued management. This can range from simply observing the patient for several hours to mechanically ventilating the patient for several days.

Respiratory patients that are sleeping and have a normal respiratory rate would most benefit from cageside observation of respiratory rate, effort, and pattern. Formerly dyspneic patients can be exhausted from the work of breathing, and waking them unnecessarily can be detrimental to their recovery. Each time the patient is handled, the technician should take the opportunity to auscultate and assess changes in lung sounds. Pulse oximetry can be a valuable, relatively noninvasive tool to assess oxygenation, but it does not need to be performed on a frequent basis unless there are patient concerns such as changes in respiratory rate or effort. Ultimately, an animal that is sleeping comfortably with a normal respiratory rate does not need a pulse oximetry measurement to tell you that it is stable at the moment. The same animal that is struggling to breathe, with a high respiratory rate and respiratory effort, does need a pulse oximetry measurement and/or more supplemental oxygen.

Long-term oxygen supplementation may need to be provided, and can have some deleterious effects. It is important to supplement oxygen only as long as necessary, and wean the level down as soon as possible. Clinical signs can be used as a judgment if other monitoring is not available. Ideally, technicians should be provided orders for oxygen supplementation based on parameters and clinical signs, rather than just set oxygen rates. This way, the technician can be providing the oxygen that the animal needs, rather than waiting for the veterinarian to assess between appointments and surgeries.

In cases of continued dyspnea after the emergent phase, it is important to note that these patients easily become hyperthermic as a result of the effort of breathing. Providing housing in roomy cages or runs with good airflow or placing mats on the cage floor may reduce overheating. Many patients may enjoy a fan to further improve airflow and heat elimination. If using an oxygen hood or cage, temperature and ventilation must be controlled to minimize overheating. Some oxygen cages have dehumidifiers that will also help to control temperature. Pyrexia may also be present, especially in cases of pneumonia, so it is important to differentiate hyperthermia from pyrexia. Cooling efforts with the pyrexic patient may result in a continued increase in patient temperature.

Other nursing considerations associated with the ongoing care of many respiratory patients include patient positioning, nebulization and coupage, removal of secretions, and management of chest drains and tracheostomy sites.

TECHNICIAN NOTE Provide respiratory patients with a large, airy cage, or floor space, rather than placing them in a cage that is confining. Maximize airflow to help avoid hyperthermia from work of breathing. A small fan can be placed in the cage with the patient.

COMMON RESPIRATORY EMERGENCIES

Numerous respiratory diseases affect our veterinary patients, and these can occur as emergency presentations, or after a patient has been hospitalized. On an emergent basis, we often see conditions such as pneumothorax, hemothorax, chest wall injuries, airway obstruction, pulmonary edema, and pneumonia. In the following sections, we will examine the features typically seen with each type of respiratory disease, and discuss common treatments that will be prescribed by the veterinarian.

TRAUMATIC CONDITIONS

Trauma to the airway, lungs, or chest wall can dramatically impair respiration, leading to respiratory distress. Patients involved in motor vehicle accidents, animal attacks, or falls are most at risk of respiratory distress secondary to trauma. Victims of house fires will have significant chemical and thermal trauma to the lungs and airways, as well as possible thermal injuries to the rest of the body. Common conditions include laryngeal or tracheal trauma, pneumothorax, hemothorax, diaphragmatic hernia, flail chest, sucking chest wound, and pulmonary contusions.

LARYNGEAL OR TRACHEAL TRAUMA

Laryngeal trauma is often caused by animal attacks, and extensive neck wounds are often present. The source of dyspnea may be due to swelling, damage to the hyoid apparatus, or damage to the larynx itself. Each of these conditions can be life-threatening, and the potential for serious blood loss is also a concern with injuries of this type because of the close proximity of the jugular veins and carotid arteries. Patients with this type of injury may not be able to breathe effectively as a result of obstruction, requiring an immediate tracheostomy tube placement and anesthesia before examination of the neck wounds.

Tracheal trauma can arise from various circumstances, including iatrogenic causes such as tracheal tears associated with intubation. With closed tracheal traumas, there is often subcutaneous emphysema, which may be extensive. When there are neck wounds present, the air often escapes and there is little to no subcutaneous emphysema. Depending on the location of the tracheal tear, treatment will differ. Often the patient will require surgery, unless it is a very small perforation. Intubation may be difficult, and may be done with a tracheostomy tube, or orally with the use of a bronchoscope. The scope can be passed through the endotracheal (ET) tube, and as the clinician is scoping the animal under an injectable anesthetic, the ET tube is slid by the tracheal tear and inflated. Then the animal can be maintained on inhalant while surgery is performed.

PLEURAL SPACE CONDITIONS

Pleural space conditions may arise following trauma, coagulopathies, ruptured bullae, or cardiac disease.

Pneumothorax occurs when an area of lung ruptures, releasing air into the pleural space. Very quickly, air will accumulate in the pleural space, and if there is no exit (such as a puncture in the chest wall), the patient will develop a "tension pneumothorax." A tension pneumothorax occurs when the pressure in the pleural space exceeds that in the lungs, causing the lungs to compress. As this happens, the patient's respirations become more and more exaggerated, often with the appearance of gasping, and then respiratory and/or cardiac failure rapidly occurs. The only treatment for a tension pneumothorax

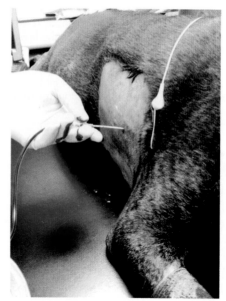

FIGURE 18-5 Thoracentesis of hemothorax in the dog, using a large-bore catheter.

is to perform a thoracentesis immediately to expel the air in the pleural space. Because the pressure is so high in this compartment, thoracentesis is best performed with a large-gauge catheter, such as a 14 gauge. Often, aspiration is not initially required because the pressure is so high, the air will literally "whoosh" out of the catheter, providing immediate relief. Once the bulk of the air is removed, a syringe is connected and air is continued to be aspirated to maintain negative pressure. Oftentimes, the rip in the lung tissue is significant, and takes time to heal, or surgical intervention. In these cases, a patient may require a continuous suction device (Figure 18-5) to maintain negative pressure.

Hemothorax occurs secondary to a ruptured vessel in the chest cavity. This can be a life-threatening emergency attributable to both dyspnea and hemorrhage, and often requires immediate thoracentesis and surgery (Figure 18-6). Blood from a hemothorax, in the absence of chest wounds or a diaphragmatic hernia, may be used for autotransfusion (returning the blood to the vascular space) when blood products are not available.

A diaphragmatic hernia occurs when there is a tear in the diaphragm, allowing the abdominal organs (often liver, stomach, intestines) to move cranially into the pleural cavity. A congenital form of this disorder can occur as well, and may be an incidental finding, or a patient may present with an acute decompensation of

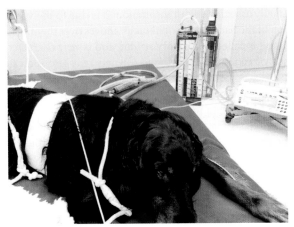

FIGURE 18-6 Continuous chest suction device, used to apply continuous negative pressure to a chest drain, withdrawing air or fluid to prevent accumulation.

the condition. The traumatic form is a surgical emergency, and may also be associated with a hemothorax or pneumothorax. Generally, thoracentesis is contraindicated in the presence of a diaphragmatic hernia, since the risk of contact of abdominal organs is high, causing contamination.

CHEST WALL DEFORMITIES

Chest wall deformities can occur following blunt or penetrating trauma to the chest. A flail segment occurs when multiple adjacent rib fractures are broken in multiple places, resulting in loss of chest wall integrity. When negative pressure is generated to initiate inspiration, the rib fractures result in an area that will move inward in response to the pressure change. The opposite happens during expiration, and the flail segment moves outward in a paradoxical pattern. Pain with each breath causes the patient to breathe very shallowly. The flail segment causes a general loss of pressure in the chest, reducing the effectiveness of each respiration. These two problems can cause significant respiratory compromise. Initially, providing adequate analgesia may encourage the patient to take deeper breaths. Analgesia may be systemic, usually with an opioid, and/or in the form of an intercostal nerve block, using lidocaine or bupivacaine. Secondly, positioning the patient affected side down will minimize movement of the flail segment. Surgery is indicated to stabilize the rib fractures in severe cases. Fixation can be performed internally or externally (most common) to stabilize the flail segment for healing.

A sucking chest wound occurs with penetrating chest trauma, causing air to rush in through the defect, when negative pressure is generated for inspiration (the sucking sound), and air may be pushed out during expiration. Again, patients require a surgical exploration of the wound, but in the emergent phase, placing an occlusive wrap over the wound (materials used are often plastic wrap or self-adhesive surgical drape) and performing thoracentesis to remove air from the pleural cavity (very important step!) will allow the patient to breathe more comfortably. If the patient has a concurrent defect in the lung, resulting in pneumothorax from within, covering the chest wall defect may result in a tension pneumothorax, and would therefore be contraindicated.

PULMONARY CONTUSIONS

Pulmonary contusions occur secondary to blunt force trauma to the chest. Contusions may not be evident initially on radiographs, but continue to develop (just like any bruise) over 24 to 36 hours following the insult. Because contusions are a result of bleeding into the lung tissue, they can worsen with excessive fluid resuscitation. Treatment usually consists of allowing time for the patient to heal and providing supportive care as necessary; however, some patients require more intensive treatments such as mechanical ventilation.

SMOKE INHALATION

Handling the animal that has survived a fire involves many factors. The owner can be experiencing a severe level of stress (having lost everything but the beloved pet). Often organizations are available to assist people in financial distress after such a catastrophe. Some veterinary facilities have established funds and specific protocols for this type of situation.

The type of injury is dependent on many factors (e.g., length of exposure, type of contents that were burned, and heat and intensity of exposure). Hypoxemia, pulmonary damage, and thermal injury are the three major concerns. The upper airway most commonly is affected by the thermal injury. Swelling and irritation to the mucosa can be severe. Lower airway complications are also common. A full physical is performed, including examination of the skin for burns or irritation, the eyes for corneal ulcers, and the nervous system for signs of abnormalities.

On presentation, immediate O_2 therapy is necessary. The animal may also have thermal injuries that need to be addressed and ash that needs to be removed from its coat to prevent further inhalation injury. Radiographs are taken once stabilized so that damage to the lungs can be reassessed during the days after the initial injury. Continued therapy includes fluid therapy, O_2 support, pain management, and care of abrasions and burn injury. Antibiotics are not recommended unless an infection develops. Nebulizing and coupaging may be indicated. Hyperbaric O_2 therapy has also been used to treat this injury.

AIRWAY DISORDERS

AIRWAY OBSTRUCTION

Airway obstruction is often secondary to a foreign object lodging in the larynx, trachea, or deeper in the lungs. It can also be caused by conformational and genetic factors, such as severe brachycephalic airway syndrome (BAS), laryngeal paralysis, and collapsing trachea, or secondary to anaphylaxis, such as a severe vaccine reaction or insect sting.

Patients with a complete airway obstruction may present in respiratory or cardiac arrest or with severe respiratory compromise. Fast identification of the obstruction is key to a successful outcome. Positioning the animal for endotracheal intubation may allow visualization of the foreign object and possibly its removal, or identification of severe swelling or laryngeal abnormalities. If the object is not readily removable, or endotracheal intubation is not possible, performing an emergency tracheostomy may stabilize the patient while the foreign body is removed or swelling is managed.

LARYNGEAL PARALYSIS

Laryngeal paralysis, often known as "Lar-Par," is a relatively common emergency in large, older dogs, most typically geriatric, male Labrador retrievers. It results from paralysis of the arytenoid cartilages of the larynx, and when viewed, the arytenoids, whose normal action is to open wide on inspiration, are found to not move or even to collapse on one another during inspiration, causing an obstruction.

Patients typically present very dyspneic, and can be cyanotic. They are frequently hyperthermic, panting, and panicked on arrival. Often they will present on a hot day, when panting to maintain body temperature causes them to become distressed. Owners may have noticed sound associated with respiration for some time, before the emergent event. This sound is very raspy and harsh, and

usually associated with inspiration; it is due to the vibration of the flaccid arytenoids as air moves over them. This sound is called inspiratory stridor, and is very characteristic of an upper airway issue. Owners may also indicate the dog's bark has changed, becoming more hoarse, raspy, or different pitched, and frequently note exercise intolerance, with increased stridor during exercise.

Paralysis may be unilateral or bilateral, and also put the patient at risk of aspiration pneumonia, as the arytenoids do not close properly to avoid aspiration. Emergency treatment is similar to other upper airway conditions: manage the airway, reduce swelling (often using corticosteroids), provide sedation (acepromazine [low dose] and butorphanol are commonly chosen), manage hyperthermia, and provide oxygen supplementation when indicated. Although medical management may be possible in patients with a mild form, in most cases surgery is recommended. Several surgeries exist to treat this condition; the most common is the unilateral arytenoid lateralization, often called the laryngeal "tieback."

BRACHYCEPHALIC AIRWAY SYNDROME

Brachycephalic airway syndrome (BAS) is another common respiratory emergency, frequently associated with hot and humid weather. Brachycephalic breeds are known to have hypoplastic (small) tracheas, elongated soft palates, stenotic nares and everted saccules, and increased resistance to airflow in the shortened nasal passages, all of which contribute to reduced airflow to the lungs. Adding a hot, humid day, or exercise, to this scenario can lead to a crisis. Similar to the other upper airway conditions, patients often present hyperthermic and tachypneic with increased respiratory effort, cyanosis, and hypercapnia. Respiratory noises include stridor (from swelling of the larynx and eversion of the tonsils and saccules) as well as stertor (the snoring sound associated with the nose and nasopharynx).

Emergency treatment hinges on active cooling of the patient to manage hyperthermia, often administration of a low dose of corticosteroid to reduce inflammation, and supplementation with oxygen (Figure 18-7). RSI is often required, and brachycephalic animals will often maintain an ET tube with minimal sedation for hours while they sleep. Aspiration pneumonia is also common in these patients and chest radiographs may be beneficial. Often, surgical revision of the airway to correct the soft palate, increase the size of the nares, and remove the saccules is indicated to minimize risk of future difficulties.

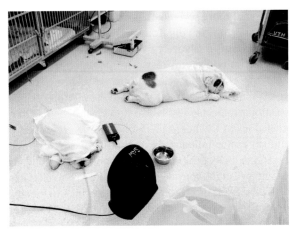

FIGURE 18-7 Two unrelated bulldogs suffering from brachycephalic airway syndrome. Active cooling (wet towels and a fan) works very well, as well as allowing to rest on a cool floor. Providing oxygen, as necessary, and administering sedation are the mainstays of therapy.

FELINE ASTHMA

Asthma is a frequent cause of cat respiratory distress. Cats present dyspneic, with open mouth, tachypnea, orthopnea, expiratory effort and/or cough, and auscultable wheezes on expiration. Occasionally it is difficult to differentiate between asthma and cardiogenic dyspnea, but generally coughing and normal or even elevated temperature can assist in differentiating asthma from cardiac causes, because cats suffering from cardiac disease generally do not cough and usually present hypothermic.

Emergency interventions include placing the cat in an oxygen-rich environment, often with mild sedation. Salbutamol is often administered as an inhaler, preferably through a feline "AeroChamber" and mask. Radiographs, once the cat is stabilized, may show the characteristic hyperinflated lungs.

PULMONARY EDEMA

A relatively common cause of respiratory distress is the development of pulmonary edema. Pulmonary edema can be cardiogenic or noncardiogenic in nature and, depending on the severity, can cause severe respiratory distress.

As the name implies, cardiogenic pulmonary edema is secondary to a cardiac condition. The underlying condition may be previously diagnosed, or may be diagnosed when the patient arrives in respiratory distress. Noncardiogenic pulmonary edema is not related to a cardiac condition and is a result of dramatic and abrupt pressure changes within the thorax. The typical presentation of pulmonary edema involves the sudden onset of dyspnea characterized by open-mouth breathing and tachypnea, serous or foamy pink nasal discharge, and hypoxia. Auscultation will usually reveal loud pulmonary crackles and wheezes.

Dyspnea associated with cardiogenic pulmonary edema is not normally acute in onset, although it may appear to be acute. Owners may have recognized a night-time cough, reluctance to lie down, harsh or rapid respirations, and general anxiety in their pet. Cardiogenic pulmonary edema is typically treated aggressively with furosemide or other diuretics, a reduced fluid rate, and oxygen therapy, although mechanical ventilation is indicated occasionally.

In contrast, noncardiogenic pulmonary edema is often a very acute event. It can be suspected in dyspneic patients following an inciting event such as a seizure, strangulation, near-drowning, or electrocution. Noncardiogenic pulmonary edema usually involves a high-protein fluid that is not responsive to diuretic therapy. It is also commonly referred to as "flash" pulmonary edema, which may give a sense of the acuteness of the onset. Supportive care includes oxygen therapy or, in severe cases, mechanical ventilation, and treatment of the causative condition.

If a pulmonary edema patient requires intubation, many times pink, foamy, edema fluid will immediately fill the tube. Suctioning the airway or "dumping" the patient (elevating the hind end and chest, to allow drainage of the fluid) will result in immediate improvement in the ability to ventilate the patient.

PNEUMONIA

Pneumonia can be a presenting condition or can occur secondary to several conditions. In general, bacterial pneumonia is the most common form in small animals. Other types of pneumonias include bacterial, fungal, viral, aspiration, and those related to irritants such as smoke, heat, and chemicals.

BACTERIAL PNEUMONIA

Bacterial pneumonia is often secondary to respiratory tract infections such as *Bordetella bronchiseptica*. Although this organism typically causes tracheobronchitis, the infection can become more invasive to the lungs, causing pneumonia. Diagnosis is typically by radiologic assessment, and the organism is often identified via diagnostic tests such as transtracheal washes (TTW) and bronchoalveolar lavage (BAL).

FUNGAL PNEUMONIA

Fungal pneumonia patients often present with a history of a worsening cough over a period of time. The fungus is usually slow growing, so respiratory signs progress gradually, until the patient is obviously having difficulty breathing. There are several fungi that can cause respiratory (as well as other systemic) illness. Most are soil organisms that are inhaled by dogs when they are exploring and sniffing the ground, although cats can also become infected. Most times, infected patients are immunocompromised, allowing the infection to take hold.

Fungi that may cause pneumonia tend to be geographically confined. The most common fungal pneumonias in North America include blastomycosis, histoplasmosis, coccidiodomycosis, and cryptococcosis. Blastomycosis is caused by the fungus *Blastomyces dermatitidis,* and is most commonly found along the Eastern Seaboard and Great Lakes regions of the United States and Canada. Histoplasmosis, caused by *Histoplasma capsulatum,* is prevalent in the Central United States, from the Great Lakes to Texas. Coccidiodomycosis, caused by *Coccidioides immitis,* is common in the Southwestern United States, California, and Mexico. Cryptococcosis, caused by *Cryptococcus neoformans,* is a ubiquitous fungus found in most environments, and spread by pigeon feces. Cats are more likely to become infected than dogs, and typically are immunocompromised with a concurrent illness.

Fungal pneumonias are typically treated with supportive care for the pneumonia, and antifungals. Infection can be severe, and mechanical ventilation may be indicated.

VIRAL PNEUMONIA

Viral pneumonia is not as common as other types of pneumonia; however, recently, canine flu has been a cause of severe pneumonia in some areas of the United States. Canine flu is caused by canine influenza virus H3N8, which mutated from a form that infects horses. It was first reported as a cause of canine flu in 2004, at greyhound racetracks, and has since been found in dogs within the community. This influenza virus acts similarly to human influenza, although it is not contagious to humans. Typical symptoms include cough, runny nose, and high fever, and just like in humans, some dogs

are affected more severely than others and may develop pneumonia, or even die from the illness.

Since this is a relatively new disease in dogs, most do not have antibodies and are easily infected. It is of the utmost importance to isolate infected, or suspected infected, dogs immediately upon arrival to the veterinary clinic. Isolation protocols must be strict to ensure the health of other dogs in the hospital. Testing can be performed to confirm canine influenza by submitting respiratory tract secretions, or two blood samples—one taken while the patient is ill and a convalescent sample 2 to 3 weeks later.

Treatment is mostly supportive; usually fluid therapy, broad-spectrum antibiotics (if indicated), and oxygen support may be required for pneumonia.

ASPIRATION PNEUMONIA

Aspiration pneumonia is a common emergency, and also common in critically ill hospitalized patients. It is usually secondary to profuse vomiting, vomiting or regurgitation while recumbent, regurgitation associated with megaesophagus or following anesthesia administration, or as a complication of laryngeal paralysis. Pneumonia occurs secondary to aspiration into the airways of contaminated, often very irritating gastric contents, causing possible airway obstruction, edema, bronchoconstriction, and alveolar collapse. It most commonly affects the right middle lung lobe but can also affect the cranial lung lobes. This pattern is usually diagnosed on radiographs as aspiration pneumonia. However, as is often the case, radiographic findings may lag behind clinical signs. Signs of aspiration pneumonia typically occur within 24 to 36 hours of the occurrence of aspiration.

Patients with pneumonia may develop pyrexia, accompanied by tachypnea or dyspnea, hypoxemia, and pulmonary crackles. Pneumonia is usually treated with antimicrobials (when indicated), oxygen therapy, nebulization and coupage, and supportive care. While mild pneumonia often carries a relatively good prognosis with appropriate care, severe cases have a guarded prognosis. The insult to the lungs can cause acute respiratory distress syndrome, which will greatly diminish the likelihood of recovery.

The technician's role in identifying and managing the respiratory emergency should not be underestimated. Veterinary technician's should be readily able to recognize life-threatening dyspnea, identify normal versus abnormal lung and airway sounds, and anticipate the needs of the veterinarian by preparing various life-saving procedures. Understanding oxygen therapy, using clinical judgment to determine need, and recognizing patient deterioration are roles with which technicians should be familiar and comfortable, and encouraged to undertake in their practice. Numerous respiratory diseases can cause profound respiratory distress in our veterinary patients. Although initial stabilization and collection of data will be similar with any distressed patient, the potential treatments can vary significantly. Having an understanding of the disease process will aid in comprehension of how the patient is treated, and ultimately the outcome of the treatment.

SUGGESTED READINGS

Byers CG, Dhupa N: Feline bronchial asthma: pathophysiology and diagnosis, *Compendium* 27(6):418–425, 2005.

King L, editor: *Textbook of respiratory disease of the dog and cat,* St Louis, 2004, Elsevier.

Lodato DL, Hedlund CS: Brachycephalic airway syndrome: management, *Compendium* 34(8):E1–E7, 2012.

Millard R, Tobias KM: Laryngeal paralysis in dogs, *Compendium* 31(5):212–213, 2009.

Steele AM: VIN/VSPN, Advanced Critical Care Nursing Course.

SCENARIO

Purpose: To provide the veterinary technician and veterinary team with the opportunity to build or strengthen the ability to quickly evaluate a typical respiratory emergency.

Stage: Emergency clinic is considered a level II facility (based on VECCS Facility Certification) and always has at least four staff members available including one ER clinician, two veterinary technicians, and one receptionist who also assists with animal handling when necessary. There is a back-up clinician on call to assist with surgeries.

Scenario

Saturday evening on the first hot day of spring
- An owner phones your clinic quite distraught. The owner's 3-year-old MN, English bulldog is panting uncontrollably, will not lie down, and is occasionally coughing, and then falling over. He immediately gets back up, and repeats the process.

Delivery
- Present the case to the staff, including receptionists.

- Using the skills of telephone triage, discuss questions to ask the owner.
- Complete the scenario with a recommendation to the owner.

Questions
- What questions should be asked of the owner?
- Consider it has been a very hot day, early in the year. Is this relevant?
- Are there any breed predispositions that must be considered?
- What major organ systems may be involved?
- Is it necessary for the owner to bring the dog immediately to the clinic, or seek veterinary care in the morning?

Key Teaching Points
- Provides a review of telephone triage of a respiratory emergency
- Allows the veterinary team to brainstorm on how best to handle this type of emergency
- Provides discussion on the major predilections, causes, and typical presentation of brachycephalic airway syndrome

MEDICAL MATH EXERCISE

A 42 kg Doberman Pinscher has presented with acute onset of weakness, syncope, and heavy breathing. On presentation, you notice his breathing is labored, he is reluctant to lie down, but is "wobbly", and his head and neck are extended. Upon physical examination, you note: HR 210 bpm with obvious pulse deficits, RR of 72 bpm, with crackles, his mucous membranes are muddy pink. You ask the client if you can take the patient to the treatment area to deliver oxygen, and have the veterinarian examine him there. The veterinarian orders pulse oximeter, ECG, and a 2 mg/kg IV dose of furosemide for suspected cardiogenic pulmonary edema. Furosemide is a 50 mg/ml solution, what volume of furosemide will you deliver to this patient?

a. 0.85 ml
b. 1.7 ml
c. 2 ml
d. 4 ml

Jennifer J. Devey

CHAPTER OUTLINE

Vomiting
Diarrhea
First Aid Measures
Physical Examination
Resuscitation of the Critical Patient
Diagnosis
Medical Treatment
Monitoring
Record Keeping
Anesthesia and Surgery
Postoperative Care

Specific Gastrointestinal
  Emergencies
  Foreign Bodies
  Esophageal Foreign Bodies
  Gastrointestinal Foreign Bodies
  Gastric Dilation and Volvulus
  Intestinal "Accidents"
  Hemorrhagic Gastroenteritis
  Pancreatitis
  Peritonitis
Conclusion

KEY TERMS

Diarrhea
Gastric dilation and
  volvulus
Nasogastric tube
Pancreatitis
Peritonitis
Vomiting

LEARNING OBJECTIVES

After studying this chapter, the reader should be able to:
- Learn how to properly characterize vomiting.
- Learn the differences between different antiemetic drugs.
- Learn the importance of nasogastric tubes in patients with gastrointestinal emergencies.
- Learn the fundamentals of managing common gastrointestinal emergencies.

Gastrointestinal (GI) emergencies are a common problem in veterinary medicine. Nausea (often in the form of drooling, gagging, or retching), vomiting, and diarrhea are usually evident in patients with GI diseases. Some of the signs associated with GI emergencies are more subtle, such as restlessness, shivering, abnormal posture, and crying. Anorexia may be the only sign in some animals, especially cats. Pain on abdominal palpation, which may or may not be present, typically indicates a more serious problem.

This chapter addresses the common emergency conditions affecting the GI system, including problems affecting the esophagus, stomach, small intestine, large intestine, and pancreas. Close attention to history, including accurate questioning of the owner, and a thorough physical examination are vital to making an early diagnosis, as well as ensuring the appropriate diagnostic tests are chosen, treatment is appropriate, and unnecessary expenses are prevented.

> **TECHNICIAN NOTE** The technician's responsibilities for the patient with GI emergencies may include taking a history, performing serial physical examination and laboratory analyses, taking radiographs, assisting with ultrasound examination, setting up endoscopy equipment, readying and assisting in the operating room, monitoring anesthesia, providing postoperative care, and ensuring treatments and supportive care are provided.

VOMITING

Vomiting (the active expulsion of GI contents) is preceded by signs of nausea (e.g., restlessness, salivation, repeated swallowing attempts), followed by forceful contractions of the abdomen and diaphragm, and expulsion of food or fluid. The act of vomiting is ultimately initiated in the medullary vomiting center, which receives input from the chemoreceptor trigger zone, higher central nervous system centers, vestibular system, and peripheral sensory receptors. Knowing which of these mechanisms is responsible for causing vomiting in the individual patient allows appropriate treatment to be instituted. For instance, if a dog is vomiting because persistent gastric distention was stimulating the peripheral sensory receptors, then it would be far better to place a **nasogastric (NG) tube** for gastric decompression than to treat the patient with a phenothiazine.

Vomiting must be differentiated from regurgitation. Regurgitation indicates an esophageal disorder. Signs of nausea do not precede regurgitation, and no active expulsion of food or fluid occurs. It often occurs soon after drinking or eating, and food is undigested.

Projectile vomiting is most commonly associated with a pyloric outflow obstruction or a complete proximal intestinal obstruction. This can be either mechanical, as in the case of a foreign body, or functional, as in the case of pyloric thickening or a mass (benign or malignant) compressing the pylorus. Vomiting of white fluid suggests a disorder of gastric or esophageal origin, and yellow fluid suggests gastric vomiting mixed with bile from the duodenum. Green fluid indicates the presence of bile that has come very recently from the duodenum. Both yellow and green fluid can be associated with pancreatitis. Brown fluid suggests reflux of fecal-like material from further down the small intestine. It usually has a fecal-like odor as well. Frank blood in the vomitus (hematemesis) typically indicates esophageal, gastric, or duodenal erosions or ulceration, although frank blood can be seen on occasion with jejunal disease. Black flecks or "coffee grounds" indicate the blood has been present long enough in the stomach for the hydrochloric acid in the stomach to denature (digest) the hemoglobin.

Vomiting should be characterized as precisely as possible in all patients (Box 19-1). The frequency and amount of vomitus being produced are important to note, because fluid therapy in these patients is adjusted largely based on the volume of ongoing losses. In addition, the timing of the episodes (as it relates to food or water ingestion, or administration of medications) is important to note because this will give clues as to the underlying disease and will help guide treatment. The presence of blood should be noted and an effort should be made to identify any foreign material that is present, because this will also help guide treatment.

DIARRHEA

As with vomiting, characterizing **diarrhea** is important in helping to determine the underlying cause (Box 19-2). The frequency and the presence of straining with the passage of feces, mucus, and frank blood (hematochezia) or black digested blood (melena) should be noted. High-frequency diarrhea is usually associated with the large intestine, as is straining and the presence of mucus. The presence of frank blood usually indicates colitis; however, patients with hypermotility disorders may have blood in the stool that is coming from the distal jejunum or ileum. The color of the stool, the presence of odor, and the presence of undigested food or foreign material should be noted, because these provide important clues about the health of the GI tract.

FIRST AID MEASURES

Owners often call veterinary hospitals indicating that their pet is showing signs of a GI disorder. They may report retching, vomiting, diarrhea, or a history of ingestion of foreign material. Some descriptions are very obvious emergencies. Nonproductive retching and abdominal distention in a 2-year-old dog are consistent with gastric dilation and volvulus; however, some problems are not so easy to diagnose.

BOX 19-1 | Assessment of Vomiting

Is it regurgitation (no nausea or active expulsion of GI contents)?

Is it vomiting (nausea and abdominal contractions/active expulsion of GI contents)?

Is it projectile vomiting?

Is it nonproductive?

What color is it (white, yellow, green, brown, red)?

Is there blood present (red, black, or chemistry strip evidence)?

How frequently is it occurring?

How much volume is being vomited?

What is the consistency (fluid, foam, fluid)?

When does it occur (after drinking, after eating, after medication)?

BOX 19-2 | Assessment of Diarrhea

How frequently does the diarrhea occur?

How much volume is being produced?

What is the consistency (e.g., watery, soft, undigested food, foreign material)?

Is there blood present (red, black)?

Does the animal have tenesmus?

Is there an odor?

TECHNICIAN NOTE In almost all situations the patient should be examined because many patients who seem to have a minor problem based on the owner's description may actually have a serious or even life-threatening problem.

If the owner declines to bring in a vomiting pet on an emergency basis, he or she should remove food for at least 12 to 24 hours and water for at least 4 hours. When water is reintroduced, ice cubes or several teaspoons to tablespoons of water (depending on the size of the patient) or electrolyte solution should be offered every 1 to 2 hours. The owner should be advised to have the pet examined immediately if vomiting recurs. If the pet does well with water for 12 hours, then several teaspoons to tablespoons of a bland diet can be offered every 3 to 4 hours. If the pet vomits after introduction of food, then examination is highly recommended. If the emergency call comes in at night and the owner refuses

to have the pet examined, then it may be appropriate to have the owner withhold all water and food and have the pet examined first thing in the morning. If the pet has severe watery diarrhea or diarrhea with blood in it and the owner declines to have the animal examined, then water should not be withheld but food should be withheld for at least 8 to 12 hours. If either of these more severe forms of diarrhea is still present after 4 to 6 hours, the owner should have the pet seen immediately. In all cases the owner should be advised that by not having the pet examined a more simple problem could become much more complicated.

If the pet has ingested foreign material or a potential toxin, it may be appropriate to have the owner induce vomiting at home and then either bring in the pet for examination and treatment or monitor the pet at home. Vomiting should never be induced if the pet has an altered level of consciousness or is having breathing difficulties. Inducing vomiting is also contraindicated with the ingestion of a caustic toxin, a petroleum-based product, or a foreign body that may get stuck or cause trauma to the stomach, esophagus, or oral cavity as it is expelled. Brachycephalic breeds also pose a high risk since their airways can be easily compromised.

TECHNICIAN NOTE If the owner is at all hesitant about inducing vomiting then the owner should be advised to bring the pet into the clinic immediately.

Refer to Chapter 25, which describes how to induce vomiting.

PHYSICAL EXAMINATION

Patients with GI emergencies may be stable, critical, or any grade in between. A complete history and physical examination including evaluation of all five vital signs (temperature, pulse, respiration, blood pressure, pain score) (Lynch, 2001) is performed in stable patients before initiating a diagnostic and therapeutic plan. In critically ill patients, rapid assessment is followed by immediate resuscitative measures; time may not be available initially to take a full history or to perform a complete physical examination.

Patients with GI diseases may have a concurrent aspiration pneumonia or metastatic disease, and close attention should be paid to the respiratory rate and effort, the ventilatory pattern, and the presence of cough. Careful bilateral auscultation of the thorax should be performed.

Assessment of the circulation should include evaluation of both the arteries and the veins. The jugular vein should be clipped and evaluated for distention and filling time when held off at the thoracic inlet. This may provide a crude estimate of venous volume, since approximately 70% of the blood volume is present in the venous side of the circulation. A completely flat, difficult to raise jugular vein is consistent with hypovolemia. Blood pressure (BP) is the fourth vital sign and should always be measured. Pulse palpation may provide a very inaccurate assessment of pressure since the finger detects pulse pressure, which is the difference between systolic and diastolic pressures rather than blood pressure per se. Normal pressure in stable patients provides a baseline in case the patient's condition deteriorates. If hypotension is evident, then it helps identify a more unstable condition that might otherwise have been missed, and aids in guiding fluid therapy. A Doppler ultrasonic blood flow detector or an oscillometric device can be used; the Doppler is preferred, because it allows flow (perfusion) and BP to be assessed. In addition, many arrhythmias can be detected with a Doppler. If the patient has any auscultable evidence of an arrhythmia or is unstable from a cardiovascular standpoint, then a lead II electrocardiogram (ECG) should be assessed. Patients with myocardial hypoxia or ischemia secondary to circulatory shock often have ventricular premature contractions or elevated T wave amplitude (greater than one fourth the R wave amplitude).

Rectal thermometers may induce a vagally mediated arrest in severely bradycardic or hypotensive patients and should be used with care in these patients. Rectal temperatures in patients with a dilated rectum may be very inaccurate because of the presence of air; the tip of the thermometer must be in contact with rectal mucosa. If there is a concern about the accuracy or safety of the rectal temperature, then axillary or auricular temperatures can be taken. If significant hypoperfusion is a concern, then toe web temperatures can be taken and compared with rectal temperatures. If the patient is perfusing normally, then the delta temperature (ΔT) should be less than 7° F (4° C).

The abdomen should be auscultated, palpated, and percussed with the goal of localizing pain and detecting fluid waves, gas-filled organs, or solid masses. Auscultation should precede palpation since palpation can cause gut sounds to diminish. A lack of gut sounds is consistent with ileus. A rectal examination should be

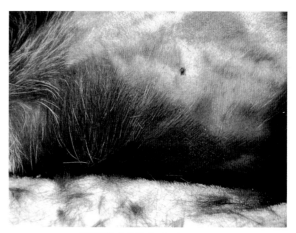

FIGURE 19-1 Ecchymoses.

performed and the presence of blood noted. The ventral abdomen should be clipped, because petechiation or ecchymoses (Figure 19-1) may indicate thrombocytopenia or a coagulopathy. Distended superficial abdominal veins are consistent with increased intraabdominal pressure, which indicates a serious intraabdominal problem and may be associated with decreased preload and decreased cardiac output.

RESUSCITATION OF THE CRITICAL PATIENT

Patients with acute abdomen secondary to GI emergencies may be unstable from a respiratory and cardiovascular standpoint; therefore, on presentation a primary survey examination (evaluation of level of consciousness, airway, breathing, and circulation) should be completed within 30 to 60 seconds, and abnormalities should be treated as indicated. For instance, an obtunded patient with shallow respiration should be intubated, and positive pressure ventilation should be instituted. Depending on the severity of the patient's condition, fluid resuscitation may need to be initiated before a complete physical examination is performed. A very brief history is obtained at this time (describe what is wrong in one or two sentences); resuscitation should never be delayed in the critical patient while a complete history is obtained. Permission to start treatment should be obtained from the owner immediately. This is frequently done by the technician while the doctor is completing the initial assessment. Resuscitation also should not be delayed while diagnostic tests are being performed unless those tests are essential to guiding resuscitation.

Oxygen (O_2) should be provided by flow-by at high flow rates (i.e., 3 to 15 L/min) to any patient showing signs of increased respiratory effort or shock. One or two large-bore peripheral catheters (14 to 16 gauge in medium and large dogs, 18 to 20 gauge in small dogs and cats) should be placed. A central line should be placed if central venous pressure (CVP) monitoring is indicated; however, this is rarely performed until the patient is more stable. Perfusion abnormalities should be corrected as quickly as possible. Fluids should be given until BP is greater than 100 mm Hg systolic, heart rate approaches normal for the breed or patient size, digital pulses are palpable, and the patient's mentation has improved. In dogs a bolus of 30 ml/kg (to a maximum of 90 ml/kg) of a buffered, balanced electrolyte solution, such as lactated Ringer's solution (Lactated Ringer's Injection USP, Abbott Animal Health, Abbott Park, IL), Normosol-R (Normosol®-R, Hospira, Lake Forest, IL), Plasma-Lyte A (Plasma-Lyte A® Injection, pH 7.4, Abbott Animal Health, Abbott Park, IL), and 5 to 20 ml/kg of a synthetic colloid (e.g., tetrastarch [Vetstarch®, Abbott Animal Health, Abbott Park, IL], pentastarch [Pentaspan®, Bristol Myers Squibb, Montreal, QC], Oxyglobin [Oxyglobin®, HbO_2 Therapeutics, Philadelphia, PA]) may be needed. Alternatively, if pressures are almost nonexistent, then 5% to 7.5% hypertonic saline (1 ml/kg) with a hydroxyethyl starch (3 ml/kg) can be given to effect. Approximately 70% to 80% of crystalloids that are infused have left the intravascular space in as little as 20 minutes intravenously, and therefore colloids are frequently needed in these patients because the volumes needed to resuscitate with crystalloids alone may lead to tissue edema (peripheral, gut, and pulmonary). Fluid volumes should be reduced by about 30% in cats, and synthetic colloids should be given over 10 to 20 minutes in this species.

Patients with SIRS (systemic inflammatory response syndrome) or sepsis secondary to a gastrointestinal problem may be hypoglycemic. The glucose level should be checked as soon as possible, and if the patient is hypoglycemic an IV bolus of 25% dextrose at 1 to 2 ml/kg (0.5 to 1 ml/kg of 50% dextrose) body weight should be given. The bolus should be diluted with crystalloid to approximately 10% to 12.5% before administration. This should be followed by immediately supplementing the fluids with dextrose, usually starting at 5% and adjusting based on blood glucose level measurements.

DIAGNOSIS

Diagnostic tests are needed to determine the extent of the disease and confirm the diagnosis. The choice of tests may vary, depending on the presenting complaint. Blood tests—including packed cell volume (PCV), total solids (TSs), blood urea nitrogen (BUN) or preferably a creatinine, and glucose—should be part of an immediate database. Ideally, electrolytes and a venous blood gas analysis are also evaluated, because these values often provide very useful information. For instance, a metabolic acidosis usually indicates altered perfusion, a hypochloremic metabolic alkalosis is consistent with a gastric or proximal duodenal obstruction, and hyponatremia often indicates significant third-spacing of fluids. All of these findings will help with treatment decisions. A complete blood cell count with microscopic evaluation of a blood smear for the white blood cell differential, red cell morphology, and platelet estimate provides important information. A more complete workup would also include serum chemistries and a urinalysis. Additional tests may be indicated depending on the underlying disease present (see Specific Gastrointestinal Emergencies). Coagulation tests (prothrombin time, activated partial thromboplastin time, or activated clotting time) should be assessed in all critical patients and all those requiring surgery. A fecal screen, including a direct smear to rule out parasites, clostridial spores, and a fecal flotation, as well as evaluation for *Giardia* should be performed on all patients with diarrhea. A parvovirus test is indicated in all young dogs with hemorrhagic diarrhea, especially if the vaccination status is uncertain.

Survey abdominal radiographs are usually indicated. A loss of serosal detail is consistent with fluid in the abdomen although upwards of 10 ml/kg needs to be present before this is consistently detectable (Henley et al, 1989). Evidence of free air indicates a rupture of the gastrointestinal tract (Figure 19-2). Contrast studies including a barium series may be needed. Barium should not be used if there is a concern for GI perforation or aspiration; water-soluble contrast material should be used instead. Abdominal ultrasound can be useful for diagnosis of some GI emergencies, but because ultrasound waves do not pass through air, the usefulness of ultrasound in patients with significant amounts of air in the GI tract can be limited. Abdominal ultrasound has been shown to be more accurate than radiographs in detecting intestinal obstructions (Sharma et al, 2011).

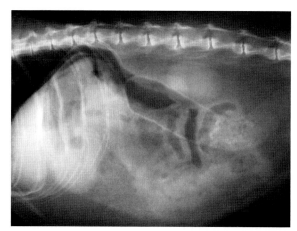

FIGURE 19-2 Pneumoperitoneum secondary to rupture of the intestinal tract.

Chest radiographs ideally should be evaluated in any patient in which esophageal disease or dysfunction, aspiration pneumonia, or metastases are a potential concern.

Four-quadrant abdominocentesis or preferably ultrasound-guided abdominocentesis is indicated if **peritonitis** is a concern. A diagnostic peritoneal lavage should be performed if the abdominocentesis is negative and there is a high index of suspicion for peritonitis. Fluid should be evaluated for PCV, TSs, white blood cell count, and chemistries (as indicated) as well as evaluated microscopically. Elevations in the levels of abdominal fluid amylase, lipase, or alkaline phosphatase relative to serum indicate small intestinal or pancreatic disease. A fluid bilirubin level measurement that is higher than the serum bilirubin level indicates a leak in the biliary tract.

> **TECHNICIAN NOTE**   A blood glucose level that is 20 mg/dl (1.1 mmol/L) higher than the abdominal fluid glucose level is consistent with peritonitis as is a blood to fluid lactate concentration difference of greater than 2 mmol/L (Bonczynski et al, 2003).

The presence of white blood cells with intracellular bacteria indicates septic peritonitis. The presence of vegetable fibers confirms GI perforation.

MEDICAL TREATMENT

Fluid therapy is essential in the management of patients with GI emergencies. IV fluid therapy is usually indicated; however, in patients that are not vomiting enteral fluid therapy may be appropriate. Fluids should be continued until the patient is drinking normally voluntarily. The type of crystalloid to be administered, the use of colloids, and the rate of administration vary depending on the patient's status and underlying disease process. Generally, replacement-buffered, balanced electrolyte solutions (e.g., lactated Ringer's solution, Normosol-R, Plasma-Lyte A) are infused; however, normal saline should be infused in patients with gastric obstructions if the patient is hypochloremic. Fluid deficits should be calculated on the basis of estimated dehydration (percent dehydration multiplied by body weight in kilograms equals the number of liters of fluid deficit). This deficit should be replaced over the first 6 to 12 hours in the stable patient; however, in the unstable patient it may be necessary to replace this deficit in 2 to 6 hours. Ongoing losses are estimated, and both the fluid deficit and the ongoing loss volume are added to the calculated maintenance rate. Glucose and potassium should be supplemented based on laboratory results. Potassium supplementation is almost always required unless the patient is receiving parenteral nutrition.

Synthetic colloids are usually indicated if the albumin level is less than 2.0 g/dl, if the colloid osmotic pressure is low, or if there is ongoing protein loss into the intestinal tract. A source of albumin may also be warranted in these patients although in larger animals the volume of plasma required to raise the albumin concentration is usually cost-prohibitive. Constant rate infusions (CRIs) of synthetic colloids of up to 20 ml/kg/day (pentastarch) or 50 ml/kg/day (tetrastarch) may be needed. Fresh frozen plasma should be provided to correct any coagulopathy. Packed red blood cells or whole blood should be administered to keep the PCV at approximately 30% in the acutely anemic dog and 27% in the acutely anemic cat.

Broad-spectrum antibiotics covering aerobic and anaerobic bacteria are indicated if infection is a concern and should be considered if patients have hemorrhagic diarrhea. Inappropriate antibiotic use should be avoided, because this can lead to bacterial overgrowth and severe diarrhea, as well as potentially creating bacterial resistance and nosocomial infection problems. Like all medications, antibiotics should be given parenterally in the vomiting patient.

Antiemetics are indicated if persistent nausea or vomiting is present. Antiemetics are classified based on the mechanism of action; therefore, knowing the cause (or possible cause) of the vomiting is important. Several classes of antiemetic medications exist. Phenothiazines (e.g., acepromazine, chlorpromazine, prochlorperazine) act at higher central nervous system centers and at the chemoreceptor trigger zone. They can cause significant hypotension, and BP should be monitored if any drugs in this class are being administered. Metoclopramide acts by enhancing gastric emptying, increasing lower esophageal sphincter tone, and acts centrally at the chemoreceptor trigger zone; clinically, metoclopramide appears to be most effective when given via CRI at 2 mg/kg/day. Anticholinergics act by decreasing GI secretions and motility; however, these agents are almost never used because even a single dose can lead to prolonged ileus. Serotonin antagonists such as ondansetron hydrochloride or dolasetron are very effective. Serotonin receptors are present in the chemoreceptor trigger zone, peripherally on vagal nerves, and in the GI tract; however, how the drug controls vomiting is unknown. Maropitant (Cerenia, Zoetis Inc., Florham Park, NJ) appears to be the most clinically effective antiemetic currently available. It is a neurokinin-1 (NK1) receptor antagonist. It inhibits binding of substance P (which helps initiate vomiting) in the chemoreceptor trigger zone and the vomiting center. Butorphanol is a fairly effective antiemetic that counteracts the nausea caused by certain medications (especially chemotherapeutic agents) and may help decrease vomiting caused by pain. Parenteral antiemetics should be used in most vomiting patients, because oral medications can cause vomiting and GI absorption is unreliable.

Ulcer prophylaxis is used in patients with evidence of hematemesis and potentially in those considered to be at risk for ulceration. This typically includes the use of an H_2-receptor antagonist or a proton pump inhibitor and sucralfate. Studies in dogs have shown that famotidine is the only truly effective H_2 blocker in dogs (Bersenas, 2005). Omeprazole and pantoprazole are two of the more common proton pump inhibitor drugs used in small animal medicine. An acid environment causes the drugs to be taken up into the parietal cells where they are trapped and converted to an active acid production inhibitor. The drug concentration increases steadily and does not reach peak concentration until 4 to 5 days into therapy; therefore, other antacids are indicated while these drugs take effect. Ideally all antacids should be tapered since rebound hypersecretion can be seen. None of these drugs have specific antiemetic properties.

TECHNICIAN NOTE Enteral feeding has been shown to be as effective as, if not more effective than, drugs at preventing ulcers in critical patients (Marik et al, 2010). Enteral feeding should be initiated early in these patients.

Many patients with GI emergencies will exhibit some degree of pain on abdominal palpation that can vary from very mild to extremely severe. The degree of pain exhibited will vary with the underlying disease or injury and the nature of the animal. Patients that are depressed may not exhibit signs of pain initially; however, once resuscitation has been instituted, the pain will often become evident. Typically the more severe the pain is, the more serious the problem. Pain should always be treated. Pure *mu* agonists such as fentanyl, hydromorphone, methadone, morphine, and oxymorphone are recommended. Butorphanol has mild analgesic properties but minimal cardiorespiratory effects and may be useful in more critical patients until they have been resuscitated. Buprenorphine is useful in cats with mild pain; however, it is not an ideal first-line drug because it has a delayed onset to peak effect and has a very high affinity for the *mu* receptor, making it difficult to override if additional analgesia is required until the drug wears off in 6 to 12 hours.

Pain medications should be given via the IV route, because absorption from subcutaneous or intramuscular sites may be unpredictable. In cases of severe pain, CRIs may be required. In the critical patient, doses of opioids may need to be reduced to 25% to 50% of normal because patients often cannot tolerate regular doses.

TECHNICIAN NOTE For those patients that are not responding as desired to systemic analgesics, a peritoneal lavage with a balanced electrolyte solution with or without local anesthetics added (lidocaine, bupivacaine) may provide significant pain relief, especially in patients with pancreatitis or serositis.

Nonsteroidal antiinflammatory drugs should not be administered because of their negative effects on splanchnic organs (and, in some cases, coagulation). Very small doses of an anxiolytic such as midazolam or acepromazine may be useful if the patient is very anxious. Acepromazine should be used with extreme caution in hypotensive patients because of its α-adrenergic blocking effects, which can lead to significant vasodilation.

Patients may be hypothermic, or may become hypothermic during resuscitation secondary to intravascular infusion of large volumes of room temperature fluids. Hypothermia interferes with normal metabolic functions, leading to altered peripheral perfusion, cardiac dysfunction, and interference with the coagulation cascade. Core rewarming should be instituted, because peripheral rewarming may lead to vasodilation and subsequent worsening of the hypothermia.

> **TECHNICIAN NOTE** Artificial-warming devices should always be insulated from the patient because they can cause burns.

Means of rewarming patients include the use of warm-water bottles, warm-water circulating blankets, oat bags, warm blankets, and hot-air circulating devices. Fluids ideally should be infused at normal body temperature in the hypothermic patient.

Appropriate catheter care is important in these patients. Peripheral venous catheters should be checked hourly to ensure they are patent and fluids are running appropriately, and veins should be checked several times daily for phlebitis. Saphenous catheters should be avoided in patients with diarrhea because it is difficult to maintain a clean, aseptic site. Central catheter sites should be inspected daily with care being taken to avoid excessive manipulation of the catheter, which can lead to irritation. If patients have indwelling urinary catheters, then the vulva or prepuce should be disinfected three times daily and antibiotic ointment should be applied around the catheter entry site.

Patients with limited mobility may require passive range of motion exercises and sling walking. Larger patients that are recumbent should be provided with padded bedding, and all recumbent patients should be turned every 2 to 4 hours. If silent regurgitation and aspiration are concerns, the head and neck should be kept slightly elevated (30 degrees) in recumbent patients.

NG tubes can be used both for decompression of the stomach and for delivery of enteral nutrition. NG tubes should be placed in all patients that are aerophagic, have a tendency to bloat, are vomiting frequently, have gastric motility disorders or megaesophagus, or are at risk for silent regurgitation and aspiration. Decompression is indicated in all patients in whom significant volumes of air or fluid are accumulating. Gastric distention is a major trigger for vomiting; if gastric distention can be prevented, then the frequency of vomiting can often be significantly reduced. Animals undergoing an exploratory celiotomy will not have normal gastric motility for at least 24 hours. Suctioning air and excess fluid not only prevents vomiting but also ensures that gastric motility will return to normal more rapidly (Moss, 1981). Suctioning is indicated every hour initially until it is determined that large volumes of air and fluid are not accumulating. Fluid volumes of up to 1 ml/kg/hr may be normal. Continuous suction devices are available if prolonged frequent suctioning is indicated. Once air is no longer being suctioned and the volume of fluid being suctioned decreases to less than 1 to 2 ml/kg/hr, then the frequency of suctioning can be reduced to every 2 to 6 hours. If large volumes of fluid are being aspirated, then electrolytes must be closely monitored because patients may develop significant abnormalities.

Enteral nutrition should be started as soon as possible based on the patient's underlying condition and clinical status. Initially, microenteral nutrition is recommended (Devey and Crowe, 2009). Microenteral nutrition is composed of electrolytes and dextrose (2.5% to 5%) given in small volumes. The fluid is infused via the NG tube starting at rates of 0.1 to 0.25 ml/kg/hr, either as a bolus or as a CRI. This rate is slowly increased up to 1 ml/kg/hr over 24 to 48 hours depending on the patient. Once this is tolerated a liquid diet can be provided via the NG tube, or gruel of small amounts of canned food can be offered orally. Microenteral nutrition can usually be started within the first 12 to 24 hours after admission. Glucose solutions delivered to the gastric mucosa have been shown to help prevent gastric ulceration, and may help improve splanchnic blood flow, thus decreasing the chance for bacterial translocation (Shorr, 1984). Clinically, the use of microenteral feeding appears to be associated with a quicker return to normal enteral nutrition. This may be in part due to preservation of GI function secondary to the early nutritional support.

When patients will not tolerate enteral nutrition, parenteral nutrition is indicated. Partial parenteral nutrition (comprised of 3% amino acids and glycerol [ProcalAmine®, B. Braun Medical, Irvine, CA] or 3% amino acids mixed with 3% dextrose) can be easily and relatively inexpensively administered. These solutions are hyperosmolar and are ideally administered via central venous catheters; however, they can also be infused via peripheral IV catheters. If peripheral catheters are used, the smallest possible gauge should be inserted to help prevent phlebitis. These solutions act primarily as protein-sparing solutions and do not provide total nutritional support. As such, they should only be used for short-term nutritional support.

MONITORING

The number of parameters being monitored, and the frequency of monitoring, will depend on the patient's underlying condition and status. If the patient's condition is critical, then parameters should be monitored every 30 to 60 minutes; in extremely critical patients, parameters may need to be monitored every 5 minutes or even continuously. In more stable patients, monitoring may be indicated every 4 to 8 hours. The technician is usually the person spending the most time with the patient; observations on how the patient is progressing as well as patient comfort are vital. As with all hospitalized patients, good communication between the technician and veterinarian helps ensure patient morbidity is minimized.

All signs should be monitored closely, including level of consciousness, respiratory rate and effort, heart rate, pulse rate, pulse strength, BP, temperature, mucous membrane color, and capillary refill time. CVP monitoring is indicated in any patient that has signs of moderate to severe shock, in any patient in whom large volumes of fluids are being used for resuscitation, and in any patient in whom fluid overload is a concern. ECG monitoring should be performed in all patients with arrhythmias or those at risk for arrhythmias. Fluid rates will need to be adjusted based on output, including ongoing losses, NG suctioning, and urine output. Intakes (ins) and outputs (outs) should be totaled on a regular basis. Patients receiving IV fluid therapy usually urinate at least every 6 to 8 hours. If this is not occurring or the patient is not producing at least 1 ml/kg/hr of urine when possible to quantitate production, then the fluid therapy is probably not appropriate.

Laboratory work consists of a minimum of measurements of PCV, TS, glucose, creatinine, and electrolyte levels, which should be repeated every 12 to 24 hours, and more frequently if the patient is critical or there are specific abnormalities that are being monitored. Ideally, a venous blood gas should be assessed at the same time,

along with serum albumin level in patients that are hypoproteinemic. IV fluids (type, rate, and supplements) should be adjusted based on these results. Complete blood cell counts and coagulation parameters may need to be monitored every 24 to 48 hours depending on the patient's status.

RECORD KEEPING

Continuous 24-hour care is ideal and should be endeavored in all GI emergency patients. The watchword is *diligent care*—from the time of arrival through the course of hospitalization. All monitoring and treatments must be recorded. A flowchart should be used to record this information in chronologic order, because accurately remembering what happened hours after the event is challenging.

> **TECHNICIAN NOTE** To decrease morbidity from factors such as inadequate fluid support, inadequate use of antiemetic drugs, and insufficient nutritional support, accurate and thorough record keeping is essential.

ANESTHESIA AND SURGERY

Some GI emergencies can be managed medically, and some warrant emergency surgery (within minutes to hours of presentation); therefore, the need for surgery must be determined rapidly. Acute abdominal conditions that warrant emergency surgery include a penetrating wound to the GI tract, a GI obstruction (e.g., foreign body, neoplasia), a GI tract accident (e.g., gastric or intestinal torsion or volvulus, intussusception), peritonitis, and vascular accidents. Valuable time can be saved if the technician always has the operating room ready in case emergency surgery is indicated. Ideally, at least three people—a surgeon, assistant surgeon, and anesthetist—are available to treat these patients. Balanced anesthesia with intensive BP monitoring (preferably with a Doppler ultrasonic flow detector) and assisted ventilation is essential. In the unstable patient, efforts should be made to use anesthetic agents that have the least negative impact on the cardiovascular system, and the anesthetist should try to keep the animal at the lightest possible level of anesthesia to minimize cardiovascular depression. Effective use of analgesia with IV or intrathecal opioids minimizes the general anesthetic needed, makes the patient more comfortable, and reduces patient morbidity both preoperatively and postoperatively. Many of these patients do not ventilate well under anesthesia and may need hand ventilation or mechanical ventilation. Positive pressure ventilation will help prevent respiratory acidosis (which can contribute significantly to hypotension), prevent atelectasis, minimize the amount of inhalant that is required, and promote a less complicated recovery.

An exploratory celiotomy consists of a ventral midline incision from the xiphoid process to near the pubis; this should be anticipated in every patient with a GI surgical emergency. The entire abdomen, including the inguinal regions and flanks and the caudal third of the thorax, should be clipped and surgically prepared to provide adequate exposure of the inguinal canals for additional venous access if necessary and extension into the chest via a parasternal approach if needed.

Every effort should be made to prevent hypothermia because hypothermia promotes vasoconstriction and poor tissue perfusion, decreases immune function, and prolongs coagulation time. This is especially important in intestinal surgery, because the intestine must often be placed outside the abdomen where it can rapidly cool to close to room temperature. Supplemental heat can be provided by various means; the patient always should be protected to ensure that burns do not occur. Patients should be placed on warmed surgical tables or on warm-water circulating blankets. Warm-air circulating blankets are effective at preventing heat loss and actively warming patients. IV fluids should be warmed before administration and kept warm during administration (by keeping them in a commercial warming unit or running the administration tubing through a warm-water circuit or warm-water bath). When the abdomen is open, the exposed organs should be covered with laparotomy pads or towels as much as possible to prevent evaporative heat and water loss.

Occasionally the technician may need to assist with surgery. An attempt should be made to set aside a set of instruments for closing (or a separate pack should be made available), because once the instruments have penetrated the GI tract, they are contaminated. Ideally, radiopaque gauze sponges and laparotomy pads should be used (Zeltzman and Downs, 2011). Sponges and laparotomy pads should be counted at the beginning of the surgery and then immediately before closure. Moistened sponges or laparotomy pads will be needed to isolate the affected area of the GI tract. Having the assistant insert a Poole suction tip into the stomach or intestine as soon as the incision has been made into the organ will help to minimize spillage of GI contents.

The abdomen should be irrigated adequately with warm sterile saline before closures. Usually 1 to 3 L is needed unless the patient has peritonitis, in which case up to 10 L may be indicated. Irrigation helps flush out any contamination, reduce adhesions, and rewarm the patient. The temperature of the irrigation fluid should be 100° F to 104° F. Neither antibiotics nor disinfectants should be added to the fluid (Schein, 1990; Schneider, 1988).

Ideally an NG tube is placed at the time of surgery, before the abdomen is closed, so that the surgeon can verify its placement. Otherwise a radiograph must be taken to confirm placement in the appropriate location. A surgically placed esophagostomy, gastrostomy, duodenostomy, or jejunostomy tube may be indicated for postoperative nutritional support.

Before extubation the oropharynx should be evaluated for signs of regurgitation. If vomitus is noted, then the oropharynx should be suctioned and strong consideration should be given to irrigation and suction of the esophagus to help prevent silent aspiration and pneumonia. Failure to remove gastric contents from the esophagus and pharynx can lead to inflammation, erosion, and possibly ulceration and stricture of these areas.

POSTOPERATIVE CARE

Postoperative monitoring should be performed as described previously except that parameters may need to be monitored more closely until the patient is normothermic and sternal. Patients ideally should not be disconnected from a ventilator until it is confirmed that the patient is able to maintain a normal end-tidal carbon dioxide concentration while spontaneously breathing. Supplementation levels of O_2 provided in the immediate postoperative period may help improve healing in patients that have undergone intestinal surgery (Pryor et al, 2004). Postoperative laboratory work in the critically ill or injured patient should consist of a minimum of measurements of PCV, TS, and glucose levels. Electrolyte, creatinine, and albumin levels also should be evaluated in more critical patients. Microenteral nutrition is started within 6 hours in the postoperative patient or as soon as the patient is sternal, normothermic, and normotensive.

SPECIFIC GASTROINTESTINAL EMERGENCIES

The following section deals with specific gastrointestinal disorders. It is assumed that the general principles discussed earlier in this chapter will be applied to these patients in addition to more specific recommendations noted in each section, based on the disease.

FOREIGN BODIES

Ingestion of foreign bodies is one of the most common reasons for the young dog or cat to present with a vomiting problem; however, animals of any age can ingest foreign material. Fortunately, many foreign bodies pass or are vomited without serious consequence; however, not infrequently these materials will cause a partial or complete obstruction of the GI tract, and endoscopic or surgical intervention is required to remove the material.

ESOPHAGEAL FOREIGN BODIES
History and Clinical Signs

Clinical signs are very important in the diagnosis of an esophageal foreign body. The animal may show signs of salivation, excessive swallowing motions, dysphagia, and apparent vomiting that on closer questioning will be determined to be regurgitation. Animals with an upper or mid-esophageal foreign body may have signs of respiratory distress, because the foreign material may be compressing the trachea. An increased respiratory rate or effort and harsh lung sounds may indicate concurrent aspiration pneumonia.

Diagnosis

Some proximal esophageal foreign bodies may be palpable. Radiographs and esophagoscopy can be used to locate the material if is not readily visible. Barium should not be used if a perforation is possible; instead, a low osmolarity, nonionic contrast material should be used. Computed tomography (CT) is more accurate for diagnosing esophageal tears than contrast radiographs, but neither will detect 100% of lesions.

Treatment

Perfusion deficits should be corrected before induction of anesthesia. The degree of hypoperfusion and dehydration present is easy to underestimate, and fluid requirements to maintain normal BP under anesthesia may be higher than expected. General anesthesia should be used, and a cuffed endotracheal tube must be in place. Suctioning esophageal fluid and contrast material will aid in observation and removal of the material, as well as in the prevention of aspiration pneumonia. Frequently the foreign material lodges at the base of the heart, and significant bradycardia may be present. Anticholinergics are often used, both to help decrease salivation and to help prevent clinically significant bradycardia.

It may be possible to remove the foreign body by the oral route using a rigid or flexible endoscope and a "mechanic's helper" (or mare uterine biopsy forceps). Generous amounts of lubrication (water-soluble jelly and water) should be provided. The lubrication can be placed at the location of the foreign body using a stiff polyethylene catheter with its tip placed at the junction of the foreign body and the esophageal mucosa. By gentle manipulation after lubrication, the foreign body is brought close to the end of the rigid endoscope, and all three objects (foreign body, grasper, and endoscope) are removed simultaneously.

If the foreign body cannot be removed orally, then it may be possible to manipulate it into the stomach, where the foreign body is removed via a gastrotomy. If it cannot be manipulated into the stomach, then the foreign material will need to be removed via an esophagotomy. After removal, a gastrostomy feeding tube may be placed to bypass the esophagus, allowing it to heal while providing enteral nutritional support. Some clinicians may prefer to use a small flexible esophagostomy tube with its tip distal to the site of injury or surgical incision.

GASTROINTESTINAL FOREIGN BODIES
History and Clinical Signs

History gathered from an owner is the most useful factor in early diagnosis of a foreign body. Early signs of a GI foreign body include nausea, vomiting, and inappetence. Vomiting usually persists until the material has been vomited, has passed, or has been removed. The character of the vomiting may help indicate the location of the problem and the degree of obstruction. Abdominal pain may or may not be present, depending on the duration of the problem and the degree of obstruction or the presence of perforation.

Diagnosis

The GI foreign body may be palpable on physical examination. Abdominal pain is a warning sign, and splinting during palpation often indicates the presence of a surgical disorder as does vomiting at the time of or at the conclusion of palpation of the abdomen. Survey radiographs will reveal radiopaque foreign bodies but radiolucent foreign bodies and linear foreign bodies that are not causing plication may not be easily seen. A significantly gas-distended loop of bowel may indicate an obstruction. Contrast radiographs may be needed to locate the material. Abdominal ultrasound is very useful at locating foreign material and has been shown to be more accurate than radiographs (Sharma et al, 2011). Loss of detail on radiographs suggests the possibility of peritonitis, and a sample of fluid should be analyzed as soon as possible.

Treatment

The patient with a foreign body may arrive in stable condition, in hyperdynamic shock, or in decompensatory (hypodynamic) shock. Fluid therapy should be guided by the patient's status. Many patients with intestinal foreign bodies cannot be stabilized completely until surgery is performed. In some patients, rehydration "lubricates" the bowel and allows the lodged material to pass.

Surgery is indicated in the vast majority of these patients and in all patients with significant clinical signs or radiographic evidence of distended bowel loops. If minimal clinical signs are present then a watch-and-wait attitude may be adopted. In these cases, serial radiographs should be taken to monitor the progress of the object. Extremely radiopaque foreign bodies should be removed immediately, because they may contain zinc, which can cause hemolytic anemia. Risk factors for dehiscence of intestinal anastomoses and development of septic peritonitis include the presence of preoperative peritonitis, low preoperative serum albumin levels (less than 2.5 mg/dl), and intraoperative hypotension (Grimes et al, 2011; Ralphs et al, 2003). Attempts should be made to avoid the latter two risk factors, and any patient with two or more of these risk factors should be closely monitored for complications. Postoperatively, enteral feeding should be instituted as soon as possible since this has been shown to improve healing, especially with intestinal anastomoses (Moss et al, 1980).

GASTRIC DILATION AND VOLVULUS
Pathophysiology

The cause of **gastric dilation and volvulus** (GDV) is not yet clearly understood. GDV has been associated with many clinical diseases and typically is seen in large, deep-chested dogs; however, it can occur in any size of dog, at any age. GDV has been observed in patients that ingest foreign material, in patients with chronic debilitating diseases, in patients with altered gastric emptying, in patients with neuromuscular diseases or respiratory difficulty, as well as in animals that are very nervous and require hospitalization.

Twisting causes a one-way valve effect at the gastroesophageal junction, allowing swallowed air to enter the stomach but not leave. Carbon dioxide may also accumulate secondary to bacterial fermentation, diffusion from trapped blood, and metabolism of gastric acid and bicarbonate from the pancreas and saliva. Normal fluid secretion into the stomach (as well as transudation from venous congestion) contributes to gastric distention. Subsequent pressure on the diaphragm from the distended stomach can lead to respiratory distress, which also may worsen the aerophagia. The gastric distention causes compression of the vena cava, resulting in a decrease in venous return that negatively affects cardiac output. Gastric distention also compromises gastric circulation, causing ischemia of the stomach. Rotation of the stomach can cause tearing of the short gastric vessels, which can lead to significant blood loss.

The distention and rotation of the stomach cause partial to complete obstruction of blood flow through the portal vein. The degree of obstruction is variable, but the liver, pancreas, small intestine, and stomach all become ischemic to some degree. Portal vein obstruction also contributes to decreased preload.

Toxic and vasoactive substances accumulate secondary to the ischemia. Ultimately, hemorrhagic, distributive, and cardiogenic forms of shock can develop. Reperfusion injury during treatment contributes significantly to the tissue damage.

History and Clinical Signs

Patients commonly have a history of attempting to vomit or having nonproductive retching. Abdominal distention may or may not be noted by the owner. The onset is usually acute. It may be associated with dietary indiscretion, such as ingestion of unleavened bread, garbage, or poorly digestible dog treats. A history of GI disease or previous episodes of "bloating" may also exist.

On presentation, dogs usually show some degree of circulatory shock. Ventilatory compromise may be evident because of pressure on the diaphragm from the distended stomach. Salivation, nausea, and nonproductive retching may or may not be present.

Diagnosis

The diagnosis is made based on the patient's history, clinical signs, physical examination, and radiographs. Abdominal distention may or may not be evident, based on the degree of gastric distention and the conformation of the breed. The gas-distended stomach will always be detectable on percussion of the cranial abdomen. Because the dog may be in hyperdynamic shock or in a stage of decompensatory shock, clinical findings vary from tachycardia, tachypnea, bounding pulses, and injected mucous membranes to collapse, respiratory distress, and weak thready pulses.

A right lateral abdominal radiograph will typically reveal a characteristic shelf sign with compartmentalization, supporting a diagnosis of a gastric volvulus (Figure 19-3). On occasion, the volvulus will not be evident on the right lateral view. If there is a high index of suspicion for a volvulus, then a left lateral radiograph should be taken in this situation. A lateral chest radiograph should be taken to help rule out aspiration pneumonia and metastases and confirm the degree of megaesophagus present. Positioning the animal in dorsal recumbency for a second view may cause cardiovascular decompensation and should be avoided.

In addition to standard blood work, a lactate level should be evaluated because an elevated lactate concentration has been shown to correlate with gastric necrosis (Santoro Beer et al, 2013). Trends in the lactate level may also provide prognostic information. GDV patients with an initial lactate concentration greater than 9 mmol/L, and whose lactate concentration did not decrease by at least 42% with treatment, were found to be significantly less likely to survive (Zacher et al, 2010).

Treatment

Treatment should be instituted before taking radiographs, unless the presence of a volvulus will lead the owner to make a decision to have the dog euthanized. Immediate treatment should consist of O_2 administration if the dog is showing any signs of shock, as well as volume replacement with crystalloids with or without synthetic colloids. Broad-spectrum antibiotics should be considered. BP should be monitored closely. A lead II ECG should be monitored, because these dogs are prone to ventricular arrhythmias (Figure 19-4). Ventricular tachycardia or premature complexes should be treated if the heart rate is greater than 160 beats/minute, if the arrhythmia is multiform, if there is R-on-T phenomenon, or if perfusion is being affected. A constant rate infusion

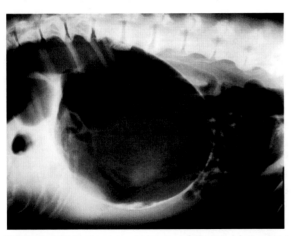

FIGURE 19-3 Compartmentalization of the stomach consistent with gastric volvulus.

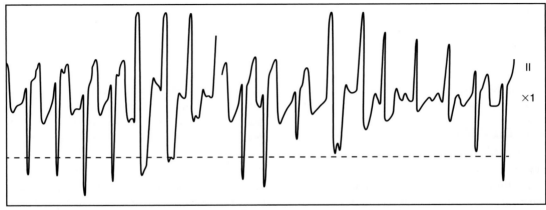

FIGURE 19-4 Multiform premature ventricular tachycardia.

of lidocaine or procainamide is typically used. Coagulation parameters should be monitored closely, because more critical GDV patients are at risk for disseminated intravascular coagulation.

The stomach should be decompressed only after volume replacement has been started because of the potential for worsening the hypovolemic shock. Gastrocentesis to decompress the stomach is performed using a 12- to 16-gauge needle or catheter. Percussion is used to identify the best insertion location.

Resuscitation is usually followed by immediate surgery; if the owner declines surgery, then gastric lavage may be indicated. Effluent that is bloody or very dark indicates the possibility of gastric necrosis. Until it is confirmed that the stomach has returned into normal anatomic position, the patient continues to be at high risk. Immediate surgery for GDV is indicated for several reasons. It can be difficult to confirm that the stomach is in its correct anatomic position without surgery. In addition, determining if gastric necrosis or active hemorrhage is present (usually from tearing of the short gastric vessels) or if the spleen is thrombosed (secondary to partial or complete torsion) is almost impossible without performing surgery. Gastric lavage can be performed before or during surgery; however, it should be remembered that passing a stomach tube through a twisted stomach is possible, so the fact that a stomach tube was able to be passed does not confirm that the stomach is in a normal anatomic position. It is also possible to pass a stomach tube through the wall of an ischemic stomach; therefore, excessive force should never be used.

INTESTINAL "ACCIDENTS"

Other intestinal disorders requiring rapid surgical intervention include intestinal intussusception, colonic volvulus, and mesenteric volvulus.

History and Clinical Signs

If seen early in the disease process these patients may only show signs of restlessness and nausea. Late in the disease they may have a history of vomiting, diarrhea (which may or may not be hemorrhagic), abdominal distention, abdominal pain, and collapse.

Diagnosis

Palpation in thin or young animals may reveal a tubular mass effect consistent with an intussusception; however, in the case of a sliding intussusception that may reduce

itself intermittently, diagnosis can be challenging. Colonic and mesenteric volvuli are not palpable. These animals generally are painful on abdominal palpation and significant splinting may be present. Gut sounds may or may not be present. Survey radiographs may reveal gas-distended loops of bowel; however, in some cases a contrast series may be required. Ultrasound is very useful for diagnosing an intussusception.

Treatment

As with all patients in shock, resuscitation should be initiated immediately. Close monitoring is required, because these patients often have a complicated preoperative, operative, and postoperative course. Surgical exploration must be done as soon as possible. Enteroplication (a procedure in which the small intestine is looped back and forth and the serosa is sutured to the adjacent serosa from the duodenum to the colon) may be performed on patients with an intussusception to help prevent recurrence. In the case of a mesenteric volvulus, endotoxic shock commonly leads to death; therefore surgery is indicated immediately on presentation if the animal is to have any hope of survival. Prognosis with mesenteric volvulus is grave but not hopeless with intensive care.

HEMORRHAGIC GASTROENTERITIS

History and Clinical Signs

The patient with hemorrhagic gastroenteritis usually is unmistakable because of the presence of blood (frank or melena) in the vomitus or diarrhea. A characteristic foul odor to the stool is also usually present. In the peracute cases, profound septic shock may be present. A bleeding ulcer (with or without perforation) may be the cause if the patient has a history of nonsteroidal antiinflammatory drug use.

Diagnosis

Because of the multiple causes of blood in the vomitus or stool, many tests may be required to obtain a diagnosis. A very dilated rectum is present on rectal examination in almost all parvovirus patients and is almost never present in other causes of hemorrhagic diarrhea in puppies. Parvovirus enteritis may appear as a surgical abdomen; fortunately, the antigen test is highly sensitive and specific. In the emergency patient the most important lab tests include those that assess the degree of anemia or hemoconcentration, a complete blood cell count, fecal parvovirus test, coagulation parameters, and radiographs to rule out the presence of a foreign body. Abdominal radiographs often reveal a small to moderate amount of gas throughout the small and large intestines, but a characteristic obstructive pattern is not observed. Free air indicates a perforation of the GI tract. A contrast series, endoscopy, and possibly exploratory surgery may be required to diagnose and treat the patient.

Treatment

The choice of IV fluid type and rate is based on the parameters noted on presentation, the degree of perfusion abnormality and dehydration, and the characteristics of underlying disease. In the patient with idiopathic hemorrhagic gastroenteritis, rapid boluses of crystalloids to restore a normal hematocrit and normal rheology may be required. Synthetic colloids frequently are needed because of the low colloid osmotic pressure often associated with this disease. In the poorly perfused parvovirus patient, colloids may be required as part of the initial resuscitation for the same reason. Because of the third-spacing of fluids into the gut that often occurs in these patients, it is easy to underestimate the volume of fluids required. Close attention must be paid to maintaining normal heart rate, normal BP, and normal venous volume. IV broad-spectrum antibiotics are usually indicated. Ulcer prophylaxis is indicated if hematemesis is evident. Plasma may be required early in the disease process to help replace albumin and to replace lost clotting factors. Red blood cell transfusions may be required if blood loss is significant. NG tubes are very effective at decreasing the frequency of vomiting in dogs with parvovirus and they allow for early institution of enteral nutrition.

In the case of severe gastric ulceration and bleeding, lavage of the stomach with ice water may be required. Some cases of GI ulceration may require surgical intervention, especially if perforation is a possibility.

PANCREATITIS

Pathophysiology

Pancreatitis ultimately is a result of activation of the pancreatic enzymes (proteases) within the pancreas, leading to autodigestion, as well as digestion of the peripancreatic tissues, and subsequent activation of the inflammatory process through neutrophil activation and production of cytokines and free radicals. If the inflammatory cascades persist unabated, then the systemic inflammatory response syndrome can result. Plasma

protease inhibitors such as the α-macroglobulins are consumed as the process continues.

Grossly, pancreatitis progresses from that of edema and saponification to abscess formation, followed by hemorrhagic pancreatitis and localized peritonitis. Secondary biliary blockage and necrosis of the ventral aspect of the duodenum can occur.

Multiple causes of pancreatitis have been identified; however, most cases are ultimately diagnosed as idiopathic. Dietary indiscretion appears to be a common predisposing factor in dogs, and cholangiohepatitis and inflammatory bowel disease appear to be involved in many cats.

History and Clinical Signs

These patients have signs similar to those of other GI emergencies. Anorexia and intermittent vomiting may be the only signs in cats. Dogs typically have a history of dietary indiscretion followed by nausea, vomiting, and anorexia. Diarrhea may be present. Abdominal pain is usually present; in mild cases, pain can be localized to the upper-right quadrant of the abdomen and in more severe cases it may be diffuse.

Diagnosis

The diagnosis of pancreatitis is not always straightforward and may be presumptive based on history, clinical signs, and physical examination findings of upper-right quadrant abdominal pain. Laboratory tests are useful but not pathognomonic. Although a leukocytosis with a left shift is commonly observed in more serious cases, there may be no changes in the white cell number or types in milder cases. Red blood cell morphology should be closely examined, especially in cats, for signs of oxidant-induced damage (suggesting depleted glutathione levels). Assays of pancreatic enzymes (amylase, lipase) do not provide any useful information in dogs and cats. Species-specific pancreatic lipase immunoreactivity (fPLI and cPLI) tests are sensitive and specific for pancreatitis in both species (Forman et al, 2004; Steiner et al, 2008) and both SNAP and Spec tests have been validated. Spec tests are quantitative and repeat tests may allow for trending of the disease process. Liver enzymes and bilirubin levels may be elevated. If the inflammatory process has progressed, then albumin levels may be decreased due to third-spacing. Blood gas abnormalities will reflect the degree of perfusion abnormalities as well as any possible secondary pulmonary involvement (aspiration pneumonia, acute lung injury, acute respiratory distress syndrome). Electrolyte abnormalities typically reflect a combination of dehydration and losses through vomiting and diarrhea. Hypocalcemia may result from calcium soap formation, intracellular shifts attributable to alterations in membrane function, or altered levels of thyrocalcitonin and parathyroid hormone. Ideally, ionized hypocalcemia should be assessed rather than total calcium level. Coagulation profiles (PT, PTT, platelet counts or estimates) are indicated in sick pancreatitis patients in order.

Abdominal radiographs often reveal loss of detail in the right cranial quadrant and displacement of the descending duodenum to the right with gas in the duodenum in dogs. Ultrasound can be very useful in diagnosing pancreatitis in dogs and cats, but false negatives are not uncommon in cats. Evaluation of abdominal fluid, obtained via abdominocentesis or diagnostic peritoneal lavage, for pancreatic enzyme concentrations and cytology can help confirm the diagnosis and rule out peritonitis. CT has not been shown to be useful.

Treatment

Fluid therapy is the cornerstone of treatment for pancreatitis. Measurement of levels of crystalloids, synthetic colloids, and plasma often is indicated. Opioids should be used as frequently as needed to control the pain. Constant rate infusions are often needed in more severe cases. Abdominal lavage clinically appears to help alleviate the pain, probably by diluting enzymes and other inflammatory mediators. The surgical management of pancreatitis is controversial. If the patient has signs of peritonitis or is not clinically improving after several days of medical management or is deteriorating, then surgery is indicated. Ideally an intestinal feeding tube is placed for nutritional support in all patients who undergo surgery for pancreatitis.

Nutritional management of pancreatitis is controversial. In the past it was recommended not to feed patients with pancreatitis for 5 to 7 days. Studies have shown that oral feeding can be provided as long as no clinical exacerbation of the pancreatitis is seen, and that by providing nutritional support early patient morbidity is decreased (Jensen and Chan, 2014; McClave et al, 2006).

PERITONITIS
History and Clinical Signs

Patients who have an acute rupture or perforation of a hollow viscus (gut, gallbladder) will often present with a history of restlessness, anorexia, vomiting, and abdominal pain. They will exhibit signs of varying degrees of shock, depending on the length of time they have been sick and the cause of the peritonitis.

Diagnosis

Peritonitis is definitively diagnosed by observation of bacteria on microscopic evaluation of fluid obtained via abdominocentesis (or diagnostic peritoneal lavage). Comparison of fluid and serum glucose and lactate concentrations is also very helpful. Abdominal ultrasound can be useful in helping to determine the underlying cause. Because patients with peritonitis may have many systemic abnormalities, complete laboratory work is recommended. Chest radiographs may be indicated to rule out concurrent injuries, aspiration pneumonia, or metastases.

Treatment

Fluid resuscitation, antibiotics, and analgesics are indicated. Antibiotic therapy is best guided by culture and sensitivity results. Before culture and sensitivity results are available, it should be assumed that a mixed infection is present. A complete exploratory surgery is indicated as soon as possible after diagnosis and initial resuscitation. Surgically placed feeding tubes are frequently indicated.

Depending on the severity of the disease process and surgeon preference, closed-suction drains might be placed or alternatively the abdomen might be left open. Open abdominal drainage allows for septic material to drain externally, allows for repeat evaluations of the intraabdominal disease, and, by permitting air to enter, decreases the survival of anaerobic bacteria. The linea alba is sutured in a continuous pattern; however, the suture is left loose, allowing a gap of approximately 2 to 3 cm (Figure 19-5). The incision is covered with sterile highly absorbent towels or laparotomy pads followed by an abdominal bandage. To facilitate changing the abdominal dressing, the laparotomy pads can be held in place by umbilical tape that has been laced from one end of the incision to the other. Suture loops are tied on either side of the abdominal incision approximately 4 to 5 cm from the edges of the incision. When it is time to change the dressing, the umbilical tape is untied, the dressing is easily removed, and a new dressing is placed. Placement of a urinary catheter attached to a closed collection system is essential in the male dog and highly recommended in the female dog. Open abdominal drainage typically is required for 3 to 5 days.

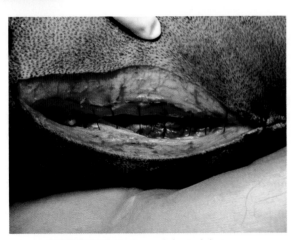

FIGURE 19-5 Open abdominal drainage.

The abdominal dressing is evaluated every 6 to 8 hours and changed between one and three times per day or when strike-through is evident. The dressing change is done aseptically and may require light sedation. General anesthesia is provided if the veterinarian intends to perform a second-look laparotomy. A second-look laparotomy typically is performed if the drainage from the abdomen does not begin to decrease in volume, becomes worse in character, when the initial repair performed or tissue viability was believed to be tenuous, or in cases in which deep intraabdominal abscesses, septic disease processes, or both are present.

Open abdominal drainage is associated with a number of complications, including significant hypoproteinemia often necessitating plasma transfusions, electrolyte abnormalities, hypothermia, ascending infection, evisceration, and additional costs associated with bandage changes and a second surgery. The amount of fluid lost through the drainage can be estimated by weighing the dressings removed and comparing this weight to that of a similar amount of dry dressings. The difference in weight of the dressings represents the amount of fluid drained, with 1 gram equaling 1 ml of fluid. The amount of protein lost can be estimated by measuring the concentration of total protein in the fluid and multiplying this number by the estimated amount of fluid drained. Fluid can be examined microscopically to trace the cellular changes within the abdominal cavity.

Closed-suction drainage provides an alternative to open abdominal drainage. After irrigation, closed-suction drains are placed in the cranial abdomen and the abdomen is closed. The drains are left in place until the amount

of fluid being produced is within physiologic limits and the fluid cytology, which is checked daily, shows no signs of active inflammation or infection. This method of drainage is effective and minimizes patient morbidity (Mueller et al, 2001).

CONCLUSION

Animals with GI disease can deteriorate very quickly, especially when vomiting, diarrhea, or both are present. Almost all calls from owners involving an animal with some form of GI distress should be considered emergencies. Evaluating this kind of problem over the phone is difficult, and what may be described by the owner as mild discomfort may be life threatening; owners should always be encouraged to have their pet examined. Surgery for GI emergencies can be very challenging; therefore the facility must be equipped with a highly skilled team to stabilize and monitor these patients throughout treatment.

REFERENCES

Bersenas AME, Mathews KA, Allen DG, et al.: Effects of ranitidine, famotidine, pantoprazole and omeprazole on intragastric pH in dogs, *Am J Vet Res* 66:425–431, 2005.

Bonczynski JJ, Ludwig LL, Barton LJ, et al.: Comparison of peritoneal fluid and peripheral blood pH, bicarbonate, glucose, and lactate concentration as a diagnostic tool for septic peritonitis in dogs and cats, *Vet Surg* 32:161–166, 2003.

Devey JJ, Crowe DT: Microenteral nutrition. In Bonagura JD, editor: *Current veterinary therapy XIV*, Philadelphia, 2009, Elsevier. (Electronic chapter: evolve.Elsevier.com/Bonagura/ Kirks/.)

Forman MA, Marks SL, De Cock HE, et al.: Evaluation of serum feline pancreatic lipase immunoreactivity and helical computed tomography versus conventional testing for the diagnosis of feline pancreatitis, *J Vet Intern Med* 18:807–815, 2004.

Grimes JA, Schmiedt CW, Cornell KK, et al.: Identification of risk factors for septic peritonitis and failure to survive following gastrointestinal surgery in dogs, *J Am Vet Med Assoc* 238:486–494, 2011.

Henley RK, Hager DA, Ackerman N: A comparison of two-dimensional ultrasonography and radiology for the detection of small amounts of free peritoneal fluid in the dog, *Vet Radiol* 30:121–124, 1989.

Jensen KB, Chan DL: Nutritional management of acute pancreatitis in dogs and cats, *J Vet Emerg Crit Care* 24:240–250, 2014.

Lynch M: Pain as the fifth vital sign, *J Infus Nurs* 2:85–94, 2001.

Marik PE, Vasu T, Hirani A, et al.: Stress ulcer prophylaxis in the new millennium: a systematic review and meta-analysis, *Crit Care Med* 38:2222–2228, 2010.

McClave SA, Chang WK, Dhaliwal, et al.: Nutrition support in pancreatitis: a systematic review of the literature, *J Parenter Enteral Nutr* 30:143–156, 2006.

Moss G: Maintenance of gastrointestinal function after bowel surgery and immediate enteral full nutrition. II. Clinical experience, with objective demonstration of intestinal absorption and motility, *J Parenter Enter Nutr* 5:215–220, 1981.

Moss G, Greenstein A, Levy S, et al.: Maintenance of GI function after bowel surgery and immediate enteral full nutrition. I. Doubling of canine colorectal anastomotic bursting pressure and intestinal wound mature collagen content, *J Parenter Enter Nutr* 4:535–538, 1980.

Mueller MG, Ludwig LL, Barton LJ: Use of closed suction drains to treat generalized peritonitis in dogs and cats: 40 cases (1997-1999), *J Am Vet Med Assoc* 219:789–794, 2001.

Pryor KO, Fahey TJ III, Lien CA, et al.: Surgical site infection and the routine use of perioperative hyperoxia in a general surgical population: a randomized controlled trial, *J Am Med Assoc* 291:79–97, 2004.

Ralphs SC, Jessen CR, Lipowitz AJ: Risk factors for leakage following intestinal anastomosis in dogs and cats: 115 cases (1991-2000), *J Am Vet Med Assoc* 223:73–77, 2003.

Santoro Beer KA, Syring RS, Drobatz KJ: Evacuation of plasma lactate concentration and base excess at the time of hospital admission as predictors of gastric necrosis and outcome and correlation between those variables in dogs with gastric dilatation-volvulus, *J Am Vet Med Assoc* 242:52–58, 2013.

Sharma A, Thompson MS, Scrivani PV, et al.: Comparison of radiography and ultrasonography for diagnosing small-intestinal mechanical obstruction in vomiting dogs, *Vet Radiol Ultrasound* 52:248–255, 2011.

Schein M, Gecelter G, Freinkel W, et al.: Peritoneal lavage in abdominal sepsis, a controlled clinical study, *Arch Surg* 125:1132–1135, 1990.

Schneider RK, Meyer DJ, Embertson RM, et al.: Response of pony peritoneum to four peritoneal lavage solutions, *Am J Vet Res* 49:889–894, 1988.

Shorr LD, Sirnek KR, Page CP, et al.: The role of glucose in preventing stress gastric mucosal injury, *J Surg Res* 36:384–388, 1984.

Steiner JM, Newman S, Xenoulis P, et al.: Sensitivity of serum markers for pancreatitis in dogs with macroscopic evidence of pancreatitis, *Vet Ther* 9:263–273, 2008.

Zacher LA, Berg J, Shaw SP, et al.: Association between outcome and changes in plasma lactate concentration during presurgical treatment in dogs with gastric dilatation-volvulus: 64 cases (2002-2008), *J Am Vet Med Assoc* 236:892–897, 2010.

Zeltzman P, Downs MO: Surgical sponges in small animal surgery, *Compend Contin Educ Pract Vet* E1–7, 2011.

SCENARIO

Scenario
A 2-year-old Great Dane that recovered from surgery for gastric dilation and volvulus has just developed ventricular tachycardia.

Questions
1. What is the difference between ventricular tachycardia and an accelerated idioventricular rhythm?
2. What four findings should be reported to the doctor as soon as they are noticed because they indicate that the dog may need immediate treatment?
3. Describe the appearance of R-on-T phenomenon on a lead II ECG strip.
4. List five treatments that are typically used to treat ventricular tachycardia. How is each administered in the ICU environment? What are common complications of each and how can each be addressed?
5. An order is given to start the patient on lidocaine at 50 mcg/kg/min. The dog weighs 70 kg. The lidocaine is a 2% solution. How much lidocaine should be added to a 250-ml bag if the rate requested is 15 ml/hr?

Discussion
1. The rate in an idioventricular rhythm is within a normal range for the breed—typically less than approximately 140 beats/min.

2. Heart rate >160 beats/min, multiform complexes, R-on-T phenomenon, significant pulse deficits or altered perfusion as a result of the arrhythmia.
3. This should be drawn with identification of the key components of the waveform.
4. Five possible treatments are oxygen, analgesics, lidocaine, procainamide, and magnesium. Other treatments are also possible.
   - Discussion should cover the various methods of oxygen supplementation (flow-by, mask, hood/collar, nasal), the pros and cons of each method, and ways to get the dog to tolerate any particular method if necessary. For example, if the dog is not tolerating nasal oxygen, then ensuring that the tip of the nasal tube is at the level of the nasopharynx, decreasing the flow rate, moving the tube to a different nostril, placing a second tube, and decreasing the flow rate or sedation might all be potential options.
   - Discussion of analgesics should cover the different opioids that are available with pros and cons of each with respect to efficacy, onset of action, duration of action, and side effects.
   - Discussion of the antiarrhythmic drugs should include how fast each is administered during the initial bolus, the serious side effects that can be seen, and ways those side effects should be treated.

Continued

SCENARIOS—cont'd

5. Various equations can be used to derive the answer. For drugs given in mcg/kg/min the following can be used:

   Convert all dosages to mcg/kg/min = Dose

   Convert body weight to kg = Weight

   Multiply dose × weight = N

N = number of mg (milligrams) of drug to place in 250 ml of diluent and delivered at 15 ml/hr

$50 \times 70 = 3500$ mg of lidocaine needs to be added to 250 ml

This is 175 ml of a 2% solution; 175 ml needs to be removed from the 250-ml bag and then the lidocaine should be added.

MEDICAL MATH EXERCISE

Patient order states: *Give 20 mg/kg cefazolin.* The patient weighs 8 kg. The concentration of cefazolin is 100 mg/ml.
   a. What dose in milligrams should be given?
   b. What dose in milliliters should be given?

20 Metabolic and Endocrine Emergencies*

Angela Randels

CHAPTER OUTLINE

Diabetic Ketoacidosis
  Definition
  Presentation
  Treatment
  Nursing Care and Monitoring
Hypoadrenocorticism (Acute Addisonian Crisis)
  Definition
  Presentation
  Treatment
  Nursing Care and Monitoring
Case Study
Hypercalcemia
  Definition and Causes

  Presentation
  Treatment
  Nursing Care and Monitoring
Hypocalcemia
  Definition and Possible Causes
  Presentation
  Treatment
  Nursing Care and Monitoring
Hypoglycemia
  Definition and Possible Causes
  Presentation
  Treatment
  Nursing Care and Monitoring

LEARNING OBJECTIVES

After studying this chapter, you will be able to:
- Provide an overall understanding of pathophysiology of commonly encountered metabolic and endocrine emergencies
- Familiarize the Veterinary Technician with common presentations of commonly encountered metabolic and endocrine emergencies
- Provide understanding of various therapeutic options and nursing care involved in treating common metabolic and endocrine patients

Patients with metabolic and endocrine emergencies are some of the most demanding and critical cases that arrive at the intensive care unit. With careful attention to details and patient monitoring, these animals can be some of the most rewarding patients to be treated. This chapter discusses diabetic ketoacidosis (DKA), hypoadrenocorticism, hypercalcemia, hypocalcemia, and hypoglycemia.

*The authors and publisher wish to acknowledge Richard W. Reid for previous contributions to this chapter.

DIABETIC KETOACIDOSIS

DEFINITION

DKA (or **diabetic ketoacidosis**) is a complicated form of diabetes mellitus that can have fatal consequences in dogs and cats. Patients with insulin-dependent diabetes mellitus have an absolute or relative insulin deficiency. Without insulin, the body's cells (except the brain, heart, and red blood cells) are unable to take up glucose via insulin-dependent glucose transport receptors (GLUT receptors) located in cell membranes. This creates an environment of cellular starvation. Starvation, or the perceived lack of glucose, initiates lipolysis (the breakdown of stored body fat into fatty acids) and promotes the conversion of the released fatty acids into glucose precursors in the liver via a process called *beta oxidation*. In states of starvation the body will convert these free fatty acids to ketones. But without insulin, the body cannot utilize the ketones as an energy source. Additionally, patients with DKA frequently experience increased secretion of the stress hormones, glucagon, cortisol, catecholamines, and growth hormone. These hormones are diabetogenic and promote increased gluconeogenesis and beta oxidation. The by-products of beta oxidation are ketoacids (i.e., acetoacetate, β-hydroxybutyrate, acetone), which eventually result in acidosis.

PRESENTATION

Diabetes mellitus in dogs can occur from 4 to 14 years of age, with most patients 7 to 9 years of age. Females are affected nearly twice as frequently as males. Diabetes seems to be common in poodles, miniature schnauzers, beagles, and dachshunds, and has a genetic basis in keeshonds and golden retrievers. There may also be a genetic basis for diabetes mellitus in cairn terriers and miniature pinschers. Diabetes mellitus can be diagnosed at any age in the cat; however, most are 6 years of age or older. No breed predispositions have been identified, but neutered males are predominantly affected.

Most cases show typical signs of diabetes mellitus for a period of time before diagnosis (Box 20-1). Polyuria, polydipsia, weight loss, and muscle wasting are common. Dermatologic signs include unkempt haircoat and flaky, dry skin. Some cats may develop diabetic neuropathy, typically in the form of a plantigrade stance, or 'hock-touching' in the pelvic limbs. Once the process of DKA begins the animal becomes severely ill quickly. A DKA

BOX 20-1	Most Common Clinical Signs Associated with Diabetes and Ketoacidosis

Anorexia
Dehydration
Dry, flaky skin
Ketotic breath
Lethargy/depression
Muscle wasting
Panting or Kussmaul type of breathing
Plantigrade stance (cats, usually)
Polydipsia
Polyphagia (nonketotic)
Polyuria
Vomiting
Weakness
Weight loss

patient will present with weakness, depression to stupor, tachypnea or Kussmaul respirations, anorexia, vomiting, and acetone smell to the breath. Table 20-1 provides a list of common clinicopathologic abnormalities. Careful evaluation for concurrent illness is essential, especially for pancreatitis (in which patients may have a painful cranial or right cranial abdomen).

TREATMENT

The major focus of the treatment of DKA involves fluid therapy and providing sufficient amounts of insulin to stabilize the patient's metabolic condition. Electrolyte, mineral, and acid-base status must be corrected concurrently. If an underlying cause is identified or concomitant infection (e.g., urogenital, skin, respiratory, abscess) is found, it must also be treated.

Intravenous (IV) fluid therapy is required in all DKA patients because of the dehydration that occurs secondary to diuresis from the hyperglycemia. If the patient arrives in shock, aggressive fluid therapy is required. Fluid deficits should be replaced over 48 hours in addition to maintenance fluids and ongoing losses. Fluid therapy improves cardiac output and tissue perfusion, provides fluid diuresis to aid in excretion of excess glucose and other retained organic acids, and helps to correct acid-base and electrolyte imbalances. IV fluids also dilute diabetogenic hormones, which will increase the effectiveness of insulin therapy once initiated. The use of an isotonic crystalloid fluid (e.g., Normosol-R,

TABLE 20-1	Common Initial Clinicopathologic Values Associated with Diabetic Ketoacidosis		
COMPLETE BLOOD COUNT	**SERUM CHEMISTRY PROFILE**	**URINALYSIS**	**BLOOD GASES**
Anemia of chronic disease	Azotemia	Bacteriuria	Acidemia
Leukocytosis (if infection present)	Decreased total carbon dioxide	Glucosuria	Decreased base excess
Polycythemia (if dehydrated)	(CO_2)	Hematuria	Decreased partial pressure
Usually normal	Hyperamylasemia (if pancreatitis	Ketonuria	of CO_2
	present)	Proteinuria	Decreased total bicarbonate
	Hypercholesterolemia	Pyuria	(HCO_3^-)
	Hyperglycemia	Submaximal urine concentration	
	Hyperlipasemia (if pancreatitis		
	present)		
	Hyperlipidemia		
	Hypertriglyceridemia		
	Hypochloremia		
	Hypokalemia		
	Hyponatremia		
	Increased liver enzyme activities		
	Increased serum osmolality		

Plasma-Lyte, lactated Ringer's solution) is preferred. Some advocate use of 0.9% sodium chloride as the initial fluid of choice, but the overall pH of saline is very low, and no buffers or additional electrolytes are present. If needed for patients with severe hyponatremia, the patient should be transitioned to a more balanced solution after 24 hours of therapy. Technicians should monitor all vital signs including lung sounds, respiration rate, and respiratory effort closely, to ensure that the patient is responding to therapy and is not becoming overhydrated. Fluid therapy should be provided for 4 to 6 hours before initiating insulin therapy in the DKA patient.

The initial insulin therapy of choice is regular IV or intramuscular (IM) insulin. Many veterinarians have a preference in the method chosen. The greatest control can be achieved with a constant rate infusion (CRI) of IV regular insulin at a rate of 0.05 to 0.5 U/kg/hr for dogs and 0.05 to 0.2 U/kg/hr for cats. An intravenous fluid pump is required for this technique. Changing the rate of the infusion will change the speed at which the blood glucose concentration deceases in the patient. Regular insulin should be placed in 250-ml bags of 0.9% sodium chloride solution at a dose of 2 U/kg for dogs, and 1.1 U/kg for cats. A buretrol may also be used. Insulin adheres to plastic, so 50 ml of the insulin solution should be allowed to flow through the line to saturate the tubing before starting the infusion. If using a buretrol, the entire contents should be allowed to flow through the line, and a new solution made. Insulin is damaged by

ultraviolet light and should be covered with UV protective bags (tin foil also is effective) and fresh infusions should be made every 24 hours. Insulin infusions are administered at slower rates than non–insulin-containing solutions used for rehydration. A double-lumen central line or a second IV catheter in another vein is preferable for this therapy (Box 20-2).

Another method to administer regular insulin is the IM route. The initial dose of 0.2 U/kg is followed by subsequent doses of 0.1 U/kg. The half-life of regular insulin is approximately 2 hours, and redosing will be needed every 1 to 2 hours initially, and then every 3 to 6 hours after glucose levels are controlled. Clinicians must consider the response to the previous insulin dose before determining when the next dose is given (i.e., if the serum glucose concentration is decreasing at an appropriate rate, then it would be inadvisable to redose the insulin, even if the patient is still hyperglycemic).

Care must be taken not to lower glucose levels too rapidly; with both IV and IM dosing, the goal is to have the serum glucose concentration decline 50 to 100 mg/dl/hr (2.7 to 5.5 mmol/L/hr). If the glucose concentration declines more rapidly, then significant complications may occur. The brain produces neurogenic osmoles (i.e., small molecules that attract water) in an effort to maintain adequate hydration in a hyperosmolar environment, preventing the brain from dehydrating or shrinking. Upon initiating treatment it takes time for these idiogenic osmoles to be removed from the brain. Rapid changes in serum glucose concentrations cause

| **BOX 20-2** | Basic Supplies Needed for Stabilization |

Selection of catheters suitable for long line or jugular vessels
Multilumen catheters
Regular insulin
50% dextrose
Potassium phosphate
Sodium bicarbonate (NaHCO₃)
Dexamethasone sodium phosphate
Desoxycorticosterone pivalate (DOCP)
Prednisone and prednisolone
Fludrocortisone acetate
Calcium gluconate 10% solution
Calcium chloride 10% solution
Furosemide
Calcitonin
Electrocardiogram (ECG; HP Pagewriter)
Infusion pumps
Syringe pumps
Blood chemistry analyzers
Blood glucose monitor

marked reductions in the osmolality of the blood. With the idiogenic osmoles, the brain then becomes hyperosmolar to the plasma and will attract water. This can cause cerebral edema, seizures, coma, and death. If neurologic signs coincide with a rapid drop in the blood glucose concentration, cerebral edema should be treated with mannitol. With either the IV CRI or IM techniques, after glucose levels drop to <300 mg/dl, dextrose should be added to the fluids to produce a 2.5% or 5% solution in order to maintain the blood glucose level in the range of 250 to 300 mg/dl (14-17 mmol/L) while continuously receiving insulin. It is vital to continue administration of physiologic doses of insulin in order to fully metabolize ketones. Since DKA patients are not eating, dextrose supplementation is necessary in order to keep blood glucose levels >200 mg/dl (11 mmol/L).

Once the patient has been stabilized, longer-acting insulin can be used. In dogs the initial dose is 0.5 U/kg once or twice daily. An initial dose of 1 to 2 U/cat once or twice daily is recommended for cats. Most dogs and cats will ultimately require lifelong, twice-daily insulin injections. Insulin glargine, a new synthetic human insulin analog, can be used once daily; along with proper nutritional management, it may induce remission of diabetes mellitus in cats.

Table 20-2 provides a comparison of insulin types and administrations. All insulin types (including regular insulin) should be refrigerated to maintain a constant temperature. Regular insulin does not settle, so it does not need to be re-suspended. Most other types of insulin will settle out and require gentle resuspension. All insulin should be protected from sunlight and ultraviolet light to prevent degradation. Bottles of insulin should be discarded after a maximum of 3 months of use, regardless of the amount left in the bottle. Most insulin is available in a concentration of 100 U/ml (U-100). Insulin syringes designed for U-100 insulin should be used, because they measure 1 U/0.01 ml more accurately than a 1-ml (tuberculin) syringe. Also available are U-40 (40 U/ml) syringes for U-40 insulin types.

Potassium supplementation is required in all DKA patients. Diabetes mellitus and especially ketoacidosis cause total body potassium depletion attributable to shifting of potassium out of the cells into the serum to replenish renal losses and to help offset acid-base imbalances. Treatment of DKA will result in a further decrease in serum potassium concentrations because of dilution from fluid therapy, insulin-mediated uptake of potassium by the body cells, correction of acidemia, and continued renal losses. The technician should measure serum concentrations of potassium before treatment, after initial fluid resuscitation, 6 to 8 hours after initiation of insulin therapy, and then following the recommendations in Table 20-3. If in-house serum chemistry measurements are not initially available, then potassium should be supplemented at a rate of 0.055 to 0.11 mEq of potassium chloride/kg/hr, or 20 mEq/L after initial fluid boluses (if needed), while waiting for pretreatment serum biochemical analysis. If hypokalemia remains refractory to high supplementation rates, magnesium level should be checked. Potassium levels will not normalize in the presence of hypomagnesemia. Potassium supplementation should be administered cautiously in patients with oliguria or anuria, hyperkalemia, hypocalcemia, or hyperphosphatemia.

Shifts in total body phosphorus concentration occur in a similar fashion as potassium. Therefore, treatment of DKA will also decrease phosphorous level via similar mechanisms as it does for potassium. Phosphorous levels may be normal initially, but will decrease rapidly after 12 to 24 hours of treatment. Therefore phosphate levels should be checked every 8 to 12 hours throughout treatment. Phosphate bonds are the main energy

TABLE 20-2	Insulin Types, Time to Maximal Effect, and Duration of Action for Cats and Dogs					
			TIME UNTIL MAXIMAL EFFECT		DURATION OF ACTION	
TYPE	ROUTE OF ADMINISTRATION	TIME UNTIL ONSET OF ACTION	CATS	DOGS	CATS	DOGS
Regular	Intravenously (IV)	Immediate	30 min-2 hr	30 min-2 hr	1-4 hr	1-4 hr
Lente	Intramuscular (IM)	10-30 min	1-4 hr	1-4 hr	3-8 hr	3-8 hr
NPH	Subcutaneous (SQ)	10-30 min	1-5 hr	1-5 hr	4-10 hr	4-10 hr
Ultralente	SQ	15-60 min	2-8 hr	2-10 hr	6-14 hr	8-24 hr
PZI	SQ	30 min-3 hr	2-8 hr	2-10 hr	4-12 hr	6-12 hr
Glargine	SQ	2-8 hr	4-16 hr	4-16 hr	8-24 hr	8-28 hr
	SQ	1-4 hr	3-12 hr	4-14 hr	6-24 hr	6-28 hr
	SQ	1-4 hr	14-18 hr	Not available (n/a)	n/a	n/a

TABLE 20-3	Potassium Supplementation Recommendations for Diabetic Patients		
	AMOUNT TO SUPPLEMENT		
SERUM KCL (mEq/L)	mEq (mmol) KCL/L*	mEq (mmol) KCL/kg/hr	
>3.5	20	0.055	
3.0-3.5	30	0.083	
2.5-3.0	40	0.110	
2.0-2.5	60	0.165	
<2.0	80	0.220	

*Amount supplemented to 1 L of fluids if delivered at a maintenance rate of 30 ml/lb/day.

storage vehicles for cells (especially red blood cells [RBCs], skeletal muscle, and brain), and phosphorus is important for the role of 2,3-diphosphoglycerol in oxygen dissociation in the RBC. Most canine and feline patients have normal serum phosphorous and phosphate concentrations and should be supplemented with 0.01 to 0.03 mmol of phosphate/kg/hr for 6 to 24 hours in the IV fluids.

> TECHNICIAN NOTE Calcium-containing fluids (lactated Ringer's) should not be used for administering phosphorus because of the risk of precipitation.

Dogs and cats with a phosphorous concentration of 1.5 mg/dl or less will require 0.03 to 0.12 mmol of phosphate/kg/hr. Close monitoring is required for these patients (see following). Phosphate supplementation should be avoided in patients with oliguria or anuria, hyperphosphatemia, hypocalcemia, or hyperkalemia. Potassium phosphate is the most common choice for phosphate supplementation, and it is important to realize this is also a source of potassium that should be considered in the supplementation plan.

IV bicarbonate (HCO_3^-) therapy is controversial. Acidosis in most DKA patients will improve with insulin and fluid therapy alone as ketones are metabolized. If the plasma HCO_3^- concentration remains 11 mEq/L or less, or total venous carbon dioxide (CO_2) concentration is 12 mEq/L or less (total $CO_2 - 1 =$ plasma HCO_3^- concentration), HCO_3^- therapy can be considered, especially if the venous blood pH is 7.1 or less. Bicarbonate therapy should only be utilized if venous blood gases can be monitored serially. The amount of HCO_3^- (in milliequivalents) needed to correct the acidosis to a plasma HCO_3^- of 12 mEq/L over a 6- to 8-hour period is as follows:

$$\text{mEq } HCO_3^- = BW_{kg} \times 0.4 \times (12 - \text{patient's } HCO_3^- \text{ [mEq/L]}) \times 0.5$$

where BW_{kg} is the body weight in kilograms. Bolusing HCO_3^- is not advised under any circumstances. The acid-base status needs to be rechecked 6 hours after starting the HCO_3^- infusion. Bicarbonate therapy should be discontinued when the pH reaches 7.2 in order to prevent iatrogenic metabolic alkalosis.

Antibiotics should be used as needed based on signs of infection. Urogenital tract infections are most common; sampling the urine for culture before antibiotic therapy is advised.

NURSING CARE AND MONITORING

Most of the monitoring of a DKA patient involves evaluating the response to treatment and identifying common complications early in the treatment process. These patients should be weighed twice daily to monitor hydration and ensure they do not gain too much weight in the form of water (more than the estimated dehydration, 1 L = 1 kg = 2.2 lb), indicating overhydration. Monitoring of respiration rate and effort and lung sounds will assist in preventing volume overload. Urine output should be closely monitored, especially if the patient is azotemic. Urine output should be 1 to 2 ml/kg/hr minimally in patients receiving IV fluid therapy. Due to osmotic diuresis that occurs in DKA patients, urine production may exceed these rates, and excess losses through urine, vomiting, diarrhea, or other causes must be replaced.

Electrolytes should be measured every 4 to 8 hours initially, and at minimum of twice a day after stabilization throughout treatment. Decreases in the potassium or phosphorous concentrations should be addressed promptly to prevent a crisis from occurring. The acid-base status should be closely monitored, and in patients with severe disturbances, venous blood gases should be monitored every 6 hours until stable, then one to two times daily.

Urine concentration (urine specific gravity [USG]) should be monitored and a packed cell volume (PCV) should be determined once or twice daily. Changes in urine or serum color should be noted and brought to the attention of the veterinarian. Severe hypophosphatemia causes the membranes of RBCs to destabilize and can result in a rapid, acute hemolysis. This will manifest as hemoglobinuria, hemolyzed serum, and a rapidly decreasing PCV. The urine should also be checked daily for ketones. The separated serum or plasma can also be used with a urine dipstick in a similar fashion to check for ketonemia. Small human blood ketone meters are now available that have been validated to monitor ketones (β-hydroxybutyric acid only) in veterinary patients. These work similarly to a blood glucose monitor. Ketones may persist for 1 to 5 days after initiating treatment. Because urinary tract infections are very common in patients with diabetes mellitus, signs of bacterial infection should be carefully noted (e.g., foul odor, cloudiness, hematuria, stranguria) on a daily basis. Urine culture is recommended on all DKA patients regardless of the presence of pyuria.

Blood glucose level should be monitored every 2 hours. Initially in some severely affected patients, taking measurements every hour may be required to ensure that the blood glucose concentration is not decreasing too rapidly. The ideal rate of decline in the blood glucose concentration is 50 to 100 mg/dl/hr. Blood glucose levels in the DKA patient should not be decreased to lower than 200 mg/dl and can be maintained by supplementation of dextrose. As previously mentioned, if the blood glucose level drops too quickly, then cerebral edema may occur; therefore careful attention must be paid to the animal's mental status. Once the patient is eating, then it should be fed. Typically once the patient is eating it may be transitioned to a long-acting insulin.

> *TECHNICIAN NOTE* If more than one blood glucose monitor is available in your practice, a glucometer should be assigned to the DKA patient, to ensure the readings are performed on the same monitor each time.

With careful monitoring and anticipation of complications, DKA patients can do quite well. No two DKA patients are the same, and nothing is routine about this disease.

HYPOADRENOCORTICISM (ACUTE ADDISONIAN CRISIS)

DEFINITION

Hypoadrenocorticism (Addison's disease) is a deficiency in the production of mineralocorticoids (aldosterone), glucocorticoids (cortisol), or both, by the adrenal glands. Destruction of the adrenal gland by immune-mediated causes is the likely etiology of most cases of primary hypoadrenocorticism. Iatrogenic hypoadrenocorticism occurs if the adrenal cortex is destroyed by mitotane (Lysodren). Secondary hypoadrenocorticism, which is decreased production of adrenocorticotropic hormone (ACTH) by the pituitary gland, causes glucocorticoid deficiency only. Iatrogenic secondary hypoadrenocorticism occurs when a sudden withdrawal of exogenous high-dose or long-term glucocorticoid therapy occurs.

Mineralocorticoids (aldosterone) are important in regulating body electrolyte status. Aldosterone promotes sodium and chloride reabsorption in exchange for potassium and hydrogen ions in the connecting segment and the collecting tubules of the renal nephron. Free water travels with the sodium. A lack of aldosterone results in sodium, chloride, and free water loss in the urine with retention of potassium, hydrogen ions, and calcium. The resultant severe electrolyte imbalances and dehydration contribute to the shock and cardiac effects seen in an addisonian crisis.

Glucocorticoids (cortisol) are important for many body systems. Gastrointestinal (GI) integrity and prevention of shock are primary functions of cortisol. Lack of cortisol results in loss of GI integrity, and lack of ability to prevent shock. Poor vascular perfusion of the intestinal mucosa, decreased mucous production, and GI ulceration may be seen. Glucocorticoids are also important gluconeogenic hormones and are one of the four primary stress hormones.

PRESENTATION

Hypoadrenocorticism is considered an uncommon disease of dogs and an extremely rare disease in the cat. Both species are treated similarly. The disease is generally seen in young dogs (mean, 4 to 4.5 years; range, 2 months to 12 years) and middle-aged cats. In dogs, 70% to 85% of those affected are female. There appear to be no breed predilections in the cat; however, with dogs, Standard Poodles, Great Danes, Portuguese water dogs, Rottweilers, West Highland white terriers, and Wheaton terriers are at increased risk. The disease appears to be inherited in Standard Poodles and Leonbergers.

Clinical signs and symptoms are variable (Table 20-4), ranging from mild signs to severe or fatal signs with acute crisis. The patient history may reveal a waxing and waning course. The most common signs in the dog are anorexia, vomiting, lethargy or depression, and weakness. Some patients also have weight loss, diarrhea, melena, shaking and shivering, polyuria, and polydipsia. In cats, lethargy, anorexia, vomiting, weight loss, polyuria, and polydipsia are the most common clinical signs.

Dogs in addisonian crisis often arrive at the clinic depressed and dehydrated. They have pale, tacky oral mucous membranes with slow capillary refill time, or they may present with hyperemic mucous membranes with a fast capillary refill time. In severely affected patients, shock, collapse, coma, and seizures can occur.

TABLE 20-4	Clinical Signs Associated with Hypoadrenocorticism and Addisonian Crisis	
MOST COMMON (50%-100% OF PATIENTS)	**FREQUENT (25%-50% OF PATIENTS)**	**INFREQUENT (<25% OF PATIENTS)**
Anorexia	Collapse	Bradycardia (<60 bpm)
Lethargy/ depression	Dehydration	Hair loss
Vomiting	Diarrhea	Melena
Weakness	Hypothermia	Painful abdomen
Weight loss	Polydipsia	Weak pulses
	Polyuria	
	Previous response to therapy	
	Shaking	
	Slow capillary refill time	
	Waxing/waning course	

Weak pulses and bradycardia, due to hyperkalemia, are a red flag of Addison's disease because a dog without adrenal compromise that presents in shock would demonstrate tachycardia. An electrocardiogram (ECG) in patients with hyperkalemia may reveal tall and spiked T waves with a narrow base (Figure 20-1). The QRS complexes become widened and the P-R interval increases as potassium levels rise. Eventually the P waves become smaller and wider and, in severe hyperkalemia, will disappear altogether (i.e., atrial standstill). Severely hyperkalemic patients may have QRS-T fusion, resulting in a wide complex idioventricular arrhythmia followed by ventricular fibrillation and asystole. A similar clinical presentation has been reported in the cat. Because many of the presenting signs of an addisonian crisis are nonspecific signs, severe GI disease, renal disease, and whipworm infestation must be ruled out. Table 20-5 provides a review of common clinicopathologic abnormalities.

TREATMENT

Patients in acute crisis or presenting with a significant number of clinical signs require hospitalization and aggressive treatment. Patients with subtle or mild signs can be treated on an outpatient basis. The primary goals are to rapidly treat shock, replace depleted fluid volume, correct electrolyte status, and provide hormone replacement therapy. (See Box 20-2 for a list of supplies required for managing a patient with hypoadrenocorticism in a well-equipped emergency facility.)

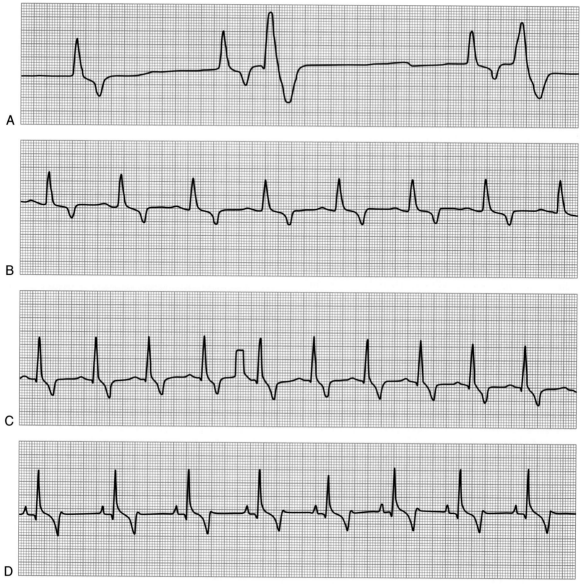

A

B

C

D

FIGURE 20-1 The ECGs of two dogs (dog 1, **A-D**; dog 2, **E-G**) with hyperkalemia caused by Addison's disease. In tracings **A** and **E,** the effects of severe hyperkalemia (8.6 and 9.4 mEq/L, respectively) exhibit a lack of visible P waves, short and wide QRS complexes, and slow heart rate. The reader should note that the T waves are not of excessive amplitude. Tracing **A** also demonstrates ventricular escape beats, which are the wide and bizarre-looking QRS complexes after the more normal-appearing QRS complexes. Hyperkalemia, hypoxia, or both may cause this. Tracings **B** and **F** were obtained after treating each dog for 1 hour with IV 0.9% saline solution as the only treatment, which lowered the serum potassium concentration to 7.6 and 7.9 mEq/L, respectively. The reader should note that the P waves have begun to return, the heart rate has increased, and the ventricular escape beats have disappeared. In addition, the prolonged P-R interval (first-degree heart block) improved, but QRS complexes still widened and the Q-T segment shortened. Tracings **C** and **G** were collected when the serum potassium concentrations were 6.2 and 5.9 mEq/L, respectively. The P-R interval and P, QRS, and T waves are of a shorter duration, and the R waves are taller. Tracing **D** demonstrates a more spiked T wave. This serum potassium concentration was 5.6 mEq/L.

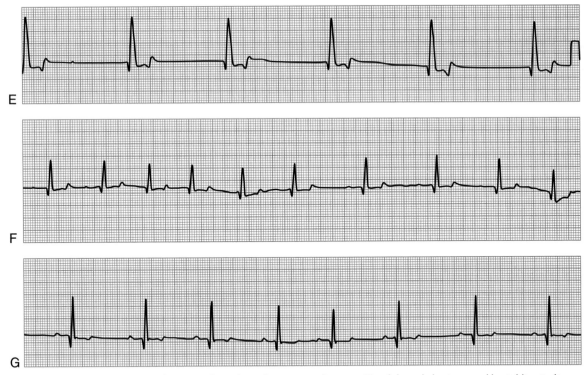

E

F

G

FIGURE 20-1, cont'd The ECGs of two dogs (dog 1, **A-D**; dog 2, **E-G**) with hyperkalemia caused by Addison's disease.

TABLE 20-5	Clinicopathologic Findings in Patients with Hypoadrenocorticism	
MOST COMMON (50%-100% OF PATIENTS)	**FREQUENT (25%-50% OF PATIENTS)**	**INFREQUENT (<25% OF PATIENTS)**
Azotemia	Anemia	Eosinophilia
Hyperkalemia	Decreased total carbon dioxide (CO_2)	Hyperbilirubinemia
Hyponatremia	Hypercalcemia	Hypoglycemia
Sodium/potassium ratio <27	Hypochloremia	Lymphocytosis
Submaximal urine concentration	Increased liver enzyme activities (alanine amino aminotransferase and aspartate aminotransferase)	

Correcting hypovolemia and hypotension and addressing electrolyte imbalances are the most important primary goals. The fluid of choice is 0.9% sodium chloride administered at a maintenance volume plus dehydration deficit volume (percent of dehydration multiplied by body weight in kilograms) over a 24-hour period. Shock doses of fluids may be required in incremental doses of 20 ml/kg (dogs) and 10 ml/kg (cats) to effect, or until maximum shock doses are reached (60 to 90 ml/kg for dogs; 40 to 60 ml/kg for cats).

TECHNICIAN NOTE As always, when administering fluid boluses the technician must be continually monitoring the response to fluid therapy. It can be positive (desired), with decrease in heart rate and improvement in perfusion parameters, or negative, with the patient becoming nauseous or uncomfortable, panting, and more distressed.

Initially, parenteral administration of glucocorticoids is advised, and electrolyte and mineral derangements can be addressed through IV fluid therapy. Once the patient is stable, oral or injectable mineralocorticoid support can be used. Dexamethasone sodium is inexpensive and readily available; therefore, most clinicians consider it the initial glucocorticoid of choice. Dexamethasone sodium phosphate is a water-soluble, rapid-onset steroid, and it does not cross-react with the cortisol assay required for the ACTH stimulation test. Table 20-6 provides glucocorticoid dose

TABLE 20-6	Commonly Used Steroid Replacement Medications and Doses
DRUG	**DOSE, ROUTE, AND FREQUENCY**
Glucocorticoids	
Prednisolone sodium succinate	11-25 mg/kg IV q2-6h
Dexamethasone sodium	1-3 mg/kg IV q12h
phosphate	1-2 mg/kg IV q8h
Hydrocortisone sodium	1-2 mg/kg IV q8h
hemisuccinate	2-4 mg/kg IV q12-24h
Hydrocortisone phosphate	1.1-2.2 mg/kg IM or SQ
Dexamethasone (Azium)	q21-30 days
Mineralocorticoids	Dogs: 0.02 mg/kg PO q24h
Desoxycorticosterone pivalate	(or divided q12h)
(DOCP)	Cats: 0.1-0.2 mg/kg PO
Fludrocortisone acetate	q24h
Hydrocortisone acetate	1-2 mg/kg PO q12h

recommendations. Once ACTH stimulation testing has been completed an alternate glucocorticoid that also provides mineralocorticoid effects may be preferable.

Once the patient has been stabilized, those with primary hypoadrenocorticism can have mineralocorticoids added to their treatment. Desoxycorticosterone pivalate (DOCP) is the most economical way to replace mineralocorticoids. DOCP (Percorten-V, Novartis) is dosed at 1.1 to 2.2 mg/kg IM every 21 to 30 days. It has no glucocorticoid activity, so supplementation with prednisone or prednisolone at a dose of 0.1 to 0.2 mg/kg/day will be required. Alternatively, fludrocortisone acetate (Florinef) is dosed at 0.01 to 0.02 mg/kg/day orally (PO) divided twice a day (bid). Fludrocortisone has some glucocorticoid activity, and only about 50% of canine patients will need oral prednisone or prednisolone supplementation. The dose of the mineralocorticoids should be based on clinical signs and electrolyte concentrations, and glucocorticoids should be dosed primarily on the presence of GI signs. The minimum dose of glucocorticoids to control clinical signs is desirable to aid in the prevention of side effects from steroid administration.

Hyperkalemia may be severe enough in some patients to warrant more than just fluid therapy. Patients with bradycardia or other serious ECG derangements will need to have their serum potassium level lowered more rapidly than what is provided by dilution from IV fluid therapy. Dextrose alone may be used with mild hyperkalemia, or in hypoglycemic patients, usually at a dose rate of 0.5 to 1 ml/kg of 50% dextrose diluted

1:2. If the patient is normo-hyperglycemic, supplementing insulin with the dextrose bolus is advisable. If using insulin and dextrose in combination, IV dextrose 50%, 2 g (4 ml)/U of insulin administered diluted 1:2 with sterile-water slow IV infusion with regular insulin (0.5 U/kg IV) will promote cellular uptake of potassium (and phosphorus). The calculated doses of insulin and dextrose can be combined in a single syringe and administered over 15 minutes as slow push. After insulin administration, a 2.5% to 5% dextrose CRI is recommended to prevent hypoglycemia. Continued monitoring of blood glucose levels is then necessary to prevent iatrogenic hypoglycemia. In life-threatening cases of hyperkalemia, 10% calcium gluconate at a dose of 0.5 to 1.0 ml/kg should be administered slowly—IV over 15 to 30 minutes, while observing the ECG for abnormalities such as bradycardia and Q-T interval shortening. Calcium does not affect serum potassium levels, but rather provides protection to the myocardium, improves function, and thereby increases cardiac output. Other methods to lower potassium levels must be instituted concurrently.

NURSING CARE AND MONITORING

Hypovolemia and shock are the most life-threatening concerns in patients with addisonian crisis. Additionally, careful monitoring of the heart rate and ECG is important, since fatal arrhythmias can occur. During initial therapy, patients with hyperkalemia should have an ECG monitored continuously if available, or at least every 1 to 2 hours. Electrolytes should be measured every 4 to 6 hours, initially. Blood work to reevaluate for resolution of azotemia, hypercalcemia, acidosis, and electrolyte balance should be performed every 12 to 24 hours.

As with any patient that is dehydrated, weighing the patient twice daily and monitoring skin turgor are important. Measuring urine output and specific gravity are good ways to determine when patients are being adequately fluid resuscitated. However, patients with Addison's disease may have a low USG despite dehydration from lack of aldosterone. Persistent azotemia after fluid resuscitation may indicate a renal insufficiency.

Fludrocortisone therapy monitoring requires measurement of the serum electrolyte, calcium, blood urea nitrogen (BUN), and creatinine concentrations on a 2- to 4-week basis, until the patient becomes stable. Once the patient is stable, monitoring every 3 to 6 months is sufficient. After the first DOCP injection, the serum electrolyte, calcium, BUN, and creatinine concentrations should be measured 3 weeks and 4 weeks after the injection to establish the duration of action of the DOCP. Most patients require injections every 21 to 30 days. Changes in the dose are based on persistent abnormalities demonstrated by the blood work. If signs of GI upset (e.g., nausea, anorexia, vomiting) occur, owners should be educated to supplement with prednisone or prednisolone as needed.

CASE STUDY

A 3-year-old, 30-kg, spayed female Standard Poodle was referred for evaluation and treatment of azotemia, polyuria, and polydipsia. The owner had noted vomiting and decreased appetite for 4 days before seeing the referring veterinarian. The referring veterinarian's initial physical examination revealed mild dehydration, and blood was drawn for serum biochemical analysis. The dog was discharged after receiving 500 ml of 0.9% sodium chloride subcutaneously (SQ).

Serum biochemistry analysis revealed blood urea nitrogen (BUN) concentration of 42 mg/dl (14.9 mmol/L) (reference range 8 to 33 mg/dl or 2.85 to 11.8 mmol/L) and a creatinine concentration of 2.1 mg/dl (185.6 mmol/L) (reference range 0.5 to 1.7 mg/dl or 44.2 to 150 mmol/L). A total serum calcium concentration of 12.1 mg/dl (3.0 mmol/L) (reference range 8.7 to 11.0 mg/dl or 2.1 to 2.75 mmol/L) was also noted. The sodium concentration was 148.2 mEq/L (mmol/L) (reference range 140 to 161 mEq/L [mmol/L]), the potassium concentration was 5.7 mEq/L (mmol/L) (reference range 3.8 to 5.4 mEq/L [mmol/L]), and the chloride concentration was 112 mEq/L (mmol/L) (reference range 105 to 121 mEq/L [mmol/L]). The referring veterinarian prescribed a low-protein diet for renal impairment. Initially the dog improved within the first 24 hours after the visit, but over the next 2 days it continued to vomit and remained polyuric and polydipsic at home. The dog was then referred for additional diagnostic and therapeutic options.

Physical examination on presentation revealed a very weak, 7% dehydrated patient with bradycardia (heart rate 60 beats per minute). A rectal examination produced dark soft stool. During the examination the dog vomited, containing small flecks of blood. Blood and urine samples were submitted for a complete blood count, serum biochemical analysis, and urinalysis. Rapid-analysis biochemical testing (venous blood gas analysis, electrolytes, and BUN and creatinine) was performed at the time of admission. An ECG was also performed.

The rapid chemistry analysis revealed a worsening azotemia (BUN 69 mg/dl [24.6 mmol/L]; creatinine 4.2 mg/dl [371.3 mmol/L]), a moderate to marked hyperkalemia (7.1 mEq/L [mmol/L]), a mild hyponatremia (136 mEq/L [mmol/L]), and a mild hypochloremia (99 mEq/L [mmol/L]). The calculated sodium/potassium ratio was 19.2. Venous blood gas analysis showed a mild acidemia (pH 7.247 [reference range 7.398 to 7.416]) with a reduced bicarbonate (HCO_3^-) concentration (15.5 mEq/L [mmol/L] [reference range 20.5 to 23.9 mEq/L]). The complete blood count produced a mild normocytic, normochromic anemia (hematocrit 35% [reference range 37% to 55%]). Additional biochemical abnormalities were a total serum calcium concentration of 12.9 mg/dl (3.22 mmol/L) and a mild increase in alanine aminotransferase (ALT) activity (121 U/L [reference range 10 to 95 U/L]). The urine specific gravity was low at 1.017 (reference range 1.015 to 1.036). The ECG was unremarkable.

A tentative diagnosis of hypoadrenocorticism was considered based on the signalment, history, hyperkalemia, hyponatremia, reduced sodium/potassium ratio, hypercalcemia, mild azotemia with suboptimal urine specific gravity, and mildly increased alanine aminotransferase activity. A central IV catheter was placed in the left jugular vein, and a rapid-rehydration protocol was initiated with 0.9% sodium chloride at a rate of 416 ml/hr (7% dehydration deficit plus 6 hours of maintenance fluid requirements) for the first 6 hours of fluid therapy. Dexamethasone sodium phosphate (0.25 mg/kg every 12 hours [q12h]) was given IV, and famotidine (1.0 mg/kg slow IV q12h) was administered to treat gastrointestinal (GI) bleeding. After the initial 6 hours, the fluid rate was reduced to 100 ml/hr (approximately 1.5 times maintenance).

An adrenocorticotropic hormone (ACTH) stimulation test was performed and submitted to the laboratory. The measurements of electrolytes and venous blood gases were rechecked after 6 hours of fluid therapy. The blood gases were within reference ranges, so HCO_3^- therapy was not required. A mild hyperkalemia persisted. The packed cell volume (PCV) was 31%, and a reticulocyte count was submitted.

On day 2 the dog was markedly improved, was no longer weak, and was very vocal. The dog's appetite was improved but still somewhat decreased. Dark formed stools were noted, and no vomiting had occurred in the past 12 hours. The electrolytes were again rechecked. The sodium and chloride levels were in the upper limits of the reference range (sodium 159 mEq/L [mmol/L]; chloride 121 mEq/L [mmol/L]), and the potassium concentration was well within the reference range (4.1 mEq/L [mmol/L]). A total of 13 mEq (mmol) of potassium chloride was added to the 0.9% sodium chloride to provide maintenance potassium needs. The reticulocyte count was 158,000/μL (reference range <50,000/μL), indicating a regenerative response. Later in the day the patient was eating and drinking normally, and the fluid rate was reduced to 50 ml/hr.

On day 3 the results of the ACTH stimulation test confirmed hypoadrenocorticism. The dog was discharged after being given desoxycorticosterone pivalate (DOCP, 1.1 mg/kg IM q28 days) for long-term management of the hypoadrenocorticism. Because it can take up to 48 hours for the DOCP to become effective, fludrocortisone acetate (0.011 mg/kg PO q12h) was prescribed in addition to the DOCP for the first 2 days. Additionally, prednisone (0.23 mg/kg) was ordered to be given if the dog's appetite waned or if the vomiting returned, or if the owner anticipated a stressful event would upset the dog. Oral famotidine (1 mg/kg PO q12h) was given for 7 days, and an oral hematinic was given for 7 days or until the PCV returned to normal.

HYPERCALCEMIA

DEFINITION AND CAUSES

Hypercalcemia is the state of increased serum total calcium concentrations. If hypoalbuminemia exists, then the calcium concentrations may be artificially low and should be corrected in dogs using the following formula:

$$\text{Corrected calcium} = \text{calcium (mg/dl)} - \text{albumin (g/dl)} + 3.5$$

or

$$\text{Corrected calcium} = \text{calcium (mg/dl)} - (0.4 \times \text{total protein [g/dl]}) + 3.3$$

These formulas do not apply to cats, although hypoalbuminemia also affects their serum calcium levels. Lipemia and hemolysis will also cause artifactual hypercalcemia. In addition, young animals with physiologic bone growth will have benign hypercalcemia.

The most common cause of persistent hypercalcemia is hypercalcemia of malignancy. Lymphoma is by far the most common malignancy causing hypercalcemia.

Other neoplasms, such as anal sac adenocarcinoma, multiple myeloma, myeloproliferative disease, and solid tissue tumors, have also been reported to cause hypercalcemia. Potentially any neoplastic disorder could cause hypercalcemia. Other important "rule outs" include renal insufficiency (most patients have normal serum calcium concentrations), primary hyperparathyroidism, and hypoadrenocorticism. Less common causes are granulomatous diseases (e.g., blastomycosis, nocardiosis), osteolytic bone lesions (e.g., primary or metastatic neoplasia, septic osteomyelitis), calciferol-containing rodenticide intoxication (e.g., hypervitaminosis D), oral calcium supplements, oral phosphate binders, thiazide diuretics, and plant intoxications (e.g., *Cestrum diurnum*, *Solanum malacoxylon*, *Trisetum flavescens*). An ill-defined syndrome of idiopathic hypercalcemia also occurs in the cat that requires further in-depth evaluation. Box 20-3 provides a list of the most frequently reported causes of hypercalcemia.

BOX 20-3	Causes of Hypercalcemia in Dogs and Cats

- Calciferol-containing rodenticides
- Chronic granulomatous diseases
  Fungal disease (blastomycosis)
  Nocardiosis
- Hypercalcemia of malignancy
  Lymphoma (most common)
  Anal sac adenocarcinoma
  Multiple myeloma
  Myeloproliferative disease
  Solid tissue tumors
- Hyperalbuminemia
- Hypervitaminosis D
- Hypoadrenocorticism
- Idiopathic
- Laboratory error
- Osteolytic bone lesions
- Plant intoxications
  Cestrum diurnum
  Solanum malacoxylon
  Trisetum flavescens
- Oral calcium supplements
- Oral phosphate binders
- Primary hyperparathyroidism
- Primary renal insufficiency
- Thiazide diuretics

PRESENTATION

Because hypercalcemia has many causes, no specific signalment is seen at the time of presentation. Table 20-7 lists the clinical signs associated with hypercalcemia.

Hypercalcemia affects primarily four body systems: (1) renal, (2) gastrointestinal, (3) neuromuscular, and (4) cardiovascular. Renal signs most commonly seen are polyuria and polydipsia, as well as signs of renal failure. Calcium inhibits vasopressin receptors in the kidney and prevents free water reabsorption, creating nephrogenic diabetes insipidus. Very severe hypercalcemia (>15 mg/dl [3.75 mmol/L]) can lead to tubular necrosis, acute kidney injury (AKI), and mineralization. Vomiting, anorexia, lethargy, and depression are common signs seen with kidney injury. On physical examination, small kidneys would suggest the kidney disease has been chronic (chronic kidney disease [CKD]) and may be the cause of the hypercalcemia. In some patients, signs of urolithiasis are present, and uroliths can be palpated in the urinary bladder or urethra.

Hypercalcemia reduces excitability of smooth, skeletal, and cardiac muscle and causes GI dysfunction. Anorexia, vomiting, and constipation are most commonly reported. Firm stool may be felt in the colon when examined. Alterations in skeletal muscle function can cause generalized weakness (common) and muscle twitching (uncommon). Cardiac conduction abnormalities may be identified with an ECG; a prolonged P-R interval, a shortened Q-T segment, and ventricular fibrillation are uncommonly seen.

The most common direct effect of hypercalcemia on the central nervous system is lethargy. Rarely this will progress to seizures, stupor, or coma.

Careful palpation of the lymph nodes and abdomen is important in the hypercalcemic patient. Lymphadenomegaly or organomegaly may support lymphoma or other neoplasia. A complete rectal examination to palpate for lymph nodes or pelvic canal tumors is essential. A waxing and waning history of clinical signs may suggest hypoadrenocorticism. Palpation of the neck may reveal a parathyroid tumor.

Hypercalcemia has many causes, and additional laboratory tests may help define the cause. Hyperphosphatemia without azotemia suggests a nonparathyroid cause. Hypophosphatemia or low-normal phosphorous levels are most commonly seen with primary hyperparathyroidism or malignancy. Combinations of hyperphosphatemia with azotemia are difficult to assess, because renal failure is both a cause and a result of hypercalcemia. Renal failure rarely causes calcium concentration to be more than 15 mg/dl. Serum ionized calcium level is high with primary hyperparathyroidism or hypercalcemia of malignancy. Low or low-normal ionized calcium level is seen in patients with renal failure. Intact parathormone concentrations are increased with primary hyperparathyroidism and renal failure, whereas low-normal or low concentrations are seen in hypercalcemia of malignancy. Other electrolyte abnormalities (e.g., hyponatremia with hyperkalemia) may be associated with hypoadrenocorticism.

Ancillary diagnostic testing such as radiography and ultrasonography can be used to evaluate kidney size and architecture, bone lesions, urolithiasis, hepatic and splenic architecture, and lymphadenopathy. Fine-needle aspirates, biopsies, and bone marrow analysis may be required. An ACTH stimulation test can be used to rule out hypoadrenocorticism.

TREATMENT

Treatment focuses primarily on removing or treating the underlying cause and on volume expansion. Care should be taken not to allow treatment to inhibit the ability to identify the underlying cause. In many cases the cause may be readily identified but not immediately treatable, and supportive care is required. (See Box 20-2 for a list of supplies required to manage a patient with hypercalcemia.)

Volume expansion with IV 0.9% sodium chloride, or another non–calcium-containing isotonic crystalloid, at a rate of 100 to 180 ml/kg/day is recommended for diuresis. Fluids containing calcium-like lactated Ringer's solution should not be used. Any dehydration deficit should be added into the fluid rate. In conditions of dehydration, the kidneys reabsorb sodium and calcium more effectively. By rehydrating and volume expanding,

TABLE 20-7	Clinical Signs Associated with Hypercalcemia	
COMMON	**UNCOMMON**	
Anorexia	Coma	
Dehydration	Constipation	
Depression/lethargy	Death	
Polydipsia	ECG abnormalities	
Polyuria	Prolonged P-R interval	
Vomiting	Shortened Q-T segment	
Weakness	Ventricular fibrillation	
	Seizures	
	Stupor	

naturesis and calciuresis can occur. To prevent iatrogenic hypokalemia, potassium supplementation is necessary. Volume expansion is sufficient in most patients to resolve the hypercalcemia; however, some patients require additional supportive care.

Calciuretic diuretics can be used following rehydration and volume expansion. Furosemide, a loop diuretic, is the diuretic of choice. Thiazide diuretics should not be used. In the acute management of severe hypercalcemia, furosemide can be dosed at 5 mg/kg IV once, followed by a CRI of 5 mg/kg/hr. Alternatively, a dose of 2 to 4 mg/kg IV, IM, or PO given bid to tid (three times a day) can be used. Maintaining adequate hydration while using diuretic therapy is important.

Glucocorticoids increase renal calcium excretion, decrease gut calcium absorption, and decrease bone resorption; they are also cytotoxic to hematopoietic neoplasms like lymphoma. Collecting all diagnostic samples before glucocorticoid administration is important if lymphoid neoplasia is a possibility. If hypoadrenocorticism is possible, then dexamethasone sodium phosphate is the preferred glucocorticoid because it will not interfere with the cortisol assay. Glucocorticoids will also help to antagonize the effects of vitamin D intoxication. In the short term, steroids may reduce inflammation and hypercalcemia associated with granulomatous disease, but high-dose, intermediate- or long-term use may cause a progression of disease, especially fungal disease. Prednisone or prednisolone can be used at a dose of 1 to 2 mg/kg PO, SQ, or IM bid. Dexamethasone can be used at a dose of 0.1 to 0.2 mg/kg IV, IM, SQ, or PO bid.

Bisphosphonates are metal-complexing compounds that also inhibit the production of calcitriol (i.e., active vitamin D) by inhibiting 1α-hydroxylase. Pamidronate is a relatively new bisphosphonate that has been described in veterinary medicine. Recent work with the medication has shown rapid reductions in serum and ionized calcium concentrations with minimal adverse reactions or signs of toxicity. Dosing in dogs is 1.0 to 2.0 mg/kg IV; dosing in cats is 1.5 to 2.0 mg/kg IV. Pamidronate is given as a single-dose, slow IV (in 0.9% sodium chloride, over 4 hours) infusion. The onset of action ranges from 24 to 48 hours, and the duration of action is days to weeks (median, 8.5 weeks). Pamidronate can be given before a definitive diagnosis, because it will not interfere with the results of additional diagnostic testing. Etidronate, another bisphosphonate, has limited use in veterinary medicine; however, oral doses of 2.5 mg/kg

PO bid for the dog and 5 mg/kg PO bid for the cat have been reported. Etidronate also is available as an IV solution. No IV dose has been reported, but most believe it to be lower than the oral dose.

Sodium bicarbonate ($NaHCO_3$) therapy is rather controversial. Most clinicians reserve this modality for management of acute crisis in the presence of metabolic acidosis. Ionized calcium concentrations decrease as serum pH rises (because the calcium binds to serum proteins and HCO_3^- ions). A dose of 1 to 4 mEq/kg as a slow IV bolus has been recommended. It may take up to 24 hours to see results. Multiple dosing may be required, but generally CRIs are not required. The clinician should refrain from using HCO_3^- if calcium and acid-base status cannot be measured. HCO_3^- seems to work best in combination with other treatments. Care must be taken to prevent iatrogenic metabolic alkalosis or paradoxical cerebral acidosis.

Bone resorption inhibitors such as calcitonin and mithramycin are much less commonly used. Calcitonin (5 U/kg IV initially, then 4 to 8 U/kg SQ every 6 to 24 hours) is a hormone that antagonizes parathormone and is used as an antidote for calciferol-containing rodenticides. It can also be used as a temporary treatment for primary hyperparathyroidism. Calcitonin is expensive, has a short duration of action, and can cause anorexia and vomiting. Mithramycin is an antineoplastic agent that is also a potent inhibitor of bone resorption. This medication has been used infrequently in veterinary medicine for treating hypercalcemia. A single dose of 25 µg/kg has been recommended, but once- or twice-weekly dosing may be required to effectively treat hypercalcemia. Significant nephrotoxicity, hepatotoxicity, and myelosuppression can occur.

NURSING CARE AND MONITORING

Evaluating changes in the patient's body weight twice daily, evaluating skin turgor, and observing urine output should be used to ensure adequate fluid resuscitation, and monitor hydration status. Ionized or serum calcium levels should be measured every 12 to 24 hours during initial therapy. Urinalysis (evaluating for presence of renal casts) and reevaluation of BUN and creatinine values need to be performed daily to monitor kidney function. Electrolytes should be monitored to identify imbalances that may occur after initiating fluid therapy. If ECG abnormalities are present, then an ECG must be continuously monitored, or at minimum, reevaluated every 12 to 24 hours. Phosphorous concentrations also should be monitored because persistent hyperphosphatemia with hypercalcemia can result in tissue mineralization (especially if the product of the calcium concentration [mg/dL] multiplied by the phosphorus concentration [mg/dL] is greater than 60).

HYPOCALCEMIA

DEFINITION AND POSSIBLE CAUSES

Hypocalcemia is the state of decreased serum total calcium concentration. If hypoalbuminemia exists, then the calcium concentrations should be corrected to confirm if hypocalcemia is real, using the following formulas for dogs:

$$\text{Corrected calcium} = \text{calcium (mg/dl)} \\ - \text{albumin (g/dl)} + 3.5$$

or

$$\text{Corrected calcium} = \text{calcium (mg/dl)} \\ - (0.4 \times \text{total protein [g/dl]}) + 3.3$$

These formulas do not apply to cats, although hypoalbuminemia also affects their serum calcium concentration. Hypoalbuminemia is the most common cause of hypocalcemia in dogs and cats. It does not cause clinical signs, because ionized calcium (i.e., physiologically active calcium) concentrations remain normal, in general. Box 20-4 provides a list of causes of hypocalcemia in dogs and cats.

Other common causes of hypocalcemia include chronic and acute kidney disease or injury, puerperal tetany (eclampsia), and acute pancreatitis. In kidney disease, mass law interactions of calcium with hyperphosphatemia result in hypocalcemia. Additionally, decreased 1α-hydroxylase activity and subsequent calcitriol (i.e., active vitamin D) production in the kidney significantly contribute to hypocalcemia. Puerperal tetany usually occurs within the first 21 days of lactation, generally in small breed females. Eclampsia causes large amounts of calcium to be diverted into milk production. Acute pancreatitis causes hypocalcemia by mineralization of traumatized tissues and precipitation of calcium salts in saponified fat.

Hypoparathyroidism is an uncommon to rare disease of dogs and cats. It can be a spontaneous primary disease or an iatrogenic result of thyroid surgery (especially

| BOX 20-4 | Most Common Clinical Signs Associated with Hypocalcemia |

- Anorexia (especially in cats)
- Disorientation
- ECG changes
  Bradycardia or tachycardia
  Prolonged S-T segment
  Prolonged Q-T segment
  Wide T waves
- T-wave alternans
- Excitation
- Facial rubbing
- Fever
- Hypersensitivity to stimuli
- Muscle tremor or fasciculation
- Panting
- Polyuria and polydipsia
- Posterior lenticular cataracts (hypoparathyroidism)
- Prolapsed nictitans gland (cats)
- Respiratory arrest
- Restlessness
- Seizures
- Stiff gait/ataxia
- Vomiting (especially in cats)
- Weakness

in cats). It can also be a result of rapid reversal of chronic hypercalcemia or after removing a functional parathyroid tumor. In all cases the lack of parathormone results in reduced gut absorption of calcium, decreased renal reabsorption of calcium, and unopposed osteoblastic activity (bone production).

Other causes include intestinal malabsorption, which is seen in patients with severe, diffuse GI diseases such as lymphangiectasia, inflammatory bowel disease, and infiltrative neoplasia (e.g., lymphoma, mast cell tumor). Ethylene glycol intoxication causes precipitation of calcium salts, usually in the urinary tract and soft tissues. Severely traumatized or necrotic tissue can absorb calcium and cause mild hypocalcemia. Phosphate enemas (Fleet® enemas) cause severe hyperphosphatemia and subsequent mass law effects with serum calcium. Phosphate enemas affect small dogs and cats more severely. Overzealous supplementation with $NaHCO_3$ or phosphate IV infusions can cause iatrogenic hypocalcemia. Dietary deficiencies in vitamin D are uncommon, as are chronic consumption of low-calcium, high-phosphorous diets (all meat).

Any condition that causes an alkalosis will cause a shift from protein-bound (measured total serum calcium) to ionized calcium.

Laboratory error should be ruled out if the patient's signs do not correlate with the laboratory data. Sampling technique should be reviewed. Citrate, oxalate, and ethylenediaminetetraacetic acid all chelate calcium and will spuriously reduce serum calcium concentrations.

PRESENTATION

Because hypocalcemia has many causes, no specific signalment is seen at the time of presentation. A careful history is extremely important in evaluating these patients (e.g., recent parturition, enemas given, toxin exposure, trauma, recent thyroid or parathyroid surgery, historic cues of kidney disease).

Hypocalcemia primarily affects the neuromuscular, cardiovascular, GI, and respiratory systems (Box 20-5). Neuromuscular excitability is increased by hypocalcemia. Clinical signs generally do not occur unless the total calcium concentration is less than 6.5 mg/dl in dogs. Acute development of hypocalcemia is associated with more severe clinical signs, whereas patients with chronic hypocalcemia may show few signs even with calcium concentrations less than 5.0 mg/dl (1.25 mmol/L) because of having time to adapt. The most common

BOX 20-5	Causes of Hypocalcemia in Dogs and Cats

- Alkalemia
- Dietary imbalance
- Hypoalbuminemia
- Iatrogenic
- IV phosphate oversupplementation
- Laboratory error
- Pancreatitis
- Phosphate enema administration
- Postoperative thyroid/parathyroid surgery
- Primary hypoparathyroidism
- Primary renal insufficiency (including ethylene glycol intoxication)
- Puerperal tetany (eclampsia)
- Sample handling (collected in calcium-chelating anticoagulant)
- Secondary renal hyperparathyroidism
- Severe intestinal malabsorptive disease
- Sodium bicarbonate ($NaHCO_3$) oversupplementation

neuromuscular signs are weakness, facial rubbing, muscle fasciculations or twitching, tetany, ataxia, and seizures. Elevated temperature may be seen in patients that have excessive muscle activity (twitching). Common cardiovascular changes present in these patients include bradycardia and ECG changes (Figure 20-2). These changes include prolongation of the S-T segment and Q-T segment, as well as wide T waves or T-wave alternans. Anorexia and vomiting are common GI signs (and are the most common clinical signs seen in cats). Panting or respiratory arrest can also be seen. Other signs less commonly seen are polyuria and polydipsia, perhaps because of nephrocalcinosis secondary to conditions that cause hypercalciuria (hypoparathyroidism). A painful abdomen may be a sign of pancreatitis.

TREATMENT

Patients with clinical signs of hypocalcemia should be hospitalized for appropriate treatment. (See Box 20-2 for a list of supplies required to manage a patient with hypocalcemia.) Hypocalcemia caused solely by hypoalbuminemia does not require treatment; instead, the cause of the albumin deficit needs to be identified and treated. Treatment focuses on parenteral calcium salt therapy. Emergency cases of severe hypocalcemia usually have primary or iatrogenic hypoparathyroidism or puerperal tetany (eclampsia), or have been given phosphate-containing enemas. However, any cause could create signs severe enough to require treatment.

The two most commonly used parenteral calcium products are calcium gluconate 10% solution and calcium chloride 10% solution. Calcium chloride is three times more potent than calcium gluconate; however, calcium gluconate is preferred because it causes much less vessel irritation and is not caustic if extravasation occurs. Table 20-8 contains dosing information that the reader will find helpful.

An ECG should be continuously monitored while calcium is being administered. Bradycardia and Q-T segment shortening are indications to temporarily stop the infusion. Acute treatment is by slow IV bolus infusion. After stabilization of serious neurologic signs, tetany, and excessive muscle activity, a CRI of calcium can be started to prevent relapse from occurring (relapse can occur from 1 to 24 hours after a bolus infusion). Patients with puerperal tetany should have the puppies removed from the dam. Long-term therapy may include oral calcium and vitamin D supplements (see Table 20-8).

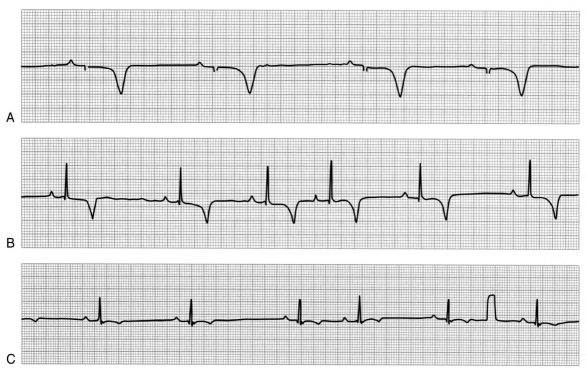

FIGURE 20-2 The ECG of a dog with hypocalcemia secondary to primary hypoparathyroidism during various stages of treatment. Tracing **A** demonstrates prolonged S-T and Q-T segments, as well as prolonged (wide) and deep T waves. The serum calcium concentration was 4.0 mg/dl, and the electrolyte concentrations were within reference ranges. Tracing **B** shows improvements in S-T, Q-T, and T-wave duration and amplitude as the serum calcium concentration has been increased to 6.2 mg/dl. Tracing **C** was taken when the calcium concentration was returned to the reference range (9.7 mg/dl). The S-T, Q-T, and T waves are normal. The three tracings also suggest diminishing R-wave amplitude and increased heart rate as the serum calcium concentration rises to normal.

TABLE 20-8	Commonly Used Calcium and Vitamin D Supplements and Doses
DRUG	**DOSE, ROUTE, AND FREQUENCY**
Parenteral Calcium	
Calcium gluconate 10% solution (9.3 mg calcium/ml)	Initial: 0.5-1.5 ml/kg slow IV
Calcium chloride 10% solution (27.2 mg calcium/ml)	Maintenance: 5-15 mg/kg/hr IV infusion or 1-2 ml/kg diluted 1:1 with saline SQ tid
Oral Calcium Supplements	5-15 mg/kg/hr IV infusion
Calcium carbonate	25-50 mg/kg/day
Calcium gluconate	25-50 mg/kg/day
Calcium lactate	25-50 mg/kg/day
Calcium chloride	25-50 mg/kg/day
Vitamin D Supplements	Initial: 0.02-0.03 mg/kg/day PO
Dihydrotachysterol	Maintenance: 0.01-0.02 mg/kg PO q24-48h
Calcitriol	2.5-10 mg/kg/day PO
Ergocalciferol	Initial: 4000-6000 U/kg/day PO
	Maintenance: 1000-2000 U/kg PO q1-7 days

Laboratory testing (i.e., complete blood count, serum biochemistry profile, urinalysis) is required to fully evaluate these patients. Azotemia and submaximal urine concentration are hallmarks of kidney injury or disease and/or ethylene glycol intoxication. Although both have increased anion gaps, ethylene glycol intoxication usually produces an anion gap of 40 or greater. Increased amylase and lipase activities and an inflammatory leukogram are seen in patients with pancreatitis. These patients may also have a secondary hepatitis as evidenced by increased liver enzymes and total bilirubin concentration. Hyperphosphatemia can be seen in patients with CKD or AKI, ethylene glycol intoxication, primary hypoparathyroidism, and those who have been given a phosphate-containing enema. Blood gases should be evaluated in these patients. The presence of increased total CO_2 concentrations supports alkalosis. Ancillary testing including ethylene glycol testing of the serum, radiography to help evaluate bone density and renal size and shape, ultrasonography of the abdomen to evaluate the kidneys, and measuring parathormone concentrations can be additionally helpful.

NURSING CARE AND MONITORING

During initial management in severely affected patients, calcium concentrations should be measured every 4 to 6 hours, if possible. The ECG should be monitored continuously if arrhythmias are present and/or throughout calcium administration. Bradycardia, Q-T interval shortening, vomiting, and cardiac arrest are indications to stop calcium administration. Neuromuscular signs may persist for 30 to 60 minutes after adequate correction of serum calcium concentrations. Repeat seizures and excessive muscle activity may cause hyperthermia severe enough to warrant cooling efforts. If the patient has kidney disease or ethylene glycol intoxication, then urine production and hydration status (i.e., body weight, skin turgor, PCV) need to be monitored closely. Monitoring the amount of intravenous fluids being administered (the "ins") and changing rates based on what the urine production and insensible losses are (the "outs") may be necessary in patients with acute kidney injury or ethylene glycol intoxication. Venous blood gases need to be initially monitored every 12 to 24 hours in patients with alkalosis. Long-term monitoring of the stable patient requires monthly calcium concentration evaluation for the first 6 months, then every 3 to 4 months until the clinician determines the underlying cause has been treated

successfully. If the underlying cause does not respond to treatment, life-long monitoring may be required.

HYPOGLYCEMIA

DEFINITION AND POSSIBLE CAUSES

Hypoglycemia is the state of decreased serum glucose concentration. Causes are usually divided into those that accelerate glucose removal and those that cause a failure of glucose production or secretion. The clinician must rule out proper sample handling and processing before pursuing a diagnostic evaluation of these patients. Red cells that are allowed to sit in the tube for longer than 1 hour before separation will have artifactual hypoglycemia. Box 20-6 lists the causes of hypoglycemia in dogs and cats.

Many disorders promote more rapid removal of glucose from the plasma. Insulinomas are rare tumors of the pancreatic beta cells that have uncontrolled insulin secretion. This is the most common tumor associated with hypoglycemia in the dog. Other tumors (e.g., hepatoma, hepatocellular carcinoma, lymphoma, leiomyosarcoma,

BOX 20-6	Causes of Hypoglycemia in Dogs and Cats

- Delayed separation of serum from red blood cells
- End-stage hepatic disease
- Extrapancreatic neoplasia
- Glycogen storage disease
- Hunting dog hypoglycemia
- Hypoadrenocorticism
- Insulinoma
- Intoxication
  - Ethanol
  - Salicylates
  - Propranolol
  - Ethylene glycol
  - Oral hypoglycemic agents
- Iatrogenic insulin overdose
- Late-term gestation
- Neonatal hypoglycemia
- Prolonged seizure activity
- Sepsis/endotoxemia
- Severe polycythemia
- Severe primary glucosuria or Fanconi's syndrome
- Starvation/malabsorptive disease
- Toy breed dog hypoglycemia

plasmacytoid tumors, oral melanoma, hemangiosarcoma, salivary gland adenocarcinoma) produce insulin-like proteins that are biologically active; however, other factors are probably involved with paraneoplastic hypoglycemia. Some patients have such a large tumor burden that it consumes a disproportionately large amount of glucose to sustain the aberrant metabolic needs. Patients with sepsis or systemic inflammatory response syndrome (SIRS) may also present with hypoglycemia attributable to consumption exceeding rate of production. Accidental iatrogenic overdose of exogenous insulin is an important consideration in all diabetic patients. Increased RBC mass (i.e., polycythemia) causes hypoglycemia by overuse of glucose to support the metabolic needs of the RBCs. Patients with Fanconi's syndrome or primary renal glucosuria will lose excess amounts of glucose in their urine. Rarely, females in late-term gestation will also experience hypoglycemia because of the demands placed on them by the fetuses. Severe prolonged seizures will cause increased consumption of glucose by the overactive skeletal muscle. (Seizures usually cause serum glucose concentration to increase, because they increase cortisol and epinephrine secretion.) Intoxications with ethanol, salicylates, propranolol, xylitol, and oral hypoglycemic agents are also reported causes.

The most common diseases associated with a failure to produce or secrete glucose are neonatal hypoglycemia and toy breed hypoglycemia. With neonatal hypoglycemia, young puppies and kittens have low hepatic glycogen stores and a reduced ability to perform gluconeogenesis. Therefore short periods of fasting can cause hypoglycemia. Starvation or malabsorptive GI diseases are associated with preexisting systemic illness that can deplete the liver of glycogen stores. After prolonged periods of physical exertion and little to no food consumption, hypoglycemia may occur, as seen in hunting dog hypoglycemia. An uncommon cause is end-stage hepatic insufficiency. Glucose homeostasis is one of the last functions to be lost with advanced liver disease.

Some diseases have a combination of causes. Sepsis, endotoxemic shock, and virulent babesiosis promote increased use of glucose by the body by altering metabolism and by increasing insulin release. These problems also deplete hepatic glycogen stores, making less glucose available for release. Patients with hypoadrenocorticism (i.e., Addison's disease) have an absence of counter-regulatory cortisol, which results in increased insulin action (increased consumption) and decreased gluconeogenesis (decreased glucose secretion). This results in mild to moderate hypoglycemia.

PRESENTATION

No specific signalment is seen in patients with hypoglycemia; however, age, breed, and breeding status (i.e., young puppies and kittens, toy breed dogs, hunting breed dogs, pregnant females) are important in evaluating these cases. Hypoglycemia primarily affects the nervous and musculoskeletal systems (Box 20-7).

Nervous tissue relies on glucose as its primary energy source, and hypoglycemia causes central nervous system depression. Typical signs include lethargy, depression, ataxia, paraparesis, and, in some cases, seizures. Abnormal behaviors like fly biting, stargazing, and staring at walls also can be seen. Hypoglycemia also stimulates appetite, and polyphagia may be a presenting sign. The skeletal muscle also requires large amounts of energy to maintain normal function. Patients with hypoglycemia will display muscle weakness, collapse, muscle fasciculations, and exercise intolerance.

Many patients will have minimal to no clinical signs. Some animals will adapt to their persistent hypoglycemia and may have few clinical signs, even with blood glucose concentrations as low as 50 mg/dl (2.8 mmol/L). Those with paraneoplastic or a large neoplastic burden usually have obvious physical examination abnormalities. Additional laboratory evaluation may show a leukocytosis and abnormalities associated with specific organs that may be affected (e.g., liver, kidneys). Animals

BOX 20-7	Most Common Clinical Signs Associated with Hypoglycemia

- Abnormal behavior
  - Fly biting
  - Stargazing
  - Staring at walls
- Ataxia
- Collapse
- Depression/lethargy
- Exercise intolerance
- Muscle fasciculation
- Muscle weakness
- Paraparesis
- Polyphagia
- Seizures

with plasmacytoid tumors can have hyperglobulinemia and proteinuria. Additional testing such as urine Bence-Jones protein, bone marrow analysis, and radiographs of the skeleton will be needed to verify the diagnosis. Animals with an insulinoma will have an inappropriately high plasma insulin concentration in the face of hypoglycemia in two thirds to three quarters of patients. A fasted (8 to 12 hours) glucose/insulin ratio should be evaluated. An amended insulin/glucose ratio can be determined using the following formula:

$$\text{Amended insulin/glucose ratio} = (\text{plasma insulin } [\text{mcU/ml}] \times 100) / (\text{plasma glucose } [\text{mg/dl}] - 30)$$

If the plasma insulin/glucose ratio is less than or equal to 30, then the denominator for the equation should be *1*. Amended ratios higher than 30 are indicative of insulin-secreting tumors. Ratios between 19 and 30 are difficult to interpret and need to be repeated. If the ratio is less than 19, then an insulinoma is unlikely. False-positive results can occur if the patient's blood glucose level is less than 40 mg/dl (2.2 mmol/L).

Patients with end-stage liver disease or portovascular anomaly often have other clinical signs. Dogs and cats with portovascular anomaly frequently have stunted growth, are thin, and have polyuria and polydipsia. Usually they are juvenile to middle-aged. GI symptoms, icterus, and ascites are signs more commonly seen with end-stage liver disease or severe hepatic dysfunction. Laboratory findings that may be observed include anemia, microcytosis (especially portovascular anomaly), decreased BUN, hypoalbuminemia, and increased serum liver enzyme activities. The fasted and 2-hour postprandial bile acid concentrations will be increased. Urinalysis may reveal urate crystals (especially portovascular anomaly), bilirubinuria, and low urine concentrations.

Septic animals are very ill when they arrive at the clinic. These cats and dogs are shocky and febrile, and have injected mucous membranes when they are in the hyperdynamic phases of septic shock. If presented in the later hypodynamic phase, then hypothermia, pale mucous membranes, and signs of circulatory collapse are seen. The leukogram can be variable from leukopenic to leukocytosis. Evidence of organ failure may be evident (liver, kidneys), and a coagulation profile may reveal disseminated intravascular coagulopathy. Blood cultures should be performed.

Dogs and cats with hypoadrenocorticism (see previous section titled Hypoadrenocorticism [Acute Addisonian Crisis]) often have a waxing and waning history. In addition to hypoglycemia, biochemical analysis may reveal azotemia, hypercalcemia, hyponatremia, and hyperkalemia. The animal also may develop a *reverse stress leukogram* (lymphocytosis, eosinophilia).

Rarely, a dog or cat will develop hypoglycemia from an uncommon cause. Glycogen storage is a rare disease and is most commonly seen in animals less than 1 year of age. Polycythemic patients have dark mucous membranes and are weak, polyuric, polydipsic, may present with seizures, and a PCV greater than 65%.

TREATMENT

The goal of therapy is to increase serum glucose concentrations by administering IV dextrose. All patients with clinical signs should be treated (see Box 20-2 for a list of supplies required to manage a patient with hypoglycemia). Patients who are able to eat (i.e., alert, not vomiting) should be fed as a part of their therapy. Some causes of hypoglycemia will require treatment of an underlying cause, whereas others will require long-term therapy. The clinician must be sure to perform diagnostic testing required to identify the underlying cause of the hypoglycemia.

IV 50% dextrose at 1 to 4 ml/kg diluted 1:1 with sterile water delivered over a 15-minute period is typically given as an initial treatment for severe hypoglycemia. Patients with an insulinoma may have an increase in insulin secretion in response to the dextrose infusion (thus driving the blood glucose level lower). Feeding them frequently using a diet high in complex carbohydrates may better treat these patients. If this is unsuccessful, then a dextrose infusion may prove better than an IV bolus of dextrose. Infusions of 2.5% or 5% dextrose solutions can be delivered at a rate that maintains blood glucose concentration high enough to eliminate clinical signs of hypoglycemia. Some patients may require dextrose concentrations of 10% or higher, which should be administered through a central, rather than peripheral, catheter. Potassium supplementation should be used as needed, based on maintenance requirements or laboratory values.

Insulinomas can be treated with surgery (e.g., partial pancreatectomy) or medically. No location predilection exists for the tumor in the pancreas. Medical management includes frequent feedings, prednisone and prednisolone (0.25 mg/kg PO bid), diazoxide (5 to 30 mg/kg PO bid, starting at the low end of dose, initially), and octreotide (10 to 40 mcg SQ bid to tid). Toy breed dogs and young puppies and kittens should be fed frequent meals high in complex carbohydrates. A bottle of corn syrup should be available in case a hypoglycemic event occurs. Hunting dogs should be fed a meal before hunting and offered snacks every 2 to 4 hours while hunting. If these dogs still have hypoglycemic events, then they should not be allowed to hunt again. If the patient is in a late term of pregnancy, then caesarian section and removal of the puppies will be required. Polycythemia requires therapeutic phlebotomy, and chemotherapy (hydroxyurea) may be required for long-term control.

NURSING CARE AND MONITORING

Monitoring the glycemic status of these patients can be difficult because of the production of counter-regulatory hormones. Single or intermittent measurement of blood glucose level is not recommended. Monitoring the blood glucose concentration every 2 hours will give a better indication of the trends in glucose control. The target blood glucose level is 60 to 150 mg/dl (3.3 to 8.3 mmol/L). Mental and neuromuscular status should be monitored frequently throughout the day, because they provide early clues to an oncoming hypoglycemic event. Septic patients need to be monitored very closely for signs of multiple organ failure syndrome, acute respiratory distress syndrome, and disseminated intravascular coagulopathy. Patients with hypoadrenocorticism should be monitored as previously described (see Hypoadrenocorticism [Acute Addisonian Crisis]). PCVs should be monitored on a daily basis in polycythemic patients. Other monitoring should be based on the patient's underlying disease.

SUGGESTED READINGS

Brady M, Dennis J, Wagner-Mann C, et al.: Abstract: evaluating the use of plasma hematocrit samples to detect ketones utilizing urine dipstick colorimetric methodology in diabetic dogs and cats, *JVECC* 13(1):1–6, 2003.

Davis H: Endocrine emergency—diabetic ketoacidosis, *Vet Tech* 22(1):14–20, Jan 2001.

DiBartola S: *Fluid and electrolyte therapy*, ed 3, St Louis, 2006, Saunders.

Engelking LR: *Metabolic and endocrine physiology, quick look series*, ed 2, Jackson, WY, 2006, Teton New Media.

Ettinger S: *The textbook of veterinary internal medicine*, vol IV, St Louis, 2004, Saunders.

Ettinger S: *Pocket companion textbook of veterinary internal medicine*, St Louis, 2004, Saunders.

Feldman EC, Nelson RW: *Canine & feline endocrinology and reproduction*, ed 3, St Louis, 2004, Saunders.

Mathews K et al.: *Veterinary emergency and critical care manual*, Guelph, Ontario, Canada, 2006, Lifelearn.

Nelson RW: *Techniques for assessing diabetic control, 2003 proceedings of the AAHA 70th annual meeting*, pp 179–182.

Nelson RW: *Hypoglycemia and the Somogyi phenomenon, 2003 proceedings of the AAHA 70th annual meeting*, pp 183–185.

Peyton J, Burkett JM: Case report: critical illness related corticosteroid insufficiency in a dog with septic shock, *JVECC* 19(3):262–268, 2009.

Plumb DC: *Veterinary drug handbook*, ed 5, Ames, 2005, Blackwell Publishing.

Plunkett S: *Emergency procedures for the small animal veterinarian*, St Louis, 2000, Saunders.

Reineke E, Fletcher D, King L, et al.: Accuracy of a continuous glucose monitoring system in dogs and cats with diabetic ketoacidosis, *JVECC* 20(3):303–312, 2010.

Silverstein D, Hopper K, editors: *Small animal critical care medicine*, St Louis, 2009, Saunders.

Wingfield WE, Raffe MR, editors: *The veterinary ICU book*, Jackson Hole, WY, 2002, Teton New Media.

SCENARIO

Purpose: To allow the veterinary technician to apply knowledge of endocrine diseases, recognition of laboratory signs, and proper course of treatment and nursing care.

Stage: Emergency or general practice. In-house chemistry, complete blood cell count, acid-base assessment, and urinalysis equipment present. Ability to monitor vital signs including blood pressure and SpO_2 should be available.

Scenario

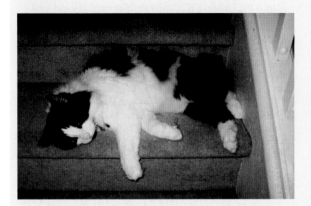

- "Oreo," a 9-year-old MN feline
- Presented for not walking—exhibited plantigrade posture when standing
- Hx: 2-wk history of PU/PD, polyphagia, and ataxia
- 8%-10% dehydrated

- HR, 150 bpm; RR, 24 rpm; MM, pink, tacky
- Labwork: glucose, 331 mg/dl; potassium, 3.0 mmol/L; sodium, 139 mmol/L; chloride, 101 mmol/L; ALT, 356 U/L; lipase, 3147 U/dl; phosphorus, 2.8 mg/dl, TBil, 3.7 mg/dl

Questions
- What would you do for the patient for initial stabilization?
- What are possible complications of disease with which the patient may present?
- Describe the pathophysiology of why this disease occurred.
- What are possible complications of treatment?
- What does continued treatment of this patient entail after stabilization?
- What labwork would you want to continue to monitor serially?
- What monitoring does this patient require?
- What nursing care is needed for this patient?

Key Teaching Points
- Focusing on understanding the pathophysiology of disease processes
- Understanding of prioritization of treatments needed
- Understanding of complications that can occur
- Understanding of nursing care required

References
- Box 20-2: Supplies needed for stabilization
- Boxes 20-1, 20-4, and 20-5 and Table 20-5: Clinical signs and causes for various endocrine diseases

MEDICAL MATH EXERCISE

'Fuzzball,' a 5-kg feline, has been in the hospital being treated for DKA for the past 3 days. Today his pH is still at 7.12 with a HCO_3^- of 10 mEq/L. The veterinarian decides to give him a dose of bicarbonate. What is the most appropriate dose?

a. 1 mEq
b. 2 mEq
c. 4 mEq
d. 6 mEq

21 | Urologic Emergencies

Andrea M. Battaglia and Andrea M. Steele

CHAPTER OUTLINE

Urinary Obstruction
  Blocked Cat
  Blocked Dog
Kidney Disease
  Kidney
  Kidney Failure
Treatment of Acute Kidney Injury
  Fluid Therapy
  Drug Therapy
  Nutritional Support
  Response to Treatment

Treatment of Chronic Kidney Failure
  Fluid Therapy
  Drug Therapy
  Nutritional Support
  Response to Treatment
  Alternative Treatments
  Peritoneal Dialysis
  Hemodialysis
  Renal Transplantation
Conclusion

KEY TERMS

Cystocentesis
Micturition
Polyuria
Renal disease
Stranguria
Urinary obstruction
Uroliths

LEARNING OBJECTIVES

After studying this chapter, you will be able to:

- Understand causes of urinary tract disease or malfunction.
- Understand different techniques in catheterization of the male and female small animal patient.
- Evaluate observations and use of diagnostics to determine if disease or trauma to the urinary tract is present.

Urologic emergencies are common veterinary emergencies, and can result from numerous etiologies including diseases, toxins, and trauma from being hit by a vehicle, gunshot wounds, bite wound injuries, or iatrogenic trauma from catheterization or surgery.

Animals with abdominal trauma from automobile collisions, fights, or physical abuse should be examined for kidney or bladder damage. Trauma also can occur during treatment for urologic emergencies. Overly aggressive palpation of the bladder or **cystocentesis** can cause the bladder to rupture. Improper catheterization techniques can cause urethral tears. The veterinary technician must understand the proper techniques for placing urinary catheters and the problems that can occur.

Urinary obstruction is common in small animals and most common in male cats and specific breeds of dogs. Immediate treatment is necessary to prevent further complications, which can lead to kidney failure and possibly death.

BOX 21-1 | Equipment for Urologic Emergency Surgery

Basic Supplies Needed for Stabilization
- IV catheters
- Fluid therapies
- Quick assessment tests (packed cell volume, blood glucose, total protein, blood urea nitrogen)
- Electrolyte analyzer
- Saline for flushing obstructions
- Rigid urinary catheters in multiple sizes (3.0 French, 3.5 French, 5-10 French)
- Flexible Foley (balloon on distal end) catheters for long-term bladder drainage in multiple sizes (5-14 French)
- Flexible feeding tubes (3.5 French) for cats
- Urinary collection system (can use sterile systems available with one-way valves or empty IV fluid bags and administration lines)

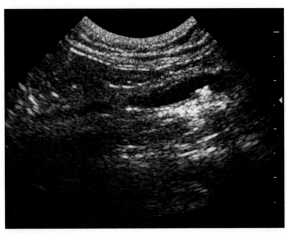

FIGURE 21-1 Ultrasound depicting a urinary obstruction caused by a stone in the urethra of a cat.

Kidney failure can be acute or chronic. Ischemic or physiologic events, nephrotoxins, or diseases may cause acute kidney injury (AKI). Chronic kidney failure (CKF) is caused by progressive congenital disease or by **renal disease** acquired during life. Appropriate treatment depends on the cause and stage of the renal failure.

Stabilization and maintenance of the patient with a urologic emergency are based on an understanding of the signs associated with the various problems that can occur and the types of treatment that can be successful. These animals may need surgical intervention and medical management (Box 21-1).

URINARY OBSTRUCTION

Urinary obstruction is the inability of urine to flow normally from the body. An obstruction can be partial or complete, resulting from a physical or functional condition of urinary outflow.

An object in the urethra, urinary bladder, ureters, or renal pelvis can cause a physical obstruction (Figure 21-1). Examples of these include urethral plugs, uroliths, ureteroliths, nephroliths, tumors, and blood clots. Uroliths are composed of very organized crystals of phosphate, urate, cystine, and oxalate and often are caused by a congenital abnormality in the metabolism or excretion of these minerals. Urethral plugs are a malleable, disorganized substance, composed of struvite crystals (most common) and a matrix, thought to be formed from excessive bladder mucus secondary to irritation. Congenital strictures or trauma to the nerves that control **micturition** can result in a functional obstruction. Urinary obstructions can be found in dogs or cats, both male and female. Urinary calculi are the more common causes of outflow obstruction in male dogs and male cats. Although obstruction in dogs is most often caused by organized uroliths, in cats (and now more recently described in dogs), the debris is much less organized and usually forms a urethral plug at the tip of the penis. The blockage in the male dog usually is found in the bladder neck or the urethra. Whether physical or functional in nature, urinary obstructions must be treated immediately because when they are untreated they can lead to kidney failure, life-threatening electrolyte abnormalities, and eventual death.

BLOCKED CAT

A urethral plug composed of mucus and crystalline material can cause physical obstructions in cats. This condition is most common in male cats, because the lumen of the urethra is small throughout its length and even smaller at the tip of the penis. The urethral plug generally is found at the tip of the penis, where the debris becomes trapped. Female cats rarely have urethral obstructions because of their shorter urethra and wider urethral lumen. Small clumps of crystals, tiny calculi, blood clots, and mucus can pass more easily during urination.

Clinical Presentation

Cats with urethral obstruction may be alert or depressed, depending on the duration and degree of obstruction. Owners may notice episodes of **stranguria** (straining to urinate) or pollakiuria (passing small amounts of urine frequently) and longer periods in the litter box. They may also find the cat urinating in unusual places outside the litter box. Hematuria (blood in the urine) also may be present in varying amounts, depending on the amount of inflammation and irritation. Cats may appear restless, vocal, and uncomfortable. They may be observed grooming the uro-genital region continuously. Owners frequently feel that these signs are associated with constipation, and will often call asking how to relieve constipation in the cat.

Cats with complete obstruction have a distended, painful bladder on palpation. Palpating the bladder may cause the cat to cry out and may induce straining to urinate and the passing of a few drops of blood-tinged urine.

Prolonged obstruction leads to depression, dehydration, vomiting, a low body temperature, and fluid volume and serum electrolyte imbalances.

Diagnosis

Typical treatment orders will include administration of analgesics, placement of an intravenous (IV) catheter or urinary catheter, and collection of a renal profile and serum electrolytes and blood gas values if available. An electrocardiogram (ECG) should be obtained to identify cardiac arrhythmias caused by hyperkalemia (Figure 21-2). If signs of hyperkalemia are present on ECG, or if the cat is bradycardic in the face of being obstructed, treatment for hyperkalemia should not wait for lab results, especially if being performed at an outside lab. Hyperkalemia will resolve once the cat is unblocked; however, this can take some time with a difficult catheterization. Initial stabilization should always be performed before relieving the obstruction.

If the cat is stable, then the bladder can be compressed carefully to check for resistance in urine outflow. Excessive or localized pressure should not be put on the bladder because it is painful and can rupture. Compressing the bladder can dislodge a urethral plug if located at the tip of the penis, and normal outflow can be obtained.

If resistance is excessive and urine outflow is not adequate, insertion of a urinary catheter and irrigation of the urethra may be necessary to dislodge the plug back into the bladder. Gentle massage of the tip of the penis may dislodge

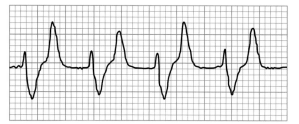

FIGURE 21-2 ECG showing hyperkalemia in a severely uremic animal.

a mucous plug and allow the passage of urine but a urinary catheter designed for this purpose may also be indicated. Before placing the urinary catheter it is usually necessary to provide adequate sedation unless the cat arrives in critical condition and obtunded. Ketamine and diazepam, or propofol, are commonly selected for this procedure.. If the cat is very painful and relaxation is difficult to achieve with injectable analgesics and sedatives, a coccygeal epidural block, using preservative- and epinephrine-free 2% lidocaine, can be performed. If a urinary catheter cannot pass easily into the bladder because of a urolith, plug, swelling, or stricture in the proximal urethra, flushing sterile saline with a gentle pulsating pressure may be necessary. Further diagnostic tests including ultrasound or radiographic imaging, which may include contrast if a tear in the urethra or bladder, or a ureterolith or nephrolith is suspected, may be indicated to define a lesion.

Cystocentesis can be performed on a palpable bladder to collect urine for urinalysis and culture or to provide decompression if the bladder cannot be catheterized. This must be done with extreme caution, because the distended bladder is also extremely friable and prone to injury. This specimen allows a more accurate assessment of bacteria, cells, crystals, the presence of blood or protein, specific gravity, and pH in the bladder. A cystocentesis should be performed with the cat in a ventral-dorsal position. The cat should be well restrained to prevent movement and possible trauma.

The collection site should be free of hair and prepared aseptically with soap and water and alcohol or a dilute solution of a tincture of benzalkonium chloride. A sterile 23- to 22-gauge needle 1 to 1½ inches long (depending on the size of the animal) is attached to a 5-ml or 10-ml sterile syringe. A larger needle should not be used because it can cause leakage from the bladder wall. The bladder is then palpated and immobilized by stabilizing with one hand, to direct needle insertion and to ensure an adequate volume for collection. The needle is inserted into the ventral midline about midway between the pelvis and dome of the bladder, with the tip of the needle pointing caudally at a 45-degree angle. If urine collection is unsuccessful because of misinsertion of the needle, then the needle should be removed and both the needle and the syringe should be replaced before the procedure is repeated.

On presentation, if the cat appears very depressed or dehydrated and has a low body temperature, then blood work should be performed immediately. These results determine the rest of the diagnostic workup and in what order treatment should be initiated, because the cat has begun to show signs of uremia.

Treatment

Treatment begins almost in conjunction with the diagnostic procedures and the efforts to relieve the obstruction. If the cat is showing signs of depression or dehydration and has a low body temperature, then the animal is probably uremic; if so, an IV catheter should be placed and fluid therapy (using a balanced, isotonic, replacement solution) should be started to correct fluid volume deficits, metabolic acidosis, and identified electrolyte disturbances. An ECG should be evaluated for evidence of arrhythmias and hyperkalemia. Hyperkalemia can cause bradycardia, diminished P waves, widened QRS complexes, and increased T waves. If abnormalities are recognized, dextrose with or without regular insulin can be administered to drive potassium into the cells and transiently correct the hyperkalemia and cardiac disturbances. Metabolic acidosis will normally correct with fluid therapy and de-obstruction; however, persistent cases may be treated with IV $NaHCO_3$ if serum pH is less than 7.2 or if the base deficit is greater than 10. IV fluids should be given at a rate of 40 to 60 ml/kg/hr in small aliquots until perfusion parameters have normalized. The use of 0.9% NaCl is no longer recommended to be the replacement fluid, but rather a balanced electrolyte solution such as lactated Ringer's or Plasma-Lyte, since this helps the metabolic acidosis resolve much more quickly.

Catheterization

The decision to use an indwelling urinary catheter should be made with an understanding of the therapeutic goals in mind. Catheters can cause injury, induce urinary tract infections, cause urethral strictures, and potentially rupture the bladder, making proper placement technique an important skill set to learn (Figure 21-3). The therapeutic

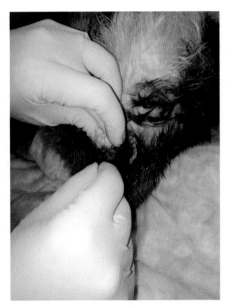

FIGURE 21-3 Feline urinary catheterization.

goals of urinary catheterization are to document the rate of urine formation in critically ill patients, prevent reobstruction during the first 24 hours after the initial obstruction has been relieved, and keep the bladder decompressed to facilitate reestablishment of normal bladder wall contractility (Boxes 21-2 and 21-3).

In 2010 Cooper and colleagues published a protocol for managing urethral obstruction in cats without catheterization, intended as an option to reduce euthanasia because of financial constraints. The study excluded systemically ill cats, or those with radiographic evidence of cystic or urethral calculi, but included relatively stable cats that the owners had declined traditional management due to finances, and were considering euthanasia. A total of 15 cats were treated using the protocol, and 11 responded favorably.

Study cats were sedated using 0.25 mg of acepromazine intramuscularly (IM) and 0.75 mg of buprenorphine IM. Once sedated, the penis was extruded, inspected for obvious trauma, and massaged gently to facilitate removal of distal obstructions. Cats then had a cystocentesis performed to relieve discomfort and bladder tension, using a 22-gauge × 1.5-inch needle on an extension with a stopcock and 20-ml syringe. Cats were then placed in a cage in a quiet, dog-free area, with a litter pan, and once recovered, their typical diet and water were offered. Buprenorphine and acepromazine doses were repeated every 8 hours, and

BOX 21-2	Technical Tip: Placing the Male Cat Urinary Catheter

Items Needed
- A sterile, soft, flexible catheter. For maximum benefit, the catheter should be the largest diameter and most flexible that will pass readily through the urethra. This prevents urine leaking around the catheter insertion site. If urine is leaking from the site, then the rate of urine production and the amount of urine collection cannot be calculated accurately. The preferred catheters are a 3.5 or 5 Fr feeding tube. Other flexible options specifically for cats include the MILA Tomcat catheters, which includes a stylet for placement
- Rigid open-ended catheters are needed for the unblocking procedure. Catheters made out of Teflon (Slippery-Sam®) are available. If it is a catheter that will remain in place following the unblocking, it should ideally be made of a material that will soften once in place
- Cotton-tipped swabs
- Suture: 3-0 Ethilon (Ethicon, Inc., Somerville, NJ)
- 1-inch tape
- Chlorhexidine soap or Betadine surgical scrub (The Purdue Fredrick Company, Norwalk, CT)
- 1000-ml sterile urinary collection bag (MILA, Erlanger, KY)
- Sterile water-based lubricant or 2% lidocaine jelly
- Sterile gloves
- Sterile needle holder and soft tissue thumb forceps
- Sterile drapes

    An indwelling urinary catheter should be placed aseptically to prevent a urinary tract infection as follows:
1. With the cat in a ventral-dorsal position, clip the hair from the prepuce and from a small area on the perineum around the preputial orifice.
2. Clean the preputial orifice with antiseptic soap and water.
3. Retract the prepuce to extrude the penis. Gently prepare the tip of the penis with antiseptic soap and water using soft cotton balls.
4. Place a sterile barrier drape under the penis to prevent contamination of the catheter with hair.
5. Put on sterile gloves.
6. Lubricate the sterile urinary catheter with sterile K-Y jelly or lidocaine jelly.
7. Retract the penis caudally to straighten the urethra, insert the catheter into the tip of the penis, and advance the catheter gently and carefully into the bladder using an aseptic technique.
8. If the catheter does not move easily, retropulsation may be required using sterile saline ± sterile lubricant.
9. Once the catheter is in the bladder, urine should flow into the catheter. Cap the catheter opening and allow the prepuce to return to a normal position.
10. Apply 1-inch tape to the catheter (making a butterfly around the catheter with the tape). Place two stay sutures on opposite sides of the prepuce, and suture each flap of the butterfly to its corresponding stay suture. A fingertrap suture tie may also be used, especially with a feeding tube.
11. Connect the catheter to a urinary drainage bag.
12. Tape the extension tubing to the tail to prevent traction on the prepuce.
13. Place the collection bag lower than the patient so that urine will flow only into the bag. Avoid having the collection bag touch the floor; wrap it in a diaper pad or place it in a plastic container. If urine does not flow properly, then it will increase the risk of urinary tract infection.

every 8 hours the bladder was gently palpated and urine output in the litter pan was monitored. After 24 hours medetomidine (0.1 mg IM) was given for additional sedation and relaxation. Treatment was considered successful if the cat was able to spontaneously urinate within 72 hours.

Managing Indwelling Urinary Catheters

Once an indwelling catheter has been placed, the cat must be monitored and the urinary catheter must be maintained properly (Box 21-4). The urinary catheter should always be connected to a collection system. Cats should not be left unobserved while catheterized, to prevent occlusion of the catheter flow from twisting the lines. Urine output should be measured every 2 to 4 hours. Elizabethan collars are often necessary to prevent the cat from pulling the catheter out.

After unblocking, approximately 50% of cats will undergo a postobstructive diuresis in which fluid administration must match the rate of urine production. The amount of crystalloid to administer can be estimated from the urine produced during the previous 2 hours; fluid input should at least match urine output, and may exceed urine output if the cat is also dehydrated or has other losses. During this time, cats produce >2 ml/kg/hr of urine, although they frequently produce up to 10 to 20 ml/kg/hr. While the diuresis is occurring, serum electrolytes should

BOX 21-3	Technical Tip: Placing the Female Cat Urinary Catheter

The list of preparatory supplies is the same as needed for male cats (see Box 21-2), with the exception of a 3.5 Fr infant feeding tube, a nasal speculum or otoscope, and a light source.

The sedated cat is placed in sternal recumbency with the hind legs hanging over the edge of the table, and the tail is retracted back toward the head. Lateral or even dorsal recumbency also will work very well in the sedated cat. Once the patient is positioned, the following procedure is recommended:

1. Clip hair from the vulvar area.
2. Gently clean the vulvar area with antiseptic soap.
3. The vestibule may be flushed with 0.05% chlorhexidine aqueous solution.
4. Place a barrier drape around the perivulvar area.
5. Put on sterile gloves.
6. Lubricate the urinary catheter with sterile K-Y jelly or lidocaine jelly.
7. Gently insert a nasal speculum or otoscope in the vagina and locate the papilla and urethral orifice. Insert the catheter into the urethra, and gently pass it into the bladder. (NOTE: A blind technique of simply running the catheter along the floor of the vagina often results in it entering the urethra.)
8. Once the catheter is in the bladder, it should fill with urine. Cap the catheter closed.
9. Attach 1-inch tape to the catheter, making a butterfly. Place two stay sutures on opposite sides of the vulva, and suture each flap of the butterfly to its corresponding stay suture. Alternatively, stabilize the catheter using a fingertrap suture tie.
10. Attach a sterile urinary collection system.
11. Attach the extension tubing to the tail to prevent tension on the catheter while allowing enough slack for a full range of tail movement.

BOX 21-4	Maintaining the Urinary Catheter*

1. Drain the urinary bag only every 2 to 4 hours to maintain a closed urinary collection system (Figure 21-4). Do not disconnect the urinary catheter from the drainage bag. Commercial urinary bags, both human and veterinary specific, are available and recommended. They are designed with antireflux chambers to prevent retrograde flow of urine into the bladder. A new IV solution set (minimum 10 drops/ml) and a "just emptied" IV fluid bag may also be used, but note that the line must be clamped anytime the bag is moved above the patient to prevent retrograde flow of urine into the bladder.
2. Cleanse the prepuce or vestibule with antiseptic soap and water.
3. The urinary catheter outside of the body and the lines are wiped with chlorhexidine tincture, from the vulva/prepuce to the bag.

*NOTE: Urinary catheter care should be performed three times a day to prevent urinary tract infections and to monitor catheter function. The catheter should be kept clean at all times and free of fecal contamination.

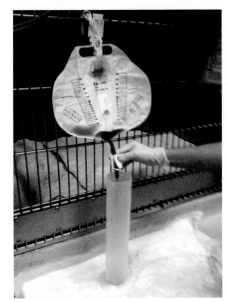

FIGURE 21-4 Emptying closed collection system.

be measured every 2 to 4 hours in a severely ill animal and every 6 to 8 hours in a stable patient. Cats should be weighed accurately every 6 to 12 hours to document net fluid balance. Serum potassium level may drop quickly during the postobstructive diuresis, and potassium supplementation may be needed to prevent hypokalemia. The diuresis period typically lasts 24 to 48 hours, and during this time, the cat will be challenged by reducing the fluids, to see if the urine production also decreases. If urine losses continue to be excessive, the fluids must continue to be matched. If the urine loss decreases, then the fluids can

continue to be decreased to maintenance levels, until the cat is producing a normal urine volume.

Occasionally, cats will not produce large amounts of urine. While this may be an indication of a very short duration of obstruction, or a result of significant dehydration, it is important to assess this critically. The cat may have sustained a tear in the bladder, resulting in a uroabdomen. While an abdominal ultrasound will easily determine free fluid in the abdomen, one can be suspicious if body weight is not matching fluid ins and outs. Clinically, hyperkalemia may not resolve, and cats with urinary obstruction frequently have concurrent urinary tract infections, and therefore may show signs of sepsis. Abdominocentesis will confirm the nature of the abdominal fluid; measurement of a fluid/blood creatinine ratio of >2:1 or a fluid/blood potassium ratio of 1.9:1 suggests uroabdomen.

Cats with cardiac problems may not tolerate fluid administration and be predisposed to fluid overload. This will require the technician to auscultate the chest for heart murmurs or gallop rhythms, and frequently listen for lung sounds and possible crackles. Maximizing water intake via a nasoesophageal tube may be necessary.

Urine output should be measured and recorded every 2 to 4 hours, and hematuria or excessive sediment should be noted. Occasionally the catheter may need to be flushed to reestablish flow, if it becomes blocked with crystals, blood clots, or mucus. This should be noted on the treatment sheet whenever flushing is required.

For cats with prolonged obstruction, serum electrolytes and venous blood gases should be measured every 1 to 12 hours to detect ongoing electrolyte and acid-base abnormalities. Blood glucose concentrations should be measured every 1 to 4 hours if the cat is being treated with dextrose and insulin, and the packed cell volume and total protein concentration should be measured in animals receiving fluid therapy every 6 hours. Measurement of blood urea nitrogen and serum creatinine should be documented every 12 to 24 hours.

Other medications that may be indicated include phenoxybenzamine to decrease urethral resistance, bethanechol to manage atonic bladder by increasing detrusor muscle contractility, or prazosin as an antispasmodic. Corticosteroids are not indicated in these patients because they can impair the immune system and make the patient susceptible to bladder infections.

The patient's bladder should be palpated every 2 to 4 hours to assess its volume. If the bladder is not emptying, then the catheter and urinary collection system should be checked for kinks or plugs. If none are noted, then the bladder may be expressed carefully to dispel urine. If the bladder remains distended, then the catheter may be obstructed and should be flushed retrograde with sterile saline. Maintenance of the urinary catheter is discussed in Box 21-4.

Response to Treatment

The indwelling urinary catheter should be removed within 12 to 48 hours of treatment if no complications occur (e.g., hematuria, atonic bladder). The next 6 to 24 hours are devoted to careful monitoring of the cat for urine production and ability to void urine. If urination is normal, all other clinical signs are stable, and the cat is eating and drinking normally, then the cat can be sent home. The owner is instructed to watch the cat for straining to urinate and for frequent trips to the litter box. The owner should observe the amount of urine produced and note whether blood is present.

The cat's diet must be monitored. Dietary recommendations include feeding canned food to increase water intake and feeding acidifying diets (e.g., Hill's Prescription Diet C/D, Waltham pH Control, Iams Low pH/S, and CNM UR), which are low in phosphate and magnesium levels, to decrease the production of struvite crystals.

The cat may also continue to receive phenoxybenzamine to reduce internal urethral sphincter tone, prazosin to decrease spasm of the urethra, and bethanechol to increase detrusor muscle tone.

If the patient does not void urine after catheter removal, a new indwelling catheter is often placed and indwelling catheter procedures are started again. Some clinicians may try the sedation protocol mentioned earlier during the assessment phase, because the additional relaxation may be all the cat needs to successfully urinate. Recatheterization usually is attempted three times. If normal urine voiding is not achieved after the third catheterization, then the urethra may be damaged and the prognosis is guarded.

Because urinary obstructions are most common in male cats, a urethrostomy, in which the penile urethra is amputated, may be performed as a salvage procedure to provide urethral patency. The urethrostomy removes the narrowest, scarred portion of the urethra to expose a larger urethral lumen, which usually prevents future obstruction.

BLOCKED DOG

Urinary obstruction in the male dog usually results from a physical blockage of urinary outflow by a urolith, but also could be a urethral plug; in the female dog the causes usually are associated with bladder tumors. Male pugs have been identified to be the most at risk for urethral plug formation.

Functional outflow obstruction occurs secondary to a traumatic event affecting the nerves that control the detrusor muscles of the bladder for micturition.

Urinary calculi and plugs are the most common causes of male dog outflow obstruction, followed by scarring in the urethra and bladder neck tumors. Usual sites of obstruction are in the middle to distal end of the penile urethra (Figure 21-5).

Uroliths form in urine supersaturated with minerals, which precipitate to form microaggregates. These aggregates can fuse, forming stones of a variety of shapes, sizes, and composition that can accumulate in the kidney or bladder and move down the urinary tract. Some examples of these mineral aggregates are magnesium ammonium phosphate (struvite), calcium oxalate, silica, and purines. Many different minerals can form uroliths, so when a urolith is removed from a site of obstruction, it should be analyzed to determine its composition. The exact composition of the stone dictates the course of medical or surgical treatment.

Clinical Presentation

Signs of **urinary obstruction** vary greatly and depend on the degree and location of the obstruction. Urethral obstruction can be associated with dysuria or anuria. If obstruction has been complete for a long time, then signs of uremia can occur, including depression, dehydration, and vomiting. The dog also may have a distended or turgid bladder. When an obstruction is located in the bladder, the dog may have signs similar to those of cystitis. Hematuria may be present, and micturition can be characterized by the frequent passage of small amounts of urine. Ureteral obstruction can lead to hydronephrosis and cause cranial abdominal pain.

Diagnosis

The diagnosis of urinary obstruction is established on the basis of a complete history and physical examination, as well as a series of diagnostic tests to determine the location and severity of the obstruction. A complete blood cell count and serum chemistry profile should be performed to identify fluid, acid-base, and electrolyte imbalances. A cystocentesis can be performed to collect a sterile sample for urinalysis and culture and to alleviate bladder distention. The technique is similar to that described for the cat. In large breed dogs, cystocentesis can be performed more easily in a standing position or in lateral recumbency as long as the bladder is palpable and the procedure is performed aseptically. Once the urine is obtained, a careful analysis of the crystals can aid in determining urolith composition.

Urethral obstruction should be considered if a urinary catheter of appropriate size cannot be passed up the urethra into the bladder.

Radiographic evaluation and ultrasound can be useful in diagnosing obstructions of the kidney ureters, bladder, or urethra. The use of contrast medium may help determine whether the obstruction is intraluminal or extraluminal (Figure 21-6).

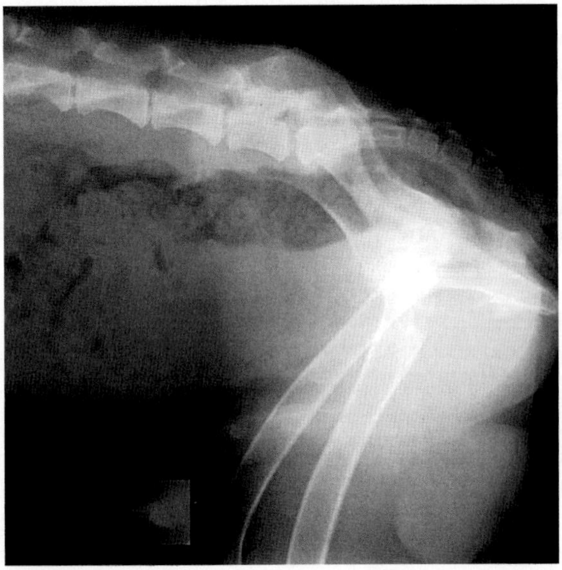

FIGURE 21-5 Urinary obstruction in the penile urethra of a male dog.

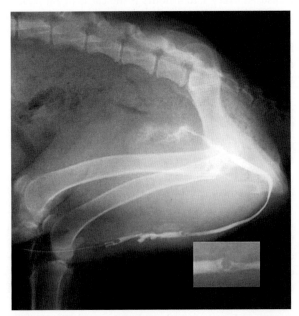

FIGURE 21-6 Use of a contrast medium to diagnose a urinary obstruction in the penile urethra of a male dog.

Treatment

If the dog is weak, hypotensive, bradycardic, dehydrated, and uremic, treatment should be initiated immediately to correct these conditions before the obstruction is corrected. An IV catheter should be placed and therapy should be started to correct fluid volume deficits, metabolic acidosis, and electrolyte disturbances. An ECG should be used to monitor cardiac arrhythmias and evidence of hyperkalemia.

Catheterization

Once the patient is stabilized, passage of an indwelling urinary catheter should be attempted to relieve the obstruction. If a catheter cannot be passed into the bladder because the urolith is blocking the urethra, then urohydropropulsion can be used in an attempt to push the stone or stones back into the bladder.

When urine outflow has been established, an indwelling urinary catheter may be placed to keep the urethra from reobstructing (Boxes 21-5 and 21-6).

Urohydropropulsion

The disposition of the animal may necessitate sedation or general anesthesia for this procedure. Choosing an appropriate sedation regimen, including analgesia, with the addition of a topical application of lidocaine may keep the animal comfortable.

With the animal in lateral recumbency, inject a liberal quantity of a 1:1 mixture of sterile saline solution and sterile aqueous lubricant through a flexible catheter into the urethral lumen to facilitate movement. An assistant should be asked to insert an index finger into the patient's rectum and firmly occlude the lumen of the pelvic urethra by applying digital pressure. Sterile saline is then injected into the urethra through the catheter; the pressure builds rapidly, causing the urethra to dilate, and the assistant releases the digital pressure placed on the pelvic urethra. Pressure should be maintained in the urethral lumen by forcing more saline forward after the assistant has released digital pressure. This technique should force the fluid and usually the uroliths into the urinary bladder.

BOX 21-5	Technical Tip: Male Dog Urinary Catheter Insertion

Equipment

- Sterile soft, flexible catheter such as a male infant feeding catheter, sizes 5, 8, or 10 French (Mallinckrodt Medical, St Louis, MO)
- Long silicone Foley catheters also an option and ideal. Balloon on Foley assists with maintaining positioning of catheter in bladder
- Cotton-tipped swabs
- Suture: 3-0 Ethilon (Ethicon, Inc.)
- Chlorhexidine antiseptic soap or Betadine scrub (The Purdue Fredrick Co., Norwalk, CT)
- Sterile urinary collection bag (MILA)
- Sterile water-based lubricant or sterile lidocaine jelly 2%
- Sterile gloves
- 12-ml syringe with a solution of 4 ml of Betadine and 250 ml of sterile water, or 0.05% chlorhexidine
- Sterile needle holder and soft tissue thumb forceps
- Sterile barrier drape

Procedure

1. Place the dog in lateral recumbency.
2. Clip hair from the prepuce and around the preputial orifice.
3. Clean the preputial orifice with antiseptic soap and water.
4. Retract the sheath to expose the entire shaft of the penis. Disinfect the tip of the penis with 0.05% aqueous chlorhexidine solution.
5. Put on sterile gloves.
6. Lubricate the sterile urinary catheter with sterile K-Y jelly or lidocaine jelly.
7. Measure the approximate length required by estimating in the air (so as not to touch the dog) the distance from the tip of penis to bladder.
8. Insert the lubricated catheter into the urethra using an aseptic technique and gently pass retrograde along the urethra into the bladder.
9. Once the catheter is in the bladder, urine should fill the catheter. Cap the catheter opening and allow the prepuce to return to a normal position.
10. Stabilize the catheter using a fingertrap suture tie, or if a Foley was used, inflate the balloon using the volume of sterile saline indicated on the Foley (typically 1-3 ml). It is recommended to apply sutures for additional stabilization even when Foley catheter is used due to potential of catheter breaking in patients that are more mobile.
11. Connect the catheter to a urinary drainage bag.
12. Tape the tubing to the hind leg or tail to prevent traction on the prepuce.
13. Figure 21-7 is a photo of a dog with closed urinary catheter system.

| BOX 21-6 | Technical Tip: Female Urinary Catheter Insertion |

Equipment
The list of preparatory supplies is the same as those needed for male dogs (see Box 21-5), with the addition of Foley catheters sizes 6, 8, and 10 French and a vaginal speculum.

Procedure
1. Clip hair from vulvar area.
2. Gently clean the vulvar area with antiseptic soap or Betadine solution.
3. Using a sterile syringe, gently flush the vestibule with a 1:60 dilution of Betadine solution, or 0.05% chlorhexidine aqueous solution.
4. If patient is awake, instill 1-6 ml of 2% lidocaine sterile jelly using a syringe (amount will depend on the size of the dog).
5. Put on sterile gloves.
6. Lubricate a sterile Foley catheter with sterile K-Y jelly or lidocaine jelly.
7. Generally a blind technique is the easiest; by inserting a gloved or well-scrubbed finger into the vulva and up into the vagina, the papilla will be evident on the midline of the vaginal floor. Palpate the papilla, and direct the catheter down underneath it. The catheter will appear to disappear if you palpate beyond the papilla. Alternatively, gently insert a gloved finger, sterile speculum, sterile laryngoscope blade, or sterile otoscope into the vagina. Locate the papilla and urethral opening and insert the catheter.
8. Once the catheter is inserted, fill the balloon of the Foley catheter with the indicated amount of sterile water.
9. Gently retract the catheter to ensure that the balloon is within the bladder, and pull the stylet.
10. Attach a sterile urinary collection system.
11. Affix the catheter to the hind leg, the base of the tail, or bring forward and attach to the abdomen, using Elastikon-type adhesive tape.

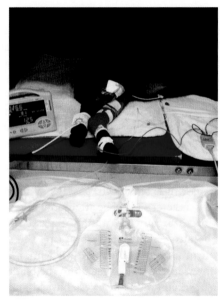

FIGURE 21-7 Indwelling urinary catheter connected to collection system.

Sometimes the urolith returns quickly to the bladder; however, it may be necessary to repeat the procedure several times until the urolith reaches the bladder.

Response to Treatment
Once urine outflow has been established, management is directed at surgical or medical removal of the uroliths and medical therapy to prevent recurrence.

Struvite is the most common mineral detected in canine uroliths. The urine must be supersaturated with magnesium, ammonium, and phosphate for struvite uroliths to form. In contrast to cats, struvite urolith formation in dogs generally is associated with urinary tract infections with urease-producing microbes, which cause alkalinization of the urine. Resolution of the urinary tract infection with antibiotics is the foundation of therapy. Dietary modifications that reduce phosphorous and magnesium excretion and urinary acidification are recommended. Hill's Prescription Diet S/D, and Royal Canine Urinary S/O are examples of diets that are low in protein, phosphorus, and magnesium. Surgical removal of existing uroliths is the preferred method of treatment, but medical dissolution with antibiotics and dietary modification has been advocated and may be indicated in animals with recurrent disease or those that are poor surgical risks.

Ammonium urate uroliths are most common in dalmatians and are managed medically. Dietary modifications reduce urine concentrations of uric acid and ammonium and hydrogen ions. The diet should be a purine-restricted, nonacidifying diet that does not contain supplemental sodium (Hill's Prescription Diet U/D or Hill's Prescription Diet K/D, Royal Canin UC 18). Besides diet changes, xanthine oxidase inhibitors (allopurinol) are given to block uric acid formation in the serum and urine. The urine should be alkalinized by the administration of $NaHCO_3$ or potassium citrate orally to achieve a urine pH of 7.0. Documented urinary tract infections are treated with appropriate antibiotics.

Calcium oxalate uroliths are managed very differently. Surgery appears to be the most effective treatment because they are very difficult to dissolve. Some dietary modifications can be effective. A diet moderately restricted in protein, calcium, oxalate, and sodium may be considered to help prevent recurrences. Ideally the diet should not be restricted or supplemented with phosphorus or magnesium. Attempts should be made to alkalinize the urine.

Some dog breeds are more susceptible to urolith production than others, and some breeds are predisposed to particular urolith types. According to the Minnesota Urolith Center, where extensive studies of canine uroliths were performed, the following uroliths were matched to a particular breed of dog. Calcium oxalate uroliths were prominent in male dogs, especially miniature schnauzers, Lhasa apsos, Yorkshire terriers, miniature poodles, and Shih tzus. Struvite uroliths were more common in female dogs, possibly because of the higher prevalence of urinary tract infections. Common breeds associated with these uroliths are the miniature schnauzer, bichon frise, Shih tzus, Yorkshire terriers, Lhasa apsos, cocker spaniels, and miniature poodles. Uroliths composed of purines were found mostly in male dogs, dalmatians, Yorkshire terriers, and English bulldogs. These breeds have normal serum uric acid concentrations but high urine uric acid concentrations.

KIDNEY DISEASE

Kidney failure is the inability of the kidneys to perform their numerous functions of excretion, metabolic regulation, and hormone production. As the disease progresses, the animal shows signs of *uremia*. Conventional and specialized treatments are available. If the disease is treated early and aggressively, then the kidney can regenerate to a degree, and recover. If left untreated, then the patient will deteriorate and eventually die.

KIDNEY

The kidneys are located in the lumbar region of the abdomen, enveloped in peritoneum and loosely attached to the body wall.

Each kidney is made up of a variety of structures that are responsible for several functions, such as fluid regulation, electrolyte balance, excretion of metabolic waste products, and hormone production.

The functional unit of the kidney is the nephron, made up of a glomerulus, proximal tubule, loop of Henle, distal tubule, and collecting duct. As blood passes through the kidney, an ultrafiltrate is formed containing water and very small molecules. This filtrate is later modified by the nephron to form final urine. Water balance and electrolyte balance is maintained in these tubules, and nitrogenous waste is excreted.

The kidneys also produce the hormones erythropoietin, renin, and calcitriol. Erythropoietin is responsible for producing red blood cells, renin is involved in controlling blood pressure (BP), and calcitriol stimulates calcium absorption from the small intestine.

KIDNEY FAILURE

When the kidneys are injured, resulting in their inability to maintain excretory function, they are considered to be in failure. Kidney failure can be an acute or chronic condition.

Acute kidney injury (AKI) is a sudden decrease in kidney function, over days to weeks. AKI is classified as either prerenal, intrinsic renal parenchymal (functional element), or postrenal. Prerenal AKI is a functional consequence of reduced blood flow to the kidneys and is completely reversible with restoration of adequate renal perfusion, although intrinsic AKI may result if prolonged. Hemorrhage, vomiting, diarrhea, dehydration, poor fluid intake, and systemic diseases such as heart failure can cause it. Intrinsic AKI results from damage to the cellular structure of the kidney by ischemic or toxic events. Postrenal AKI results from an obstruction or diversion of the outflow of urine from the animal. Obstructions can be located in the urethra, bladder, ureter, or renal pelvis, and urine can be diverted into the abdominal cavity or soft tissue with rupture of the ureters, bladder, or urethra. All of these conditions are potentially reversible if diagnosed early and treated aggressively, and they constitute a urologic emergency.

Chronic kidney failure (CKF) develops over an extended period of time, usually several months to years. The kidney injury is not reversible; however, in its early stages the animal can be supported with proper diet and medication; CKF rarely is considered an emergency condition.

BOX 21-7 | Causes of Acute Kidney Injury

- Ischemia
- Shock
- Hypovolemia
- Hemorrhage
- Decreased cardiac output
- Heart failure
- Renal thrombosis
- Nephrotoxins
- Organic compounds such as ethylene glycol (antifreeze) and pesticides
- Antimicrobials such as cephalosporins, aminoglycosides, and tetracyclines
- Anesthetics
- Heavy metals such as lead
- Analgesics or nonsteroidal antiinflammatory drugs, including aspirin and phenylbutazone
- Snake venom
- Lyme disease
- Infectious diseases
  Leptospirosis
  Bacterial infections, including pyelonephritis
  Immune-mediated diseases (e.g., glomerulonephritis, systemic conditions, hypercalcemia)

Acute-on-chronic kidney failure, defined as an acute decompensation of a preexisting chronic kidney failure, can also occur, often secondary to other disease processes, or iatrogenic causes such as lack of water, causing the patient to rapidly dehydrate. This is a common emergency that often requires treatment such as fluid therapy to resolve the acute kidney injury.

Causes of Intrinsic Acute Kidney Injury

AKI most commonly results from ischemic or physiologic (prerenal) events, nephrotoxins, or other diseases. Ischemic injury occurs with profound or prolonged decreases in renal blood flow. Prolonged ischemia causes the epithelial cells of the kidney to be deprived of oxygen, lose cellular function, and die (Box 21-7).

Clinical Presentation of Acute Kidney Injury in Animals

The presenting complaints typically are vague and nonspecific for renal disease and may include the following:
- Anorexia
- Vomiting
- Listlessness
- Diarrhea
- Halitosis
- Ataxia
- Seizures
- Known toxin exposure
- Oliguria
- Anuria
- Polyuria

The physical examination may demonstrate the following:
- Normal body condition and hair coat, which help differentiate AKI from CKF.
- Dehydration or overhydration. Dehydration is most commonly caused by a decrease in fluid intake, vomiting, or diarrhea; overhydration may be seen if the animal has been given parenteral fluids.
- Oral ulceration or necrosis of the tongue, halitosis, hypothermia, or fever. Most uremic animals have low body temperature proportional to their azotemia; however, if the condition is caused by infection, then the temperature may be elevated. A normal temperature in a uremic animal may suggest the presence of fever and infection.
- Scleral infection; nonpalpable urinary bladder; tachypnea; bradycardia; large, painful, firm kidneys.

Causes of Chronic Kidney Failure

With CKF, the injury to the kidney is cumulative over months to years, and there is little or no potential for repair. Surviving nephrons compensate maximally for those that have been lost. As the CKF progresses and renal function deteriorates, the animal becomes polyuric and progressively azotemic and eventually develops uremia. CKF may result from congenital diseases that progress or from kidney disease acquired through life. The animal may be able to compensate for the loss of renal function initially, but over time, as more kidney function is lost, the signs of kidney failure materialize.

Clinical Presentation of Patients with Chronic Kidney Failure

Some telltale signs of CKF include weight loss, prior episodes of illness, **polyuria,** polydipsia, pale mucous membranes, small irregular kidneys, low body temperature, and poor hair coat and body condition.

Diagnosis of Acute and Chronic Kidney Failure

The diagnosis of kidney failure is confirmed with laboratory tests that document the extent of renal impairment and distinguish between AKI and CKF. These tests may include the following:

- A complete blood cell count may reveal changes in hematocrit depending on hydration levels. If the kidney failure is caused by an infection, then an increase in the white blood cell count will be seen. A complete blood cell count can distinguish regenerative from nonregenerative anemia. Anemia usually is not present in AKI but is present in CKF.
- A chemistry panel demonstrates progressive increases in serum urea nitrogen, creatinine, phosphate, and potassium levels. Serum bicarbonate level usually is decreased, and serum calcium concentration may vary. The chemistry panel also helps determine whether other organ systems are involved. If blood gases are available, the patient will tend to have a metabolic acidosis, associated with a high anion gap.
- Urine specimens should be obtained by cystocentesis to prevent contamination by the lower urogenital tract and to provide a clearer interpretation. In AKI, urine specific gravity ranges from 1.007 to 1.017, representing an inability to concentrate urine. A more concentrated urine predicts a prerenal component. Mild proteinuria is often present. Casts, white blood cells, red blood cells, bacteria, and crystals usually are present. The presence of calcium oxalate crystals suggests ethylene glycol toxicity.
- Radiographs typically reveal normal to large kidneys with smooth contours or may show small, irregular kidneys in animals with decompensated CKF. Ultrasound may confirm ethylene glycol toxicity, which appears as brightness of the cortex secondary to calcium oxalate crystal deposition. Ultrasound can further define the shape and size of the kidneys and alterations in intrarenal architecture.
- Renal biopsy confirms the diagnosis of AKI and may establish its cause. Renal histopathology can define the severity of the disease and its potential reversibility and is an excellent indicator to distinguish between AKI and CKF. The procedure is invasive, with inherent risks such as hemorrhage and further renal damage.
- Ethylene glycol levels should be assessed in cases of known antifreeze exposure or when calcium oxalate crystals are present in the urine of an animal with AKI.

- Leptospirosis titers must be evaluated in animals with AKI. Leptospirosis is highly suspected in young dogs with AKI of unknown origin. Animals with signs of systemic infection including fever and an increase in white blood cells also must be evaluated for this disease. Leptospires are spirochetes that infect humans and animals; urine from the infected host is the common source of contamination. The staff working with these animals should wear gloves and use other measures to prevent contamination.

TREATMENT OF ACUTE KIDNEY INJURY

Once the diagnosis of AKI or CKF has been established, the goals of treatment are to minimize further injury to the kidney, quickly correct renal hemodynamics, and reestablish water and solute balances. The sooner treatment is implemented, the greater the chances for renal regeneration and recovery.

If a patient arrives to the clinic after a nephrotoxin has been ingested, gastric lavage should be instituted or vomiting induced, and activated charcoal should be administered within 30 to 60 minutes to absorb any residual toxin. When the toxin has been identified, specific treatments or antidotes can be given to reverse the effects. For example, ethanol or methylpyrazole is given to treat ethylene glycol toxicity.

AKI treatment can be divided into three areas: (1) fluid therapy, (2) drug therapy, and (3) nutritional support.

FLUID THERAPY

Animals with AKI can be dehydrated because of vomiting, diarrhea, and anorexia or may be overhydrated if they are anuric and have no way to excrete excessive fluid loads. If a fluid deficit is present, then fluid volume to be replaced is calculated by multiplying the estimated percentage of dehydration by the body weight in kilograms. Fluids should be given via IV catheter (peripheral or central venous catheter). Using a jugular catheter is preferable, because other diagnostic sampling or testing can be performed easily through this site. During the period of rehydration, the animal should be monitored to determine urine output and detect signs of overhydration (i.e., changes in body weight, arterial pressure, and central venous pressure, packed cell volume, and total solids). If blood losses are also detected, then transfusion should be given to restore packed cell volume and BP.

Animals who are oliguric or anuric must be monitored closely because they have a greater potential of becoming fluid overloaded, hypertensive, and edematous.

DRUG THERAPY

If oliguria or anuria persists, additional treatment is needed to induce diuresis. Furosemide, an osmotic diuretic, is most commonly used. Furosemide may be administered as a bolus, and then often will proceed to a continuous rate infusion (CRI) to maintain diuresis, if the initial bolus is effective. Urine output should improve within 1 to 2 hours if treatment is likely to be effective.

BP should be monitored with changes in fluid balance. Oscillometric techniques or ultrasonic Doppler can measure BP indirectly. Normal BP of the dog should be 148 mm Hg systolic, 87 mm Hg diastolic, and 102 mm Hg mean. Normal BP of the cat should be 125 mm Hg systolic, 75 mm Hg diastolic, and 100 mm Hg mean. Systemic hypertension develops from either fluid overload or uremia and may warrant antihypertensive therapy to prevent retinal detachment and cerebral hemorrhage.

Animals with AKI also have severe hyperkalemia and acidosis. Hyperkalemia is the most life-threatening electrolyte abnormality associated with ARF. Acidosis may resolve with fluid therapy, but if serum bicarbonate concentration is less than 10 to 15 mEq/L, then treatment with $NaHCO_3$ may be initiated. Blood gases and total carbon dioxide levels should be reevaluated to determine whether additional therapy is needed.

Hyperkalemia can cause cardiac disturbances such as bradycardia, ventricular tachycardia, and fibrillation. ECG changes include peaked T waves, loss of P waves, and wider QRS complexes. If the ECG changes are severe, then immediate therapy is needed to decrease serum potassium level. The effects on the heart can be counteracted with calcium gluconate, which antagonizes the cardiotoxicity of high serum potassium concentrations. Glucose and insulin can be given in an emergency to promote the shift of potassium into the cells, where it is safe. If this therapy is used, then monitor the animal for hypoglycemia, and place the animal on a dextrose CRI of 2.5% to 5% following the initial dextrose and insulin doses.

Gastrointestinal complications such as vomiting, diarrhea, anorexia, and severe ulceration of the gastrointestinal tract and mouth are some of the most common signs of AKI. Histamine blockers such as cimetidine, ranitidine, or famotidine may reduce gastric pH and reduce nausea. Gastrointestinal protective medications such as sucralfate are given to promote gastric ulcer healing and prevent formation. Oral ulcerations are managed effectively by rinsing the mouth frequently with a 0.1% chlorhexidine solution.

NUTRITIONAL SUPPORT

Many animals with AKI cannot tolerate oral food intake because of vomiting, nausea, or ulcerations. Their diet should be low in protein, phosphorus, and sodium while providing adequate amounts of calories, vitamins, and minerals. Unfortunately these diets are often not palatable and often not ingested willingly. The basal energy expenditure in kilocalories per day can be determined by the following formula: 70 × body weight in kilograms to the 75th power. If an animal is critically ill, the basal energy expenditure should be multiplied by 1.5. If the animal is under minimal stress and has a low activity level, the basal energy expenditure is multiplied by 1.25. When the patient is catabolic or has a very severe disease, the basal energy expenditure should be multiplied by 1.75 to 2.0.

Animals that will not eat enough can be fed by a nasogastric (NG) or nasoesophageal (NE) tube, with an esophagostomy tube (E-tube), or through a percutaneous endoscopically placed gastric tube (PEG tube). Feeding can be achieved by blending therapeutic diets (Hill's Prescription Diet K/D, Waltham Low Protein Diet) or by using formulated liquid diets (Renal Care). Percutaneous endoscopically placed gastric tube feeding should be provided three or four times daily. Each meal should not exceed half the animal's stomach volume (60 ml/kg in cats, 90 ml/kg in dogs). Feedings should be introduced slowly in anorexic animals, taking up to 3 days to reach desired intake.

RESPONSE TO TREATMENT

Appropriate therapy should improve renal hemodynamics and water and solute imbalances as predicted by a decrease in azotemia, normalization of serum potassium and serum bicarbonate levels, control of vomiting, resolution of oral and gastric ulceration, and a stabilization of body weight.

If medical management fails to increase urine production and the clinical complications associated with ARF cannot be controlled, alternative approaches must be initiated to stabilize the animal.

TREATMENT OF CHRONIC KIDNEY FAILURE

CKF is irreversible and progressive. No cure exists, but medical and dietary management can minimize the progression of CRF. Acute-on-chronic kidney failure is treated similarly to AKI, with the understanding that the underlying kidney failure is simply being managed.

FLUID THERAPY

In CKF, urine production is increased. Therefore, to maintain fluid balance and prevent dehydration, water consumption must be increased orally, subcutaneously, or intravenously. Some owners are able to give their pets fluids subcutaneously at home. Other owners may prefer the placement of an E-tube or PEG tube to allow for increased oral intake, which is an excellent, less invasive long-term option than subcutaneous fluids.

DRUG THERAPY

Animals with prolonged CKF become progressively azotemic and eventually develop uremia. Laboratory tests reveal changes in the serum blood chemistry, complete blood cell count, and fluid and electrolyte balances. These can include increases in serum bicarbonate levels, increases in serum phosphorous concentrations, and a nonregenerative anemia caused by the failure of the kidney to synthesize erythropoietin. BP monitoring can reveal systemic hypertension.

Metabolic acidosis can be treated with oral $NaHCO_3$. Hyperphosphatemia can be controlled with a dietary phosphate restriction and oral phosphate binders (aluminum hydroxide or sucralfate). Nonregenerative anemia can be supported with blood transfusions of compatible packed red blood cells or recombinant human erythropoietin (EPO). EPO stimulates red blood cell production.

Systemic hypertension can be treated with a combination of sodium-restricted diets and antihypertensive drugs such as enalapril, hydralazine, or diltiazem. Treatment depends on the severity and causes of the systemic hypertension.

NUTRITIONAL SUPPORT

Dietary therapy plays an important role in managing CKF. Some of the benefits of appropriate diet for animals with CKF include preventing clinical signs of uremia, minimizing the excess or loss of electrolytes and minerals, slowing the progression of CKF, and maintaining adequate nutrition.

Diets should be low in protein, phosphorus, and sodium. Numerous veterinary diets exist to manage mild, moderate, and severe CKD. The diets should be fed according to the animal's caloric needs. Appropriate measures should be taken if the animal is showing signs of an acute onset of uremia such as vomiting and anorexia.

RESPONSE TO TREATMENT

The animal with CKF should be reevaluated at regular intervals to check for therapeutic response. Monitoring these animals regularly allows treatment of the changing needs that develop over time. If conservative medical management cannot support the patient with CKF, then alternative treatments are available.

ALTERNATIVE TREATMENTS

When conventional therapy fails to restore renal function or the clinical consequences of uremia, dialysis or renal transplantation must be considered. In veterinary medicine, there are two broad types of dialysis available: peritoneal dialysis or hemodialysis.

PERITONEAL DIALYSIS

Peritoneal dialysis (PD) is a procedure that utilizes the patient's own peritoneum as a semipermeable membrane across which waste products, glucose, and albumin are removed from the blood of the patient. PD is used in AKI to allow the kidneys time to repair themselves. It is usually only indicated with oliguria and anuria.

To perform PD, dialysate (an isotonic fluid) is instilled in the abdomen through a special catheter and allowed to "dwell" for a prescribed period (often up to 1 hour). During the dwell, solutes are exchanged across the membrane, at varying rates, depending on the osmolarity of the solution instilled. In veterinary medicine, the osmolarity is typically adjusted using 1.25%, 2.5%, or 4.25% dextrose. Once the prescribed dwell time is complete, a stopcock is turned, allowing fluid from the abdomen to flow into a second bag, via gravity; then the process is repeated. PD can be performed at any clinic that offers 24-hour veterinary care. The only specialized equipment is the peritoneal catheter (many substitutes are described in the literature), and cautious, aseptic technique.

PD is very intensive, requiring around-the-clock nursing care to ensure, for example, that the dialysis

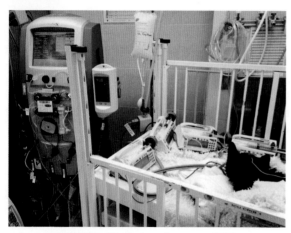

FIGURE 21-8 Animal receiving CRRT.

is well timed, the patient is comfortable, and the catheter is functioning properly. Serial blood work will be obtained at a minimum of once per day, but often blood gases and electrolytes must be monitored several times per day. PD can continue for days, until the patient's creatinine level normalizes. Then PD will be slowed, and urine production and creatinine level will be closely monitored as the kidneys take over more of the workload. PD is discontinued once the kidneys are able to maintain creatinine levels in the normal range and urine production has increased.

HEMODIALYSIS

Hemodialysis is a sophisticated renal replacement therapy instituted on a temporary or permanent basis when conventional therapies fail. In veterinary medicine, like human medicine, we have options: continuous renal replacement therapy (CRRT) or intermittent hemodialysis (IHD). In AKI, CRRT is most often used, and most available of the two therapies. It is initiated at an early stage to stabilize the animal and provide excretory supplementation until renal injury is repaired and adequate renal function returns (Figure 21-8). IHD, while less common, can be used in combination with conventional medical therapy in animals with severe CKF that cannot be managed with medications and diet alone. This is most frequently performed in acute-on-chronic kidney failure situations, to manage the patient through a difficult time.

The major difference between IHD and CRRT is the length of time required to clear creatinine and urea and normalize the patient. IHD does this very rapidly, in a few hours, but since it is used primarily in CKF, this requires the patient to return every few days. CRRT runs continuously, often for 48 to 96 hours or longer, slowly removing wastes from the patient and taking over the function of the kidney.

Hemodialysis incorporates an artificial kidney or dialysis filter to reduce the azotemia and correct life-threatening fluid, electrolyte, and acid-base imbalances. The filter uses a biocompatible membrane that removes nitrogenous waste products, excess water, and other solutes from the animal's blood down gradients from high to lower concentrations without permitting diffusion and ultrafiltration of larger constituents such as blood cells and proteins.

To perform hemodialysis, a special double-lumen catheter is surgically placed into the external jugular vein for access to the animal's blood for delivery to the dialysis machine. Blood is carried to and from the dialysis delivery system and dialyzer by extracorporeal tubing. Liters of blood, many times the total blood volume of the animal, are processed to normalize the serum creatinine and blood urea nitrogen levels, the concentrations of electrolytes, and water balances.

Many therapeutic options are available for animals with AKI. If treatments are initiated early enough, then the chances of kidney regeneration and recovery increase. The animal may go on to lead a normal life with or without supportive care and nutritional management for many months to years.

RENAL TRANSPLANTATION

Renal transplantation can be used to treat cats with AKI or CKF if regeneration and recovery of the existing kidneys is unlikely (Figure 21-9). Dogs have undergone successful transplantation procedures; however, the success rate is low and no veterinary teaching hospitals currently offer the procedure.

The owners of the animal with a transplanted kidney must be dedicated to treating their pet for life with medications to prevent donor kidney rejection. These medications are immunosuppressive drugs that are combined for optimum effect, such as cyclosporine and prednisone. Transplant recipients must be examined periodically to assess their renal function and cyclosporine levels. Most centers that offer transplants also require that the clients adopt or find a home for the donor cat. Transplanted patients can lead a normal life, and the new kidney can function for many years.

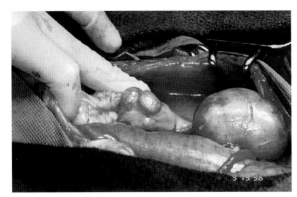

FIGURE 21-9 Kidney transplant. The left organ is a diseased kidney; on the right is the newly transplanted kidney. (Photograph courtesy Dr. Lili Aronson, University of California–Davis, Veterinary Medical Teaching Hospital, 1997.)

CONCLUSION

Treatment of the urologic emergency depends on the stage of disease or degree of trauma that has occurred. Monitoring equipment and blood analyzers must be available.

The veterinary technician plays a very important role in treating these patients by recognizing the progression of symptoms in the declining patient and understanding the tools used to evaluate the patient's condition.

SUGGESTED READINGS

Anderson RB, Aronson LR, Drobatz KJ, et al.: Prognostic factors for successful outcome following urethral rupture in dogs and cats, *JAAHA* 42:136–146, 2006.

Cooper ES, Owens TJ, Chew DJ, et al.: A protocol for managing urethral obstruction in male cats without urethral catheterization, *JAVMA* 11:1261–1266, 2010.

Cowgill LD: Renal failure, acute. In Tilley LP, Francis WK, Smithe JP, editors: *The five minute veterinary consult, canine and feline*, Baltimore, 1997, Williams & Wilkins.

Cowgill LD, Langston CE: Role of hemodialysis in the management of dogs and cats with renal failure, *Vet Clin North Am Small Anim Pract* 26(6):1347, 1996.

Finco DR: Obstructive uropathy and hydronephrosis. In Osborne CA, Finco DR, editors: *Canine and feline nephrology and urology*, Baltimore, 1995, Williams & Wilkins.

Lees GE: Management of voiding disability following relief of obstruction. In August JR, editor: *Feline internal medicine*, ed 2, Philadelphia, 1994, Saunders.

Ling GV: *Lower urinary tract diseases of dogs and cats. Diagnosis, medical management and prevention*, St Louis, 1995, Mosby.

O'Hearn AK, Wright BD: Coccygeal epidural with local anesthetic for catheterization and pain management in the treatment of feline urethral obstruction, *J Vet Emerg Crit Care* 21(1):50–52, 2011.

Osborne CA et al.: Feline lower urinary tract disease: relationships between crystalluria, urinary tract infections and host factors. In August JR, editor: *Feline internal medicine*, ed 2, Philadelphia, 1994, Saunders.

Osborne CA, et al.: Canine and feline urolithiasis: relationships of etiopathogenesis to treatment and prevention. In Osborne CA, Finco DR, editors: *Canine and feline nephrology and urology*, Baltimore, 1995, Williams & Wilkins.

Rieser T: Urinary tract emergencies, *Vet Clin Small Animal Pract* 35(2005):359–373, 2005.

SCENARIO

Purpose: To provide the veterinary technician with an opportunity to discover different approaches providing stabilization and nursing care to the patient with a urologic emergency.

Stage: Level III emergency clinic is open Monday through Thursday 6 PM to 8 AM, weekends 24/7 beginning Friday night at 6 PM, and closing Monday morning at 8 AM. All patients are transferred to the referral practice in the morning except on weekends.

Scenario

2-year-old male Labrador arrives lethargic and with a history of inappetence and vomiting for 2 days. Owners noted an increase in drinking and urinating. He also has been quieter during their walks in the woods and unwilling to swim in the nearby stream—something he enjoys regularly.

The exam reveals the following: HR, 140 bpm; RR/pattern, 44/tachypnea; pulses bounding; temp, 103.0° F (39.4° C). Quick assessment tests show: Azo, 50-80 mg/dl; BG, 120 mg/dl (6.6 mmol/L); PCV, 32%; TS, 7.0 g/dl. Further diagnostics reveal neutrophilia, creatinine 4.0 g/dl (353 μmol/L), phosphorus 3.5 mg/dl (1.13 mmol/L). Urine analysis: SG, 1.010, + protein, no cells or cast on sediment.

Questions

1. What would be the initial differentials?
2. What would be some causes for the condition?
3. How would you proceed?

Discussion

1. Acute kidney injury.
2. Acute kidney injury in a young dog could be due to toxicity or dehydration, or be infectious in origin.

   Considering this dog has a history of being exposed to streams and is very active outdoors, leptospirosis should be suspected. Careful consideration of how to avoid contact with urine must be included in nursing care plan including wearing proper PPE and disinfecting areas in which patient is housed.

MEDICAL MATH EXERCISE

A patient with AKI is hospitalized on fluids and you have been tasked with closely monitoring his urine output. What would be the normal expected urine volume for a 25-kg patient on fluids?

 a. 25-50 ml/hr
 b. 50-100 ml/hr
 c. 2.5-5.0 ml/hr
 d. 5.0-10.0 ml/hr

22 Reproductive Emergencies

Amy Breton

CHAPTER OUTLINE

Four Phases of Ovarian Cycle
  Proestrus
  Estrus
  Diestrus
  Anestrus
Reproductive Emergencies in Females
  Stages of Parturition
  Dystocia
  Uterine/Vaginal Prolapse

  Mastitis
  Pyometra
  Uterine Torsions
  Eclampsia
Reproductive Emergencies in Males
  Prostate Disorders
  Paraphimosis
  Testicular/Scrotal Disorders
  Penile Trauma
  Urethral Prolapse

KEY TERMS

Caesarean section
Canine
Dystocia
Eclampsia
Emergency
Feline
Female
Male
Mastitis
Neonatal
Parturition
Penis
Prostate
Pyometra
Reproduction
Testicle
Urethral

LEARNING OBJECTIVES

After studying this chapter, you will be able to:

- Understand the different reproductive emergencies that occur in both the male and female dog and cat.
- Understand the unique nursing care that patients experiencing reproductive emergencies require.

There are numerous life-threatening emergencies that can affect both the **male** and the **female** reproductive tract. Legitimate breeders are often well-versed and educated about the latest advances. A good breeder must be concerned for all of their dogs, including the female, the litter (which represents their financial return), and the male (for which they must be concerned about future fertility). In both male and female patients, stabilization and treatment depend on disease severity, age, and breeding potential. Treatment of these emergencies requires knowledge of the **reproduction** system and its pathophysiology as well as understanding of the options that are available.

FOUR PHASES OF OVARIAN CYCLE

PROESTRUS

The duration of this phase is usually 6 to 11 days (Noakes et al, 2009). During this phase vaginal bleeding begins. In addition, males are attracted to the female but she is not receptive to breeding. Hormonal activity in the proestrus phase is dominated by estrogen that is being produced by developing ovarian follicles. Peak plasma estrogen levels are achieved 24 to 48 hours before the end of proestrus and the beginning of estrus. Anatomic changes include enlargement or swelling of the vulva, growth of the mammary glands, thickening of the oviducts and endometrium, increased glandular activity in the endometrium, elongation of the uterine horns, increased myometrial sensitivity, enlargement of the cervix, and edema and elongation of the vagina along with a thickening of the vaginal walls (Noakes et al, 2009).

ESTRUS

The duration of estrus is usually 5 to 9 days (Noakes et al, 2009). Vaginal bleeding stops and the female shows signs of behavioral estrus allowing breeding. Hormonal activity during estrus changes from estrogen to progesterone. Follicular cells begin producing progesterone. Ovulation occurs within 24 to 72 hours of the beginning of this phase (Noakes et al, 2009). The uterus increases in size and thickness and may be palpable during abdominal examination. The appearance of the vulva is more flaccid.

DIESTRUS

The duration of this phase averages 56 to 58 days in the pregnant female and 60 to 100 days in the nonpregnant female (Noakes et al, 2009). Diestrus begins when the female no longer allows breeding. Hormonal activity is still progesterone dominant with concentrations reaching 15 to 90 ng/ml (Noakes et al, 2009). Pregnant females have higher levels of progesterone than nonpregnant females. Individual variations do exist. The uterus continues to respond to progesterone production by maintaining glandular secretions and vascularity required for pregnancy regardless of mating. The vulva returns to normal size.

ANESTRUS

Transition from diestrus to anestrus is not easily detectable because of the variations in duration of the nonpregnant female. Typically, the female begins proestrus about every 6 to 7 months. Therefore, anestrus is approximately 4 to 5 months in duration (Noakes et al, 2009). In the pregnant female, anestrus begins with whelping and ends when proestrus begins. Anestrus is the quiet phase in which the uterus undergoes repair. Progesterone levels remain low during anestrus.

REPRODUCTIVE EMERGENCIES IN FEMALES

STAGES OF PARTURITION

In order to fully understand **dystocia,** it is important to remember what constitutes normal **parturition.**

> **TECHNICIAN NOTE**   The length of pregnancy is between 62 and 67 days in cats and 64 and 66 days in dogs. Most literature will cite that a bitch or queen is considered late after 70 to 72 days of pregnancy.

There are three official stages of parturition; using the dog as an example, these are the following:

Stage 1 of parturition is usually noticed when the female becomes restless, possibly pacing and nesting (building a bed in which to whelp) (Noakes et al, 2009). In a normal pet, signs at this stage may include behavioral changes such as nesting behaviors, seeking seclusion, panting, and anorexia, vomiting, and sometimes shivering. Although not usually visible, uterine contractions begin in this stage. This stage lasts from 6 to 24 hours. Lactation and a transient temperature drop of approximately 2° F (≈1° C) (usually less than 100° F/37° C) occur about 24 hours before delivery (Noakes et al, 2009).

Stage 2 of parturition consists of visible uterine contractions, cervical dilation, rupture of the chorioallantoic fluid, and expulsion of the fetus (Figure 22-1).

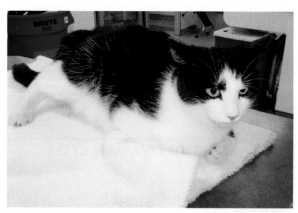

FIGURE 22-1 Female having active contractions and straining to push.

The actual onset of parturition occurs when plasma progesterone levels decrease to <2 ng/ml (Macintire, 2008). There may be green mucoid vaginal discharge before, during, and even after parturition. Once strong contractions are occurring and the animal is pushing and fluid discharge has been seen, the time of delivery should be less than 1 hour for the delivery of the first fetus. A puppy should be whelped, every 10 to 60 minutes, but this can extend up to 3 hours in some cases. Both resting and straining phases occur between individual fetuses. The resting phase may last up to 3 hours. The size of the litter and the quality of the labor are factors in the length of time between delivery of the first and last puppy.

Stage 3 of parturition is the expulsion of the fetal membrane, known as the allantochorion or placenta. This stage actually is interspersed with stage 2. The placenta should be seen 5 to 15 minutes after each fetus. Passage of the placenta may occur after each fetus or after two or three fetuses. The female should be monitored to ensure that a placenta is delivered with each fetus. Retention of placentas may cause endometritis later. A green to reddish brown vaginal discharge can occur for up to 2 weeks after whelping, and light spotting can occur for 8 weeks.

There are several in-house tests that can be used to measure the level of progesterone of dogs. Although there is not one specific to cats, there have been several reports of using the **canine** progesterone tests on cats with success. One of the most accurate is the ICAGEN-Target canine ovulation timing diagnostic test, which has been proven to accurately detect progesterone levels in dogs with an 85% accuracy (Manothaiudom et al, 1995). This test can be used to time both ovulation and parturition.

DYSTOCIA

Dystocia is defined as abnormal labor or birth, which could mean anything that is not considered normal.

> *TECHNICIAN NOTE* The consequences are numerous and include the following: increased stillbirth rate; increased mortality of fetuses; increased neonatal morbidity; increased mortality for the female; reduced fertility and increase of sterility in the female. There are several key indicators that a female is experiencing dystocia (Box 22-1).

There are two types of causes of dystocia: maternal or fetal (Noakes et al, 2009). Maternal causes include uterine inertia (e.g., heredity, systemic illness, hormones, senility, intrinsic weakness) or an anatomic abnormality (e.g., pelvic fracture, vaginal stricture or mass, uterine torsion). Fetal causes include giant fetuses, death, and malpositioning (Macintire, 2008). A study performed in 1994 of 155 bitches that suffered dystocia showed that 75.3% were due to maternal causes and 23.7% were fetal causes (Noakes et al, 2001).

Dogs tend to experience dystocia more than cats. It is more common in brachycephalic (large heads and wide shoulders, such as bulldogs, pugs, Boston terriers) and achondroplastic breeds (Macintire, 2008). Achondroplasia (dwarfism) causes a reduction in dimension from the sacrum to the pubic bone and thus reduces the pelvic canal (basset hounds, dachshunds). In one of the few studies involving cats, dystocia was reported in only 5.8% of cats. Pedigree breeds had a slightly higher incidence, such as the Devon Rex, which was reported to have an 18.2% frequency. In dogs this number is increased to 15% to 20%. Brachycephalic and achondroplastic breeds have a significantly higher frequency, with some reports being as high as 50% (Noakes et al, 2001).

In livestock, prevention of dystocia begins by trying to eliminate fetomaternal disproportion (condition in which the fetus is too large, relative to the diameter

BOX 22-1	Eight Signs of Dystocia

1. If no signs of labor are present within 24 hours of a decrease in rectal temperature or a decrease in progesterone levels
2. If no puppy is produced after 30 to 60 minutes of hard labor
3. Crying, biting or injuring the vulva area
4. Abnormal vaginal discharge (hemorrhage, odorous, mucopurulent)
5. Resting for more than 4 hours between fetuses without contractions
6. Presence of a fetus or fetal membranes in the vulva for >15 minutes
7. Weak or absent contractions for more than 2 hours
8. Signs of illness on the female (major exhaustion, fever, tremors, multiple vomiting)

From Macintire D: *Reproductive emergencies*, Atlantic Coast Veterinary Conference Proceedings, 2008.

BOX 22-2	Screening for Potential Dystocias

- What is the female doing now?
- What concerns prompted the owner to call?
- What is the age and breed of the female?
- What is the breed of male who bred with her?
- Is the due date known? If not, then when was the female bred?
- When was the last time the female was in season?
- Does the owner know how many puppies/kittens exist (by radiograph or ultrasound)?
- Does the female have any discharge? If so, what is the color of the discharge? Is there a foul odor?
- Have any fetuses been delivered? How many were born alive? How many were stillborn?
- Is the female actively pushing now? If so, for how long?
- If the female is not pushing, how long has it been since the last fetus was born?

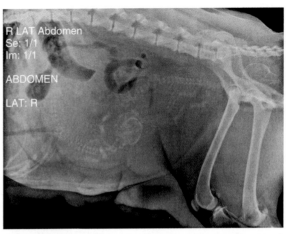

FIGURE 22-2 Radiograph of a fetus stuck in the pelvic canal.

of the dam's pelvic canal) (Noakes et al, 2001). Prevention can occur by simply breeding smaller size males to larger size females. Unfortunately, this does not always occur and the variety of dog breeds has caused this to be impossible at times. There have been studies showing an increase in obesity linked to an increase in dystocia. Therefore, ideally only well-conditioned females should be bred (Noakes et al, 2001). This is why overweight achondroplastic and brachycephalic females typically require a cesarean section.

Diagnosis is based on a thorough history and physical exam of the patient (Box 22-2). Sometimes this can be difficult if the owner is not a legitimate breeder. Often owners have no idea when their female was bred or sometimes even that it is pregnant. Radiographs should be taken to check for fetal positioning, number and size of fetuses, maternal pelvic abnormalities, signs of fetal death (spinal collapse, interfetal gas patterns, overlapping skull bones), and loss of abdominal detail and free gas (uterine rupture) (Macintire, 2008). Ultrasonography and Doppler may allow for auscultation of fetal heartbeats (Figure 22-2).

Treatment options depend on many different issues including the owner's wishes, the viability of the female, and the viability of the fetuses (Noakes et al, 2009). Three treatment options are available: (1) manual manipulation, (2) medical intervention, and (3) surgical management.

If radiographs reveal no abnormalities, then a vaginal exam should be performed. If a fetus is detected in the birth canal, attempts should be made to remove it with gentle steady traction and copious lubrication. Instruments should be avoided because they can cause serious injury to the fetus. If necessary, an episiotomy can be performed (Macintire, 2008).

If no obstruction is present, then medical management should be attempted. Before the administration of oxytocin or the performance of a C-section, the female should have her blood glucose and calcium levels tested. Both a low blood glucose level and a low calcium level may cause dystocia. Neither dextrose nor calcium should be given to the pet unless there has been blood work performed to conclude the pet is deficient. If blood work is not possible, then either drug can be given as long as there is obvious physical evidence that the female is showing signs of hypoglycemia or hypocalcemia. Pets with hypoglycemia will be lethargic, shaking/twitching, and ataxic, or they will develop seizures. Hypocalcemic pets will exhibit nervousness, seizures, focal muscle cramping, tetany, ataxia, weakness, lethargy, panting, and facial rubbing. Compared to cats, it is more common in dogs for them to develop hypocalcemia and is a particular risk in smaller dog breeds (Macintire, 2008). Intravenous calcium gluconate should always be given with caution and the patient should be monitored with an electrocardiogram (ECG) when it is given. If given too rapid intravenously (IV), calcium can cause hypotension, cardiac arrhythmias, and cardiac arrest. A good rule of thumb is to administer 1.0 ml over 2 minutes. If you notice any arrhythmias on the ECG or bradycardia, administration of the drug should be immediately discontinued and the patient reevaluated. Veterinarians experienced in this area have suggested that calcium gluconate be given subcutaneously 15 minutes before oxytocin administration and that intravenous calcium be reserved for cases of **eclampsia;** they believe that the oxytocin will stimulate contractions and the subsequent dose of calcium will strengthen them.

Oxytocin is the drug of choice to help increase contractions. Most of the time, unless hypoglycemia or hypocalcemia has been diagnosed, it is the first drug that will be administered. It is a drug specific to help with inertia issues. There are two types of uterine inertia. Primary uterine inertia is where the uterine muscles do not contract normally at parturition. This is generally attributable to a failure of the muscles to respond to hormonal stimuli or a failure of the actual release of hormonal stimuli. It may also be a lack of the development of receptors. In females with primary uterine inertia, oxytocin will likely be ineffective (Shaw, 2007). In these cases, a cesarian section is indicated. Secondary uterine inertia is where the female has experienced prolonged dystocia or where normal labor ceased after the delivery of fetuses even though more fetuses are in the uterus. Oxytocin will help those females experiencing secondary uterine inertia. Because it is usually impossible to differentiate between primary and secondary uterine inertia, oxytocin is typically given in both cases to see if it is efficacious. Lower doses have been proven just as effective as higher doses (0.25 to 5 units/kg intramuscularly) (Macintire, 2008). Oxytocin can be given IV, but it is important to not overdose because it can lead to tetanic uterine contractions (sustained muscular contraction without intervals of relaxation), which can impair placental blood flow (Noakes et al, 2009). After IV administration, uterine response should occur almost immediately while intramuscular (IM) administration response generally takes about 3 to 5 minutes. The effects last between 10 and 20 minutes.

A C-section should be performed if it has been longer than 24 hours after the rectal temperature drop, the radiograph reveals fetal oversize or inadequate pelvic diameter, more than two doses of oxytocin have been given with no contractions, or the female appears in inappropriate distress (Noakes et al, 2009). Although there are certainly risks involved, a study in 1994 revealed a 75% success rate in all dog neonates and a 42% success rate in all cat neonates following a C-section (Noakes et al, 2001). In approximately 60 to 80% of dystocia cases in the bitch and queen, surgical intervention is required (Traas, 2009).

The goal of any C-section is to minimize anesthesia time and still provide adequate analgesia to the female. It is important to determine whether the client wishes to preserve the life of the mother, the offspring, or both. Despite continued debate, there are no data that suggest that local versus general anesthesia is superior (Carroll, 2004). However, one could argue that having an awake patient may be very difficult to handle, so likely the use of an inhalant may be a more practical technique (Carroll, 2004; Pascoe, 2004). The longer it takes for the neonates to be removed from the female, the more time they will have to absorb drugs and therefore it will take a longer time to resuscitate them. Drug time can be reduced by shaving the patient and performing a rough-scrub before any administration of drugs or inhalant anesthesia. Current data suggest that anesthesia time may not influence neonatal survival; however, until further research is performed, it is best to decrease the amount of time the neonates have to absorb drugs (Pascoe, 2004).

Remember that pregnant animals are not generally fasted, so aspiration is a concern. A rapid induction technique should follow preoxygenation because of the increased potential for regurgitation and aspiration during induction (Pascoe, 2004). Using face masks or strong-acting opioids may be inappropriate because of the delay in intubation that they may cause. However, mask induction may be chosen because it will have the least effect on the neonates since the inhalant can be breathed off rapidly and does not need to be metabolized (Pascoe, 2004). Progesterone decreases the MAC (minimum alveolar concentration) of an inhalant (Carroll, 2004). Isoflurane has been associated with improved **neonatal** survival compared with older inhalants. Sevoflurane has a greater effect on uterine muscle relaxation than isoflurane, but no studies have been performed yet indicating it is a superior choice (Pascoe, 2004).

Pregnant females also have an apparent sensitivity to anesthetics (Carroll, 2004).

Almost all drugs cross into the placenta and will likely need to be metabolized by the fetus. The fetus is not able to metabolize most drugs on an adult level, which may cause them to be sedated for a longer period of time (Pascoe, 2004). Propofol is interesting because it initially is rapidly absorbed by the female and therefore the fetuses initially experience a very high concentration. However, eventually the drug crosses back from the fetuses to the bitch/queen (Pascoe, 2004; Traas, 2009). It has been suggested that the optimal time to remove the puppies/kittens would be about 15 to 20 minutes after the induction with propofol since this would allow them to metabolize most of the propofol back to the female. Propofol-isoflurane as a combination has been shown to have minimal effects on neonatal survival (Pascoe, 2004). There is no advantage to maintaining anesthesia only with propofol. Maintaining only with propofol would cause greater concentrations in the neonates, which would have to be metabolized rather than exhaled (Pascoe, 2004).

Thiopental has been widely used in human obstetric medicine because it has more of a rapid onset of action than propofol (Pascoe, 2004). The dose used in people is considerably lower than that needed in a dog or cat. Neonates take a long time to metabolize thiopental so it is not an ideal choice (Pascoe, 2004).

Ketamine and diazepam (or midazolam) help to increase blood pressure, cardiac output, and uterine blood flow in the female (Pascoe, 2004). In several studies ketamine combinations did not affect puppy survival, but ketamine can cause a major depressant effect, causing the neonates to need intensive resuscitation (Pascoe, 2004; Traas, 2009).

Alpha-2 agonists (xylazine, romifidine, and medetomidine) are definitely not recommended for C-section (Pascoe, 2004). They have all been associated with higher mortality after C-section. Bradycardia, hypertension, and hypoxemia have all been reported. Even at low doses (1 mcg/kg IV) medetomidine has been shown to decrease cardiac output 60% to 70% and cause a 200% increase in systemic vascular resistance (Pascoe, 2004).

Pregnant females, in general, are often volume depleted and exhausted (Carroll, 2004). In severely ill females, etomidate may be a safe but expensive induction agent (Pascoe, 2004). Etomidate is fast acting with a short duration of action and still provides good cardiovascular support (Pascoe, 2004). There is not a lot of research in veterinary medicine available regarding etomidate. If the female has any preexisting cardiac dysfunction, etomidate would likely be the drug of choice.

In humans the FDA classifies etomidate as a Class C drug, meaning "Animal reproduction studies have shown an adverse effect on the fetus and there are no adequate and well-controlled studies in humans, but potential benefits may warrant use of the drug in pregnant women despite potential risks." While it has not been reported in dogs and cats, etomidate has caused embryocidal (death of a fetus) effects in rats and maternal toxicity in rabbits and rats. Despite concerns, etomidate may be the drug of choice in severely ill females.

Hypotension and hypoxia may be a problem when the patient is placed in dorsal recumbency position (Macintire, 2008). Blood flow to the fetus is not auto-regulated. Uterine perfusion depends on the blood pressure of the rest of the body (Carroll, 2004). To help with pressure, the patient may need to be slightly tilted toward the surgeon (Noakes et al, 2009). Aggressive cardiovascular support is needed. Mean arterial pressure should ideally be maintained greater than 80 mm Hg (Carroll, 2004).

Pain medication must be used once the neonates are delivered, as well as postoperatively. All opioids (e.g., fentanyl, morphine, oxymorphone, butorphanol) have been used in human obstetric anesthesia. Oxymorphone has been shown to be more of a depressant than the other opioids to human neonates (Pascoe, 2004). In humans, fentanyl has been shown to cause no change in neonatal Apgar scores (score assessing condition of newborn child), blood gases, or uterine blood flow. Both oxymorphone and hydromorphone can be used for pain and both allow for minimal transmission into the milk. Nonsteroidal antiinflammatory drugs may also be used because they do not appear to cross into the milk in high quantities. In general, opioids are not considered a major risk factor in dogs or cats during C-section, and, if there is concern, depression may be reversed with naloxone (Pascoe, 2004).

Once the neonates are delivered, resuscitation should begin immediately. Fetal membranes should be cleared from the face and nasal passages by using gentle suction. Flinging the neonate in a downward motion should be avoided because this has been shown to cause head trauma or accidental injury by dropping. Oxygen and warmth should be administered immediately. A large face mask with oxygen flowing into it on top of a warm pad makes a nice place to put the neonates. If a face mask is not available, flow-by oxygen can be administered (Figure 22-3).

Doxapram given under the tongue can be used to help stimulate breathing. However, more literature suggests that doxapram is of little to no benefit to the neonate. There is some evidence that it causes the neonate to require an increase in oxygen demand, something that their body cannot handle. There is no evidence showing that the death rates change with the use or nonuse of doxapram. It is the decision of the veterinarian on duty whether doxapram should be integrated into the resuscitation of the neonates. Umbilical cords should be ligated with absorbable suture. As soon as the female is fully recovered, she should be allowed to nurse.

Care of the Neonates

Puppies that remain in the hospital to be with the bitch are considered separate patients. Color-coded neck bands or ribbon can be used to differentiate between multiple puppies and will eliminate confusion when attempting to maintain records of assessments on individual puppies.

Owners are encouraged to take the bitch home soon after recovery (owners sometimes choose to take puppies home while the bitch recovers). Instructing owners on how and when to feed their animals as well as how and when to stimulate them to urinate and defecate is important. Puppies are not to be fed unless their temperature is 96° F or higher.

Puppies that remain in the hospital are not to be left in the cage with the bitch unsupervised (having one of the puppies fall through the bars of the cage or become trapped in a blanket is too great a risk). The bitch must be introduced to the puppies slowly and cautiously. She is a postoperative patient and uncomfortable; therefore the technician should assume that she is unpredictable. To ensure their safety, puppies should be placed in an incubator between feedings.

The clinician should do the following when filling out the patient's treatment sheet:

- Document behavior, strength, nursing ability, and increase or decrease of urine and/or defecation when stimulated.
- Assess ventilatory nature, respiration rate, heart rate, and environmental temperature every 30 minutes for the first 90 minutes postoperatively, then every 2 hours afterward. (The doctor will order rectal temperatures if necessary.)
- Encourage puppies to latch on every 1 to 2 hours; stimulate the animals to urinate and defecate.
- Check the umbilical cord site for excessive bleeding.
- Record examination on the puppy's individual form when the doctor examines for cleft palate and heart murmurs.

UTERINE/VAGINAL PROLAPSE

Although it is extremely rare, uterine prolapse usually occurs during or within 48 hours of parturition when the cervix is open. Uterine prolapse is more common in cats than in dogs (Traas and O'Connor, 2009). Both horns or one of the horns of the uterus can prolapse. If fetuses remain, surgery will be needed immediately to offer the best chance of survival (Figure 22-4).

Even rarer is a vaginal prolapse in the dog or cat (Noakes and Parkinson, 2001) (Figure 22-5). It generally occurs during the period of estrus, but also can occur

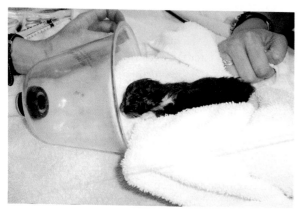

FIGURE 22-3 Oxygen support and warming of neonates are important during resuscitation.

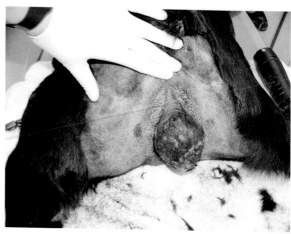

FIGURE 22-4 Uterine prolapse.

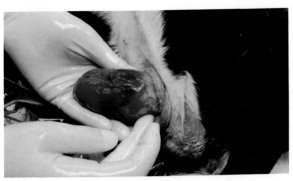

FIGURE 22-5 Vaginal prolapse.

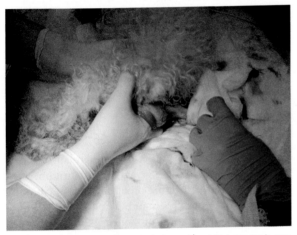

FIGURE 22-6 Digital manipulation without instruments is preferred when there is a trapped fetus.

during dystocia or forced extraction of the male's **penis** during mating (Ettinger and Feldman, 1993; Noakes and Parkinson, 2001). If a vaginal prolapse has occurred, a uterine prolapse may occur secondarily (Ettinger and Feldman, 1993).

Digital manipulation under general anesthesia may be attempted to replace the uterus or vagina as soon as possible to help reduce tissue necrosis and edema (Figure 22-6). Applying hyperosmotic fluids (50% dextrose/ mannitol) may reduce swelling and allow for easier replacement (Traas and O'Connor, 2009). If successful, oxytocin should be given IM to aid in uterine contractions (Macintire, 2004). If digital manipulation is unsuccessful, then a laparotomy may be needed. There is a high risk of infection, trauma (uterine vessel rupture, hemoabdomen), and necrosis with a vaginal or uterine prolapse. Usually an ovariohysterectomy is the simplest option unless the pet is a breeding animal. While reoccurrence may

happen with future litters, females have been reported to have successful pregnancies following uterine or vaginal prolapse (Traas and O'Connor, 2009).

MASTITIS

Mastitis is an inflammatory process in one or more mammary glands within the nipple, usually in a lactating female. Mastitis causes the nipple to become hard, swollen, and painful. Mastitis can range from galactostasis (cessation of lactation) to septic shock.

> *TECHNICIAN NOTE*   While it is not always an emergency, it should be treated in a timely manner to ensure it does not become an emergency. Neonates should be allowed to nurse as long as the female will tolerate. This will allow for continued drainage and help to avoid galactostasis (Macintire, 2004).

If the nipples become necrotic or the female is systemically ill (such as fever or vomiting), the neonates should be transferred to bottles. The most common bacteria are *Escherichia coli, Staphylococcus aureus,* and beta-hemolytic *Streptococcus* (Macintire, 2004). The nipples should be cultured and hot-packing, antibiotics, and pain medications should be started. In very severe cases, the nipples may need to be lanced, drained, flushed, and debrided (Macintire, 2004). Females with very high fevers may need IV and nutritional support until the fever has subsided and the patient is eating again.

PYOMETRA

Pyometra generally occurs in middle-aged females during diestrus (Macintire, 2004). It can also be seen up to 10 weeks after estrogen therapy for mismating in female dogs and in cats or dogs receiving progestins. Normally during diestrus the cervix begins to close and the inner lining begins to return to normal. Unfortunately, cystic endometrial hyperplasia (CEH) may occur during this time for some females attributable to an inappropriate response to progesterone (Macintire, 2004). If this occurs, bacteria (usually *E. coli*) that migrated from the vagina into the uterus find the CEH favorable for growth. Unfortunately, progesterone also causes mucus secretion, aids in closing the cervix, and decreases uterine contractility, which makes the

environment even more favorable for bacterial growth. The condition of the cervix is a major factor in the severity of the condition. If the cervix remains open, the infected material can leave the body, making it far easier and safer to treat (open pyometra). If the cervix becomes fully closed, the uterus may rupture, causing a septic abdomen (closed pyometra).

Signs generally include vaginal discharge (open pyometra), vomiting, diarrhea, dehydration, lethargy, anorexia, depression, polyuria, and polydipsia. Clinical signs may be subtle in cats. Because of their grooming habits, vaginal discharge may not be seen.

A diagnosis is generally made by radiographs or ultrasound. Radiography is used to confirm the presence of an enlarged uterus. Loss of abdominal detail may suggest peritonitis secondary to uterine rupture. Ultrasonography is used to differentiate pyometra from pregnancy or hydrometra.

Blood work generally reveals leukocytosis. The pet may also have prerenal azotemia because E. coli interferes with Na^+ and Cl^- absorption in the loop of Henle and also blocks the action of antidiuretic hormone (ADH) on the collecting ducts. This results in polyuria and subsequent polydipsia (Macintire, 2004). It is important not to perform a cystocentesis if a pyometra is suspected because you may rupture the uterus. E. coli can produce an endotoxin upon bacterial death that can result in endotoxemia. This can cause a severe shock reaction and death (Romagnolli, 2002). Vaginal cytologic and culture results may be helpful in diagnosing pyometra and selecting antibiotics. Determination of blood gas and electrolyte levels will help in developing a fluid therapy plan.

Any emergent signs should be stabilized (hypotension, decreased blood glucose levels, high fever). Closed pyometras should be managed surgically because it offers the best chance of survival for the female (Figure 22-7). Surgical complications include sepsis and peritonitis. In Europe the drug aglepristone may be used instead of surgical intervention. Aglepristone works by blocking the progesterone receptors and thus impedes the adhesion of bacteria on the surface of the endometrium. It also allows for the opening of the cervix, which then allows for emptying of the uterine contents. For many patients that are very critical where surgery may not be an immediate option, aglepristone can be given to start alleviating the infection. This may also be indicated when the female is prized breeding stock.

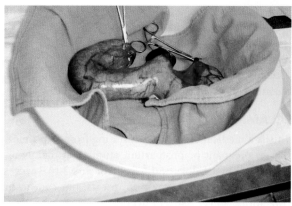

FIGURE 22-7 An overiohysterectomy is always the safest option for a female who has a pyometra.

Open pyometras may be managed medically. Low-dose oxytocin can be administered to help empty the discharge from the open pyometra. However, if the cervix is only partially dilated or the uterus is fully dilated with purulent material, then inducing contractions may cause a rupture to occur. If there is a large amount of material, then prostaglandins can be used (dinoprost, cloprostenol, alphaprostol) two to three times a day for about 2 to 3 weeks (Romagnolli, 2002). The prostaglandins have a direct stimulating effect on uterine smooth muscle, causing contraction and a relaxant effect on the cervix. Side effects of prostaglandins are usually short in duration and include anxiety, vomiting, diarrhea, tachypnea, and tachycardia (Noakes et al, 2009). Antibiotics should be administered for 2 to 4 weeks for either an open or a closed pyometra. Ultimately, there are pros/cons on whether to medically manage or surgically manage a pyometra. Owners generally make the decision on treatment based on finances and whether it is a valuable breeding animal.

UTERINE TORSIONS

Rarely do uterine torsions occur. If it does occur, it could be a partial or full torsion. Some reasons they may occur could be jumping or running late in the pregnancy, very active fetal movement, partial abortions, or abnormalities of the uterus. Uterine torsions are life threatening and can result in severe hemorrhage if the uterine artery becomes damaged (Noakes et al, 2009). Signs include severe pain, collapse, and abdominal distention.

It is often difficult to determine if the problem is torsion versus dystocia. On radiograph you may see a large fluid- or air-filled tubular structure in the abdomen (Noakes et al, 2009). Ultrasound generally provides a better diagnostic. An ovariohysterectomy is always recommended.

ECLAMPSIA

This is a medical **emergency** resulting from hypocalcemia in pregnant or postpartum animals. It mainly affects small breed dogs and usually occurs 2 to 3 weeks after delivery. It is uncommon in cats, but can occur (Macintire, 2004). Signs of hypocalcemia include tremors, panting, stiffness, pacing, whining, salivation, and restlessness. As the condition progresses, the pet can experience muscle spasms, fever, tachycardia, seizures, miosis, and death.

Hypocalcemia is defined as total calcium levels <7 mg/dl or ionized calcium levels <0.6 mmol/L (Traas and O'Connor, 2009). Diagnosis is made by running in-house calcium levels. If in-house testing is not available then hypocalcemia should be suspected if the female is showing signs and is pregnant or in the postpartum period. Although not ideal, treatment should begin on females if in-house testing is not available if symptoms are present since it is a life-threatening emergency.

Treatment must be started immediately. The treatment of choice is 10% calcium gluconate, and should be administered slowly with the patient monitored on ECG (Traas and O'Connor, 2009). The patient's other signs (fever, tachycardia) should be treated with IV fluids. A second dose of calcium gluconate can be given subcutaneously (SQ) as long as it is mixed in saline at a 50:50 dilution (Macintire, 2004; Traas and O'Connor, 2009). Calcium chloride can also be administered, but can only be given IV since other routes of administration cause tissue necrosis and skin sloughing. The animal should be sent home with oral calcium, which should be continued through lactation. Puppies should be removed from the female and bottle fed if the problem recurs (Traas and O'Connor, 2009).

REPRODUCTIVE EMERGENCIES IN MALES

PROSTATE DISORDERS

The **prostate's** function is to store and secrete a slightly alkaline fluid, milky white in appearance, which usually comprises about 25% to 30% of the volume of the semen. It also aids in helping to control the flow during ejaculation.

Cancer

In humans, a prostate-specific antigen (PSA) in a secretary protein can be evaluated to look for evidence of prostatic carcinoma (O'Connor and Traas, 2009). In dogs and cats there is currently no protein that has been found to be diagnostic (O'Connor and Traas, 2009). The most common prostate cancer results from adenocarcinoma (O'Connor and Traas, 2009). Other types of neoplasia include hemangiosarcoma, lymphosarcoma, and squamous cell carcinoma (O'Connor and Traas, 2009).

Abscesses/Cysts

Prostatic cysts and abscesses can also occur. The cause of cysts is unknown. The cause of most abscesses is due to benign prostatic hypertrophy (BPH). A prostate abscess can lead to sepsis and septic shock. Prostatic abscess occurs in dogs with an acute or chronic form of prostatitis. Clinical signs include lethargy, fever, vomiting, dysuria, abdominal pain, and **urethral** discharge. The animal may also experience signs of shock if the abscess has ruptured. A prostatic abscess can be confirmed by the use of radiography, ultrasonography, and prostate fluid analysis.

Surgical drainage of the prostatic abscesses or prostatectomy is performed once the dog has been stabilized. Castration also is recommended. Antimicrobials are continued postoperatively (Figure 22-8).

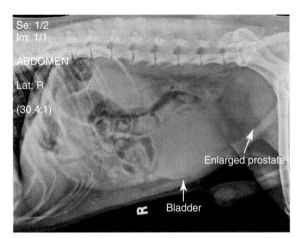

FIGURE 22-8 Radiograph of an enlarged prostate.

Benign Prostatic Hypertrophy

Benign prostatic hypertrophy (BPH) is the most common prostate disorder in intact male dogs and can cause an emergency to the pet. A metabolite of testosterone (5α-dihydrotestosterone) reaches the prostate in extremely high concentrations and promotes the accelerated growth of prostate cells (O'Connor and Traas, 2009). BPH is caused by the hyperplasia of prostatic stromal and epithelial cells that results in the formation of large nodules in the periurethral region of the prostate. When these nodules become significantly large, they can compress the urethral canal, causing partial or even complete obstruction of the urethra and resulting in the animal barely able to urinate. The most common complaint is bloody urine. Other signs include abdominal discomfort, straining to urinate, and dysuria (though more common in humans than in dogs). Dogs may have BPH and be asymptomatic. Although rarely an emergency, if an owner is not observant, the dog may experience the same signs and symptoms as a blocked male cat.

Acute bacterial prostatitis is common in dogs with BPH and occurs when bacteria grow in the prostate parenchyma. It is an acute inflammation of the prostate gland with gram-positive or gram-negative bacteria. The infection commonly results from bacteria ascending through the urethra. The bacteria also can be introduced through the bloodstream or reproductive tract. Older, intact male dogs are most commonly affected.

Clinical signs include lethargy, fever, dehydration, bloody discharge, and abdominal pain (Macintire, 2008). The dog may walk with a stiff gait and arched back because of the pain. A diagnosis usually is made based on the examination, routine laboratory evaluation, and response to treatment. A radiograph and ultrasound should be performed to rule out other diseases. Caudal abdominal radiographs may show an enlarged prostate.

Evaluation of the prostatic fluid including culture and cytology would be another tool for diagnosing bacterial prostatitis. Obtaining prostatic fluid from a dog experiencing prostatitis is painful and difficult, because ejaculation is necessary. Prostatic washes are an option but must be performed very carefully because of the risk of sepsis.

An antimicrobial is chosen based on the urine culture and administered for 4 to 6 weeks. Stabilization and fluid therapy may be necessary for more severe cases. Castration is recommended once the animal is stabilized.

PARAPHIMOSIS

> *TECHNICIAN NOTE* Paraphimosis is one of the most common reproductive emergencies in males.

It is the inability for the dog or cat to retract their penis. Causes include small prepubital orifice, a ring of fur encircling the penis, ineffective preputial muscles, preputial hypoplasia, trauma, infection, and neoplasia; alternatively, it could be an idiopathic cause. Exposure of the penis should always be treated like an emergency because of the risk of penile necrosis or injury, which may result in the need for a penile amputation (O'Connor and Traas, 2009). Generally, replacement of the penis can be done manually with some lubrication. Sedation may be needed. If edema is present then a hyperosmolic solution (dextrose, mannitol) may be used (O'Connor and Traas, 2009). Rarely, surgical intervention is needed. The pet should be monitored to ensure no self-mutilation occurs. Placement of an Elizabethan collar is usually necessary for a short time immediately after the incident.

TESTICULAR/SCROTAL DISORDERS

Orchitis (inflammation of one or both testicles) and epididymitis (inflammation of the long coiled tube attached to the upper part of each **testicle**) are more common in younger dogs. Signs include fever, lethargy, hunched posture, scrotal edema, or purulent penile discharge (O'Connor and Traas, 2009).

There are numerous diseases that can cause the testicles to become inflamed. If it results in a stud dog, antibiotics can be tried. If it is unilateral infection, a castration of the infected testicle may still allow the dog to be fertile. In general, if both sides are affected, infertility usually results and a full castration is recommended. Reasons for orchitis and epididymitis include trauma (laceration, hit by car, or burns, for example), neoplasia, vasculitis, spermatic cord torsion, and infection with *Brucella canis* (O'Connor and Traas, 2009).

Spermatic cord torsions are very uncommon, but should be considered in dogs with acute abdominal pain, vomiting, lethargy, anorexia, dysuria, hematuria, and fever. Torsion is more common in dogs where both testicles are retained (O'Connor and Traas, 2009). Treatment includes castration of the testicle(s) (Noakes et al, 2009).

Neoplasia should be considered whenever there are changes to the size or shape of the testicles. The most

common tumor is the Sertoli cell tumor. Scrotal neoplasia can also occur, and the three most common types of scrotal neoplasia are squamous cell carcinoma, melanoma, and mast cell (O'Connor and Traas, 2009). While generally these do not result in an emergency department visit, if they are left to spread and grow the symptoms may certainly cause a life-threatening condition (fever, sepsis, pain).

PENILE TRAUMA

Penile trauma can be common in both young and older dogs. It is rarely seen in cats. The actual fracture of the os penis is rare, but certainly a radiograph should be taken to rule it out (O'Connor and Traas, 2009). If the penis is injured, a urethral injury should also be suspected and contrast radiography may be indicated to rule out a tear in the urethra. Injury to the penis can occur during breeding, but the penis can also be injured during a traumatic event (hit by car, jumping a fence, bite wounds). Severe hemorrhage may occur because the penis is cavernous and very vascular. Treatment depends on the extent of the injury. Os penis fracture may result in a surgical reduction (O'Connor and Traas, 2009). Wound repair, antibiotics, indwelling urinary catheters, pain management, and penile amputation may all be indicated.

URETHRAL PROLAPSE

Urethral prolapses are generally seen in young brachycephalic breeds.

> *TECHNICIAN NOTE* Owners generally report excessive licking of the prepuce, blood dripping from the prepuce, or a fleshy mass protruding from the penis.

Usually only about 3 to 4 mm of urethra protrudes from the urethral orifice. Causes include repeated sexual arousal or urethral infection. Often the cause is unknown. Neoplasia should be ruled out.

Urethral prolapses are as much of an emergency as is paraphimosis. Treatment includes reducing the prolapse and preventing a reoccurrence by suturing the area closed. An indwelling urinary catheter should not be used because it can cause irritation to the surgical site, hemorrhage, and urinary tract infection. Occasionally amputation of the prolapsed portion of the urethra may be required. Placement of an Elizabethan collar is usually necessary for a short time immediately after the incident.

REFERENCES

Carroll G: *Anesthesia for C-section: what's safe and effective?* Western Veterinary Conference Proceedings, 2004.

Ettinger S, Feldman E: *Textbook of veterinary internal medicine, Chapter 304: Vaginal disorders*, St Louis, 2010, Saunders Elsevier, p 1933.

Macintire D: *Reproductive emergencies I: dystocia, acute metritis, eclampsia*, Western Veterinary Conference, 2004.

Macintire D: *Reproductive emergencies II: mastitis, pyometra, prolapses and mismating*, Western Veterinary Conference, 2004.

Macintire D: *Reproductive emergencies*, Atlantic Coast Veterinary Conference Proceedings, 2008.

Manothaiudom K, Johnston S, Hegstad R, et al.: Evaluation of the ICAGEN-Target canine ovulation timing diagnostic test in detecting canine plasma progesterone concentrations, *J Am Animal Hosp Assoc* 31(1):57–64, 1995.

Noakes D, Parkinson T, England G: *Veterinary reproduction & obstetrics*, ed 8, Philadelphia, 2001, Saunders.

Noakes D, Parkinson T, England G: *Veterinary reproduction & obstetrics*, ed 9, Philadelphia, 2009, Saunders.

O'Connor C, Traas A: *Male reproductive emergencies*, IVECCS Proceedings, 2009.

Pascoe P: *Cesarean section anesthesia*, Western Veterinary Conference Proceedings, 2004.

Romagnolli S: *Canine pyometra: pathogenesis, therapy, and clinic cases*, WSAVA Congress Proceedings, 2002.

Shaw S: *Dealing with reproductive emergencies*, IVECCS Proceedings, 2007.

Traas A: *Surgical management of dystocia*, IVECCS Proceedings, 2009.

Traas A, O'Connor C: *Postpartum emergencies*, IVECCS Proceedings, 2009.

SCENARIO

Purpose: To provide the veterinary technician with the ability to think about how he or she would handle a telephone call from a client with a pregnant female.

Stage: Emergency clinic is a 24-hour facility. Veterinary technicians are required to perform telephone triage.

Scenario

Female dog, 5 years old, first time pregnancy. Owner believes the female was mated with an unknown male about 2 months ago, but is not sure. The female had gone missing during this time. Owner brought in bitch to her own veterinarian about 6 weeks ago and

SCENARIO—cont'd

a radiograph was taken that confirmed nine fetuses at that time.

Today female started delivering puppies. So far, four have been delivered. The last fetus was delivered 90 minutes ago. The owner would like to know if she should be worried at this point.

Delivery
- Staff divides into groups and has **10 minutes** to discuss options.
- Discussion should continue without goal being to find the right answer.

Questions
- What questions should be asked of this owner over the phone?
- List some answers the owner may give and what you should then instruct the owner to do.

Key Teaching Points
- Provides veterinary technicians the opportunity to discuss how they would handle triage of a pregnant female over the telephone.

Discussion
Some questions to ask the owner:
- What is the breed of male who bred with her?
- Does the female have any discharge? If so, what is the color of the discharge? Is there a foul odor?

- How many fetuses were born alive? How many were stillborn?
- Is the female actively pushing now? If so, for how long?
- Do you see a fetus protruding?
  - If the owner answers that there was a possibility the female was bred with a significantly larger male the owner should watch the female more closely for signs of dystocia.
  - If the owner answers there is a discharge other than green or slightly brown/red in color or that there is an odor, the owner should be instructed to bring the animal to the clinic.
  - If there are stillborn fetuses that were delivered this may indicate she is now having an issue.
  - If the female is actively pushing and has been for more than 60 minutes she should be taken to the clinic because she is likely to have a dystocia.
  - If the owner can see a fetus and it has been more than 15 minutes since she saw it, then she should come into the clinic immediately.

References
- Box 22-1 should be used as a reference for the eight key signs of a dystocia.
- Box 22-2 should be used as a reference on questions to ask the owner.

MEDICAL MATH EXERCISE

Patient order states: *Give 0.25 unit/kg oxytocin IM.* The concentration of oxytocin is 20 units/ml. The dog weighs 23.5 kg.
  a. How many units of oxytocin does the dog need?
  b. How many milliliters of oxytocin will the dog receive?

23 Ocular Emergencies

Pam Dickens

KEY TERMS

Blepharospasm
Globe
Miosis
Ulcers
Uveitis

CHAPTER OUTLINE

Globe   Anterior Chamber
Eyelid   Lens
Cornea   Conclusion

LEARNING OBJECTIVES

After studying this chapter, you will be able to:
- Introduce common conditions of the eye seen in an emergency clinic.
- Identify different parts of the eye.
- Understand the terminology commonly used in ophthalmology.
- Introduce commonly used items and supplies used in an emergency involving the eye.

The eye is a sensitive organ that, when irritated may cause an animal a great deal of pain. Animals may express this discomfort in various ways such as squinting, rubbing or scratching at the eye, hiding in dark places, becoming aggressive or anorexic. A mild inflammation or infection may change to a serious condition in a short period of time. When an owner calls with a concern involving a pet's eye, the animal should be seen to rule out a serious condition and provide pain relief as soon as possible.

There are also breed predispositions to certain conditions of the eye (Table 23-1).

TECHNICIAN NOTE All brachycephalic breeds should be seen as soon as possible when any signs of blepharospasm are present (squinting of the eyelids).

The emergency facility must be equipped to deal with eye problems. Instruments used only for eyes should be stored in a separate pack; ointments and eyewash also should be available. Pain relievers and restraints are used to prevent the animal from damaging the eye after treatment. A variety of Elizabethan collars should be available to meet the needs of each patient.

The following is a list of suggested items.

Equipment:
- Welch Allyn ophthalmoscope or pan ophthalmoscope for direct ophthalmoscopy
- Condensing lenses (20-28 diopter) for indirect ophthalmoscopy

- Finoff transilluminator with blue light attachment
- OptiVISOR for magnification
- Tono-Pen/Tono-Vet (does not require topical anesthetic)
- 4-0 or 5-0 silk suture with P-3 or G-3 needle
- 8-0 Vicryl suture

Surgical pack with the following instruments:
- Nasolacrimal cannula (23 gauge)
- Bishop-Harmon dressing forceps
- Barraquer cilia forceps
- Troutman-Barraquer corneal utility forceps
- Hartman curved hemostatic mosquito forceps

TABLE 23-1	Breed Predisposition for Ocular Disease		
BREED	**CONDITION**	**BREED**	**CONDITION**
Dogs		Gordon setter	Entropion, ectropion
Akita	Entropion	Great Dane	Glaucoma, entropion, ectropion
Alaskan malamute	Glaucoma	Greyhound	Pannus
American Staffordshire terrier	Entropion	Irish setter	Entropion
		Japanese chin	Entropion
Australian cattle dog	Anterior luxating lens	Labrador retriever	Entropion, ectropion
Basset hound	Glaucoma, entropion, ectropion	Lhasa apso	Cherry eye
Beagle	Glaucoma, cherry eye	Mastiff	Entropion, ectropion
Belgian sheepdog	Pannus	Newfoundland	Entropion, ectropion, cherry eye
Belgian tervuren	Pannus		
Bloodhound	Entropion, ectropion, cherry eye	Norwegian elkhound	Glaucoma
Border collie	Anterior luxating lens	Old English sheepdog	Entropion
Boston terrier	Glaucoma	Pekingese	Entropion
Bouvier des Flandres	Glaucoma	Pomeranian	Entropion
Boxer	Ectropion, corneal ulcers	Pug	Entropion
Brachycephalic breeds	Corneal ulcers	Rottweiler	Entropion
Brittany spaniel	Anterior luxating lens	Saint Bernard	Entropion, ectropion
Bulldog (English)	Entropion, ectropion, cherry eye	Samoyed	Glaucoma
Bull mastiff	Glaucoma, entropion, ectropion	Shih Tzu	Entropion, ectropion
Burmese mountain dog	Entropion	Siberian husky	Glaucoma, entropion
Cairn terrier	Glaucoma	Smooth fox terrier	Glaucoma
Chesapeake Bay retriever	Entropion	Terriers	Anterior luxating lens
Chinese Shar Pei	Glaucoma, anterior luxating lens, entropion, cherry eye	Tibetan spaniel	Entropion
		Viszla	Entropion
Chow chow	Glaucoma, entropion	Weimaraner	Entropion
Clumber spaniel	Entropion, ectropion	Welsh Springer spaniel	Glaucoma
Cocker spaniel	Glaucoma, entropion, ectropion, cherry eye	Wire-haired fox terrier	Glaucoma, anterior luxating lens
Dachshund	Pannus	Yorkshire terrier	Entropion
Dalmatian	Glaucoma, entropion	**Cats**	
English Springer spaniel	Entropion	Burmese	Corneal sequestrum, keratoconjunctivitis sicca (KCS)
English toy spaniel	Entropion		
Flat-coated retriever	Entropion	Himalayan	Corneal sequestrum
German shepherd	Pannus	Persian	Corneal sequestrum
Golden retriever	Glaucoma, entropion	Siamese	Corneal sequestrum

- Barraquer eye speculum (pediatric and adult sizes)
- Catalano needle holder, curved with or without lock (8-0 Vicryl)
- Westcott curved or straight tenotomy scissors
- Stevens straight tenotomy scissors
- Derf needle holder

Table 23-2 provides a list of ophthalmic drugs that should be stocked.

Any pet owner calling with concerns related to the eye should be seen because of the potential for devastating outcomes. The globe, eyelids, cornea, anterior chamber, and lens are the areas covered in this chapter (Figure 23-1).

TABLE 23-2	Ophthalmic Drugs to Have in the Pharmacy
Antibiotics	
Aminoglycosides (neomycin, gentamicin, tobramycin)	Triple antibiotic solution and ointment; ideal for treatment of eyelid, conjunctival, and corneal infections
Tetracycline (Terramycin)	Broad spectrum, active against many gram-negative and gram-positive bacteria, antibiotic of choice for *Mycoplasma* sp. and *Chlamydia* in cats, inhibits corneal metalloproteases associated with collagenase (melting) ulcers
Fluoroquinolones (ofloxacin, norfloxacin, ciprofloxacin)	Bactericidal against gram-negative and gram-positive bacteria and *Mycoplasma* sp. and *Chlamydia* sp.
Antivirals	
Idoxuridine solution 0.1% solution or ointment or cidofovir compounded	Virostatic
Antiinflammatories	
Steroids	
Hydrocortisone	Lower surface penetration, most useful for eyelid and conjunctival disease
Prednisolone acetate 1% suspension	Penetrates ocular surface well; can be used for surface, stromal, and intraocular inflammation
Dexamethasone 0.1% suspension or ointment	Slightly less corneal penetration than prednisolone; use same as prednisolone acetate
Nonsteroidals	
Cyclosporine 0.2% ointment or compounded higher concentration 1% solution	Effective in surface ocular diseases such as pannus, KCS
Diclofenac 0.1% (Voltaren) /flurbiprofen 0.03% (Ocufen)/ketorolac 0.5%	NSAIDs inhibit prostaglandin synthesis
Tear Replacements	
Methyl cellulose (Genteal extreme gel) and polyvinyl alcohol (Systane) solutions	Intermediate in viscosity while petrolatum ointments are the most viscous
Hyaluronate drops (iVet)	Modified to provide a longer contact time on the cornea
Glaucoma	
Prostaglandins	
Latanoprost, travoprost, bimatoprost	Effective for lowering IOP via increasing uveoscleral outflow, causes extreme miosis, contraindicated in cases of lens luxation because malignant glaucoma may result
Beta-adrenergic antagonists (betaxolol, timolol, demecarium bromide [compounded])	Used in the contralateral eye as prophylactic therapy to delay or prevent the onset of glaucoma
Hyperosmotics	
Mannitol 20%	Osmotic diuretic, given at a rate of 1-2 g/kg IV slowly over 10-20 min; avoid use in dogs with cardiovascular, renal, respiratory, and CNS disease

TABLE 23-2	Ophthalmic Drugs to Have in the Pharmacy—cont'd
Mydriatics/Cycloplegics	
Parasympatholytics (atropine 1%, tropicamide 1%)	Inhibit iridal sphincter contraction and relax the ciliary body musculature; atropine is preferred for anterior uveitis because of its prolonged duration, solution or ointment (ointment is preferred in cats to prevent bitter taste causing hypersalivation)
Sympathomimetics (epinephrine 1%, phenylephrine 2.5% and 10%)	Used for the diagnosis of Horner's syndrome
Anti-Proteinases/Anti-Coallagenases	
Autologous serum	Contains growth factors, fibronectin, vitamin A, and anti-proteinases; can be drawn up and kept frozen for 6 months; once thawed, should be kept refrigerated and is viable for 7 days; inexpensive
Acetylcysteine 2-5% (Mucomyst)	Can be mixed with topical antibiotics; keep refrigerated
EDTA 0.2-2%	Inhibits certain metalloproteinases (MMPs); chelates calcium, zinc, and other ions

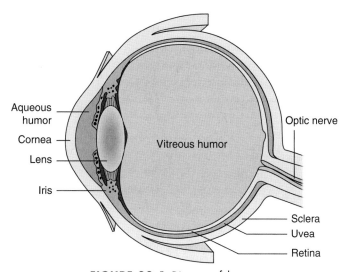

FIGURE 23-1 Diagram of the eye.

GLOBE

Exophthalmos (i.e., the protrusion of a normal-sized **globe** from its usual position) may be seen with retrobulbar abscesses and tumors, as well as trauma from proptosis and some immune-related diseases. Exophthalmos should not be confused with buphthalmos, which is actual globe enlargement.

Glaucoma may present with a dilated pupil, corneal edema, and conjunctival congestion (hyperemia). The pupillary light reflex may or may not be present.

Glaucoma can be caused by inherited predisposition, trauma, anterior luxating lens, or infection.

Treatment begins by determining whether vision is present and whether the glaucoma is a chronic or acute condition. If the condition is chronic and vision is not apparent, then pain relief is the goal. Pain relief is accomplished medically or surgically. Medical therapy can include topical drugs, prostaglandins, beta-adrenergic antagonists, topical carbonic anhydrase inhibitors, and/or hyperosmotic intravenous therapy. Surgical procedures used to relieve the pain in the blind eye include enucleation, ciliary body ablation, and intrascleral prosthesis.

If the glaucoma is acute, the vision may be preserved with immediate treatment. Intraocular pressures in the 40 to 60 mm Hg range respond to intravenous mannitol, which can be administered (1 to 2 g/kg) slowly to shrink the vitreous humor. Elevated intraocular pressure responds well to intravenous Mannitol or Latanoprost drops; however, Latanoprost is contraindicated in cases of anterior lens luxation due to the secondary effect of miosis/uveitis!

Cyclophotoablation (laser therapy) and gonio implants are used to decrease intraocular pressure.

Surgical removal of the lens is an option to relieve the pressure and preserve vision if a luxated lens is the cause of the glaucoma.

Intraocular tumors may present as an acute onset of pain. Hyphema, melanosis (a change in the iris color, most common in cats), buphthalmia, inability to retropulse the eye, and medial or lateral strabismus are other signs associated with tumors. Pupillary light response may or may not be present. Cats with a history of previous trauma to an eye can have acute onset of uveitis, glaucoma, and hyphema. Affected cats have a potential for posttraumatic ocular sarcoma, which is highly malignant. Treatment is enucleation or exenteration; but even with surgery, the prognosis is poor due to metastasis.

Panophthalmitis is inflammation of all structures or tissues of the eye. It presents as an acute onset of pain, conjunctival congestion, or hypopyon (i.e., pus in the chamber). Panophthalmitis can be a secondary sign of a systemic illness, especially if hypopyon is present. Aggressive oral/intravenous and topical antibiotic therapy is necessary. Antiinflammatory medications are also used. Enucleation often is necessary to relieve the pain (Figure 23-2).

Retrobulbar masses may be caused by trauma, tumors, or abscess. Skull radiographs, chemistry profiles, and a complete blood cell count are performed to determine the underlying cause. The protrusion of the globe, inability to blink, and inability to retract the eye are common presenting signs. Once the underlying cause is determined, treatment can begin. The cornea must be protected from drying with a lubricating ointment.

Animals with proptosis, the forward displacement of the globe, may have conjunctival hemorrhage, hyphema,

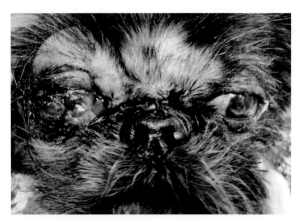

FIGURE 23-2 Panophthalmitis secondary to corneal rupture OD, KCS OS.

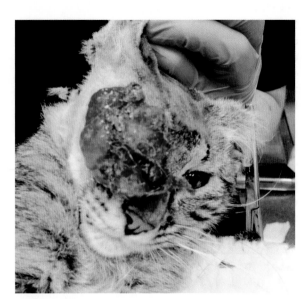

FIGURE 23-3 This feral cat was presented to a TNR clinic for neuter. Unknown history. Eye was enucleated and sent for pathology. It was a proptosed eye that then formed granulation tissue (granuloma).

or both. The common causes include trauma or tumors. Intravenous (IV) dexamethasone is used to decrease inflammation in the optic nerve. The eye can be replaced with or without a lateral canthotomy; then a temporary tarsorrhaphy is performed to protect the cornea. Topical antibiotic is used to protect the cornea. Oral antibiotics and cortisone are continued after surgical intervention. Lids are closed for 2 weeks minimally, and an Elizabethan collar is used to prevent rubbing. Lateral strabismus may be observed after proptosis (Figure 23-3).

Animals with enophthalmos, the backward displacement of the globe into the orbit, have a retracted eye, prolapse of the third eyelid, **blepharospasm,** miotic pupil, or epiphora. Corneal ulcers, a foreign body, Horner's syndrome, acute glaucoma, trauma, and entropion are possible causes of this condition. Determining the underlying cause is important (if possible). Topical anesthetic (Ophthaine) is used to relieve the blepharospasm. Horner's syndrome should be considered a possibility if the topical anesthetic provides no relief.

Horner's syndrome involves the sympathetic nervous system. The sympathetic nerves are located close to the surface of the skin, and consistent pressure applied to this area (e.g., by a choke collar) can damage these nerves. Drops of 2.5% to 10% phenylephrine are used to test for this disorder. A positive response occurs when the pupil dilates, the third eyelid goes down, and the eyeball comes forward. If the underlying disorder is not determined, then this treatment can be used as needed. Some animals recover without treatment; however, when the underlying disorder is determined, it must be treated appropriately.

EYELID

The animal with entropion (i.e., inward displacement of the lid) experiences squinting, third-eyelid protrusion, epiphora, and blepharospasm. An inherited form and a spastic form of entropion exist. The spastic form is usually caused by trauma or corneal ulceration, and loss of the fat pad. If a corneal ulcer is present, then enophthalmia can result from pain, relaxing the eyelids to cause entropion. Treatment for spastic entropion includes temporary tacking of the eyelids and applying lubricating ointment. Antibiotic ointment may be necessary if an infection is present.

Age is an important factor in the inherited form of entropion. Many dogs grow out of the defect, and surgical intervention in young dogs is to be avoided if possible. Temporary eyelid tacking may be necessary until the animal is fully grown.

Ectropion, the outward displacement of the lids, can cause epiphora and mucopurulent discharge. Horner's syndrome, enophthalmia caused by trauma, and lagophthalmos can cause this condition. Ectropion is an inherited disorder. Lubricating ointment is used to protect the corneal surface, and an Elizabethan collar is placed to prevent further trauma.

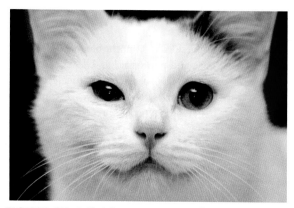

FIGURE 23-4 Eyelid agenesis upper eyelid OD. This cat was being treated for conjunctivitis with no response due to the misdiagnosis.

Meibomian gland abscess or adenoma (chalazion) is the chronic or acute swelling of one or more meibomian glands along the upper and lower eyelids. Crusting or bleeding along the eyelids may be observed. Inflammation caused by an abscess or benign growth of the glands is a common cause of this condition. Treatment includes lancing the swelling if an abscess is present and surgical excision of the growth if a tumor is present. Topical antibiotic ointment is applied after the surgical intervention, and an Elizabethan collar is placed on the animal to prevent rubbing.

Symblepharon is the adhesion of the conjunctiva to the lid and the eyeball. This condition occurs in utero and is caused by a virus (i.e., herpes, calici, chlamydia). Treatment includes surgical removal of the conjunctiva from the cornea or topical antiviral medication. Note: no specific treatment is guaranteed and these cases usually need lifetime monitoring but do very well.

Eyelid agenesis (lack of an eyelid) is a congenital defect that may affect any eyelid. Most common in felines, surgical correction is required (Figure 23-4).

Cherry eye, or prolapsed gland of the third eyelids, can appear very red and irritated. Trauma, curved cartilage of the nictitans, and breed predisposition are the common causes of this condition. The gland can be replaced manually after the use of a topical anesthetic. Steroid ointment controls the inflammatory response. Surgical intervention may be necessary if the gland continues to prolapse. Removing the gland is not recommended because of the risk of causing keratoconjunctivitis sicca (KCS). Surgical correction utilizing the "pocket" technique is preferred.

CORNEA

Corneal ulcers can cause epiphora, blepharitis, muco-purulent discharge, and photophobia. Ulcers can be superficial, recurrent, collagenase, descemetocele, or viral; they occur when chemicals, foreign bodies, ectopic cilia, or trauma has irritated the cornea. Breed predisposition also can be a factor. Treatment varies according to the type of ulcer present. An Elizabethan collar should be placed and other necessary measures taken to prevent further trauma for all types of ulcers (Figure 23-5).

Superficial ulcers are commonly treated with an antibiotic solution or ointment. Recurrent erosions present as chronic ulcers that did not respond to previous therapies. Additional treatment or medication is needed, and a grid keratectomy is usually necessary. Topical and general anesthesia may be needed before the procedure. First, a cotton swab is used to débride the ulcer; then a 25-gauge needle is used to make a grid. This allows attachment of new epithelial cells to the cornea. A sodium chloride ointment (Muro 128 ophthalmic ointment) can be used to promote attachment of new epithelial cells.

Collagenase ulcers, or melting ulcers, are the most difficult to treat. Brachycephalic breeds are commonly affected. The cornea is made of collagen, and the ulcer produces a collagenase that eats through the cornea. Intensive medical therapy is necessary. Serum can be used from the patient (as an eye drop) to stop the collagenic activity. Acetylcysteine may be used hourly to stop collagenic activity in some cases. Conjunctival grafting can be performed if the medical therapy fails.

Descemetocele is an ulcer that has progressed to the last layer of the cornea. The cornea will rupture if it progresses. Topical therapy may be indicated if blood vessels are present and no leakage occurs. Medical therapy must be attempted with caution. Sometimes just a sneeze will rupture the cornea. Do not use ointments if a rupture is present or suspected as this is irritating to intraocular structures! A topical antibiotic, autologous serum, EDTA, or acetylcysteine can be used to treat along with atropine to dilate the pupil and relieve pain. Surgery is recommended to preserve vision and prevent rupture of the eye. Surgical correction may include conjunctival grafting or corneoscleral transposition (Figure 23-6).

Viral ulcers commonly occur in cats with a history of upper respiratory tract infection. Treatment includes a systemic antibiotic for a bacterial infection and topical antiviral medications (Figure 23-7).

KCS can cause purulent discharge, blepharitis, keratitis, and a dull cornea. Thickened eyelids may result from rubbing. Cats may have very mild signs, but Burmese cats are more susceptible. Cherry eye removal, conjunctivitis, congenital defects, anesthesia, drug therapy (i.e., sulfa drugs), and hypothyroidism can cause KCS. Treatment involves (Optimmune Ophthalmic Ointment) or compounded Cyclosporine or Tacrolimus solutions (Figure 23-8).

Keratitis can cause a cloudy or pigmented cornea and blepharitis; chronic exposure, KCS, virus, lagophthalmos, pannus, trichiasis, distichia, and facial nerve paralysis can cause this condition. The underlying problem must be determined and treated appropriately.

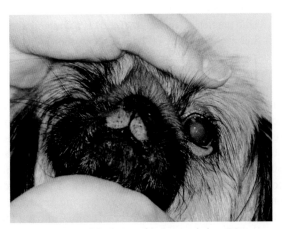

FIGURE 23-5 Superficial corneal ulcer OS.

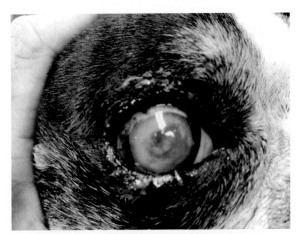

FIGURE 23-6 Desmetocele, ruptured, iris prolapse, corneal vascularization OD.

Pannus, the superficial vascularization of the cornea with infiltration of granulation tissue, is most common in certain breeds and believed to be an immune-mediated disease. Depigmenting of the third eyelid, granulation tissue, superficial blood vessels, and pigment on the cornea are common presenting signs. Optimmune ophthalmic ointment and corticosteroids are used to treat pannus.

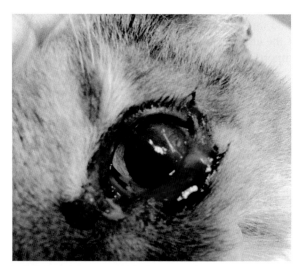

FIGURE 23-7 Eosinophilic keratitis with secondary viral conjunctivitis OS.

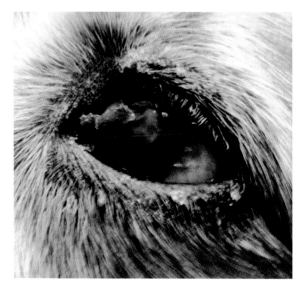

FIGURE 23-8 Keratoconjunctivitis sicca (KCS) OS.

A corneal foreign body can cause acute blepharospasm, epiphora, and conjunctival hyperemia. The object usually can be removed with topical anesthetic. A small-gauge hypodermic needle or ophthalmic surgical forceps is used for this procedure. The ulcer is treated with topical antibiotics, and an Elizabethan collar is placed around the patient's head to prevent further damage. If the injury is deep, then autologous serum may be needed.

Corneal sequestrum occurs when an area of the cornea has become sequestered and dies. Brown or black areas can be seen on the cornea; epiphora and blepharospasm also can be observed. The animal usually has a history of corneal injury. It can also be caused by a virus or breed predisposition in cats. Topical therapy is used to prevent infection and lubricate the eye. Surgical excision is usually necessary to remove sequestered tissue.

ANTERIOR CHAMBER

Uveitis, inflammation of the vascular layer of the eye, can cause blepharospasm, **miosis,** iritis, iris color change, photophobia, hypopyon, and epiphora. It can be idiopathic or caused by a virus, systemic illness, or trauma. Diagnosing and treating any underlying problems is important. Topical therapy can include nonsteroidal or steroidal antibiotics or a combination thereof.

Hyphema, blood in the anterior chamber, can cause blepharospasm, epiphora, and glaucoma. Trauma, retinal detachment, iris tumors, and ciliary body bleed are possible causes. Topical cortisone can be used if the cornea is intact. IV dexamethasone and intraocular injection of tissue plasmin activator is used to dissolve clots and reduce the chance of adhesion. Oral steroid therapy and topical therapy are continued until the clot is absorbed and the intraocular structures can be viewed.

LENS

Anterior lens luxation can cause corneal edema, blepharospasm, and lethargy. The resulting glaucoma causes severe pain in acute cases. Breed predisposition, trauma, and glaucoma are the most common causes of this condition.

IV mannitol 20% is administered (1 g/lb, 2 g/kg) over 30 minutes to relieve intraocular pressure. Mydriatics can be used to dilate the pupil and allow the lens to fall behind the iris. Antiinflammatories and antiglaucoma medications also may be needed to control the pressure.

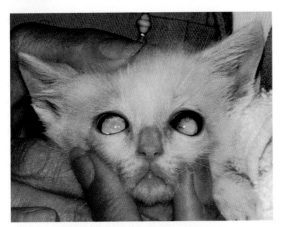

FIGURE 23-9 Juvenile cataracts OU, hyper mature cataract with iris adhesions OS, immature cataract OD.

Latanoprost is contraindicated in cases of anterior lens luxation due to extreme miosis that can trap the lens in the anterior chamber. It may be necessary to remove the lens to restore vision and relieve pressure and the inflammatory reaction in the acute cases.

Cataracts can cause epiphora, uveitis, blepharospasm, hypopyon, miosis, and vision loss in acute cases. Trauma, diabetes, and chronic uveitis are possible causes of this condition; cataracts can also be hereditary, congenital, or age related.

The goal in acute onset is to control the reaction caused by the changing lens. Medications can control the reaction caused by the cataract but will not cure the condition. Topical steroids and nonsteroidal medications are used to control lens-induced uveitis. Mydriatics are used to dilate the pupil and prevent synechia (adherence of the iris to the lens). The cataract is removed once the lens-induced uveitis is controlled (Figure 23-9). Research is ongoing to develop drugs to dissolve developing cataracts.

Nuclear sclerosis is the hardening of the nucleus; it may be confused with cataracts because it produces a graying of the lens. Depth perception and limited visual capabilities in various lighting may be observed.

CONCLUSION

Determining the severity of an ophthalmic emergency over the phone is not easy. If the animal is experiencing pain around or on the surface of the eye (as evidenced by squinting, epiphora), then it must be examined. A mild infection can quickly turn into a severe problem if the animal rubs or scratches the area. Pain relief is important.

Many problems of the eye are a secondary sign of a primary infection. Other tests should be conducted to determine whether any other underlying medical problems exist.

REFERENCES

Abarca E: *Feline ophthalmology; things are just different*, Gainesville, Fla, 2014, North American Veterinary Community.

Ford R, Mazzaferro E: *Handbook of veterinary procedures and emergency treatment*, ed 8, St Louis, 2006, Elsevier.

Mags D: *What drugs should I have in my pharmacy?* Gainesville, Fla, 2014, North American Veterinary Community.

Martin C: *Ophthalmic disease in veterinary medicine*, ed 1, London, 2005, CRC Press.

Miller P: Ocular emergencies, ed 5, *Slatter's fundamentals of veterinary ophthalmology*, St Louis, 2013, Saunders Elsevier.

Plummer C: *Ophthalmic pharmacology—the best and the rest, canine glaucoma—medical and surgical therapies*, Gainesville, Fla, 2014, North American Veterinary Community.

Torres Caballero M: *Neuro-ophthalmology, recurrent corneal lesions—medical and surgical approach*, Gainesville, Fla, 2014, North American Veterinary Community.

SCENARIO

Purpose: Provide the veterinary technician with an opportunity to evaluate common ocular emergencies seen in the emergency room and determine proper response.

Stage: Level III emergency clinic open only evenings and weekends. One veterinarian is present at all times with a swing shift during weekends. Two veterinary technicians, one animal attendant, and one client care representative constitute the support staff provided for most of the shifts.

Scenario

An owner calls stating that his/her 2-year-old male pug's eye has popped out and the dog also has a bleeding toenail. He had been at the local groomers when the incident occurred. It was stated the pug tried to jump from the tub. It was confirmed when the pug arrived there was a proptosis of the globe OD and subconjunctival hemorrhage OS.

Initial assessment included the following: temp, 102.5° F (39.2° C); HR, 166 bpm; RR, pant. Dog is very agitated and difficult for owner to subdue. He continues to rub face along the side of the owner's leg.

Answer the following questions:
1. What advice would you give to the owner over the phone?
2. What would be the most important thing to address immediately once the patient has arrived?
3. How would you assess the globe?
4. What would be the recommended treatment?

Discussion

1. Eye must be kept moist using saline (contact lens solution is fine for temporary use), sterile artificial tears, or sterile water soluble-ointment. Water can also be used if nothing else available. Important to make sure further injury to eye does not occur and preventing dog from rubbing is important.
2. Immediately place an E-collar to prevent further injury to globe and apply sterile ointment on globe.
3. Pupil response and any further damage (lacerations) to globe are evaluated, as well as the contralateral eye; globe position will be laterally strabismic in the proposed eye, but will accommodate with replacement.
4. Ideally, immediate surgical repositioning of eye should occur under general anesthesia. Dexamethasone, if no corneal ulcer is present, is recommended (0.1 mg/kg IV) to control secondary anterior uveitis, retinal/optic nerve inflammation.

MEDICAL MATH EXERCISE

A 5-year-old 12-kg female Cocker spaniel presents with glaucoma. The order states to administer 2 g/kg IV mannitol over 20 minutes. Mannitol is a 20% solution.
  a. How many milliliters of mannitol will be used?
  b. What will be the rate (milliliters/hr)?
  c. Should there be any special considerations for administering this medication?

24 Neurologic Emergencies

Fiona James and Jennifer Collins

CHAPTER OUTLINE

Seizures
*Diagnostic Procedures and
    Treatment Plans*
Vestibular Disorders
*Diagnostic Procedures
    and Treatment Plans*
Spinal Cord Injury
*Diagnostic Procedures
    and Treatment Plans*
**Peripheral Nervous System
  Emergencies**

*Diagnostic Procedures and
    Treatment Plans*
Head Trauma
*Diagnostic Procedures and
    Treatment Plans*
Rabies
*Diagnostic Procedures and
    Treatment Plans*
Conclusion

LEARNING OBJECTIVES

After studying this chapter, you will be able to:

- Components of the neurologic examination
- Understanding neurolocalization
- Taking a thorough history
- Prioritizing common neurologic emergencies
- Learning important history components
- Recognizing common therapeutics for neurologic emergencies

Veterinary technicians are commonly presented with patients exhibiting neurologic disease or impairments, making it vitally important that the technician be comfortable handling neurologic emergencies. When clients complain that their animal is either behaving strangely or is moving oddly, these concerns are frequently neurologic in origin. The first task is to determine whether these situations are truly emergencies, and triage the situation. Does the pet need to see a veterinarian immediately? Can the pet wait until the next morning for assessment? Was there trauma associated with the pet's change in condition? Distinguishing the emergent from the urgent helps in two ways—it minimizes the cost of veterinary emergency care for the owner and focuses appropriate attention to the true emergencies. It is hoped that this chapter can improve and play an active role in triage, assessment, diagnosis, and treatment of neurologic emergencies for the veterinary technician.

A thorough history-taking, careful observation, and physical testing of reflexes and responses can localize the problem to a specific anatomic region within the nervous system. As a result, neurologic emergencies may be diagnosed and treated rapidly without having to await the results of ancillary laboratory tests or diagnostic imaging procedures. Therefore accurate observation and monitoring of neurologic patients is crucial in a busy veterinary clinic. It is important that veterinary technicians understand both how to perform a neurologic examination and how to interpret their findings.

The neurologic examination is outlined in Table 24-1, along with the corresponding region to which each neuroanatomic test relates. The findings of the neurologic examination result in a **neuroanatomic diagnosis,** which, when considered with the patient's signalment and history, allows the veterinary medical team to generate a list of differential diagnoses and then a diagnostic and treatment plan.

SEIZURES

Consider three main causes of acute episodes of animals behaving strangely: intoxications, seizures, and metabolic illnesses. Intoxications are the subject of a separate chapter (see Chapter 25: Toxicologic Emergencies). Seizures are more likely to be transient episodes, whereas metabolic illnesses tend to present as more prolonged episodes.

Seizures originate in the brain (thalamocortex). Epilepsy, at its most basic level, is a disorder of multiple seizures. Definitions of this term, and other seizure-related terms, can vary among veterinary neurologists because there is a lack of standardization of veterinary epilepsy terminology, contrary to human epileptology.

TABLE 24-1	Components of the Neurologic Examination and Related Neuroanatomy		
Mentation		**Postural Reactions**	
Behavior/personality	Thalamocortex	Proprioceptive placing (knuckling), hopping, hemiwalking, wheelbarrowing	Spinal cord, brainstem, thalamocortex
Level of alertness	Brainstem (reticular activating system)		
Gait and Posture		**Spinal Reflexes (Commonly Evaluated)***	

Muscle tone (limb and anal), atrophy	Lower motor neuron	Thoracic limbs:
		  Flexor*
		  Extensor carpi radialis*
		  Biceps
		  Triceps
		  Cross-extension
			C6-T2 spinal cord segments, spinal nerves, brachial plexus

Paresis/paralysis	Lower vs upper motor neurons (spinal cord/brainstem)		

Ataxia	Cerebellar vs vestibular vs proprioceptive	Pelvic limbs:
		  Patellar*
		  Flexor*
		  Cranial tibial
		  Gastrocnemius
		  Cross-Extension
			L4-S1 spinal cord segments, spinal nerves, lumbosacral plexus

Cranial Nerves (CNs)			
Pupillary light reflex (PLR)	CN II and III		
Menace response	CN II, thalamocortex, cerebellum, CN VII	Cutaneous trunci (sometimes called *panniculus*)	Thoracolumbar spinal cord segments, C8-T1 spinal nerves, brachial plexus
Physiologic nystagmus	CN III, IV, VI, VIII, brainstem	Perineal	S1-S3 spinal cord segments, spinal nerves, cauda equina
Palpebral reflexes	CN V, VII		
Muscles of mastication	CN V		
Nasal septum response	CN V, thalamocortex		
Facial symmetry	CN VII		
Head tilt	CN VIII		
Swallowing	CN IX, X, XII		
Voice change	CN X		
Tongue muscle	CN XII		

*Most reliable.

TABLE 24-2	Descriptors of Seizure Manifestations
DESCRIPTOR	**DEFINITION**
Tonic	Increased muscular rigidity, usually extensor muscles
Clonic	Rhythmic jerking movements
Atonic	Flaccid muscles
Myoclonic	Brief twitch of a muscle or muscle group
Absence	"Spaced out" or "staring into space"

BOX 24-1	Four Neurologic Tests for the Thalamocortex

Mentation
Menace response
Nasal septum response
Postural reactions

There are several ways to classify seizures and epilepsies; these classifications are not mutually exclusive. One way to classify seizures is by their physical manifestations (Table 24-2). Obtaining these descriptions can help to determine whether the episode was truly a seizure. A video-recording is better than a description, but is not always available. Such a description would include the preictal signs (i.e., the signs that precede the onset of the actual ictus or seizure) as well as the postictal recovery period. During the postictal period, the patient may display signs of disorientation, confusion, aggression, restlessness, and/or varying levels of responsiveness. These patients might be found to be blind (absent menace response in both eyes) and might have decreased or absent nasal septum responses and postural reaction deficits with delayed proprioceptive positioning (knuckling) and/or hopping (Box 24-1). The postictal period may last minutes, hours, or days. Deficits found during this period result from the seizure(s) and do not necessarily represent the true neurologic state. Postictal deficits are transient. Persistent, unilateral, or asymmetric deficits imply a true neurologic lesion. Complicating this are the effects of anticonvulsant medications used to stop the seizures—these effects may range from weakness and depression to obtundation ("floor mat") and have the potential to last for days, depending on the medication. Consequently, conclusions about the cause of a patient's seizures may be delayed until the medication effects dissipate or the patient improves.

Borrowing from the International League Against Epilepsy, the authority on human epileptic conditions, the definition of a seizure is "a transient occurrence of signs and/or symptoms due to abnormal excessive or synchronous neuronal activity in the brain." In the veterinary literature, the various definitions of a seizure are similar. There are two types of seizure and epilepsy that are recognized—"focal" and "generalized." Historical synonyms for **focal seizures** include "petit mal" and "simple or complex partial" seizures (the latter are not practical distinctions in small animals because they involve assessing how mentation may be altered). Similarly, **generalized seizures** have also been referred to as "grand mal" seizures. Focal seizures arise from abnormal neurons in one hemisphere of the thalamocortex. Typically, this results in abnormal movements on the contralateral side of the body, with or without altered mentation. Focal seizures can spread to excite neuronal networks in both hemispheres of the thalamocortex, which can be described as "secondary generalization." Generalized seizures originate in neuronal networks that extend bilaterally through both hemispheres, and may not have a consistent physical onset. The classic generalized seizure involves loss of consciousness with tonic-clonic whole body movements and possibly autonomic signs such as salivation, urination, and defecation. However, generalized seizures may also present as "absence" seizures, where there is a transient alteration in consciousness with or without an external manifestation, such as a myoclonic jerk.

Other terms that clients might use to describe such a seizure include *convulsion* or *(epileptic) fit.* However, it must be recognized that there are many acute episodic disorders that might be confused with seizures by the client, and it is the responsibility of the veterinarian and veterinary technician to rapidly and accurately distinguish between them. A list of things easily mistaken for seizures is provided in Box 24-2.

Another way to classify seizures and epilepsies is their etiology. Certain breeds of dogs have a genetic predisposition to epilepsy, based on pedigree analysis or genetic mutation identification. These include, among others, Australian shepherds, beagles, Belgian shepherds, Border collies, English Springer spaniels, German

BOX 24-2 Other Conditions Easily Mistaken for Seizures

Behaviors
  Feline estrus
  Obsessive-compulsive disorders
Cataplexy and narcolepsy (extremely rare)
Metabolic disorders
  Hepatic encephalopathy (e.g., from portosystemic shunts)
  Hypoadrenocorticism (Addison's disease)
  Hypoglycemia
  Electrolyte disturbances (e.g., calcium)
Other neurologic syndromes
  Acute-onset vestibular signs*
  Cerebrovascular accidents* (strokes)
  Shakers syndrome (also known as "Little White Shakers Syndrome")
Pain
  Neck pain* (e.g., from intervertebral disk herniation)
Peripheral nervous system diseases
  Myasthenia gravis
  Polyneuropathies
  Polymyopathies
Syncope*

*Common conditions.

shepherds, golden retrievers, Labrador retrievers, Shetland sheepdogs, standard poodles, and vizslas. In these breeds, the first seizure tends to occur between 1 and 5 years of age, with generalized seizures as the most common manifestation. The interictal neurologic examination is normal, as are most diagnostic tests. This type of epilepsy has been referred to as *idiopathic,* but with ongoing advances in genetics research it would be more correct to refer to these cases as *genetic epileptics.*

The interictal neurologic examination may also be normal in some cases of metabolic or systemic disease, or in instances of early structural brain disease. For example, liver disease (causing hepatic encephalopathy) or hypoglycemia may present with normal neurologic examinations and a history of altered mentation. Many metabolic or systemic causes can be identified on routine blood work. Early structural brain disease is hard to detect on the neurologic examination, especially if it affects certain portions of the brain. For example, a tumor in the olfactory bulbs or frontal lobes may be referred to as "quiet" structural disease. For these cases, advanced diagnostic testing is required to identify the cause of the seizures, such as magnetic resonance imaging (MRI) of the brain, computed-assisted tomography (CT, also known as a "CAT scan") of the brain, and cerebrospinal fluid (CSF) collection and analysis ("spinal tap").

If the seizures occur in the younger or older patient (younger than 1 year or more than 5 years of age), or if there are persistent or asymmetric neurologic deficits, then structural or metabolic (symptomatic) causes for the epilepsy should be suspected (Figure 24-1). In these cases, abnormalities might be found on diagnostic testing. In the younger patient, consider hypoglycemia or hepatic encephalopathy (e.g., from a portosystemic shunt) or infectious causes (e.g., viral or bacterial disease). Occasionally, in one of these suspected symptomatic epileptic patients, nothing is found on diagnostic testing, including brain MRI/CT and CSF analysis. These cases are truly idiopathic; however, given the meanings associated with the term, it would perhaps be better to refer to these as epilepsies of unknown origin.

Feline seizures may be approached similarly. Approximately 40% of cats have epilepsy with no discernible cause and appear to do well with therapy. Otherwise, they have structural or metabolic causes for the epilepsy. This is especially true if they present in **status epilepticus** (defined as seizure activity continuing for 20 minutes or more), or if they are older than 7 years of age, or if they have an abnormal interictal neurologic examination.

DIAGNOSTIC PROCEDURES AND TREATMENT PLANS

Emergency treatment is indicated to stop seizure activity and manage any secondary effects of seizures. The paramount emergency is *status epilepticus,* or *clusters* of seizures where the patient does not regain consciousness between seizures. High-frequency seizures (3 or 4 seizures in 30 minutes or large numbers in 12 to 24 hours) should also be treated aggressively. From the client's perspective, any seizure lasting longer than 5 minutes should necessitate emergency veterinary attention. Prolonged or high-frequency seizure activity may result in serious systemic effects; these include hyperthermia, cardiovascular and renal compromise, neurologic damage, and metabolic derangements. The first choice for stopping active seizures is usually diazepam. Depending on the patient's presentation and the expertise of the technician, diazepam may be given intravenously (IV) or per rectum for the first dose. Additional medications, if diazepam is insufficient, may involve constant rate infusions

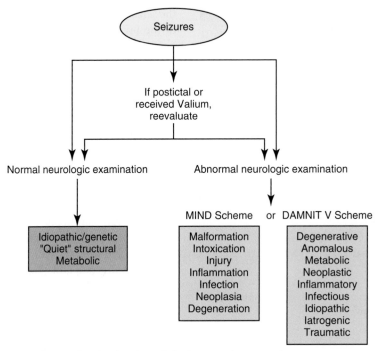

FIGURE 24-1 Algorithm to help determine the cause of seizure activity.

(CRIs), other injectable anticonvulsants, (levetiracetam or phenobarbital), or anesthetics.

The therapeutic approach depends on whether these are a patient's first seizures or whether this is a previously diagnosed epileptic patient under treatment with usually good control. Box 24-3 describes a step-by-step approach for the diagnosis and initial therapy of a first-time seizure patient versus patients with previously diagnosed epilepsy, status epilepticus, or cluster seizures. Previously diagnosed epileptics usually do not require extensive diagnostic testing unless it has been some time since their last routine monitoring blood work or if there is a sudden change in the frequency or severity of their seizures. Check if there has been a recent weight or diet change because these factors can affect dosage.

After stopping the seizure activity, management of the secondary seizure effects must begin. Most of these effects are due to high-intensity prolonged muscle activity, with hyperthermia being the most common side effect. Body temperatures may rapidly rise higher than 40° C (104° F), requiring frequent or continuous rectal temperature monitoring. Active cooling is recommended for body temperatures greater than 39.5° C (103° F) and should be discontinued once the temperature drops

below 39° C (102° F). This is because extreme hyperthermia may interfere with normal thermoregulation, resulting in accidental hypothermia. Hyperthermia may also result in disseminated intravascular coagulation (DIC), organ failures (renal and hepatic), and muscle necrosis (which also contributes to renal failure). Inspect the patient carefully and regularly for petechiation resulting from thrombocytopenia or DIC.

Seizures may also result in dehydration, hypoglycemia, and respiratory difficulties. The respiratory difficulties result from **noncardiogenic (neurogenic) pulmonary edema,** believed to be a direct result of seizure activity affecting the autonomic (sympathetic) system. These patients will display rapid shallow breathing; some cases develop into dyspnea, cyanosis, severe hypoxia, or respiratory arrest. Thoracic auscultation can reveal crackles. Pulse oximetry or arterial blood gas analysis will identify hypoxemia. Thoracic radiographs will show interstitial to alveolar lung patterns primarily affecting the caudodorsal lung fields. The same therapy should be offered as for other causes of noncardiogenic pulmonary edema, including supplemental oxygen via mask, nasal cannula, or oxygen tents/cages. Chapter 7 discusses Oxygen Therapy Techniques.

BOX 24-3	Diagnosis and Treatment in First-Seizure, Cluster Seizure, or Status Epilepticus Patients, or in Established Epileptics

1. Place IV catheter.
2. Give IV medication to stop seizures if in active seizure:
   Diazepam (typical first choice*): 0.25-1 mg/kg (repeat × 3 PRN)
   Quick-dosing suggestions (diazepam 5 mg/ml, 2-ml vials):

Cat/toy dog	0.5 ml (quarter vial)
Small dog	1 ml (half vial)
Medium dog	2 ml (whole vial)
Large dog	3 ml (vial and a half)
Giant dog	4 ml (two vials)

   Initiate CRI of diazepam if indicated—give successful dose in mg/kg/hr (usually 0.5-1 mg/kg/hr).
3. Measure TPR (temperature, pulse, respiration rate) and blood pressure.

FIRST TIME SEIZURE

4. Draw blood for initial database:

   Quick Assessment Tests
   Blood glucose
   Electrolytes
   Packed cell volume and total protein (PCV/TP)
   Blood gas analysis
   Blood urea nitrogen (BUN)
   Coagulation testing (if indicated)
      Activated clotting time (ACT)
      Prothrombin time (PT)
      Partial thromboplastin time (PTT)
      Thromboelastography (TEG)

   Complete blood count (CBC) and peripheral blood smear
   Serum biochemistry profile
   Urinalysis
   Lead levels (if indicated)
   Serology for infectious diseases (if indicated)
   Thyroid profile (if indicated)

5. Start maintenance seizure therapy:
   A. Doses for rapid induction of therapeutic serum concentrations (as adjunctive medication if diazepam CRI insufficient to control seizure activity):
      • Phenobarbital as IV bolus, IV CRI, PO, IM, or PR up to 20 (to 30) mg/kg in 24 hr (stop if very groggy)
      • Levetiracetam as IV 5-min bolus, IM, PO, or PR 60 mg/kg in 24 hr
      • Potassium bromide as PO or PR up to 600 mg/kg in 24 hr (will make very groggy; use as final option; **not for cats**)
   B. Maintenance doses:
      Phenobarbital 2-3 mg/kg PO q12h
      Levetiracetam 20 mg/kg PO q8h
      Potassium bromide 30 mg/kg/day PO **(not for cats)**
      Zonisamide 5-10 mg/kg PO q12h

ESTABLISHED EPILEPTIC

Draw blood for initial database:

Quick Assessment Tests
Blood glucose
Electrolytes
Packed cell volume and total protein (PCV/TP)
Blood gas analysis
Blood urea nitrogen (BUN)

Blood for anticonvulsant serum levels to adjust dosing

Continue any maintenance drugs.

Continued

BOX 24-3	Diagnosis and Treatment in First-Seizure, Cluster Seizure, or Status Epilepticus Patients, or in Established Epileptics—cont'd

FIRST TIME SEIZURE   **ESTABLISHED EPILEPTIC**

6. Consider starting adjunctive maintenance anticonvulsant drugs if diazepam + maintenance drugs are not giving adequate control:
   A. Doses for rapid induction of therapeutic serum concentrations (as adjunctive medication if diazepam CRI insufficient to control seizure activity):
      • Phenobarbital as IV bolus, IV CRI, PO, IM, or PR up to 20 (to 30) mg/kg in 24 hr (stop if very groggy)
      • Levetiracetam as IV 5-min bolus, IM, PO, or PR 60 mg/kg in 24 hr
      • Potassium bromide as PO or PR up to 600 mg/kg in 24 hr (will make very groggy; use as final option; **not for cats**)
   B. Maintenance doses:
      Phenobarbital 2-3 mg/kg PO q12h
      Levetiracetam 20 mg/kg PO q8h
      Potassium bromide 30 mg/kg/day PO **(not for cats)**
      Zonisamide 5-10 mg/kg PO q12h

*Give per rectum or intranasally at higher dose if IV is not accessible.

While hospitalized, ongoing seizure management should include maintenance anticonvulsant medication to reduce the future frequency and severity of seizures. This maintenance therapy should be initiated during acute seizure treatment and continued beyond discharge. Medications like phenobarbital may be administered via various routes, including intravenous (IV), intramuscular (IM), oral (PO), and per rectum (PR) infusions. For the latter, a red rubber polyethylene or polyvinyl chloride (PVC) feeding tube and large syringe is recommended to ensure the medication is deposited rostrally in the colon, with subsequent flushing with water to ensure complete dosing.

Patient monitoring and care are intensive. If they are receiving multiple CRIs of drugs, monitoring can be similar to that needed for anesthesia, with some patients requiring endotracheal intubation to protect the airway. This includes charting temperature, pulse, and respiration rates (TPRs); measuring blood pressure and pulse oximetry values; and performing regular arterial blood gas analysis. Lubrication of the eyes should be performed regularly to prevent corneal injury. Frequent position changes of the patient are necessary to prevent atelectasis and decubital ulcers. Bladder care might include regular expression or (closed, indwelling) urinary catheterization. Routine management would also include IV maintenance and oral care, along with administration of other medications such as maintenance anticonvulsants.

VESTIBULAR DISORDERS

Vestibular syndromes often present as emergencies because of their alarming clinical signs, but fortunately are rarely life-threatening. The vestibular system mediates the body's sense of balance. Clinically, a distinction is made between the peripheral and central vestibular systems. The peripheral vestibular system comprises the inner ear sensors and the vestibulocochlear nerve (cranial nerve VIII). The rostral medulla and cerebellum make up the central vestibular system. This distinction is helpful in neurolocalization and for generating differential diagnoses. Although some clinical signs are common to both peripheral and central vestibular systems, others may be used to distinguish between them. Table 24-3 highlights the differences and commonalities between central and peripheral vestibular clinical signs.

TABLE 24-3	Clinical Signs Associated with Peripheral and Central Vestibular Disorders		
	PERIPHERAL	COMMON TO BOTH	CENTRAL
Mentation	Normal		May be abnormal (depression, somnolence, stupor, coma)
Cranial nerve deficits		VIII ± VII: head tilt, facial paresis/paralysis	± V-XII
Nystagmus		Pathologic nystagmus (resting, positional, rotary, horizontal)	Pathologic nystagmus (vertical, shifting phase)
Eye position		Positional strabismus (ventrally deviated eye on side of head tilt when head is elevated)	
Postural reactions	Normal postural reactions		Postural reaction deficits
Gait and posture		Vestibular ataxia (wide-based stance, leaning, falling, circling, rolling)	
Sympathetic innervation	± Horner's syndrome		Rarely Horner's syndrome
Other			Paradoxical vestibular syndrome (head tilt away from lesion)

Differentiating between central and peripheral vestibular disease is important for prognostication because central lesions tend to carry a worse prognosis.

The most common vestibular syndrome seen as an emergency is *idiopathic old dog (geriatric) vestibular syndrome*. This is a peripheral vestibular syndrome of no known cause that affects dogs typically more than 8 years of age. These dogs tend to present with severe clinical signs, including head tilt, resting nystagmus with the fast phase away from the direction of the head tilt ("the eyes run away from the lesion"), severe vestibular ataxia possibly with falling or "log-rolling," and no postural reaction deficits. However, postural reaction deficits can be hard to test when the patient is rolling and nonambulatory. While definitely alarming for the clients, this condition improves in the majority of patients over 2 to 4 weeks, often with only a head tilt remaining. Improvement usually begins within 2 to 3 days and patients mostly require supportive care (discussed in the following section).

Feline idiopathic vestibular syndrome is another common peripheral vestibular syndrome. It is seen in cats with outdoor access (never in indoor-only cats). It has a temporal peak in the north-eastern regions of North America, occurring during summer through autumn months (no such association elsewhere). This seasonal timing might be associated with *Cuterebra* larval migration in those regions. Similar to idiopathic vestibular

BOX 24-4	Clinical Signs of Horner's Syndrome in the Dog and Cat

Miosis (minimum clinical sign)
Ptosis
Enophthalmos
Protruding nictitans

syndrome in dogs, this usually resolves over 2 to 4 weeks with only supportive care, beginning within 2 to 3 days of onset.

Otitis media/interna is one of the more common causes of peripheral vestibular syndrome in both dogs and cats. There may or may not be evidence of otitis externa on examination. Because both cranial nerve VII (the facial nerve) and the sympathetic innervation to the eye travel through the petrous temporal bone surrounding the tympanic bulla, both ipsilateral facial **paresis/paralysis** and Horner's syndrome are commonly associated with this syndrome. The clinical signs of Horner's syndrome are listed in Box 24-4. Both unilateral and bilateral otitis may occur, but unilateral is more common. Otic cleansing to visualize the tympanum should be performed only with gentle saline irrigation. If other products are used and the tympanum is not intact, their entry into the middle ear may worsen the vestibular signs and possibly also cause permanent deafness. Prognosis is good with appropriate antibiotic therapy, although the head tilt may persist. Chronic infections may require draining of the middle ear via a surgical procedure called a bulla osteotomy. Occasional infections ascend into the brainstem, resulting in central vestibular signs. In cats (rarely dogs), *nasopharyngeal polyps* may contribute to otitis media/interna by blocking the eustachian tube that drains the middle ear. Polyps require some sort of visualization (direct otoscopic, endoscopic, or indirect via MRI) for diagnostic confirmation. Polyp growth may also passively cause peripheral vestibular signs. Polyps require removal for improvement of the otitis.

Common causes of emergency presentations of central vestibular syndromes in dogs include cerebrovascular accidents (strokes) and encephalitis (inflammatory brain disease). While a stroke patient will begin to recover in 2 to 3 days and continue to improve over 3 months with supportive care, encephalitis requires much more aggressive diagnostic tests and therapy. A cause for the stroke might be identified via diagnostic tests in approximately 50% of cases. Cats also present for encephalitis, with infectious causes most commonly including feline infectious peritonitis (FIP–the dry form), toxoplasmosis, and cryptococcosis.

DIAGNOSTIC PROCEDURES AND TREATMENT PLANS

Emergency treatment may be required to treat dehydration secondary to protracted vomiting from the nausea associated with vestibular disturbance. However, these cases are usually stable such that immediate attention and therapy are not often warranted. Diagnostic investigation usually involves careful otic examination and/or other visualization methods, including radiographs. Labwork should be considered, similar to the initial database listed in Box 24-3 (row 4).

To treat the nausea, antinauseants, antiemetics, and gastrointestinal prokinetics may be used. Maropitant citrate is commonly used, as are meclizine and dimenhydrinate. Metoclopramide may be used for intractable vomiting. With persistent nausea and/or profound head tilts, patients may be unable to eat and drink, therefore requiring parenteral fluid supplementation. Sometimes sedation is required (e.g., with diphenhydramine or diazepam) to control the rolling and flailing. Well-padded cages will also help prevent self-injury by rolling or nonambulatory patients.

Antibiotics are indicated for cases of otitis media/interna and if bacterial encephalitis is suspected. Some viral and all noninfectious encephalitides benefit from immunosuppressive doses of corticosteroids (e.g., dexamethasone).

SPINAL CORD INJURY

There are two neurolocalizations that might present as an animal moving oddly—spinal cord injury or peripheral nervous system diseases. Spinal cord injury is by far the more common cause of emergency presentations. These animals often walk oddly ("drunk"/ataxic) or weakly (paretic) or not at all (paralyzed). The neurologic examination should have normal mentation and cranial nerves. Key deficits found include abnormalities of gait and spinal reflexes, as well as the presence or absence of spinal pain. The finding of proprioceptive (spinal) ataxia almost guarantees a spinal cord neurolocalization. **Proprioceptive ataxia** is a condition in which the animal does not know the location of its paws or body in space. It is characterized by erratic paw placement while walking or standing, crossing the limbs (tripping over its own paws), dragging the paws, spontaneous knuckling over on the paws, and truncal or pelvic swaying or tipping. Weakness, also known as paresis, results from the loss of either upper or lower motor neuron instructions to the muscles. This manifests as sinking while standing or walking, a crouched stance, difficulty rising, scuffing the paws while walking, or decreased or complete loss of voluntary movements. In the worst cases of spinal cord injury, sensory pathway disruption results in the loss of all sensation caudal to the level of injury. Therefore, the patient will no longer be able to feel its toes. The loss of **nociception** (perception of noxious stimuli) is tested by clamping on a toe with a pair of hemostats and observing the head for reaction (turning, snapping, vocalizing, blinking, etc.). Loss of pain is a significant prognostic indicator; the longer nociception has been lost, the less likely there will be return of function despite intervention. The order of loss of function in spinal cord injury follows a rule of thumb (Box 24-5). Recovery of function returns in the opposite order and worse injuries result in greater loss of function. The neurologic exam findings will depend on where the spinal cord injury occurred, as outlined in Figure 24-2.

Causes of spinal cord injury can be divided into those intrinsic versus extrinsic to the animal. Intrinsic causes include compression of the spinal cord from intervertebral disc herniation (via extrusion or protrusion of the disc), vascular accidents (fibrocartilaginous embolic myelopathy [FCEM]), neoplastic compression of the spinal cord (from outside the cord or inside the cord), compression of the cord from bony malformations (e.g., congenital malformations like atlanto-axial subluxation or developmental malformations such as wobbler syndrome), and other benign structural lesions (e.g., cysts).

BOX 24-5	Order of Appearance of Clinical Signs in Acute Spinal Cord Injury*

Spinal pain
Proprioception
Paresis/paralysis
Urination/defecation
Nociception

*Function returns in the opposite order.

Extrinsic causes are most commonly fractures or luxations resulting from trauma such as patients hit by a car, gunshot wounds, bite wounds, abuse, and/or falls.

The most common of all of these causes is intervertebral disc herniation (IVDH). Intervertebral discs are located between the vertebral bodies from C2 to the first sacral vertebra (Figure 24-3). The intervertebral disc acts as a shock absorber, contributes to spinal flexibility and structural integrity, and is constructed as a gelatinous filling (nucleus pulposus) contained within a tough fibrous outer covering (annulus fibrosus). As seen in Figure 24-3, the annulus is thinnest dorsally, just ventral to the spinal cord, and this is where it usually ruptures as a result of trauma or disc degeneration.

There are three ways that a disc can impinge upon the spinal cord. The first is via degenerative changes affecting the nucleus pulposus, whereby the gel dehydrates and calcifies. The disc loses its elasticity, and ruptures dorsally through a weakened annulus fibrosus, compressing the spinal cord, or dorsolaterally, compressing a spinal nerve.

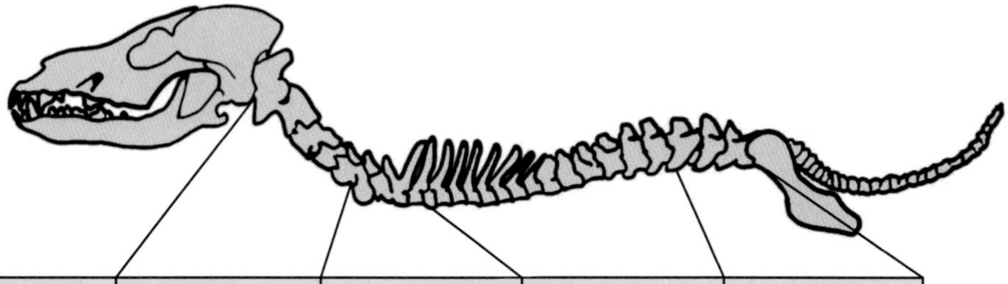

Spinal Cord Segment	C1 - C5	C6 - T2	T3 - L3	L4 - S2
Strength				
Thoracic Limbs	Paresis/Paralysis	Paresis/Paralysis	Normal	Normal
Pelvic Limbs	Paresis/Paralysis	Paresis/Paralysis	Paresis/Paralysis	Paresis/Paralysis
Reflexes				
Thoracic Limbs	Hyper	Hypo	Normal	Normal
Pelvic Limbs	Hyper	Hyper	Hyper	Hypo
Tone				
Thoracic Limbs	Hyper	Hypo	Normal	Normal
Pelvic Limbs	Hyper	Hyper	Hyper	Hypo
Postural Reactions				
Thoracic Limbs	Decreased	Decreased to Normal	Normal	Normal
Pelvic Limbs	Decreased	Decreased	Decreased	Decreased to Normal

FIGURE 24-2 Neurologic findings associated with injury of a particular spinal cord segment. (Illustration by A.D.K. James.)

This type of IVDH occurs most commonly in chondrodystrophic dogs, such as dachshunds, shih tzus, Lhasa apsos, and basset hounds. It most typically affects these breeds at the thoracolumbar junction (85% of the time), between T10 and L2 vertebrae, resulting in spinal pain, proprioceptive deficits, and pelvic limb gait abnormalities. However, it can occur in the neck 15% of the time, most commonly causing profound neck pain, possibly accompanied by neurologic deficits in all four limbs.

The second type is degeneration that involves a weakening and thickening of the annulus fibrosus, resulting in a dorsal bulge that compresses the spinal cord. This is less commonly an emergency since it tends to have a more chronic history. It is most often seen in large breed dogs.

The third type is an acute nucleus pulposus extrusion wherein a small jet of nucleus is propelled at the spinal cord with high velocity through an annulus rupture.

It occurs often secondary to trauma, like falling off the bed or colliding with another dog at the park. The neurologic deficits are secondary to spinal cord bruising and concussive injury; sometimes there is so little nucleus pulposus extruded that there is no compression. In addition to traumatic disc herniation, fractures may also result from traumatic forces applied to the spine (Figure 24-4).

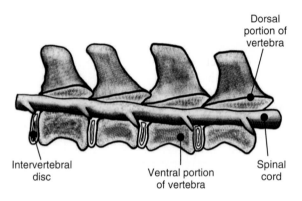

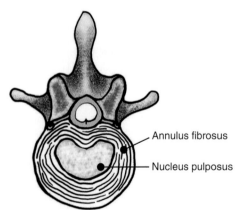

FIGURE 24-3 *Upper,* Sagittal section through the vertebral canal. *Lower,* Transverse section through a vertebra showing the relative positions of spinal cord and intervertebral disc. (Illustration by A.D.K. James.)

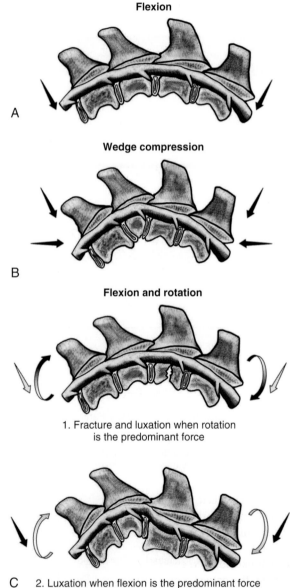

FIGURE 24-4 Types of injury and forces associated with trauma to the vertebral column (arrows indicate direction of force). (Illustration by A.D.K. James.)

Severe vertebral fractures may not be apparent on visual inspection of a patient. Appendicular skeletal injuries (e.g., fractures or degloving injuries) might mask neurologic dysfunction. Therefore, it is important to perform a complete neurologic examination once a trauma patient is cardiovascularly stable; the neurolocalization not only identifies neurologic problems but also minimizes the risk of inadvertent worsening of spinal cord injury by the emergency care team. As previously mentioned, neurolocalization also helps in generating the differential diagnoses and appropriate diagnostic testing.

Fibrocartilaginous embolic myelopathy (FCEM) is a fairly common emergency in medium to large breed dogs. This is a vascular accident ("stroke") that occurs in the spinal cord secondary to a plug of cartilage blocking the spinal cord blood vessels. The cartilage is thought to come from a nearby nucleus pulposus through unknown mechanisms. The typical history for these patients is that they are doing something active (e.g., chasing a ball or retrieving a stick) when they cry out and go down. The onset is therefore very acute. The neurologic deficits are usually asymmetric and nonprogressive, and spinal pain does not typically persist beyond the first 12 to 24 hours.

DIAGNOSTIC PROCEDURES AND TREATMENT PLANS

After initial stabilization of the patient, a complete neurologic examination is essential for neurolocalization, even for parts of the patient that might seem undamaged. If there is no voluntary movement, nociception should be tested in all limbs and the tail. For practical purposes, the spinal cord is divided into four functional segments, as described in Figure 24-2, allowing fairly specific neurolocalization. Neurolocalization thus defines the regions of the spine that should be imaged with radiographs (to rule out fractures/luxations) or more advanced diagnostic imaging options like myelography, computed tomography (CT), or MRI. The latter allows the most complete characterization of the form of spinal cord injury, whereas myelography and/or CT helps to determine whether there is a surgically approachable spinal cord compression or fracture. For example, if a patient had suffered an FCEM at T13-L1 while playing Frisbee, the patient would have pelvic limb neurologic deficits with intact pelvic limb spinal reflexes and no spinal pain, and the lesion would only be detected by MRI of the thoracolumbar spine.

There are two exceptions to the findings outlined in Figure 24-2. The most commonly encountered is known as Schiff-Sherrington syndrome. This occurs when a severe lesion affects the spinal cord segments between L1 and L4. Cells in this region facilitate coordination of movement between the pelvic limbs and the thoracic limbs. Loss of these cells and/or their axons results in disinhibition of the extensor muscles of the thoracic limbs. When these patients are placed in lateral recumbency, severe extensor rigidity of the thoracic limbs results. Schiff-Sherrington syndrome does not carry any prognostic implications. The other exception is spinal shock, but this is seen less commonly. Spinal shock occurs with severe spinal cord trauma and results in a transient loss of reflexes and muscle tone caudal to the injury instead of the hyperreflexia and spastic paresis that might be expected. It is more common to see a loss of muscle tone. These findings resolve within 12 to 36 hours of the injury, eventually presenting clinical signs as outlined in Figure 24-2.

Transport of a patient with a possible vertebral fracture should be done cautiously, whether transferring to the emergency clinic or transferring between clinics. The patient should be carefully secured to a flat board (e.g., door or piece of plywood) with tape, belts, rope, or any other tie-down necessary to ensure the patient remains immobilized. Clients should be warned of the extreme pain associated with vertebral column injury (the most painful tissues are bone, nerve roots, and meninges) such that even their faithful pet may bite or scratch. A physical and neurologic examination should be performed upon arrival without unnecessarily disturbing the support structure. Stabilization of the respiratory and cardiovascular systems should also be performed with minimal movement of the patient.

Analgesia should be provided if the patient is in pain. Opioids may be used judiciously with close monitoring to avoid respiratory depression. Hydromorphone (0.05 to 0.1 mg/kg IV, IM, or subcutaneously [SC]) or buprenorphine (0.01 to 0.03 mg/kg IV or IM) is a good option. Sedation may be necessary to reduce anxiety and flailing—diazepam is another good option at 0.2 to 0.4 mg/kg IV.

The use of corticosteroids for spinal cord injury is still controversial. Human research suggests that high-dose methylprednisolone sodium succinate (30 mg/kg bolus IV over 15 minutes, followed by a maintenance infusion of 5.4 mg/kg/hr over 23 hours), if administered within

8 hours of injury, might improve neurologic outcome up to 1-year post-injury. There are no comparable veterinary studies. Some veterinary neurologists use a dosing protocol similar to the human one, or substitute two boluses of 15 mg/kg IV at 2 and 6 hours after the initial bolus. The boluses must be given slowly over 15 minutes; otherwise, vomiting or hypotension may occur. Despite little evidence, dexamethasone is sometimes used instead of methylprednisolone at doses up to 1 mg/kg IV at initial presentation. Adverse effects may result from the use of corticosteroids, including gastrointestinal hemorrhage and septic or infectious complications. When corticosteroids are used, concomitant gastroprotectant administration is advised. Subsequent to initial treatment, spinal cord injuries are treated medically or surgically, depending on the cause. Medical management may include splinting, enforcing cage rest, performing analgesia, and administering antiinflammatories. For patients with FCEM, medical management in the form of supportive care and physiotherapy is all that is required. These FCEM cases have a fair prognosis depending on the severity of initial deficits. Surgical interventions for spinal trauma include spinal cord decompression or vertebral column stabilization, determined on a case-by-case basis.

PERIPHERAL NERVOUS SYSTEM EMERGENCIES

These patients typically present with weakness and the most emergent is the acutely floppy patient. This is life-threatening if the respiratory muscles become paralyzed. One of the first signs of respiratory weakening may be an elevated temperature (pyrexia) attributable to the increased work of breathing. Because of weakness, increased respiratory effort may not be apparent in these patients.

Although peripheral nervous system diseases in general are less common than other presentations, there are four that the emergency clinic might see: myasthenia gravis, polyradiculoneuritis, botulism, and tick paralysis. All of these involve disruption of lower motor neuron communication with the muscles. This results in flaccid paralysis and loss of reflexes that typically start in the pelvic limbs and ascend to involve thoracic limbs, facial weakness, and respiratory muscles. Esophageal muscles may be affected, resulting in megaesophagus, with concomitant risk of regurgitation and aspiration pneumonia.

Acquired myasthenia gravis is the result of antibodies generated against the acetylcholine (neurotransmitter) receptors on a muscle's surface at the neuromuscular junction. It can manifest three ways: (1) focal, involving megaesophagus and facial weakness; (2) generalized (most common form), involving megaesophagus and slowly progressive ascending generalized weakness; and (3) fulminant (least common form), involving megaesophagus and rapidly progressive generalized weakness resulting in respiratory failure. The cause is most often idiopathic (immune-mediated of no known cause). It can be seen secondary to neoplasia (e.g., thymoma) in both dogs and cats.

Polyradiculoneuritis may also be seen in both dogs and cats. In North America, exposure of dogs to raccoons (and their saliva) in the 2 weeks preceding onset of the clinical signs has led to this condition, also being known as "Coonhound Paralysis." Analogous to a "raccoon saliva allergy," immune-mediated inflammation develops in the motor nerve roots. Signs will progress for several days before reaching a plateau, which might include respiratory paralysis. Urination and defecation are preserved, and some dogs will develop hyperesthesia.

Tick paralysis is more commonly seen in dogs than cats, but can occur in both species. The paralysis in these cases is due to salivary neurotoxins introduced by the bite of a tick. The genera of tick vary geographically, with *Ixodes, Dermacentor,* and *Amblyomma* being the main ones implicated worldwide, and with cats susceptible to *Ixodes holocyclus,* in particular in Australia.

Botulism is a rapidly ascending motor paralysis in dogs resulting from ingestion of the botulinum toxin produced by *Clostridium botulinum* type C. The organism and the toxin can most often be found in decomposing animal tissue (e.g., chopped raw meat or fish). The toxin prevents release of the neurotransmitter acetylcholine at the neuromuscular junction, disrupting signals from the lower motor neuron to the muscle.

DIAGNOSTIC PROCEDURES AND TREATMENT PLANS

The first concern is respiratory stability, especially in the acutely floppy patient. Cases of respiratory weakening will require intubation and ventilation (for more information see Chapter 8: Mechanical Ventilation). Neurologic examination, as previously mentioned, will reveal loss of spinal (and possibly palpebral) reflexes in all but the not-yet-paralyzed myasthenic patients. In myasthenic patients, reflexes may fatigue with repeated testing and exercise intolerance will be noted. Once myasthenic patients become paralyzed, the reflexes will become absent. Thoracic radiographs may reveal megaesophagus with or without aspiration pneumonia. In some myasthenic patients, a mediastinal mass (likely a thymoma) may also be visible—this may be the causative agent.

Diagnostic confirmation of acquired myasthenia gravis requires acetylcholine-receptor antibody titer testing. This test must be sent to an outside laboratory, and takes a few business days for results to be returned. For quicker, but less reliable results, an anticholinesterase trial can be attempted to see if the weakness rapidly resolves. These drugs leave more acetylcholine neurotransmitter available to stimulate the muscles. If edrophonium hydrochloride (0.1 to 0.2 mg/kg IV) is available, it has the shortest half-life of its class, making it suitable for a therapeutic trial. Other drugs in the class have longer half-lives (pyridostigmine and neostigmine) and are used for maintenance treatment of myasthenia. Overdosing a patient with an anticholinesterase results in exacerbated weakness and a cholinergic crisis. Signs include **s**alivation, **l**acrimation, **u**rination, **d**efecation, **g**astrointestinal upset (i.e., diarrhea), and **e**mesis (this forms the often-used acronym SLUDGE).

Diagnostic confirmation of tick paralysis involves finding and removing the tick. If a tick cannot be found, a dose of an acaricide may provide the solution. Recovery begins within hours of tick removal, with the exception of Australian ticks, in which patients may continue to worsen for a further 24 hours before improving.

There are no emergency clinic diagnostic tests that will help to immediately diagnose either botulism or polyradiculoneuritis patients. In these instances, a careful and thorough history may help raise the clinical suspicion for these diseases. There are also no specific treatment requirements beyond supportive nursing care (corticosteroids do not help to resolve polyradiculoneuritis). This includes using padded bedding and performing frequent position changes to avoid decubital ulcers, performing bladder care to avoid urine scalding, and using frequent eye lubrication if patients are unable to blink because of facial nerve paralysis. Daily physical therapy is helpful to maintain mobility of joints and prevent muscle contracture. Muscle atrophy can occur rapidly and will take months to improve.

To minimize the risk of aspiration pneumonia, patients with megaesophagus should be fed in an upright position, and then maintain the position for 10 to 15 minutes after eating. Some cases might benefit from a gastrostomy tube. Antibiotics will be necessary for those with radiographic evidence of aspiration pneumonia.

HEAD TRAUMA

This is a fairly common emergency presentation, usually with a history of being hit by a car or other object, or falling from a height. The inciting injury might have been witnessed or suspected from external injuries such as abrasions, visible fractures, and bleeding from or around the eyes, ears, mouth, or nose. On closer examination, **anisocoria** (unequal pupil size) may also be seen. All causes result in the same pathophysiology of brain injury.

The actual neurologic exam findings will depend on the site of brain injury, that is, whether one or both cerebral hemispheres are affected, or the thalamus or the brainstem (and which parts of the brainstem). Behavior and mentation changes can be seen, including altered levels of consciousness (depression, dullness, stupor, obtundation, or coma), aimless or compulsive pacing, circling, or seizures. As previously mentioned, abnormal pupil size or symmetry can be seen. Vestibular imbalance, nystagmus, and/or cerebellar tremors, paresis, or paralysis may occur, suggesting a caudal fossa (cerebellum, pons, medulla) lesion.

The brain injury occurs in two stages—there is the primary brain injury as a direct result of the trauma, and the secondary injury as a sequel. The primary brain injury involves the concussive forces resulting in shearing or tearing of brain tissue, or tissue disruption from skull fractures or hemorrhage pressing on the brain or within the brain parenchyma. Secondary injury occurs as a result of either systemic or intracranial effects. Systemic effects include ischemia (decreased blood flow and perfusion), hypotension, hypoxia, anemia, hyper/hypoglycemia, and acid-base and electrolyte disturbances. Intracranial effects include increased intracranial pressure (ICP), cerebral edema, or mass effect from bone fragments or hemorrhage.

DIAGNOSTIC PROCEDURES AND TREATMENT PLANS

The patient should be fully and carefully evaluated. Head trauma is often accompanied by systemic injuries that may affect the ability of the respiratory and cardiovascular systems to support the brain. The first neurologic examination should be carefully and thoroughly performed. This not only allows lesion localization (to direct diagnostic testing, treatment, and prognostication) but also provides a baseline for future neurologic examinations, allowing the care team to serially monitor trends in the neurologic state. Deterioration would be seen as losing brainstem (cranial nerve) reflexes, decreasing responsiveness of mentation, and decreasing responsiveness of pupillary light reflexes (PLRs). Although ocular trauma can result in pupil size changes, the pathways that determine pupillary light reflexes pass through the thalamus to the midbrain and back to the eye under the control of upper motor neurons in the cortex. As ICP increases, compression anywhere along this pathway can alter the control and responsiveness of the PLRs. Initially, disinhibition of the lower motor neuron results in miosis. With increased swelling of the brain, it shifts out of place (herniates) and pressure on the lower motor neuron results in loss of function and mydriasis—the pupil becomes dilated and nonresponsive on checking the PLR. This allows monitoring for changes in ICP, and should be interpreted together with mentation (which should be severely altered if the brain is herniating). The most common direction for the brain to herniate as pressure increases is through the foramen magnum. As it does so, compression of the descending fibers from the upper motor neurons results in paralysis, known as **decerebrate rigidity.** This characteristic recumbent posture involves opisthotonus with extensor rigidity of all limbs. Respiratory paralysis may eventuate.

As primary injury occurs at the time of the trauma, nothing can be done to lessen its effects. However, the extent of secondary injury can determine the outcome in humans. Thus therapeutic intervention is directed at ameliorating the effects of secondary injury. Systemic changes must be addressed, including the normalization of blood pressure and hypoxia.

Cerebral perfusion pressure equals the mean arterial pressure minus ICP. Therefore, monitoring and maintaining a normal mean arterial pressure (approximately 90 mm Hg) will directly affect cerebral perfusion. Intravenous fluid therapy can be used to treat hypotension via commonly used crystalloids (lactated Ringer's solution or Plasma-Lyte A), or more rapidly via hypertonic saline or colloid solutions. Hypertension should be avoided to minimize increases in ICP. Proper physiologic resuscitation should be performed for all extracranial organ systems.

Hypoxia may be a result of concurrent trauma to other organ systems (e.g., thoracic trauma or hemorrhage). Blood transfusions (e.g., packed red blood cells) can help to maintain adequate red blood cell counts. Chest injuries such as pneumothorax, hemothorax, and pulmonary contusions should be assessed via radiographs and treated appropriately. Monitor oxygenation via arterial blood gas analysis or pulse oximetry. Aim to maintain oxygen saturation higher than 98% via oxygen supplementation and other therapies.

A direct therapy to reduce increased ICP and improve cerebral blood flow is mannitol. Increasing intravascular volume and reducing blood viscosity immediately improve cerebral blood flow upon administration of a rapid IV bolus (2 ml/kg/min). It also works as an osmotic diuretic to dehydrate the brain, thus reducing interstitial edema. Mannitol's osmotic diuretic effects can last up to 6 hours, with a dose dependency ranging from 0.25 to 1 g/kg of a 25% solution; this may be repeated every 4 to 8 hours up to three doses in 24 hours. The addition of furosemide (0.7 mg/kg) approximately 15 minutes after the mannitol administration may extend the duration of the diuretic effect. As mentioned previously, mean arterial blood pressure must be maintained, so ensure that the patient does not become dehydrated while mannitol is being administered. There is risk that administration of mannitol during active intracranial hemorrhage may increase the amount of blood outside the blood vessels and thus increase ICP. Do not give either mannitol or furosemide to a dehydrated, hypovolemic, or hypotensive patient—hypertonic saline would be the more appropriate agent to give in these instances. In humans, evidence suggests that a bolus or continuous infusion of hypertonic saline is more effective than mannitol at controlling elevated ICP, but there are varied recommendations as to the optimal concentration of hypertonic saline. In veterinary medicine, the recommendation is saline 7.5%, 3 to 5 ml/kg IV (dog) and 2 ml/kg IV (cat) over 2 to 5 minutes.

Mechanical ventilation may be required if the patient is unable to guard his or her airway (e.g., severely obtunded or in a coma). Ventilation will require endotracheal intubation, which may require sedation in some cases. Ventilation allows control of arterial carbon dioxide partial pressure ($PaCO_2$) via hyperventilation. There is some controversy regarding the use of hypocapnia in severe acute brain injury. Hypocapnia can quite potently lower ICP via cerebral arterial vasoconstriction; however, sustained hypocapnia causes or worsens cerebral ischemia and subsequent normocapnia can cause rebound cerebral hyperemia and consequent increased ICP. Therefore, it is recommended to normalize $PaCO_2$ as quickly as possible.

Other techniques may help to reduce ICP. Placing the patient on an incline with the head and forebody elevated 30 degrees will help venous blood drain from the brain. Compression of the jugular veins should be avoided for the same reason. Patients may flail around because of pain or altered mentation, with self-injury worsening the situation. Sedation may be required for these patients (e.g., diazepam 0.2 to 0.4 mg/kg IV). Analgesia can be provided with opioids such as fentanyl (2 to 6 mcg/kg/hr IV continuous rate infusion).

Steroids have been recommended historically for head trauma. Evidence in people with severe head trauma indicates that steroids lack efficacy and may be detrimental. There is no convincing evidence to support their use in veterinary medicine; however, many veterinarians still use them as a last resort (e.g., using methylprednisolone succinate in doses similar to those listed earlier for spinal cord injury).

RABIES

This viral encephalitis warrants mention because of the zoonotic risk it presents to humans. Its rarity in developed countries is a result of thorough vaccination of the pet population. Viral reservoirs remain in various populations of wildlife (e.g., foxes in Canada or Europe, skunks and raccoons in the United States, or bats in Latin America). Dogs and cats are the main cause of transmission to humans after the pet comes into contact with the saliva of infected wildlife. The virus first replicates at the site of inoculation, and then travels up the peripheral nerves to reach the central nervous system (CNS). From there, it spreads outwards again via peripheral nerves to reach the salivary glands (and other organs). Depending on the site of exposure, amount of virus transmitted, host immune status, and many other factors, rabies has a variable incubation time before CNS signs are visible (e.g., 3 weeks to 6 months in dogs).

Initial clinical signs are nonspecific, including behavior or temperament changes (anxiety, fear, and restlessness), anorexia, and vomiting. Hypersalivation may also be noted. These signs are then followed by the dumb or furious form of rabies, although they can be hard to differentiate. Clinical signs of the furious form (seen in

approximately a quarter to a third of cases) include aggression, restlessness, wandering, vocalizing, panting, drooling, and, occasionally, seizures. The dumb form manifests as progressive ascending paresis or paralysis of the limbs and paralysis of the face, lower jaw, pharynx, or tongue (resulting in difficulty eating and drinking, as well as drooling). Either form will result in death within approximately 7 days of the onset of CNS signs.

DIAGNOSTIC PROCEDURES AND TREATMENT PLANS

Because clinical signs of rabies can be extremely variable, diagnosis is by laboratory confirmation. The most common tests are histopathologic examination of brain tissue samples and immunofluorescent antibody staining (that can also be performed on skin biopsy of tactile facial hair follicles). Many jurisdictions require reporting of suspected rabid animals. If there is clinical suspicion of rabies, isolation protocols should be followed and the patient handled cautiously.

There is no treatment for rabies. Unvaccinated exposed animals should be euthanized. Exposed animals with a current rabies vaccine status (and the owners do not wish euthanasia) should be revaccinated and closely confined and monitored for up to 3 months or as instructed by your local jurisdiction.

CONCLUSION

Regardless of the particular neurologic emergency, the basic approach to these patients is taking a meticulous history, performing a complete neurologic examination, and paying careful attention to detail in patient care. The veterinary technician is the first observer of changes in a patient's neurologic state. The awareness of how the neurologic examination relates to the anatomy will ensure that the appropriate alarms are raised and addressed properly.

REFERENCES

Braund KG: *Clinical syndromes in veterinary neurology*, ed 2, St Louis, 1994, Mosby.

de Lahunta A, Glass E: *Veterinary neuroanatomy and clinical neurology*, ed 3, St Louis, 2006, Saunders.

Lorenz MD, Kornegay JN: *Handbook of veterinary neurology*, ed 4, St Louis, 2004, Saunders.

Wheeler SJ: *Manual of small animal neurology*, ed 2, United Kingdom, 1995, BSAVA.

SCENARIO

Purpose: To provide the veterinary technician with the opportunity to build, or strengthen, the ability to quickly evaluate and respond to a neurologic emergency, as well as plan ahead for emergency drug use.

Stage: Emergency clinic is considered a low level facility. Three staff members are usually available (one veterinarian, one veterinary technician, and one receptionist, who also assists with animal handling when necessary).

Scenario

Friday night. A 3-year-old Border Collie is carried into the clinic by a very upset owner, who describes the dog as abnormal after having bumped into a coffee table, falling to the floor, and thrashing around while trying to stand. The dog had done something similar about a month previously. This time the dog had urinated and defecated while thrashing, and had been thrashing intermittently on the floor for the last 3 hours. Initial assessment: dog is unconscious, tachypneic (60 breaths/min), tachycardic (160 beats/min), and hyperthermic (39.9° C/103.8° F); mucous membranes are tacky and pink, with a capillary refill time of 2 seconds.

While you are taking the temperature, the dog starts thrashing again.

Delivery: This is a self-assessment exercise or can be discussed with colleagues.

Questions

- What do you think might be happening?
- Make a prioritized list of what you would do next.
- Consider what drugs you might want to get for your veterinarian to administer to the collie—what does your clinic carry? What are you authorized to give? What routes should they be given? What amounts would you give for a 20-kg Border Collie versus a 2-kg Chihuahua?
- What would you discuss with the owner?

Key Teaching Points

- Provides veterinary technicians the opportunity to review clinic procedures and guidelines on how to approach emergency receiving, as well as emergency drugs.
- Provides veterinary technicians the opportunity to consider their first responses to a neurologic emergency and to plan ahead.

References

See Box 24-4.

MEDICAL MATH EXERCISE

A patient arrives at your clinic and promptly has a generalized seizure. You are asked to get a 0.5 mg/kg dose of diazepam STAT. The dog is 22 kg, how much 5 mg/ml diazepam will you draw up?

a. 1.1 ml
b. 2.2 ml
c. 4.4 ml
d. 11 ml

25 Toxicologic Emergencies

Jessica D. Davis

CHAPTER OUTLINE

Fundamentals of Treatment
Decontamination: Prevention of
 Further Absorption
 Dermal/Topical Exposure
 Ocular Exposure
 Ingested Toxins
Activated Charcoal
 Antidotes
 Enhanced Elimination Techniques
Lipids
Supportive Care
Specific Types of Toxicities
 Plants
 Foods

Pesticides/Antiparasitics
 Rodenticides
Environmental Toxins
 Ethylene Glycol
 Less Toxic Environmental Toxins
Pharmaceuticals
 Acetaminophen
 Nonsteroidal Antiinflammatory
  Drugs
Metals
 Zinc
 Lead
Toxicology in the Veterinary
 Hospital
Conclusion

KEY TERMS

Adsorption
Antidote
Decontamination
Supportive care
Toxin

LEARNING OBJECTIVES

After studying this chapter, you will be able to:

- Gain understanding of fundamentals of treatment of toxicities.
- Recognize some of the most commonly encountered toxins and how they should be treated.
- Understand supportive care for different types of toxicities.

Toxicologic emergencies can occur in any type of veterinary practice. Potential toxicants are found in the home, garden, community, and even the veterinary clinic. Pet owners may witness exposure to **toxins** or simply present with a sick animal that has clinical signs suggestive of toxin exposure.

A hospital and staff need to be prepared to provide information to pet owners calling with questions about toxin exposure as well as provide care for animals suffering from toxin exposure. A good basic database and access to further information through reference materials, online resources, and poison call centers will help facilitate timely and appropriate treatment for animals that have encountered toxic substances. The list of potential toxins is extensive; however, there are some commonly encountered themes. Box 25-1 lists the top 10 **toxins** published by the ASPCA Animal Poison Control Center.

Although many substances that animals encounter can cause serious illness, some exposures are of limited toxicity or not toxic at all. One common example is ant bait stations. Most contain a very small amount of a safe insecticide (in many cases, avermectin, which is commonly used as a heartworm preventative), but many cautious pet owners will call poison control centers—or the veterinary office—in search of advice if they believe their pet has been exposed to or ingested ant baits. Knowledge of what is toxic can help guide pet owner's decisions to seek veterinary care when necessary.

Toxicology/pharmacology: Toxicology and pharmacology are intricately linked. Knowledge of how a toxin is absorbed, distributed throughout the body, metabolized, and excreted, as well as the mechanism of the toxin and its expected clinical signs is necessary for treatment. Although it is beyond the scope of this chapter, it is worth remembering that an understanding of pharmacology and physiology is necessary for successful treatment of animals exposed to toxins.

All organ systems are interrelated, and toxins may affect many organs. Gastrointestinal (GI) symptoms are common, for example, in many toxicities, even those that do not directly affect the GI tract. Treating the symptoms is as important as treating the specific toxin. Supportive care in addition to careful monitoring can alleviate many symptoms of intoxication, even when the toxicant is unknown.

The liver and kidneys are largely responsible for the majority of metabolism and excretion of most toxins. Animals with preexisting diseases that impair function of either organ can present challenges to treatment. Additionally, particular characteristics of metabolism and excretion should be well understood for successful treatment. In particular, enterohepatic recirculation is a common complication of ingested toxins that requires particular decontamination regimens. Enterohepatic recirculation occurs when a toxin is excreted from the liver via the bile, which is then deposited in the small intestine, where it can be reabsorbed, sometimes repeatedly, effectively extending its toxic effects. Repeated doses of activated charcoal may be necessary to account for this recirculation.

Distribution of toxins can be important, as well. The blood-brain barrier (BBB) has an important role in limiting distribution of drugs and toxins to the central nervous system. When its function is altered, the distribution of potentially harmful substances is also altered.

In order to limit exposure to certain compounds, the capillaries in the brain have tight junctions that restrict passage to particles that are small, uncharged, lipid soluble, and unbound to plasma proteins. Genetic variances can play a role in the permeability of the BBB. The *ABCB1-1Δ (mdr-1)* gene controls P-glycoprotein, a crucial component of the BBB. P-glycoprotein is a drug transporter on the luminal surface of brain capillaries, responsible for transport of substances from brain tissue back into the capillary lumen, limiting brain exposure to drugs and toxins. Certain breeds of dogs (notoriously white-footed breeds such as collies, although other breeds can be affected) lack full expression of the *ABCB-1Δ* gene and are susceptible to toxic brain exposure to these drugs at normally therapeutic doses (hence, the old adage "white feet, don't treat"). Additionally, sufficiently high doses of a drug or toxin can overwhelm the BBB's selective ability and permit absorption into the cerebral circulation. Young animals have an undeveloped BBB, and may experience increased sensitivity to drugs or toxins as a result. Inflammatory disease, intracranial disease, and many drugs can alter BBB function.

FUNDAMENTALS OF TREATMENT

Toxicity should be a differential when an animal arrives at the clinic in an emergent state of unknown cause. Clinical signs may include abnormal behavior, neurologic dysfunction, coagulopathies, lethargy, or gastrointestinal (GI) disorders. Diagnosis of poisoning usually is made by a confirmation from the owners that the animal was exposed to the toxin, as well as by clinical signs exhibited by the animal and chemical analysis. Possible underlying disease processes must be ruled out. Animals with metabolic diseases can have many of the same clinical signs as a poisoned animal. Clinical signs alone must not be used in diagnosing toxicity.

Toxicity can result from ingestion, inhalation, injection, ocular, cutaneous, or topical exposure. Ingestion is the most common and occurs accidentally, when the animal eats something or when uninformed owners give an animal a toxin in the form of food or an over-the-counter medication. Occasionally toxicity may occur at a hospital when a drug dose is miscalculated.

In cases of toxicity the animal should be brought to the veterinary hospital immediately. In general, owners should not treat the animal at home because of the increased risks to the owner and the animal. For topical exposures, the owner can wash the animal (if stable) in a mild dishwashing detergent before bringing it into the hospital. Box 25-2 lists instructions for owners over the phone, before presentation to the hospital.

Equipment list:
- The basics (intravenous [IV] catheters and wrap materials, IV fluids, electrocardiograph, oxygen, crash cart)
- Emetics
- Activated charcoal (with and without sorbitol)
- Stomach tubes of various sizes
- Diazepam and other muscle relaxants
- Consider stocking Intralipid 20%
- Reversal agents: naloxone, flumazenil, atipamezole
- Dishwashing detergent

The goals of treating the poisoned animal are to treat the patient, evaluate its condition, and stabilize vital signs. This includes checking the airway, breathing, and circulation. These patients may arrive in various stages of toxicity and have very mild clinical signs (e.g., anxiety) or very serious clinical signs (e.g., seizure, coma).

BOX 25-2	Advice to Give to Owners Over the Phone

- Owners should protect themselves from exposure by wearing gloves or other protective clothing before handling the animal if it experienced a topical exposure.
- Owners should protect themselves from injury when handling the animal, because poisoned animals may not behave normally.
- Owners should protect the animal from further exposure to the toxin by removing the pet from the potential source.
- Owners should bring samples of the animal's vomit, feces, and urine after exposure, as well as any container or package that the toxin was in and a sample of the possible toxin (e.g., plant material, rat bait).

A thorough history should be obtained. This may be difficult if a recreational drug is involved, because owners may be embarrassed or fear that law enforcement agencies will become involved. Many times treatment begins based on clinical signs because the toxin cannot be identified.

The veterinary team is at risk when treating the poisoned animal. For example, what has been ingested can convert to poisonous gases. When emesis is induced, the gas is emitted. Zinc phosphide (used in rodenticides, most commonly in gopher baits) is converted to phosphine gas when ingested. Therefore, these animals should be treated in a well-ventilated area.

The team must protect themselves from coming into contact with topical exposures by wearing gloves and protective clothing. Protective eyewear is highly recommended before bathing the animals to avoid the spread of contaminants should they shake during the bathing procedure.

Toxins can cause behavioral abnormalities and hypersensitivity. The team must be focused on the patient to avoid any unnecessary injury.

DECONTAMINATION: PREVENTION OF FURTHER ABSORPTION

Decontamination consists of removal of any toxin and prevention or reduction of absorption. Depending on the type of exposure, patients may require bathing, emesis, lavage, and activated charcoal as part of decontamination.

DERMAL/TOPICAL EXPOSURE

Toxic agents on the skin or fur should be removed to prevent further exposure and absorption. This type of exposure may carry risks to owners and hospital staff, so protective clothing should be considered when removing topical agents. Patients should be bathed in tepid water and a mild dishwashing detergent (not dishwasher detergent). Solvents should not be utilized to remove adhesives or paints because they are often as, if not more, harmful as the original substance. Exposure to strong acids or bases may require extended bathing or lavaging of up to 20 to 30 minutes. An ocular protective agent like artificial tears should be applied before bathing, unless ocular exposure is suspected (see Ocular Exposure).

OCULAR EXPOSURE

Chemical exposure to eyes can occur as a result of chemicals splashed, sprayed, or aerosolized. Exposure to any caustic substance should initiate immediate decontamination because continued exposure will worsen damage. Decontamination with copious lavage with sterile saline or tap water for as long as 20 to 30 minutes may be necessary, especially for alkaline chemicals, because damage can continue to occur after initial exposure. Eyes should be rinsed from the medial to lateral canthus, to avoid contaminating the other eye. Frequent breaks may be necessary for patient comfort.

Alkalis and strong acids penetrate tissues rapidly, causing severe pain and blepharospasm. Chemical burns from alkalis can also cause a rise in intraocular pressure, inflammation, and epithelial erosion. Weak acids do not penetrate tissues well and may self-limit due to precipitation of epithelial proteins. Provide analgesia—systemic or topical or both—as needed. Often an Elizabethan collar is necessary until relief can be provided to prevent self-trauma.

Cycloplegia, antibiotics, carbonic anhydrase inhibitors for secondary glaucoma, and treatment for epithelial erosions may be necessary. Topical lubricants should be applied as needed, usually every 4 to 6 hours.

INGESTED TOXINS

Emesis, gastric lavage, and use of adsorbents, cathartics, and enemas are all methods of gastrointestinal decontamination.

Inducing emesis is a technique of administering a substance to the animal so that it will vomit. This procedure is preferred over gastric lavage for removing stomach contents, although vomiting typically only removes 40% to 60% of stomach contents, and seldom provides complete decontamination. In most cases, additional treatment is required. Vomiting should not be induced during a seizure or if the animal is comatose, dyspneic, hypoxic, or lacking normal pharyngeal reflexes. It also is contraindicated if the animal has ingested a caustic substance or a central nervous system (CNS) stimulant. Caustic substances can permanently damage the mucosa of the GI system. If the toxin is a CNS stimulant, then inducing vomiting may increase the risk of seizures. The technician should not attempt to induce vomiting in rabbits or rodents, because they lack the natural ability to vomit.

If gastric decontamination is required in patients at risk of aspiration, anesthesia, intubation with a cuffed endotracheal tube, orogastric intubation, and gastric lavage may be necessary. See Box 25-3 for a gastric lavage technique. In the case of caustic or corrosive substances, small amounts of water or milk can be administered to dilute the substance. In general, for other toxins rapid dilution with large amounts of milk or water is not recommended because it may enhance the absorption of toxins into the GI tract.

Several emetic substances are available. Emetics work by two different mechanisms: (1) local gastric irritation or (2) central nervous system (CNS) stimulation. Some work by both mechanisms. Emetics are most effective when administered quickly and some food is in the stomach.

The most common emetics include hydrogen peroxide, apomorphine, and xylazine. Syrup of ipecac, salt, and dishwashing detergent have also been used to induce vomiting but can carry significant risks. Side effects of ipecac include cardiotoxicity, hemorrhagic diarrhea, and skeletal muscle weakness. Activated charcoal absorbs ipecac well and can be used if any side effects are observed from the use of ipecac. Salt acts as a pharyngeal stimulator and is not recommended because of the risk of sodium toxicity. Salt is also unreliable as an emetic. Dishwashing detergent has been used primarily in humans and only in dogs experimentally, and is not recommended because of its questionable efficacy and potential for side effects.

Hydrogen peroxide (3%) induces emesis by gastric irritation. The recommended dose is 1 tablespoon per 20 lb (1 ml/10 kg) and can be repeated if emesis has not occurred within 10 minutes. This product is not a reliable emetic.

BOX 25-3	Technical Tip: Gastric Lavage Technique

- A large-bore stomach tube and large amounts of tepid water are necessary for the lavage.
- The animal is lightly anesthetized so intubation with a cuffed endotracheal tube is possible; this reduces the patient's risk of aspirating any of the fluid.
- The tube is premeasured from the tip of the nose to the xiphoid cartilage, lubricated, and then introduced into the stomach. The stomach tube must be passed with care, and the lavage should be done with very little pressure. The toxin may weaken the stomach wall, and lavaging could push the toxin into the duodenum.
- Once the lavage has been completed, activated charcoal should be given.
- The tube should be kinked at the end before removal to prevent excess fluid from running into the mouth, which increases the risk of aspiration.

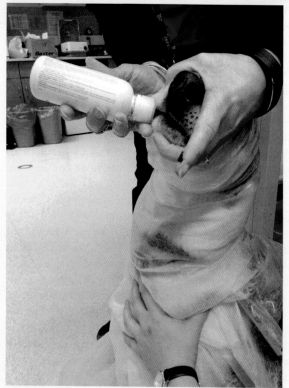

Administration of activated charcoal using the sleeve of a disposable gown to keep the patient clean.

Apomorphine is considered the most reliable emetic in the clinical setting and is a morphine derivative that stimulates dopamine receptors in the chemoreceptor zone (which activates the vomiting center). The recommended dose for apomorphine is 0.03 to 0.04 mg/kg IV or 0.08 mg/kg intramuscularly (IM). The dose for topical conjunctival or subcutaneous (SQ) application is 0.03 mg/kg. Apomorphine is poorly absorbed after oral administration. If using apomorphine topically on the conjunctiva, then the conjunctiva should be rinsed thoroughly with physiologic saline after the animal vomits to alleviate some of the irritation that will occur. Side effects that can occur with apomorphine include lethargy or restlessness and protracted vomiting. Vomiting usually occurs within 10 minutes of IV injection and within 20 minutes of administration via other routes. Some consider apomorphine use in cats to be contraindicated.

Xylazine hydrochloride is an α_2-agonist that has sedative, analgesic, and muscle relaxant properties and is commonly used as an emetic for cats. The dose for cats is 0.44 mg/kg IM or SQ. For dogs the recommended dose is 1.1 to 2.2 mg/kg IM or SQ or 1.1 mg/kg IV. The animal must be monitored closely when this drug is used because of the possibility of increased respiratory depression and bradycardia. Vomiting usually occurs within a few minutes. If needed, xylazine can be reversed with yohimbine or atipamezole.

A gastrotomy or endoscopy should be considered in animals that have ingested metal objects (e.g., pennies, lead weights), which can be confirmed radiographically.

Whole bowel irrigation may be necessary for ingestions of large amounts of toxins or those that have delayed or prolonged effects (such as sustained-release medications).

ACTIVATED CHARCOAL

Activated charcoal (AC) is commonly used as an adsorbent, drawing substances to its surface and binding them to prevent absorption into the bloodstream through the gastrointestinal tract. The very large surface area (1000 m^2/g) allows effective **adsorption** of many toxicants, although it is not effective with all toxins. Metals, ions, and very small molecules are not well attracted to activated charcoal and for those intoxications it is not generally considered beneficial. Activated charcoal can be used with a cathartic (usually sorbitol) to increase gastrointestinal motility and shorten absorption time; generally a cathartic should be used only once. AC can be used multiple times to prevent enterohepatic recirculation. Some toxins that have already been absorbed may diffuse into the GI tract from the bloodstream with the use of activated charcoal; once trapped, they can be safely eliminated. The osmotic characteristics of AC can also result in potentially life-threatening electrolyte imbalances, so electrolytes should be monitored, especially when repeated doses of AC are administered.

Obtunded or vomiting patients have a high risk of aspiration and caution should be used when considering oral administration of any medication in these animals. If administration of AC to at-risk patients is necessary, endotracheal intubation with a cuffed tube is recommended. A nasogastric tube may be placed to facilitate AC delivery; however, this can become an exercise in frustration because the tube is likely to clog.

Food can affect the rate of adsorption with activated charcoal, and adding dairy or oil-based products is not recommended. Although dog food can aid in palatability, it can reduce adsorption. However, the adsorptive ability of AC is extensive and a small amount of food is unlikely to significantly reduce adsorption. The choice to add food should be weighed with the risks of less voluntary methods of administration such as via a syringe or an orogastric tube.

ANTIDOTES

When available, **antidotes** offer a specific and often very successful treatment option. When used expediently, they can offer in some cases full reversal of disease. Antidotes work in a number of different ways: they can function as specific receptor antagonists or as antioxidants to scavenge oxygen-free oxygen radicals, or they

TABLE 25-1	Common Antidotes and Toxins
ANTIDOTE	**INDICATION/TOXICANT**
N-Acetylcysteine	Acetaminophen
Atropine	Organophosphate, carbamate insecticides
CaNa$_2$EDTA	Lead, zinc
Calcitonin	Cholecalciferol
Ethanol	Ethylene glycol
Flumazenil	Benzodiazepines
4-Methylpyrazole (4-MP, fomepizole)	Ethylene glycol
Vitamin K$_1$	Anticoagulant rodenticides
Pralidoxime chloride (2-PAM)	Organophosphate insecticides
Naloxone	Opioids
Yohimbine	Xylazine, Amitraz

can provide metabolic support for detoxification. Table 25-1 lists some common antidotes and their use.

ENHANCED ELIMINATION TECHNIQUES

Enhanced elimination can be obtained by the use of forced diuresis (the use of high rates of IV fluids to enhance renal excretion) and ion trapping (the use of acidifying or alkalinizing agents that may trap ions and facilitate excretion), although these methods carry risks that may outweigh the benefits. Peritoneal dialysis, hemodialysis, or hemoperfusion can be employed to enhance elimination of some toxicants, or to support renal function until the kidneys have recovered sufficiently. Although these treatments may not be available at many facilities or may be prohibitively expensive for some pet owners, they can be extremely effective treatments for intoxication.

LIPIDS

A new and still mostly experimental treatment is the use of lipids for fat-soluble toxins; it has been well documented in human medicine that the use of intravenous lipids can reduce the toxic effects of lipid-soluble drugs such as lidocaine and bupivacaine. In animals, lipids have shown to be effective in the treatment of local anesthetic toxicity, permethrins, ivermectin, baclofen, and some antidepressant medications. Although not fully understood, it is theorized that the lipid infusion provides a "sink" where fat-soluble toxins can be bound and held, inactive, in the plasma component of the intravascular space. This prevents exposure of tissues to the toxin and allows excretion. This new therapy can be miraculous in its effects but it should be noted that the lipid "sink" is not selective, and therapeutic lipid-soluble drugs can be affected as well. A typical dosing protocol is 1.5 to 2.5 ml/kg of a 20% solution as an initial bolus over 1 to 10 minutes, then 0.25 ml/kg/min for 1 to 2 hours. Lipid infusions should be administered through a dedicated catheter (peripheral vessels can be utilized). Treatment can be repeated every few hours as needed; before subsequent dosing, a blood sample should be evaluated for lipemia; if the sample is lipemic then dosing should not be repeated until the serum is clear. IV lipid infusions are excellent media for bacterial growth and should be handled aseptically; unused portions should be refrigerated and discarded after 24 to 36 hours.

SUPPORTIVE CARE

As is the case for all illnesses, the aim is to treat affected systems and provide appropriate **supportive care.** Cardiovascular monitoring, intravenous fluids for cardiovascular support, and diuresis, analgesia, and nutritional support can be just as valuable to successful treatment as any antidote. Close monitoring and attentive nursing care are essential to the treatment of toxicosis because secondary organ damage is a common result of severe poisonings.

SPECIFIC TYPES OF TOXICITIES

PLANTS

Plants are found in almost every environment, and are encountered by all species of animals. Most toxic plants, if ingested, provide local irritation and exert their effects primarily on the gastrointestinal tract, resulting in self-limited illness. Vomiting is a common response in many species, thereby self-decontaminating. Often, no further treatment is necessary; in more severe cases supportive care for GI upset is sufficient and seldom life-threatening. However, some plants are highly toxic or even deadly.

Plant identification can often be challenging and in many cases supportive care is the mainstay of treatment without a definitive toxin. In some cases, the utilization of local plant nurseries or universities may be useful in correct identification in order to best direct treatment. Although many owners may have non-native and exotic plants in their gardens and homes, it is important for the veterinary staff to be aware of native toxic plant species.

Some of the most common plants ingested by companion animals are from the Araceae family (dumb cane, split-leaf philodendron). These plants contain calcium oxalate crystals and histamine releasers. Common clinical signs include hypersalivation, oral mucosal edema, and local pruritus. More severe signs may be observed if a large amount of the plant has been ingested and can include vomiting, dysphagia, dyspnea, abdominal pain, vocalization, hemorrhage, gastritis, and enteritis.

The oral cavity should be rinsed with milk or water to remove the calcium oxalate crystals, and GI decontamination and supportive care may be necessary. The prognosis for this toxicity is usually very favorable.

Lilies

Lily toxicity is commonly reported in cats. Accurate identification of the plant as a true lily can be challenging, since not all commonly-called lilies are toxic or may have different toxic qualities; there are many species of lily, and not all common-name lilies are truly lilies. The following focuses on the *Lilium* and *Hemerocallis* genera, which cause acute renal failure in cats. These include tiger lily, Easter lily, stargazer lily, and some daylilies.

The toxic principle of lilies is unknown. All parts of the plant are toxic, including the leaves, flowers, and pollen. Small quantities (less than one leaf) are required to cause toxicosis. Cats can become exposed to lilies that are brought into the home for decorative purposes or grown in the yard.

Symptoms of lily toxicosis develop within 12 hours of exposure, although delayed reactions have been reported as long as 2 to 5 days postexposure. Initial symptoms are generally a response to gastric irritation and include vomiting and depression. Acute renal failure results in 24 to 72 hours; clinical signs are consistent with acute renal failure and include polyuria, oliguria, anuria, dehydration, vomiting, and depression. Central nervous system signs can also be observed, including head pressing, ataxia, tremors, and seizures. Serum chemistry findings show evidence of severe azotemia; creatinine level can be disproportionately elevated. Urinalysis may reveal epithelial casts and glucosuria.

Treatment consists of decontamination with emesis, activated charcoal, and supportive care. In cases where ingestion is observed, vomiting can be induced in stable and awake patients, followed by activated charcoal at 1 to 2 ml/kg with a cathartic. Intravenous fluid therapy instituted and maintained for at least 48 hours will induce diuresis, protecting the kidneys. Serial monitoring of renal values and electrolytes can help direct fluid and electrolyte therapy. Aggressive diuresis may be necessary in patients in which treatment has been delayed; patients in oliguric renal failure may require careful measuring of central venous pressures and urine output. Histopathologic examination of the kidneys reveals that despite severe renal damage, the basement membrane generally remains intact, and if hemodialysis or peritoneal dialysis is available, even severely affected cats can recover given enough time and aggressive treatment.

Cardiac Glycosides

Cardiac glycosides are present in *Kalanchoe,* oleander, laurel, dogbane, foxglove, lily of the valley, and some milkweeds. The highest concentration of the toxin is generally found in the flowers. Glycosides are bitter tasting; as a result, large amounts may not be consumed; water in which plants were placed can cause poisoning as well. Cardiac glycosides inhibit sodium/potassium ATPase: potassium accumulates outside the cell, preventing calcium release. Positive inotropy is decreased, and heart block can occur. Additional digitalis glycosides in some plants can cause decreased atrioventricular (AV) conduction, skipped beats, changes in the S-T segment, escape beats, and ventricular arrhythmias. Vagal stimulation occurs within the first 24 hours, resulting in bradycardia and hypotension; beta/sympathetic stimulation occurs after 24 hours and can result in tachycardia and hypertension.

With large doses, onset of signs can occur within 1 hour; in smaller doses, 8 to 12 hours may elapse before symptoms are seen. Gastrointestinal and central and peripheral nervous system effects can be observed, including salivation, polyuria, depression, diarrhea, and inappetence. Chemistry changes include increased levels of blood urea nitrogen (BUN), creatinine, blood glucose, and carbon dioxide.

Treatment involves repeated doses of AC to prevent enterohepatic recirculation, administration of IV fluids without potassium unless hypokalemia is noted, and avoidance of calcium-containing fluids. Cardiac arrhythmias can be treated with atropine, propranolol, or lidocaine. Inotropic and/or pressor therapy may be necessary if hypotension is present.

Autumn Crocus

Colchicines and other alkaloids constitute the toxic component of autumn crocus. These toxins arrest mitosis, leading to cell death. Clinical signs include inappetence, vomiting, diarrhea, salivation, depression, abdominal pain, hemorrhagic gastroenteritis, weakness, ataxia, paresis, collapse, and renal failure; as intestinal mucosal crypt epithelium swells, malabsorption can occur. Increased levels of BUN, erythrocytosis, leukopenia, and myelosuppression can occur.

Treatment is symptomatic; fluid therapy, GI protectants, and cardiac monitoring are recommended. Antibiotic therapy is generally indicated for myelosuppression and to prevent bacterial translocation from compromised gastrointestinal integrity.

Cycad (Sago) Palm

Found all over the world in tropical and subtropical areas, Sago palms can also be brought into the home as decorative plants. Palm-like in appearance, they can be attractive ornamental plants that also produce large cones of seeds. All parts of the plant are toxic, with the highest concentrations in the seeds. Cycads have three toxicants: methylazoxymethanol (MAM); β-methylamino-L-alanine (BMAA, a neurotoxic amino acid); and an unidentified toxin.

Cycasin is a gastrointestinal irritant and a hepatotoxin, causing hepatic necrosis. Cycasin poisoning can potentially cause necrosis of the cerebellum, with resulting ataxia. As little as two seeds can cause symptoms, which occur within 12 to 24 hours of ingestion. Neurologic signs may require chronic exposure. Clinical signs include vomiting, with or without blood, depression, diarrhea, and anorexia. Seizures can occur but are thought to be secondary to hepatic damage.

Labs do not routinely test for cycasin or BMAA; fragments of plant or seeds in the gastrointestinal tract can lead to a diagnosis.

Emesis and activated charcoal will help reduce adsorption. There is no antidote, so treatment is supportive with gastrointestinal protectants (H$_2$ blockers, sucralfate), intravenous fluids, and electrolyte support. Gastric hemorrhage can be severe, and blood transfusions may be necessary. Prognosis is good if decontamination can be performed before clinical signs are present, and guarded if signs have developed. Even successfully treated toxicosis may require life-long hepatic support.

Castor Beans

Castor bean plants are tropical and subtropical plants often found as ornamental plantings in yards and gardens. The toxic compound in castor beans is ricin, a type of lectin. The toxin is found in all parts of the plant, but is most concentrated in the bean. Lectins are found in many beans, and in particularly high concentrations in castor beans. Castor oil if properly extracted does not contain ricin because lectins are destroyed by moist heat. The bean coat must be broken to release ricin; as a result, multiple ingestions of whole beans result in little absorption through the gastrointestinal tract. However, ricin is considered one of the deadliest substances known, so any ingestion should be considered potentially lethal. The mechanism of action is due to the cellular toxin, which is contained in A and B glycoprotein chains; chain B facilitates endocytosis of the toxin by binding to proteins on the cell surface, allowing absorption of the toxin. Glycoprotein A inhibits protein synthesis and causes cell death. It also disturbs calcium homeostasis by decreasing calcium uptake, resulting in an increased sodium/calcium exchange and disturbance of cardiac nerve conduction. Ingestion of even small amounts of any part of the plant can cause clinical signs.

Clinical signs most often occur within 6 hours of ingestion and are consistent with damage to the intestinal mucosa and include vomiting, diarrhea, abdominal pain, and hemorrhagic gastroenteritis. There is no (readily available) antidote to ricin. Decontamination and supportive care are the primary treatment. Emesis, activated charcoal, gastrointestinal protectants, and antibiotics are recommended. Frequent feeding is recommended to maintain the health of intestinal villi. Hepatic failure may occur.

The death rate of ingested castor bean seeds is low because of the tendency of most animals to swallow the seeds whole; however, if the seed coat is broken, and especially if clinical signs are present, prognosis is guarded.

Less Toxic or Nontoxic Plants

Many plants when ingested produce very mild symptoms that seldom require veterinary care. Poinsettia plants are commonly brought into the house during winter holiday months and owners may be concerned about toxicity to dogs and cats. Poinsettia is a mild GI irritant that is self-limiting due to vomiting of plant parts. Christmas cactus and Christmas trees are of limited toxicity and seldom cause clinical signs.

FOODS

Pet owners are often unaware that foods or food additives present in the home can pose a threat to animals.

Grapes, Raisins, and Currants

Once considered a low-fat, healthy treat, grapes, raisins, and currants are now known to cause acute renal failure in dogs. The toxic principle of raisins and grapes is unknown, and the amount required varies among animals; some appear to be more sensitive than others. The lowest concentration reported to be toxic is 0.32 to 0.65 g/kg. Both red and white grapes may have toxic properties.

Symptoms include vomiting (usually occurring within the first 2 hours), diarrhea, anorexia, lethargy, and polydipsia, progressing to renal failure in 24 hours to several days. Signs are consistent with acute renal failure: vomiting, lethargy, anorexia, diarrhea, abdominal pain, and dehydration. Serum chemistry results are consistent with acute renal failure; hypercalcemia is also a frequent finding.

Treatment consists of decontamination with emesis, activated charcoal, and supportive care. Early diuresis may prevent renal failure. Renal chemistry values should be monitored for 72 hours. Furosemide, dopamine, and mannitol may be of use in anuric renal failure; hemodialysis or peritoneal dialysis may also be of benefit, where available. The renal basement membrane remains intact in many cases, and renal damage can be reversed given enough time and supportive treatment.

Onions

Allium species include onions, garlic, leeks, shallots, chives, and a number of ornamental flowering plants. Animals can become exposed to *Allium* species through ingestion of plants in gardens or grown in the home, by onions or garlic fed directly to the pet, or by consumption of food additives. Garlic is sometimes advocated as a dietary supplement to deter flea infestation. *Allium*s are toxic regardless of whether the consumed plant is raw, cooked, or dehydrated. The toxic component in *Allium* plants is propyl disulfide, which exerts its effects through the metabolism of disulfides, producing oxygen-free radicals.

Erythrocytes are sensitive to oxidative injury, and cell membrane damage and intravascular hemolysis result. Disulfides also denature hemoglobin, which precipitates and binds to the interior of the cell membrane, forming Heinz bodies, which are then removed from circulation by the reticuloendothelium and hemolysis. Methemoglobin is also produced.

The time between ingestion and the presentation of clinical signs is dose dependent, and can be as long as 7 to 10 days. Raw onions at a dose of 11 to 15 g/kg cause clinical signs; dehydrated onions can cause signs at 5.5 g/kg. Cats fed baby food with as little as 0.3% onion powder exhibited increased Heinz body formation.

Clinical signs include inappetence, ataxia, lethargy, recumbency, tachycardia, tachypnea, dyspnea, pale or icteric mucous membranes, vomiting, and diarrhea. Laboratory tests may reveal Heinz bodies, Howell-Jolly bodies, regenerative anemia, hemoglobinemia, hemoglobinuria, and elevations in bilirubin and lactate levels. There are no diagnostic tests specific to *Allium* poisoning, although a distinctive odor of onions or garlic can often be detected in the breath.

Treatment involves supportive care with intravenous fluids and blood products if the anemia is severe.

Methylxanthines

Methylxanthines stimulate the heart and respiratory muscles and cause minor diuresis. Caffeine, theobromine, and theophylline can be found in coffee, tea, stimulants, medications, and chocolate.

Chocolate (Theobromine)

Theobromine is found in cocoa beans, cocoa bean hulls, chocolate, colas, and tea. The cocoa bean contains three methylxanthine compounds: (1) caffeine, (2) theophylline, and (3) theobromine. Theobromine is toxic to dogs and cats. Cats are less likely to experience this type of toxicity because of their selective eating habits. The toxic dose of theobromine is 250 to 500 mg/kg. Milk chocolate contains 44 mg/oz of theobromine, and baking chocolate contains 390 mg/oz of theobromine.

Clinical signs include anxiousness, vomiting, diarrhea, tachycardia, cardiac arrhythmias, urinary incontinence, ataxia, muscle tremors, abdominal pain, hematuria, seizures, cyanosis, coma, and sudden death caused by cardiac arrhythmia.

Diagnosis is based on the history and clinical signs and the presence of xanthines in serum, plasma, tissue, urine, or stomach contents. Theobromine is stable in serum and plasma for 7 days at room temperature.

Treatment includes inducing vomiting (if not contraindicated) and performing gastric lavage with either charcoal or cathartics. It may be beneficial to induce vomiting even if the ingestion occurred more than 2 hours earlier, because chocolate melts and forms a semisolid mass in the stomach. Diazepam may be necessary to control seizure activity, as well as antiarrhythmics to control arrhythmias. Catheterizing the bladder frequently is also recommended, because methylxanthines can be reabsorbed from the urinary bladder.

Caffeine

Caffeine can be found in coffee, tea, chocolate, colas, and stimulant drugs. The lethal dose is 140 mg/kg. The clinical signs include vomiting, diuresis, restlessness, and hyperactivity. Tachypnea and tachycardia may be present. Ataxia, cyanosis, cardiac arrhythmias, and seizures also may be observed. Death is not common in caffeine toxicity but can result from cardiac collapse. Diagnosis and treatment are the same as those for theobromine toxicity.

Xylitol

Xylitol has had growing popularity in the United States as a sweetening agent because it contains two-thirds the calories of sugars, and causes little insulin release in people; this, in addition to the fact that it does not require insulin to enter the cell, makes it a good sugar substitute for diabetic humans, as well as an emergency energy source. In dogs, however, xylitol causes insulin release that is up to six times greater than an equal dose of glucose. Additionally, it is rapidly and completely absorbed in the GI tract. Found in sugar-free gums, mints, oral rinses, chewable vitamins, and granulated for cooking, xylitol has a toxic dose as low as 0.1 g/kg. An estimated 0.3 g can be found in a stick of gum; a cup of granulated xylitol equals approximately 190 g.

Xylitol causes a rapid drop in blood glucose concentration in dogs. The resulting signs of severe hypoglycemia (depression, ataxia, and seizures) can mimic other central nervous system disorders. Clinical signs can be rapid in onset because of its ease of absorption and can appear within 30 to 60 minutes, although delayed symptoms as late as 12 hours have been reported. Vomiting and lethargy secondary to hypoglycemia can progress rapidly to ataxia, collapse, and seizures.

Rarely, hyperglycemia can be observed, thought to be Somogyi-type effect. Hypokalemia secondary to an intracellular uptake of potassium with insulin is a common finding. Hypophosphatemia is also a common finding. The effect of xylitol on cats is unknown. Liver failure can develop in 12 to 24 hours, in some cases without initial hypoglycemia. Clinical and laboratory findings include a coagulopathy with increases in prothrombin time (PT), activated partial thromboplastin time (APTT); severely increased level of alanine transaminase (ALT); moderately increased bilirubin level; and, less commonly, mild thrombocytopenia and a mild increase in phosphorous concentration. The presence of phosphatemia is a poor prognostic indicator. In general, a dose of >0.5 g/kg is considered hepatotoxic. As a result of the rapid onset of clinical signs, decontamination is often not an option. Emesis should only be induced in asymptomatic patients; activated charcoal is of little use because the xylitol molecule is small and rapidly absorbed. A baseline measurement of blood glucose, serum potassium, and phosphorous levels should be obtained; additionally, liver enzymes and coagulation status should be assessed. Dextrose-containing fluids may be indicated even if hypoglycemia is not present. Liver protectants and antioxidants may be of use, such as *N*-acetylcysteine and *S*-adenosylmethionine.

Garbage

Garbage toxicity is more common in dogs, and those allowed to roam freely are at greatest risk. Enterotoxemia can occur if the animal ingests decomposed food, carrion, or compost. The small bowel pH may increase to greater than 6, which results in an absence of hydrochloric acid (achlorhydria). Hydrochloric acid promotes normal digestion and prevents multiplication of bacteria. Achlorhydria increases the risk of enterotoxemia. Common enterotoxin-producing bacteria associated with enterotoxicosis include *Streptococcus, Salmonella,* and *Bacillus* species.

Clinical signs can begin within minutes to a few hours after ingestion. The signs include anorexia, lethargy, vomiting, diarrhea, ataxia, tremors, and anxiousness. This can progress to endotoxic shock and death. The tremors can be mild to severe.

Diagnosis is based on the history and clinical signs. Treatment includes fluid therapy, broad-spectrum antibiotics, and intestinal protectants. Muscle relaxers or diazepam may be necessary to control tremors.

Mold

Tremorgenic mycotoxins are produced as the result of fungal metabolism. Mold is frequently encountered in garbage and composted food remains. Penitrem A and roquefortine are the two most commonly encountered tremorgenic mycotoxins associated with spoiled food and are found in moldy foods, compost, and grains. They primarily affect the central nervous system, and are produced by the fungi genera *Penicillium, Aspergillus,* and *Claviceps*. Both penitrem A and roquefortine mycotoxins are readily absorbed and excreted primarily in bile, making them prone to enterohepatic recirculation. They are lipophilic and therefore cross the blood-brain barrier and have multiple effects on neurotransmitter release mechanisms at central and peripheral levels. Clinical signs occur within 30 minutes, although they can be delayed as long as 2 to 3 hours. Early signs include vomiting, hyperactivity, panting, irritability, weakness, muscle tremors, and rigidity. Later signs include severe tremors, opisthotonos, seizures, nystagmus, and recumbency with paddling. Increased muscle activity can result in hyperthermia, exhaustion, metabolic changes, rhabdomyolysis, and dehydration.

Treatment entails stabilization of vital signs: control tremors, seizures, and resulting hyperthermia. Decontaminate asymptomatic patients with emesis, and activated charcoal. Full gastrointestinal lavage and multiple doses of activated charcoal may be necessary because of enterohepatic recirculation. Seizures can be treated with diazepam and phenobarbital. Muscle relaxants such as methocarbamol and guaifenesin may be beneficial. Intravenous lipid therapy may be of benefit because of the toxin's lipid solubility.

Prognosis is good when decontamination occurs early, and guarded when clinical signs are already present.

PESTICIDES/ANTIPARASITICS
Permethrins and Pyrethroids

Permethrins are derived from chrysanthemum flowers and are available over the counter as sprays, dusts, gels, dips, shampoos, spot-on treatments, and more. Pyrethroids—synthetic analogs of permethrins—are more potent, more toxic, and more stable than permethrins. Available for use in the garden, in the home, and on livestock and pets, pyrethrins and pyrethroids account for 25% of the world insecticide market.

In small animals, permethrins are most often utilized as over-the-counter flea treatments. Cats are more sensitive to the neurologic effects of permethrins and toxicities are often the result of inadvertent or intentional use of products intended for dogs. Cats can also become intoxicated after physical contact with treated dogs. Cats that are weak or debilitated because of high flea burdens are especially sensitive to the compound.

Absorption is rapid, with 40% to 60% absorbed after oral exposure and less than 2% after dermal exposure. Pyrethroids can be stored in the skin and slowly released over time.

Permethrins and pyrethroids work by binding to the membrane lipid phase of nerve cells, slowing the opening and closing of neural sodium channels. This leads to repetitive discharge and membrane depolarization, with a direct action on sensory nerve endings, causing repetitive firing. Less than 1% of sodium channels must be affected to produce neurologic signs. Clinical signs include paresthesia, hyperesthesia, ear twitching, tail flicking, and twitching of the skin on the back; these can progress to tremors and seizures. Onset can be minutes to hours.

Initial treatment consists of decontamination by bathing in dishwashing detergent, with care taken to keep the patient dry and warm. Thermal regulation and support may be necessary since patients may present with high temperatures that plummet once tremors are controlled, and hypothermia can worsen tremors. Muscle relaxants such as methocarbamol are often more helpful than anticonvulsant drugs, although both may be required to control muscle tremors and seizures in more severely affected animals. Methocarbamol can be administered at 55 to 220 mg/kg IV; give ⅓ to ½ dose, and then to effect, not to exceed 2 ml/min. There is a published maximum daily dose of 330 mg/kg; exceeding this dose may be necessary in some cases. Atropine is not antidotal and is contraindicated in treatment of permethrin toxicity.

Unfortunately, because of rapid absorption, activated charcoal is not likely to be of benefit. IV fluid support is provided to prevent myoglobinuric-induced renal failure, and manage hyperthermia. Hypoglycemia is possible secondary to increased muscle activity, especially if the patient is young or unable to eat as a result of toxicity. As a lipid-soluble toxin, permethrin toxicity can be responsive to IV lipid therapy. Results can be rapid and remarkable, with resolution of tremors within an hour of initiating lipid therapy.

Generally, no permanent sequelae result from intoxication unless hyperthermia or hypoxia was severe during seizures, but symptoms can persist for 3 to 5 days (typically less if lipid therapy is utilized).

Organophosphates

Organophosphates and carbamate insecticides inhibit cholinesterase activity, interfering with autonomic nervous system function. These insecticides are highly fat-soluble and are well absorbed from the skin and GI tract. Carbamates are found in dusts, sprays, shampoos, and flea and tick collars. Organophosphates are commonly found in dips, pet sprays, dusts, yard and kennel sprays, premise sprays, and systemics. Toxicity usually occurs after one of these preparations has been applied to the animal's skin or if the animal has ingested the preparation during licking while grooming. Cats, animals that have been previously exposed to an anticholinesterase insecticide, and animals who are malnourished are more susceptible to this toxicity.

Clinical signs of carbamate and organophosphate poisoning may include excessive salivation, vomiting, diarrhea, muscle twitching to fasciculations, and miosis. Signs can progress to seizures, coma, respiratory depression, and death. Diagnosis is based on the history and clinical signs. The response to a dose of atropine (0.2 mg/kg) also supports the diagnosis.

Treatment of this toxicity includes washing the animal in a mild detergent if a topical exposure has occurred and administering activated charcoal if ingestion has occurred. Atropine also is recommended to control the muscarinic signs at a dose rate of 0.2 to 0.4 mg/kg, half IV and half IM or SQ. This dose can be repeated; however, caution must be taken not to induce an atropine intoxication, signs of which include tachycardia, ataxia, and lethargy. Pralidoxime chloride is recommended for organophosphate poisoning; it reactivates cholinesterase that has been inhibited. The dose is 20 mg/kg IM twice a day for several days or until clinical signs of the toxicity are no longer observed. Exposure to another anticholinesterase insecticide should be avoided until 4 to 6 weeks after recovery.

Metaldehyde

Metaldehyde and methiocarb are two types of snail or slug killers. The baits are very palatable to dogs and cats. Metaldehyde's mechanism of action is unknown; methiocarb is a carbamate and parasympathomimetic. Both cause a rapid onset of severe neurologic symptoms that include hypersalivation, incoordination, muscle fasciculations, hyperesthesia, tachycardia, and seizures.

Hyperthermia and severe acidosis also are common, and cats display nystagmus. Bradycardia, respiratory and neurologic depression, and pulse irregularities may be noted in severely affected animals.

Diagnosis is based on the history and presentation of clinical signs. The odor of acetaldehyde (resembles formaldehyde) in the stomach contents may be noted.

The treatment includes inducing emesis and administering adsorbents. Anticonvulsants or muscle relaxants may be necessary to control CNS hyperactivity. Supportive care includes correcting acidosis.

Ivermectin

Ivermectin is a broad-spectrum antiparasitic derived from the bacterium *Streptomyces avermitilis* used in the treatment of endo- and ectoparasites in dogs and cats. It is available as a liquid for injection or oral administration in small and large animal concentrations, as well as a paste for large animals. It is available over the counter and owners may purchase the drug in an attempt to save money, but frequently overdose their pets.

Ivermectin works in invertebrates by inhibiting chloride channels, causing a flaccid paralysis and death. In vertebrates at high enough doses, it can overwhelm the BBB drug transport and enter the CNS. Here it acts similarly as a gamma-aminobutyric acid (GABA) agonist, hyperpolarizing cell membranes and preventing neuronal depolarization. This results in a flaccid paralysis, which can progress from ataxia to stupor and even coma and death. Animals lacking full expression of the *mdr-1* gene and P-glycoprotein synthesis show an increased sensitivity to ivermectin.

Absorption is rapid via SQ or oral routes, and the half-life of the compound (in dogs) is up to 2 days. The toxic dose for dogs is 2.5 mg/kg and 1.3 mg/kg in cats although this dose varies among individuals. Sensitive dogs may show clinical signs of toxicity with doses as low as 100 to 500 mcg/kg. Young animals possess an undeveloped BBB and may exhibit clinical signs with doses as low as 300 mcg/kg.

Clinical signs include ataxia, agitation, vocalization, disorientation, mydriasis, blindness, weakness, and bradycardia. More severe intoxications may cause the animal to develop seizures and become stuporous or comatose. Hypoventilation and aspiration are a concern with more markedly depressed animals.

Treatment revolves around supportive care and decontamination. Ivermectin undergoes enterohepatic recirculation and multiple doses of activated charcoal may be indicated. Treatment of CNS effects with anticonvulsant therapy may be needed; there is some concern that benzodiazepines may share a close enough receptor on GABA to warrant avoiding the use of these agents. Phenobarbital, propofol, and etomidate can be utilized to control seizures. Physostigmine has been shown to counteract the CNS effects of ivermectin for short periods of time although the potential hypotensive effects of this drug may be detrimental. Mechanical ventilation may be indicated if the patient is hypoventilating or has respiratory compromise secondary to aspiration.

Ivermectin is a lipid-soluble toxin and IV lipids can be utilized as part of treatment. In some patients, the use of lipids can precipitate a very rapid recovery, shortening hospital stays and markedly decreasing the severity of symptoms.

Spinosad is another antiparasitic that can be found in some flea and heartworm preventives. Spinosad is a P-glycoprotein antagonist, which means it can lower the toxicity threshold for ivermectin by permitting more ivermectin to remain in the central nervous system. This can exacerbate or potentiate ivermectin toxicity when high doses of ivermectin are used concurrently with Spinosad.

Ant Traps

Ant traps are available as discs, chambers, baits, and trays; some formulations contain arsenic; most contain boric acid, avermectin, fipronil, hydramethylnon, propoxur, or sulfuramid. Because of the low concentration of insecticide and the small size of the bait, toxicosis is not expected; risk of foreign body contamination from the plastic container is greater. Signs are usually limited to mild GI symptoms and generally do not require treatment.

RODENTICIDES

When exposure to rodenticides is suspected, instruct clients to bring packaging whenever possible to aid in identification. There are numerous types of rodenticides, and many are manufactured in similar-looking formulations. Proper identification is essential for appropriate treatment.

Anticoagulant Rodenticides

Anticoagulant rodenticides work by depleting stores of vitamin K_1, impairing coagulation. Although toxicosis can be severe and life-threatening, exposures can be treated with a high success rate, especially if treatment is initiated before coagulopathies develop. These anticoagulants work by binding the vitamin K factor, which then inhibits the synthesis of prothrombin (factor II), as well as factors VII, XI, and X. The depletion of these factors slows all coagulation pathways. This effect can occur within 6.2 to 41 hours in a dog and is very dependent on the type of anticoagulant ingested. (For more information, see Chapter 16: Hematologic Emergencies.)

The most common rodenticides consist of first- and second-generation warfarin-based toxicants, with the second-generation drugs having been developed for enhanced toxicity. A few first-generation rodenticides include warfarin, pidone, diphacinone, and chlorophacinone. They can depress clotting factors for 7 to 10 days. The second-generation rodenticides (capable of killing warfarin-resistant rats) include brodifacoum and bromadiolone, and can depress clotting factors for 3 to 4 weeks.

Formulations include cakes, granules, and grains; most contain a nondigestible, blue-green dye, which can aid in identification of ingestion. Although primary exposure via ingestion of rodenticides is the most common route of intoxication, relay toxicosis can occur when poisoned rodents are ingested by pets.

The lethal dose varies with many factors, including the species of the animal that has been exposed, age, preexisting disease conditions such as renal failure or liver failure, number of ingestions, and concurrent drug (e.g., aspirin) use. Because they are highly protein bound (warfarin 90% to 95%), these toxicants can interfere with other medications that are also protein bound and enhance their toxicity.

Most are metabolized by the liver and excreted renally; brodifacoum has some hepatic excretion and enterohepatic recirculation can occur. The duration of action varies by compound and species; in dogs, the duration of action of warfarin is 14 days; brodifacoum, 30 days to as long as 6 weeks.

Clinical signs occur after the depletion of active clotting factors (1 to 7 days after ingestion) and include lethargy, vomiting, anorexia, ataxia, diarrhea, hemorrhage, melena, dyspnea, epistaxis, scleral or subconjunctival hemorrhage, bruising, and pale mucous membranes. Sudden death may result from hemorrhage into the pericardium, thorax, mediastinum, abdomen, or cranium.

Diagnosis is based on the history of exposure to the toxin, prolonged bleeding times, and the response to vitamin K_1 therapy, which occurs 24 to 48 hours after the initiation of therapy. Dye-colored feces may be present if a rodenticide has been ingested.

Treatment includes inducing vomiting (if not contraindicated) and administering activated charcoal and cathartics. Fresh whole blood transfusions or component therapy may be necessary to replace clotting factors and red blood cells if the patient is anemic. Fresh frozen plasma (10 to 20 ml/kg) can be used for animals in need of the clotting factors but not red cells (for more information, see Chapter 5: Transfusion Medicine). Vitamin K_1 (3 to 5 mg/kg) should be administered every 24 hours until toxic concentrations of the anticoagulant are no longer in the animal. Vitamin K will begin the synthesis of new clotting factors 6 to 12 hours after administration. Clotting factors should return to normal within 24 to 36 hours. Oral administration with canned dog food is the preferred route unless there is concern for GI dysfunction or if activated charcoal has been administered. Because vitamin K_1 is fat soluble, the fat in the dog food will increase the absorption rate. SQ administration is the next best route unless the animal is hypovolemic. IV administration may cause anaphylaxis, and IM injections may cause hemorrhage.

Vitamin K_1 therapy should be continued in accordance with the duration of action of the rodenticide. Clinical signs can develop within 48 hours if vitamin K_1 is discontinued too soon; generally, testing coagulation factors 48 hours after vitamin K_1 therapy has been discontinued to ensure that the treatment duration has been sufficient.

Bromethalin

Bromethalin has a name similar to brodifacoum and bromadiolone, but is not an anticoagulant rodenticide. It is available in forms identical to other rodent baits, including the tell-tale green tablets that are commonly identified as brodifacoum.

The minimum lethal dose in dogs is 2.5 mg/kg; cats are more sensitive at 0.45 mg/kg. Bromethalin acts by disrupting cellular ATP production; as a result, the sodium/potassium pump loses function. Cells lose their ability to maintain osmotic control and swell with water. Signs are most pronounced in the central nervous system as intracranial pressure increases due to fluid shift into the CNS.

After ingestion, peak plasma concentrations occur in 4 hours; onset of signs occurs in 1 to 4 days. Symptoms include ataxia, seizures, coma, and paralysis, and are usually classified as either paralytic or convulsant, which is dose dependent. If the amount ingested is less than the LD50 (lethal dose 50%) but greater than the toxic dose, a paralytic syndrome occurs in 1 to 4 days and includes hind limb weakness and ataxia that progresses to depression, tremors, upper motor neuron paralysis in the hind limbs, loss of deep pain reflexes, and decreased conscious proprioception. Vomiting, anorexia, nystagmus, anisocoria, opisthotonos, seizures, and coma may also be observed. Signs can progress over 1 to 2 weeks. In doses greater than the LD50 a convulsant syndrome occurs within 4 to 36 hours of ingestion and includes hyperexcitability, hyperthermia, tremors, and seizures. Cats exhibit a paralytic syndrome regardless of dose, including upper motor neuron paralysis; patients in the final stages of toxicity may exhibit a decerebrate posture.

Diagnosis can be challenging if the exposure was not observed, because there are no pathognomonic lab abnormalities and therefore diagnostics may not help to rule out other toxicologic causes of neurologic dysfunction.

Treatment consists of emesis in nonsymptomatic animals; multiple doses of activated charcoal are recommended as metabolites undergo enterohepatic recirculation and continued absorption can occur. Supportive care and anticonvulsants may be required in affected animals. Traditional treatment for increased intracranial pressure consisting of corticosteroids and osmotic agents is largely ineffective and transient; once treatment is discontinued, the intracranial pressure (ICP) can rise again.

The severity of symptoms and the low effectiveness of treatment require early and thorough decontamination. Animals presenting with paralysis or seizures have a poor prognosis.

Cholecalciferol

Cholecalciferol is an active vitamin D_3 derivative used in the rodenticides Quintox, Rampage, and Rat-B-Gone. The baits contain 0.075% active ingredient and usually are in a cereal or pellet form. The mechanism of action is calcium reabsorption from the bone and intestine into the blood; then increased calcium absorption by the kidneys occurs. Hypercalcemia (more than 11.5 mg/dl) is the result. If not treated appropriately, hypercalcemia can result in soft tissue calcification and nephrosis. Death is caused by hypercalcemic cardiotoxicity. The toxic dose can range from 1 g/kg to 100 g/kg.

Clinical signs usually occur 12 to 36 hours after ingestion and include anorexia, vomiting, muscle weakness, and constipation, and may progress to hypertension, ventricular fibrillation, seizures, polyuria, and polydipsia. Calcium deposits can be found on postmortem examination in soft tissues, aorta, tendons, and muscle if long-term exposure has occurred.

The diagnosis is based on the history of exposure and the clinical signs (most often discovered when a routine serum chemistry panel is performed and the serum calcium concentration is greater than 12 mg/dl).

Inducing vomiting and administering activated charcoal and cathartics are recommended if ingestion has occurred within 2 hours of presentation. Correcting the electrolyte balances with IV physiologic saline (not lactated Ringer's solution, because it contains calcium) is also recommended. The following drugs are commonly used to reduce and prevent hypercalcemia. Furosemide (5 mg/kg IV followed by 2.5 mg/kg orally three or four times a day) increases calcium excretion from the kidneys. Prednisone (2 to 3 mg/kg orally once or twice a day) helps decrease calcium reabsorption from the bone and intestines. Calcitonin, a peptide hormone that functions in hypercalcemia to lower the calcium concentration, also is administered (4 to 6 IU/kg SQ every 2 to 3 hours initially) until serum calcium levels stabilize (less than 11.5 mg/dl). Decreasing the calcium and phosphorous mobilization from bone and increasing phosphate movement into bone from extracellular fluid accomplish this. Calcitonin also increases renal calcium and phosphorous excretion. Furosemide and prednisone treatment is continued for 2 to 4 weeks, and a low-calcium diet is recommended.

Zinc Phosphide

Zinc phosphide is a widely-used rodenticide. It can be found in such colorfully named products such as Sweeney's Toxic Peanuts, ACME Gopher Killer Pellets, and Mole Guard. In acidic conditions such as the stomach, zinc phosphide forms phosphine gas. Heavier than air, phosphine gas is highly toxic and has been described as having an odor of rotten fish or acetylene. Once absorbed, zinc phosphide inhibits oxidative phosphorylation, interrupting cellular energy and producing processes in the mitochondria that result in cell death, peroxidation, and cellular oxidative damage.

Many formulations contain additives to induce vomiting in nontarget species; this helps to reduce morbidity.

The lowest reported lethal dose in dogs and cats is 40 mg/kg. Relay toxicosis can occur commonly as rodents tend to die in the open with this rodenticide. Clinical signs appear rapidly after ingestion and include vomiting, anorexia, and depression; rapid, deep, wheezy respirations; vomiting, with or without blood; ataxia; weakness; and hypoxia. Emptying the stomach early can delay signs.

Zinc phosphide can be detected chemically, but it degrades rapidly, making testing less practical.

Treatment involves rapid decontamination with emesis, lavage, and activated charcoal. Increasing the gastric pH with sodium bicarbonate will slow the hydrolysis into gas. Intravenous fluid support is essential. Care must be taken to avoid exposure of personnel or owners to phosphine gas that may be present in vomitus; the toxic level is lower than 2 ppm, which is the threshold at which human noses can detect the gas. Induction of vomiting should be performed in a well-ventilated area to prevent human exposure to zinc phosphide gas.

The prognosis is good when decontamination occurs early, and guarded when clinical signs are already present.

ENVIRONMENTAL TOXINS

ETHYLENE GLYCOL

Ethylene glycol is found in antifreeze, hydraulic fluid, transmission fluid, airplane deicers, detergents, lacquer, polishes, cosmetics, pharmaceuticals, and industrial humectants, and as a solvent in paints and plastics. Colorless, odorless, and sweet-tasting, ethylene glycol is frequently found in and around the home and garage.

Increased exposures are noted in March through May, and most occur in the home. Dogs are reported more frequently than cats. Only a small amount is required for toxicity; the lethal dose in the dog is 4.4 ml/kg, and lower in the cat (due to a higher baseline production of oxalic acid) at 0.9 ml/kg.

It is rapidly absorbed through the GI tract after ingestion and through the lungs after inhalation, and it is metabolized by the liver and kidneys within 24 hours; most ethylene glycol and metabolites are excreted within 24 to 48 hours. Metabolism is primarily in the liver and follows several pathways; the clinically significant pathway is via alcohol dehydrogenase to glycoaldehyde, which is further metabolized to glycolic acid, glyoxylic acid, and oxalic acid. Oxalic acid is the most toxicologically significant metabolite, and is excreted renally. Severe metabolic acidosis and renal damage result from these metabolites.

The most common clinical signs observed within 12 hours after ingestion include CNS depression (the animal may appear intoxicated), vomiting, ataxia, lethargy, polydipsia, polyuria, seizures, coma, and death. Tachypnea and tachycardia may be observed 12 to 24 hours after ingestion. Severe lethargy, vomiting, diarrhea, oliguria, isosthenuria, azotemia, uremia, and death usually are observed 12 to 24 hours after ingestion.

Diagnosis begins with the history and presentation of clinical signs. An increase in serum osmolality, hypocalcemia, a high ion gap, and metabolic acidosis are considered a strong indication of ethylene glycol poisoning.

In-house ethylene glycol testing is available but is not specific to ethylene glycol; false positive results can be encountered with propylene glycol, glycerol, or metaldehyde exposure. These tests are sensitive to the parent compound and will only yield a positive result before biotransformation of ethylene glycol; therefore early testing is necessary and negative results in the face of clinical signs do not preclude a diagnosis of ethylene glycol poisoning. Quantitative tests for ethylene glycol may be performed at some labs or human hospitals. Calcium oxalate monohydrate crystals can be observed from urinalysis but cannot confirm ethylene glycol poisoning unless clinical signs exist. This type of crystal also can be found in the urine of normal dogs and cats. More commonly, these crystals are seen in dogs that have been poisoned with ethylene glycol than in cats.

Treatment is aimed at reducing absorption and blocking metabolism. Decontamination with emesis and AC may be recommended; administer AC within 4 hours because of the rapid absorption of ethylene glycol. Because ethylene glycol is rapidly absorbed within the GI tract, induction of vomiting may have limited value. Ethylene glycol may also have limited adsorption by AC, limiting efficacy of decontamination. Hemodialysis and peritoneal dialysis remove ethylene glycol and metabolites; hemoperfusion can also be used if such treatments are available. Fluid diuresis is essential and increases urinary excretion and maintains renal perfusion; monitor urine output. In nonvomiting patients, water should be available ad libitum. If oliguria is present, IV fluids without potassium should be administered.

Ethanol is an antidote, and competes with ethylene glycol for the active site of alcohol dehydrogenase;

alcohol dehydrogenase has a much higher affinity for ethanol than ethylene glycol. The ethanol dose in dogs is 5.5 ml of 20% ethanol/kg IV every 4 hours for five treatments, then every 6 hours for four treatments; for cats, 5 ml of 20% ethanol/kg IV every 6 hours for five treatments, then every 8 hours for four more treatments. Ethanol administration is titrated to stupor while avoiding severe CNS depression. Disadvantages are the resulting CNS depression and the exacerbation of osmotic diuresis and plasma hyperosmolality. 4-Methylpyrazole (4-MP, fomepizole) is a specific, and more effective, inhibitor of alcohol dehydrogenase and is associated with few to no adverse effects. A loading dose is administered at 20 mg/kg IV as a 5% solution, then 15 mg/kg at 12 hours, 10 mg/kg at 24 hours, and 5 mg/kg at 36 hours. It should not be given with ethanol since fatal alcohol toxicosis will result. For cats, off-label use of 4-MP has been reported at 125 mg/kg IV at 1, 2, and 3 hours after ethylene glycol ingestion; then 31.25 mg/kg IV at 12, 24, and 36 hours after ingestion with fluid therapy. Acidosis can be treated with sodium bicarbonate; calcium gluconate can be administered for hypocalcemia.

Prognosis varies according to time elapsed between exposure and treatment. If less than 8 hours have elapsed and treatment with fomepizole is initiated, the prognosis is good. If 24 to 48 hours have elapsed and renal azotemia is present, the prognosis is poor.

LESS TOXIC ENVIRONMENTAL TOXINS
Bleach
Household bleach formulations are generally 3% to 6% sodium hypochlorite. Nonchlorine bleaches are generally formulated from sodium peroxide, sodium perborate, or enzymatic detergents.

Commercial bleaches with higher concentrations of the active ingredient can cause severe burns, but household formulations are not generally associated with severe tissue destruction. Skin and eye irritation can occur, as well as oral and esophageal burns and gastrointestinal irritation. Treatment can often occur at home and consists of rinsing the affected areas and offering milk or another bland liquid to drink. Induction of vomiting is contraindicated.

Glow Jewelry
Glow necklaces, bracelets, or sticks are bright, colorful objects that attract the attention of curious pets that may bite into them. The toxic compound dibutyl phthalate lends luminescence to most types of glow jewelry. It has a low toxicity and is present in very small concentrations; the contents of an entire necklace would not provide the minimum toxic dose in a small dog or cat. The fluid is also extremely bitter and deters animals from ingesting more than a small amount. Ingestion can cause agitation, salivation, and vomiting. Brief, transient CNS signs may occur including hyperesthesia and ataxia; these resolve rapidly and complete recovery occurs within minutes.

Adhesives
Sticky substances pose a special dilemma for fur-covered animals. Sticky rodent traps, paint, tape, and glue can be encountered, with messy results. Owners may be tempted to remove sticky substances with solvents that are far more toxic and hazardous than the initial material. Most adhesives and paints can be removed with vegetable oil, which then can be removed through bathing with dishwashing detergent. Glues should be identified as nontoxic because some can present a hazard. In some cases it may be advisable to clip or shave fur to remove large amounts of adhesives; care should be taken to avoid inadvertently cutting the animal while doing so; scissors should not be used.

PHARMACEUTICALS

ACETAMINOPHEN
Acetaminophen is a commonly used pain and fever reliever in humans and is found in many homes. Most owners have it in the house and believe it is a safe medication to give dogs or cats. It is rapidly absorbed from the GI tract and metabolized by the liver via sulfation and glucuronidation. Cats lack sufficient glucuronyl transferase to safely metabolize acetaminophen and instead produce the toxic metabolite N-acetyl-p-benzoquinoneimine (NAPQI), which in turn causes oxidative damage to red blood cells and liver cells. Dogs have greater capacity for nontoxic metabolism but these pathways can still become overwhelmed in cases of overdose. Cat red blood cells are more susceptible to oxidative injury and therefore the first clinical signs in this species are of methemoglobinemia: dyspnea, cyanosis, and dark mucous membranes. There is no safe dose of acetaminophen for cats and toxicity can be seen at doses as low as 10 mg/kg. Additional clinical signs can be observed 1 to

2 hours after ingestion and include vomiting, salivation, facial and paw edema, depression, increased respiratory rate, dyspnea, and pale mucous membranes.

The minimum toxic dose for dogs is 75 mg/kg. Clinical signs are consistent with hepatic injury and include lethargy, anorexia, vomiting, and abdominal pain. Dogs can recover spontaneously within 48 to 72 hours in cases of moderate toxicity; more severe toxicity may result in hepatic necrosis, icterus, weight loss, hemolysis, and hemoglobinuria. Without treatment death can occur within 2 to 5 days after the onset of clinical signs.

Treatment consists of decontamination by emesis and prevention of absorption with activated charcoal. *N*-Acetylcysteine (NAC) can be utilized as an antidote by providing a substrate for glutathione, allowing inactivation of toxic metabolites. Acetylcysteine can be given orally or intravenously, and is most effective when initiated within 8 hours of ingestion. NAC is given at an initial loading dose of 140 to 280 mg/kg orally or IV, then at a maintenance dose of 70 mg/kg orally or IV four times a day for 2 to 3 days. IV NAC is available in a sterile 10% to 20% solution, and should be diluted with D_5W or sterile water before IV administration.

Ascorbic acid (30 mg/kg orally four times a day) can be used for methemoglobinemia in affected cats. Blood transfusions also may be necessary to treat animals with a packed cell volume less than 15% or to aid in the treatment of methemoglobinemia. Supportive care including fluid therapy is necessary. Cytochrome P-450 inhibitors such as cimetidine or ranitidine may be administered to slow metabolism of acetaminophen. It has been recently discovered that cats utilize the CYP pathway to convert methemoglobin to hemoglobin and therefore inhibition of CYP in cats is contraindicated. Prognosis is poor in animals exhibiting clinical signs.

NONSTEROIDAL ANTIINFLAMMATORY DRUGS

Nonsteroidal antiinflammatory drugs (NSAIDs) are commonly prescribed or over-the-counter analgesic drugs for both human and animal use. This is a large group of drugs that include ibuprofen, naproxen, aspirin, carprofen, and meloxicam. As a result, ingestion of high doses of NSAIDs—particularly by dogs—occurs frequently. NSAIDs work by inhibiting the cyclooxygenase (COX) system. COX enzymes are responsible for inflammation: the release of inflammatory cytokines at tissue injury sites results in pain. By inhibiting the production

of these enzymes and reducing inflammation, pain can be controlled. COX enzymes, in particular prostaglandins, are also crucial mediators in maintaining stasis. Central nervous system function, hemostasis, renal tubule function, renal perfusion, and gastric mucosal function and perfusion all depend on COX enzymes to maintain proper function.

Toxicity is dose-dependent and varies by drug. At low doses, primary toxic effects are to the GI tract. Besides being a direct irritant, the anti-prostaglandin effects of NSAIDs result in a decrease in epithelial mucous production, local bicarbonate secretion, mucosal blood flow, and overall mucosal resistance to injury. Gastrointestinal distress in the form of pain, vomiting, diarrhea, gastrointestinal ulceration, hemorrhage, and even perforation can occur secondary to NSAID toxicity.

At higher doses, renal injury can occur because renal perfusion decreases as a result of the inhibition of prostaglandin. In either case, decontamination, activated charcoal, and GI protectants are generally recommended. Misoprostol, a prostaglandin analog, can be administered to protect against GI ulceration. IV fluids at high rates for 48 hours maintain renal perfusion and can protect the kidneys from the effects of NSAID overdose. At very high doses CNS depression can occur. Naloxone (0.04 mg/kg IV) can be utilized to reverse neurologic effects.

Chronic use or overdose of NSAIDs can result in liver damage; although this mechanism is not fully understood, any animal receiving long-term NSAID therapy should be regularly evaluated for liver function. Liver support with *S*-adenosylmethionine and silymarin can be initiated in patients with impaired liver function.

METALS

ZINC

Zinc is a commonly encountered substance and can be found on galvanized surfaces such as pet cages, some topical ointments, and some paints. Pennies (United States) minted after 1982 contain 98% zinc, and are often easily accessible to pets.

Zinc is rapidly absorbed from the small intestine, with high concentrations accumulating in the liver. The mechanism of action in this toxicant is not established but it is believed to be similar to that of toxicosis. Inhibition of red blood cell enzymes, direct damage to red cell membranes, or increased erythrocyte susceptibility to oxidative damage all may play roles in this toxicity. The acidic environment of the stomach causes rapid release of zinc from metallic objects. The toxic doses in dogs and cats have not been established; in the case of penny ingestion, even one penny can cause symptoms in a small sized dog.

Clinical signs include vomiting, diarrhea, lethargy, inappetence, depression, pale or icteric mucous membranes, tachycardia, tachypnea, and dyspnea. Clinical pathology includes severe intravascular hemolysis with a regenerative but often severe anemia; hemoglobinemia; red blood cell changes, including basophilic stippling, polychromasia, target cells, nucleated red cells, and Heinz bodies; and leukocytosis and neutrophilia with a left shift. Increases in the levels of serum protein, alkaline phosphatase, and bilirubin as well as azotemia can be observed. Urinalysis may reveal hemoglobinuria and casts. The cause of renal failure in zinc toxicosis is unknown; other heavy metals can cause direct damage to renal tubular epithelial cells; hypoxia and hemoglobinemia are other potential causes.

Diagnosis can be made by measurement of serum zinc levels; care should be taken to utilize the proper blood collection tubes because rubber-topped tubes contain zinc and can contaminate blood samples. Royal blue topped tubes with plastic stoppers should be used.

Treatment for zinc toxicosis includes supportive therapy with intravenous fluids and electrolytes. Oxygen-carrying capabilities of hemoglobin can be adversely affected secondary to hemoglobinemia; this combined with anemia can cause life-threatening hypoxia. Oxygen and blood transfusions may be necessary. Removal of gastrointestinal metallic foreign bodies can be very efficacious when the patient is stable enough for anesthesia and surgery since serum levels are shown to drop rapidly after removal of the source. Increasing the gastric pH with H_2 blockers may help slow the absorption of zinc. Activated charcoal is not effective in the adsorption of metals. The use of chelating agents such as CaEDTA is generally not recommended, as removal is curative, and failure of zinc levels to drop after removal either indicates that there remains a source of zinc or indicates there is a renal insufficiency. In either case, chelation may be contraindicated, because it may cause an increase in the absorption of zinc, and the chelated metal is potentially nephrotoxic. Prognosis is fair with treatment.

LEAD

Lead is a common toxicity in companion animals, more commonly in dogs than cats because of their selective eating habits. Lead toxicity may be observed more frequently in young animals less than 6 months of age because of their chewing habits and because the blood-brain barrier is not fully developed, permitting toxins to enter the central nervous system.

The most common source for lead poisoning is lead-containing paint, which was used before the 1950s. Other sources include batteries, linoleum, plumbing supplies, ceramic containers that were not glazed properly, lead pipes, fishing sinkers, and shotgun pellets. Lead poisoning usually results from a recent exposure but can result from chronic exposure and accumulation. The most common signs involve the GI and nervous systems.

Anorexia, vomiting, abdominal pain, diarrhea, megaesophagus, and constipation usually are observed before neurologic signs. Anxiousness, behavioral changes (e.g., whining, barking, continuous running, snapping), tremors, seizures, ataxia, opisthotonos, and blindness also are seen, and may be associated with a higher level toxicity.

Diagnosis begins with a history and clinical signs. Blood smears containing large numbers of nucleated red blood cells, with increased numbers of cells with basophilic stippling and a packed cell volume of 30% or more, support the possibility of lead poisoning. To confirm the diagnosis, whole blood is submitted for lead levels. Concentrations of 35 mcg/dl or more are supportive, but a concentration of 60 mcg/dl is diagnostic.

Treatment includes removing any lead from the GI tract, which may be accomplished through a magnesium or sodium sulfate cathartic, or surgery may be indicated if the object is made of lead. The following chelators are commonly used to treat lead poisoning: Thiamine is given IM or SQ at 2 mg/kg to alleviate the clinical signs; however, it can cause muscle soreness at the injection site. Commercial calcium ethylenediaminetetraacetic acid (CaEDTA) is used to help remove lead from the body stores. The drug is given IV or SQ 100 mg/kg/day divided into four daily doses for 2 to 5 days (10 mg of EDTA in 1 ml of 5% dextrose). NOTE: CaEDTA can cause renal toxicity and should not be used in anuric patients. Hydration must be maintained throughout this treatment to promote renal function and the proper excretion of the chelated lead. D-Penicillamine is another drug commonly used as a chelation treatment in animals less severely affected by the lead poisoning or as a treatment after the calcium EDTA therapy. The recommended dose is 110 mg/kg/day divided into three or four oral doses given 30 minutes before feeding for 1 to 2 weeks. Adverse side effects include vomiting, anorexia, and lethargy. Antiemetic medications can ease GI symptoms.

TOXICOLOGY IN THE VETERINARY HOSPITAL

Intoxications can occur anywhere, including the veterinary hospital. Inadvertent overdoses from drug miscalculations, drug interactions or incompatibility, and idiosyncratic responses to drugs can result in illness. A detailed pharmacologic reference and well-trained staff can avoid many errors and allow for expedient therapeutic responses when they do occur.

One uncommonly encountered toxin that can potentially poison patients within the hospital as a direct result of treatment is cyanide.

Cyanide can be found in the pits and seeds of fruits like apricots and apples, and can be released as a result of combustion of many substances like nylon and natural fabrics. Generally ingestions of toxic amounts of cyanide are rare, but pets exposed to smoke from house fires may suffer from cyanide toxicity. Cyanide is also a byproduct of sodium nitroprusside metabolism. Sodium nitroprusside can be used therapeutically as a potent vasodilator to treat hypertension and to reduce afterload and work of a failing heart. Small amounts of cyanide are present in the environment, and cyanide detoxification occurs via hepatic metabolism. However, these enzyme systems are easily overwhelmed. Ongoing administration of nitroprusside at doses greater than 2 mcg/kg/min may result in amounts of cyanide greater than metabolic capabilities. Cyanide exerts its toxic effects by inhibiting cellular respiration and by displacing oxygen from the hemoglobin molecule by converting hemoglobin to cyanohemoglobin, which cannot carry oxygen. Clinical signs of cyanide toxicity include respiratory distress and tachycardia, progressing to loss of consciousness and death. Mucous membranes and skin may appear a bright pink or cherry red color. Unfortunately, these respiratory signs are nonspecific and can occur with cardiac and respiratory disease. Patients receiving sodium nitroprusside for heart failure may already be exhibiting these signs, so recognition of cyanide toxicity can be challenging. The recognition of pink mucous membranes in the face of respiratory distress may aid in diagnosis.

Treatment involves decontamination (or discontinuation of nitroprusside) and initiation of oxygen supplementation. Sodium nitrate (except in smoke inhalation), sodium thiosulfate, and hydroxycobalamin can be utilized as antidotes.

CONCLUSION

Toxins are ever present in our environments and the explorative nature of cats and dogs can result in exposure to dangerous substances too numerous to list. A well-equipped veterinary hospital includes not only the basic equipment needed to treat intoxicated patients but also a knowledgeable staff who is up to date on the newest treatment options and has access to databases such as poison control centers and in-house reference material. Rapid treatment, supportive care, and attentive monitoring provide intoxicated patients with the support necessary to recover from many toxic exposures.

REFERENCES

Boothe DM: Adverse reactions to therapeutic drugs in the CCU patient. In Wingfield WE, Raffe MR, editors: *The veterinary ICU book*, Jackson, WY, 2002, Teton NewMedia, pp 1049–1080.

Boothe DM: Changes in drug disposition and drug interaction. In Wingfield WE, Raffe MR, editors: *The veterinary ICU book*, Jackson, WY, 2002, Teton NewMedia, pp 1081–1105.

Bough MG: Castor bean toxicosis—one mean bean, *Vet Tech* 498–499, 2002.

Cope RB: *Allium* species poisoning in dogs and cats, *Vet Med* 562–566, 2005.

Dalefield R: Ethylene glycol. In Plumlee KH, editor: *Clinical veterinary toxicology*, St Louis, 2004, Mosby, pp 150–154.

Dunayer E: Bromethalin: the other rodenticide, *Vet Med* 98:9, 2003.

Dunayer EK: New findings on the effects of xylitol ingestion in dogs, *Vet Med* 101:791–797, 2006.

Enberg TB, Braun LD, Kuzma AB: Gastrointestinal perforation in five dogs associated with the administration of meloxicam, *J Vet Emerg Crit Care* 16(1):34–43, 2006.

Galey FD: Cardiac glycosides. In Plumlee KH, editor: *Clinical veterinary toxicology*, St Louis, 2004, Mosby, pp 386–388.

Klein BG, Cunningham JG: Cerebrospinal fluid and the blood-brain barrier. In Klein BG, Cunningham JG, editors: *Textbook of veterinary physiology*, St Louis, 2007, Saunders Elsevier.

Kuo K, Odunayo A: Adjunctive therapy with intravenous lipid emulsion and methocarbamol for permethrin toxicity in 2 cats, *J Vet Emerg Crit Care* 23(4):436–441, 2013.

Mazzaferro EM, et al.: Acute renal failure associated with raisin or grape ingestion in 4 dogs, *J Vet Emerg Crit Care* 14(3):203–212, 2004.

McKnight K: Grape and raisin toxicity in dogs, *Vet Tech* 135–136, 2005.

Means C: Anticoagulant rodenticides. In Plumlee KH, editor: *Clinical veterinary toxicology*, St Louis, 2004, Mosby, pp 444–446.

Means C: Colchicine. In Plumlee KH, editor: *Clinical veterinary toxicology*, St Louis, 2004, Mosby, p 352.

Poppenga R: Treatment. In Plumlee KH, editor: *Clinical veterinary toxicology*, St Louis, 2004, Mosby, pp 13–20.

Reineke EL, Drobatz KJ: Cyanide. In Silverstein DC, Hopper K, editors: *Small animal critical care medicine*, St Louis, 2009, Saunders Elsevier, pp 366–368.

Richardson JA, Gwatlney-Brant SM, Villar D: Zinc toxicosis from penny ingestion in dogs, *Vet Med* 97, 2002.

Roder JD: Pharmaceuticals. In Plumlee KH, editor: *Clinical veterinary toxicology*, St Louis, 2004, Mosby, pp 282–336.

Rosendale ME: Glow jewelry (dibutyl phthalate) ingestion in cats, *Vet Med* 94(8):703, 1999.

Schildt JC, Jutkowitz LA: Approach to poisoning and drug overdose. In Silverstein DC, Hopper K, editors: *Small animal critical care medicine*, St Louis, 2009, Saunders, pp 326–329.

Scott NE: Ivermectin toxicity. In Silverstein DC, Hopper K, editors: *Small animal critical care medicine*, St Louis, 2009, Saunders, pp 392–394.

Smith G: *Kalanchoe* species poisoning in pets, *Vet Med* 99:933–936, 2004.

Spoo W: Concepts and terminology. In Plumlee KH, editor: *Clinical veterinary toxicology*, St Louis, 2004, Mosby, pp 2–6.

Spoo W: Toxicokinetics. In Plumlee KH, editor: *Clinical veterinary toxicology*, St Louis, 2004, Mosby, pp 8–12.

Steenbergen V: Acetaminophen and cats: a dangerous combination, *Vet Tech* 43–45, 2003.

Volmer PA: Easter lily toxicosis in cats, *Vet Med* 94(4):331, 1999.

Wilson HE, Humm KR: In vitro study of the effect of dog food on the adsorptive capacity of activated charcoal, *J Vet Emerg Crit Care* 23(3):263–267, 2013.

SCENARIO

Purpose: Learn to recognize common toxicants and their associated clinical signs while gaining triage assessment skills.

Stage: Emergency clinic with veterinarian and sufficient technicians to rapidly assess emergent patients.

Scenario

A 6-year-old male neutered feline is presented for lethargy and dyspnea. The owner reports that her purse had been knocked over sometime in the past 4 hours and some medications may be missing, some of which contained acetaminophen. Upon initial assessment the cat has a respiratory rate of 60 breaths/min, with increased effort. Its mucous membranes are cyanotic to brown in color, and some facial swelling is noted. HR is 220 bpm and blood pressure is 100 mm Hg systolic.

Questions

Students should discuss answers to following questions:
- What is your primary concern based on initial assessment?
- What is your first therapy or intervention that you would offer?

Activity: The clinician orders the following treatments. Prioritize them according to your patient's status:
- IV catheter and crystalloids at 60 ml/kg/day
- Oxygen-enriched environment (oxygen cage)
- Activated charcoal
- Acetylcysteine loading dose of 200 mg/kg PO

Key Teaching Points
- Importance of triage according to clinical signs (respiratory distress must be addressed first, then diagnostics and decontamination).
- Oral administration of antidote will delay decontamination or vice versa.

MEDICAL MATH EXERCISE

Patient's orders state: *Calculate the dose of theobromine ingested by a 22-kg Labrador retriever.* The owner reports the dog ingested 22 ounces of semi-sweet baking chocolate.

a. Calculate the dose of theobromine, if there is 390 mg/oz of theobromine in semi-sweet chocolate.

26 Avian and Exotic Emergencies

Jody Nugent-Deal

CHAPTER OUTLINE

Hospital Preparedness
Preparing for CPR for the Avian, Reptilian, and Small Animal Exotic Patient
  Rabbit V-Gel Device
Avian Emergencies
  The Avian Physical Examination
  Common Avian Emergencies
Exotic Small Mammal Emergencies
  The Exotic Small Mammal Physical Examination

Common Ferret Emergencies
Canine Distemper Virus
Rabbit and Rodent Emergencies
Common Emergencies in Rabbits
Common Emergencies in Rodents
Reptile Emergencies
  The Reptilian Physical Examination
  Common Snake Emergencies
  Common Reptilian Emergencies
  Common Chelonian Emergencies

LEARNING OBJECTIVES

After studying this chapter, you will be able to:

- Describe how to capture and restrain exotic animal patients.
- Perform physical exams and note species-specific anatomic areas that should be addressed.
- Describe common emergencies associated with different exotic animal species.
- Describe the best options for venous access.
- Explain treatment options for the exotic animal patient.

KEY TERMS

Air sac cannula
Airway management
Exotic small animal
Husbandry
Intraosseous catheters

Exotic animals have been kept as pets for several decades, but their popularity has vastly grown over the last 20 years. The need for veterinary care continues to increase as these animals become more popular. Poor **husbandry** is widespread and generally the most common reason an exotic pet is seen for veterinary care; in many cases, these patients present in a critical state and need to be stabilized.

These unique patients will present a variety of challenges. Understanding the basics of how to proceed with stabilization and medical management of a critically ill or injured exotic animal patient will assist the veterinary technician in providing the best care possible for a successful outcome.

Exotic species provide an exciting challenge in emergency medicine, because the clinical syndromes they have are often unique to each species. It is also important for emergency clinics to be prepared to receive a variety of species.

HOSPITAL PREPAREDNESS

Basic equipment used for puppies and kittens can be used on many exotic patients. Many of these animals are small and therefore pediatric equipment is ideal. For example, the normal heart rate for many exotic small mammals and birds can easily be greater than 250 to 300 beats per minute. In mammalian species this would be considered tachycardic, but for most of the exotic small mammals and birds, this is considered normal. It is difficult to find machines such as an electrocardiograph (ECG), pulse oximeter, or oscillometric blood pressure monitor that measure values high enough to produce accurate readings in most exotic animals. The author has found one multiparameter monitor manufactured by Digicare®. The ECG on this multiparameter monitor reads up to 999 beats per minute and works well with exotic animals and canine and feline patients.

Safe housing is another important consideration for hospitalized exotic patients. In some cases, the average metal small dog or cat hospital cage will not be adequate, because small birds, reptiles, rodents, and ferrets can easily maneuver their way through the cage door front and escape, or become trapped and injured. If these standard cages are going to be used, a plastic cage front that screws onto the metal cage door can be constructed from Plexiglass. Plastic cage fronts will keep the patients safe as well as keep the cage warm and draft-free. It is important to remember that ventilation is important, and easy to provide with appropriately sized holes drilled through the plastic.

Incubators can also be used for housing and are often preferred since they provide both heat and oxygen. There are many commercial incubators on the market, and in general, if an incubator will work for a kitten or puppy, it will probably work for most exotic animals. Species-specific cages are available and should be considered if the clinic cares for a large volume of exotic animal patients.

PREPARING FOR CPR FOR THE AVIAN, REPTILIAN, AND SMALL ANIMAL EXOTIC PATIENT

The basic ABCs of emergency medicine are used with the understanding that establishing an airway can be difficult. With the exception of ferrets, many exotic small mammals can be difficult to intubate. Reptiles and birds are much easier to intubate than most exotic small mammals. They do not have an epiglottis and the tracheal opening is located directly at the base of the tongue. It is important to have pediatric endotracheal tubes available because most of the exotic patients will require a size 3.5-mm tube or smaller. The exception is large birds and large rabbits. Some large macaws may require up to a 6.5-mm uncuffed tube. Even though intubation may be impossible in some situations, it is still attempted. Several techniques can be used to aid in successful endotracheal intubation. Common techniques used for exotic small mammals include, but are not limited to, the use of a traditional laryngoscope, passage of an endotracheal tube over a flexible stylet, blind endotracheal tube placement, the use of rigid endoscopy, and placement of a laryngeal mask airway (LMA) or V-gel® device.

> **TECHNICIAN NOTE** Birds have complete cartilaginous tracheal rings. Because the trachea lacks distensibility, noncuffed endotracheal tubes should be used instead of cuffed tubes. Pressure placed upon the trachea can lead to trauma and the formation of transtracheal membranes.

Rabbit V-Gel Device

The rabbit V-gel device is a veterinary species-specific supraglottic airway that can be used for **airway management** during anesthesia and resuscitation. The rabbit V-gel can be a lifesaving product (Figure 26-1). In the author's opinion, the rabbit V-gel device is not a complete and total replacement for endotracheal intubation, but it serves many important purposes. The author uses it specifically for three purposes: establishing an airway

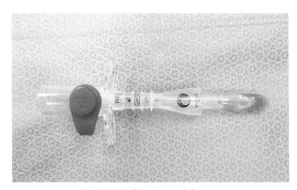

FIGURE 26-1 V-gel device.

during cardiopulmonary resuscitation (CPR), performing a difficult intubation, and executing an accidental extubation where it is nearly impossible to reintubate the patient (e.g., due to apnea or patient positioning).

The rabbit V-gel device is species-specific so it cannot be used for anything other than rabbits. It takes about 10 seconds to place; therefore, you can establish an airway very quickly. Like any other product, the V-gel has pros and cons. You cannot use the V-gel for oral surgery or dental procedures because it is too large. You cannot provide long-term intermittent positive pressure ventilation (IPPV) via a mechanical ventilator, but you can provide very light IPPV via manual ventilation when necessary. This means that use of advanced analgesic techniques, such as fentanyl constant rate infusions, can be difficult when mechanical IPPV is needed. If the head or neck is manipulated a lot, the V-gel can become dislodged and fill the stomach with air. Capnography is used to ensure proper placement.

After the patient is intubated, oxygen is administered and manual IPPV is provided as needed. When performing CPR, the number of breaths per minute has not been established in exotic small mammals; therefore, 10 breaths per minute are employed (same rate and technique used during CPR in dogs/cats). Circulation is also addressed while attempting intubation. This will include performing chest compressions as well as placing an intravenous (IV) or intraosseous (IO) catheter and starting fluid therapy. Chest compressions may be impossible in some species like turtles and tortoises. Moving the limbs in and out of the shell may be beneficial, but is often very unproductive. The sternum or large keel bone in birds also hinders the effectiveness of chest compressions in avian species. Ideally intubation and catheter placement should take place at the same time. Effective chest compression techniques have not been established in exotic small mammals. At this time, these patients are treated in the same manner as a cat or kitten. Patients are first placed in lateral recumbency. The dominant hand is cupped around the area of the heart with the thumb on one side of the thorax and the remaining fingers on the other side of the thorax. If the patient is very small, one or two fingers can be used instead of all four. Compression rates generally range from 100 to 120 per minute.

Emergency drugs such as epinephrine, atropine, and glycopyrrolate should be available and ready to use at any time during a critical situation. Atropine is the anticholinergic drug of choice for emergency situations because it has a shorter onset of action compared to glycopyrrolate. It is estimated that about 30% to 50% of rabbits have endogenous atropinase enzymes. These endogenous enzymes block the effectiveness of injectable atropine. In an emergency situation, atropine is always administered to rabbits first, but if there are not any changes in heart rate, glycopyrrolate is then administered. When possible, it is helpful to have everything pre-drawn once it is apparent the patient may be in distress. Flow charts with correct doses can be made available for quick reference or a spreadsheet program can be created. Spreadsheets are helpful because one can be created for each major group of animals commonly seen in practice (e.g., chinchillas, birds, snakes). The spreadsheet should remain simple and contain the common drugs used during emergency situations. Spreadsheet programs are convenient because they can be adapted to individual patients by inserting the patients' weight. The program automatically calculates the proper drug doses.

> **TECHNICIAN NOTE** Your clinic can make a species-specific spreadsheet that will quickly and easily calculate dosages of emergency drugs. If you know a critical patient is en route to the clinic, an emergency drug sheet can be printed and drugs prepared ahead of time.

AVIAN EMERGENCIES

Supplies
- Avian mouth speculum (or paper clips and tape stirrups)
- 25-gauge and 27-gauge needles
- Intraosseous (IO) catheters (22-gauge 1½-inch and 20-gauge 2½-inch spinal needles) (If the previous sizes are not available, then a 25-gauge 1½-inch needle can be inserted as a stylet inside a 20-gauge 1-inch needle.)
- Microtainer® blood tubes
- Incubator cage (heated)
- Oxygen (O_2) cage
- Nebulizer
- Rubber and metal feeding tubes (various sizes)
- Emeraid or Kaytee Exact hand-feeding mixture
- Basic emergency drugs
- Insulin syringes

THE AVIAN PHYSICAL EXAMINATION

Birds have maintained their wild instincts throughout evolution. They are prey species and hide their illnesses to avoid being preyed upon in the wild. These instincts will also be present in the clinic. The owner will report the bird is looking fluffy, at the bottom of the cage, and eyes closed at home, but when it arrives to the clinic it will suddenly look "normal." The bird feels safe at home and will let its guard down, revealing illness. In the clinic it will appear to perk up since it is not in what it perceives as a safe place. If the bird does not have an improved behavior change when it arrives, this usually indicates the illness is severe and immediate stabilization is necessary (Figure 26-2).

Before the bird is handled, it should be observed in the cage. The following are observations that should be recorded in the medical record: mentation, respiratory rate, signs of a tail bob, interactions in the cage, droppings, types of toys, food and substrate used. It is important to inquire what food the animal is being offered, and what the animal is actually eating. Owners will often state that their pet eats fruits and veggies, but when further investigated it is discovered the bird is not ingesting the food offered.

If the actual cage cannot be taken to the clinic, ask the owners for pictures. This will assist in a thorough evaluation of the environment and will allow the healthcare team to suggest changes if necessary. It is important to gain a full history; however, this may not be possible during the initial stabilization process. Either this form is emailed to the clients before their appointment or the clients can complete it in the waiting room. This becomes a permanent part of the patient's record (Figure 26-3).

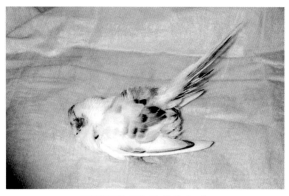

FIGURE 26-2 Fluffy bird.

> **TECHNICIAN NOTE** It is important to remind clients to bring their bird into the clinic in an enclosed carrier or cage. It is dangerous to have the bird free on the owner's shoulder or arm, or even attached to a harness. In an ideal world, the clinic would have a separate waiting room for the exotic animal clients coming into the hospital. This is not possible in many situations, but you can try to reduce the stress of the exotic patient by placing it away from barking dogs.

Restraint

The key to good avian restraint is to accomplish procedures as quickly and easily as possible to reduce stress on the patient. Many birds are well trained and will step up to their owners when out of the cage. The bird can then be taken from the owner. If it becomes necessary to remove a bird from its cage, perform the following:

- Take out all perches and bowls that can be easily removed.
- Place the cage in a closed, dimly lit room if any chance exists that the bird may escape.
- Use a paper towel for small birds such as budgerigars and towels for larger birds.
- Slowly enter the cage, and attempt to immobilize the head first.
- Bring the bird out of the cage, gently but firmly keeping control of the head and gaining control of the wings and body with the other hand.

> **TECHNICIAN NOTE** To hand off a bird to another staff member, one should allow the other person to gain control of the head by placing the thumb under the mandible and elevating the head; then the other hand should be used to gain control of the wings and body (Figure 26-4).

Needed supplies for an avian physical examination include a penlight, infant or pediatric stethoscope, towel, and tape stirrups to open the mouth (paper clips for small birds work well). Obtaining the patient's weight should be the first part of the physical examination. Since many avian patients are very small, it is best to use a scale that weighs to the nearest gram. The patient should be weighed every time it is brought into the clinic (once to twice daily if they are staying in the hospital). A loss of a few grams can be a concern in small patients.

AVIAN HISTORY FORM

UC Davis School of Veterinary Medicine
Companion Avian and Exotic Pet Medicine Service
One Garrod Drive
Davis, CA 95616
(530) 752-1393

General History

Bird's Name_____ Sex: M_____ F_____ UNK_____
How was bird sexed?   Blood Test_____ Surgical?_____
Any Specific Identification? (i.e: tatoo, band, microchip) _____
If bird is female, has she produced eggs in the past? (if yes, please describe)_____
Bird is a: Pet _____ Breeder_____
How did you acquire the bird? Store_____ Breeder_____ Other (describe)_____
Date acquired? _____
Do you have any other pets? Y_____ N_____
If yes, please specify including ages and when acquired _____

Housing

Is this bird kept: Indoors_____ Outdoors_____ Both _____ (if both, please specify % time in
each)_____
How is your bird housed? Cage_____ Aviary_____ Free in the house_____
Is the bird housed alone? Y_____ N_____ If no, describe_____
If bird is caged, what type of cage? _____
What do you use on the bottom of the cage?_____
How often is the cage cleaned?_____
Method/frequency of cleaning food/water dishes _____
Any toys in the cage? Y_____ N_____ If yes, describe_____
Has the bird's environment changed recently? Y_____ N_____ If yes, describe_____
At night, do you cover the bird? Y_____ N_____
How many hours of darkness does the bird have each day? _____

Diet:

What foods are offered to your bird/in what total percentages? (ie: 50% seed,
etc)_____
What percentages of these foods do you remove from the cage at
night?_____
Any supplements offered? Brand name? _____
Any treats offered? Type? How often?_____
Any recent diet changes or new foods? Y_____ N_____ If yes, describe_____
How is water offered? (i.e: sipper bottle, bowl) _____

Reason For Today's Visit:

What signs have you noticed that prompted today's
visit?_____
_____
How long have you noticed the problem?_____
Has your bird been sick previously? _____
Has the bird ever been seen by any other veterinarian? Y_____ N_____ If yes, when/
why?_____
Have any tests been performed previously on your bird? Please circle all that apply:
Psittacosis; CBC; Psittacine Beak and Feather Disease; Polyoma Disease; Parasites; Other blood work; Other
(please describe)_____

Additional comments (your comments regarding the reason for this visit):

CAPEward folder/CAPE History Client Forms/2003/kph

FIGURE 26-3 Example of patient history form.

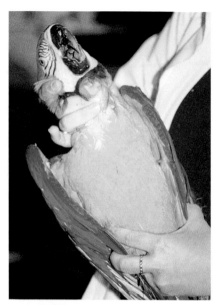

FIGURE 26-4 Avian restraint.

If a 100-gram bird lost 5 grams, then it has lost 5% of its body weight.

The exam is performed systematically from head to tail. Look at the eyes, ears, and nares. They should be symmetrical, clean, clear, and free of discharge. The mouth is ideally opened atraumatically. The oral cavity should be pink (although some birds have pigmented mucous membranes) and free of debris. The mucous membranes are often normally dry. The choanal slit is located on the roof of the mouth and should have sharp papillae protruding from the slit. The choana is an opening at the roof of the mouth that connects the trachea to the sinuses and the nares.

The crop, neck, limbs, and body should be palpated. Look for signs of trauma, swelling, ectoparasites, and masses. The uropygial gland is located at the base of the tail and should be examined. There should be a small amount of yellow "grease" around the gland. This "grease" helps birds preen and waterproof their feathers. It is important to note that some companion species such as Amazon parrots lack a uropygial gland. The legs and wings should extend normally. Examine the feather quality and make notation of any abnormalities. The pectoral muscle should be palpated and the patient should be assigned a body condition score (BCS). A BSC of 1 is emaciated and a body condition score of 9 is grossly obese. A 4 to 5 BCS is ideal.

The coelom should be palpated. You will only be able to use one or two fingers to palpate most bird species. The coelom should be concave and primarily empty feeling. It is normal to feel the pubic bones, some gastrointestinal (GI) tract, and the caudal end of the ventriculus (or an egg or other space-occupying mass if present). It is abnormal to feel the liver, masses, and extreme distention. The cloaca, also referred to as the "vent," should be examined for accumulation of fecal material and urates, hyperemia, and elasticity. The cloaca should be clean and free of debris. The feet should be checked for signs of trauma and pododermatitis.

Hydration should be assessed by looking at skin turgor around the eyes and keel. The skin over the keel can be gently "tented" or pulled to the side of the keel bone. The skin should return to its normal position almost instantly. The longer the skin takes to return to normal, the more dehydrated the animal is. Capillary refill time is hard to assess in birds. Generally, venous refill time is observed by depressing the cutaneous ulnar vein. The vein should refill instantly. The patient is considered dehydrated if the vein does not refill instantly.

The bird should be auscultated using an infant or pediatric stethoscope. Note any potential abnormalities or murmurs present. Auscultation is performed by placing the bell of the stethoscope on both the left and the right sides of the pectoral muscle as well as over the back. The lungs should be clear and free of wheezes, crackles, or harsh sounds. The lungs are auscultated over the patient's back while the heart is auscultated over the pectoral girdle and keel.

Due to the large sinuses over the skull, the top of the head should be auscultated as well. Little to no sound should be heard in normal birds. Bacterial and fungal infections can occur and often harsh sounds can be noted when an infection is present.

Obtaining a temperature can be challenging in a bird and is not done on a regular basis in the awake patient. Cloacal temperature can be attempted using a digital thermometer (unless the patient is just too small—most birds weighing less than 200 grams).

Venipuncture

Drawing blood from the avian patient can be challenging but a skill set that can be learned. Common venipuncture sites in birds include the jugular, cutaneous ulnar (basilic vein), and medial metatarsal veins. The medial metatarsal vein (commonly used in species larger than 150 to 200 grams) crosses the medial surface of the leg just

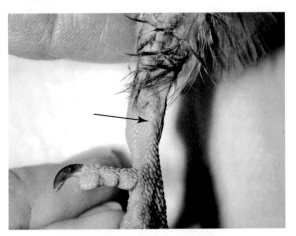

FIGURE 26-5 Medial metatarsal vein.

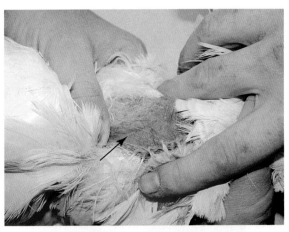

FIGURE 26-6 Avian jugular vein.

above the tarsal (hock) joint (Figure 26-5). The jugular vein is generally largest on the right side of the neck and is located in a featherless tract within the jugular groove. This vessel is often used when large samples of blood are needed or in very small species such as finches, canaries, and cockatiels. The right jugular vein is usually larger in most species of birds and is more often chosen over the left jugular vein. The cutaneous ulnar vein crosses a featherless tract at the ventral surface of the elbow joint. This vessel can be used in larger species of birds, but it is hard to bandage and often forms a large hematoma. Special care should be taken when dealing with anxious or fractious birds because the wing can be fractured with rough or improper restraint during venipuncture.

To obtain blood from the jugular vein, the bird should be placed in lateral recumbency. The vessel is found in the featherless area of the lateral neck (Figure 26-6). It is very easy to visualize. The assistant will need to restrain both the wings and the legs. Restraint can be difficult in some species; therefore, a towel is often used to gently wrap around the body, keeping the wings from flapping around and making the bird feel more secure. The phlebotomist will hold the head with one hand and draw the blood sample with the other. Once the sample is obtained, the assistant will place his or her thumb over the vessel, to prevent hematoma formation, while holding the bird upright.

Obtaining a blood sample from the cutaneous ulnar vein can be challenging. The vessel runs across the proximal radius/ulna and the distal humerus and is very easy to visualize. The bird is usually placed on its back with the wing extended out. Because birds are prey species, being placed on the back is stressful. Excessive flapping can also lead to injuries such as fractures. Birds are often wrapped in a towel to secure the legs and the wing that is not being used for venipuncture. The other wing should be gently pulled away from the body and restrained during blood sampling.

The medial metatarsal vein is located on the medial aspect of the metatarsal region. The vessel is easy to visualize. The assistant will restrain the head, body, wings, and the leg not being used for venipuncture. The use of a towel will help facilitate proper restraint. The phlebotomist will hold the leg with one hand and draw blood with the other.

Selecting the proper syringe and needle size is very important. A syringe that is too large can easily collapse the vessel due to the amount of negative pressure applied. A 27- to 25-gauge needle with a 1- or 3-ml syringe attached is used for medium to large birds. A 27-gauge needle attached to a 1-ml syringe or an insulin syringe is used for venipuncture in small birds.

> **TECHNICIAN NOTE** In birds, blood can be obtained from both the left and right jugular veins. The right vessel is often chosen over the left because it is larger and often easier to obtain the sample.

> **TECHNICIAN NOTE** It is safe to draw up to 1% of the bird's body weight in grams. For example, in a 450-g Amazon parrot, it is safe to draw about 4.5 ml (450 × 0.01), although this volume is rarely necessary.

TABLE 26-1	Common Catheterization Sites in the Avian Patient	
BIRD	**COMMON VESSELS**	**CATHETER SIZE (GAUGE)**
All species	Jugular Medial metatarsal: most common Cutaneous ulnar (basilic)	26 to 20 IV catheter; depends on size of patient

IV Catheter Placement

The patient should first be properly restrained and positioned. Positioning will vary based on catheterization site. Common IV catheterization sites are summarized in Table 26-1.

The medial metatarsal vein is one of the easiest sites to catheterize in medium to large birds. (This vessel is usually too small in species like cockatiels and small conures.) The medial metatarsal is often the preferred site because it is easy to secure and maintain. The patient should be restrained in left or right lateral recumbency and wrapped in a towel to help secure the wings. The patient can also chew on the towel during catheterization, which can help reduce the overall stress of restraint. Some patients can overheat if wrapped in a thick towel for long periods of time. It is the responsibility of the handler to monitor the patient's overall well-being and communicate concerns with the person placing the catheter.

Once the patient has been properly restrained, the person restraining the patient can then hold off the vessel using the thumb and index finger. The area over the vessel is then plucked if necessary and aseptically prepared before catheter placement. The catheter should be held at about a 20-degree angle to the leg and vessel. Once the vessel is stabilized, the catheter can be inserted and advanced into place. If the leg is scaled, the catheter should be inserted between the two scales and not through the scales. An injection port or a pediatric T-port should be placed onto the hub of the catheter. The catheter should be flushed with heparinized saline and taped into place. Taping is done in the same manner as for a dog or cat. Once the catheter has been taped into place, a sterile 2 × 2 inch gauze sponge or sterile adhesive bandage should be placed over the insertion site. Roll gauze followed by an elastic wrap should be used to stabilize and cover the catheter. All IV catheters, regardless of site, are covered and stabilized in a similar manner.

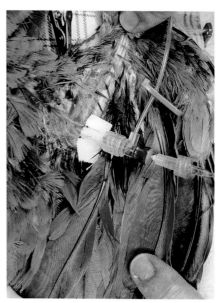

FIGURE 26-7 Cutaneous ulnar vein catheter.

The cutaneous ulnar vessel (also called the basilic vein) is also commonly used for IV catheter placement in small, medium, and large birds. This vessel is easy to catheterize, but must be sutured in place and is harder to maintain. The bird should be placed on its back with the wing of choice gently pulled away from the body. Flapping of the wing in an awake bird can cause it to fracture; therefore, extreme care must be taken in awake patients (Figure 26-7).

The area is aseptically prepped as mentioned previously. The catheter should be held at about a 20-degree angle to the wing and vessel. Once the vessel is stabilized, the catheter can be inserted and advanced into place. A small piece of "butterfly" tape is then placed around the hub of the catheter and a simple interrupted suture is used to tack each side of the tape down to the skin. In general, a figure-of-eight bandage works best to protect the catheter site.

The jugular vessels are not commonly used for IV catheterization, but certainly can be used if necessary. In most species of birds, the right jugular vein is larger than the left, but either can be used. Jugular catheter placement is done under heavy sedation or anesthesia. The bird is placed in lateral recumbency and positioned in the same manner as you would if drawing a blood sample. The person placing the catheter will position the head and neck and the restrainer will help position the body and hold off the vessel.

The catheter should be held at about a 20-degree angle to the neck and jugular vessel. Once the vessel is stabilized, the catheter can be inserted and advanced into place. A small piece of "butterfly" tape is placed around the hub of the catheter and a simple interrupted suture is used to tack each side of the tape down to the skin. The jugular catheter site is bandaged in the same manner as a dog/cat jugular catheter site.

> **TECHNICIAN NOTE** The medial metatarsal, cutaneous ulnar, and jugular veins can be used for intravenous catheterization in the avian patient, although the medial metatarsal vein is the easiest to secure and maintain for longer periods of time.

Intraosseous Catheter Placement

In some cases, an IV catheter may be impossible to place. Such instances include poor perfusion, phlebitis, hematomas, or vessels that are too small. Under these circumstances, an intraosseous catheter should be considered. **Intraosseous (IO) catheters** are most commonly placed in the ulna and tibial crest. A regular hypodermic needle can be used as an IO catheter, but the author suggests using a spinal needle. Spinal needles have a stylet through the middle of the needle that helps keep the needle from becoming clogged with bone.

IO catheters are placed using aseptic technique. The area should be plucked and aseptically prepared before catheter placement. Sterile gloves should also be worn when placing the catheter.

Placing an IO catheter is painful and should be performed under anesthesia or, at minimum, heavy sedation with analgesia. The catheter can be quickly placed without the aid of any drugs when the patient is in need of immediate stabilization. In these cases, prepping the site for placement could be detrimental due to time limitations. Placement needs to be performed immediately to begin lifesaving therapies.

> **TECHNICIAN NOTE** Never place an IO catheter in the avian humerus or femur. The humerus and often the femur (depending on the species) are pneumatic bones with direct communication to the air sacs. Fluid administration into a pneumatic bone can result in the drowning of an avian patient.

> **BOX 26-1** Technical Tip: Suggested Intravenous and Intraosseous Bolus Volumes
>
> - Budgerigar, 0.25-0.5 ml
> - Cockatiel, 1-2 ml
> - Cockatoo, 5-10 ml
> - African grey/Amazon, 5-10 ml
> - Large Macaw, 15-25 ml (Olsen, Orosz)

Disadvantages of IO catheters include risk of bone contamination and difficulty maintaining the catheter. However, IO catheters do offer quick placement and excellent fluid absorption.

Key Point: An initial IV or IO fluid bolus (1% of the body weight in grams) may safely be given to a critical avian patient. For example, a 100-g cockatiel is given the following (Box 26-1):

$$1\% \times 100\,g = 1\,ml$$

Tube Feeding

Tube (or gavage) feeding is used only if the bird needs supplemental feeding and will not eat on its own. The decision to tube feed a critically ill avian patient must be weighed against the potential stress of the tube-feeding procedure.

Products such as Emeraid (Lafeber) or Exact (Kaytee) or homemade formulas can be tube fed. The formula should be mixed thoroughly to remove lumps so that the solution will pass easily through the tube. Formulas should be warm to the touch. Temperatures exceeding 110° F (43.3° C) can result in serious crop burns.

> **TECHNICIAN NOTE** Approximately 5% of the bird's body weight (in grams) can be fed at one time. For example, a 30-g budgerigar can be fed 1.5 ml; a 100-g cockatiel can be fed 5 to 6 ml. Because individual requirements may vary, one should always pay close attention during the procedure.

Feeding tube sizes vary based on the size of the patient. For example, an 8-French red rubber feeding tube works well for a parakeet or Quaker parrot; a 14-French tube for an African grey; and a 16- to 18-French tube for a large macaw. The author prefers metal feeding tubes over rubber feeding tubes in birds. Rubber feeding tubes can be bitten in half fairly easily.

The bird's mouth should be carefully opened with the feeding tube (generally only suggested in smaller species because of the potential trauma that could occur from a large beak biting down on the feeding tube), with a speculum (paper clips work well in smaller birds), or with tape stirrups. The glottis, which opens at the base of the tongue, should be located before insertion of the feeding tube. The esophagus opens caudal to the glottis and to the right of the trachea. The tip of the feeding tube should be lubricated and then placed into the oral cavity and passed gently from the right side of the bird's mouth into the crop. Palpate the feeding tube and the trachea as two distinct tubes in the bird's neck to ensure proper placement of the feeding tube. The tube can also be seen and felt in the crop area when moved in and out at the mouth. The formula should be fed slowly and the oral cavity watched. If the formula backs up in the mouth, tube feeding should be stopped, the tube removed, and the patient released so that it can swallow or shake out any excess food remaining in the oral cavity. The more swiftly this is done, the more likely the bird will clear any formula from the airway. The patient should be fed two to three times daily (Figure 26-8).

Fluid Administration

The decision to administer fluids and the route chosen depend on the condition of the patient and the degree of dehydration. IV fluids can be supplied to birds in shock or to those suffering significant blood or fluid loss. Subcutaneous (SQ) fluids may be administered to moderately dehydrated patients. A fairly large volume may be given SQ, and the slow absorption rate makes cardiac overload unlikely. Oral fluid supplementation alone is reserved for the noncritical patient but is the preferred route if the patient is able to stand, can swallow, and is in the condition to metabolize food.

> **TECHNICIAN NOTE** Fluid volume should always be estimated conservatively. Volume overload is a frequent complication when fluids are administered too rapidly via the IV or IO route. The patient can always be reevaluated in 1 or 2 hours, and more fluids administered at that time if necessary.

Key Point: Maintenance fluids are calculated at 50 to 60 ml/kg/day. Locations for SQ fluid administration

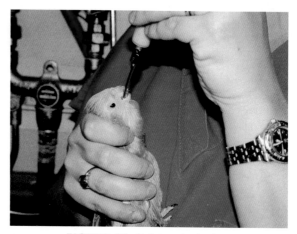

FIGURE 26-8 Avian tube feeding.

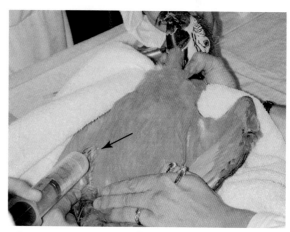

FIGURE 26-9 Avian SQ fluids. The arrow is pointing to the inguinal area where the needle is inserted under the skin for SQ fluid delivery.

include the inguinal web, wing web, and the skin over the back. The inguinal web offers the largest SQ space and is safer compared to the wing web. Improper wing restraint during fluid administration can lead to iatrogenic fractures (Figure 26-9).

Fluids may be supplied primarily by tube feeding in the noncritical patient. If the patient is being fed a slurried diet, then the clinic may provide approximately 100% of the fluid requirement by the oral (PO) route (Box 26-2).

The volume of fluid administered can generally be decreased as the hydration approaches normal and especially as the bird begins eating and drinking on its own.

- Total amount of fluids to be administered/day = daily maintenance + one-half fluid deficit
- Daily maintenance = 50-60 ml/kg/day
- Fluid deficit (ml) = body weight (grams) × percent dehydration
  For example, a 500-g African grey is 10% dehydrated:

  Maintenance = 50 ml/kg × 0.5 kg = 25 ml

  Fluid deficit = 500 × 0.10 = 50 ml

  Administer one half of fluid deficit = 25 ml

  Total volume to be administered on day 1 = 50 ml

Types of fluids commonly used include lactated Ringer's (for shock or dehydration), normal saline (for shock or hypercalcemia), and hypertonic saline (for hypovolemic shock or sepsis). Solutions of 5% dextrose provide energy for birds that have been off-feed for 24 hours.

Anesthesia

Isoflurane and sevoflurane are the anesthetic gases of choice for avian patients. Very small birds may need to be maintained via masks, which can be fashioned from plastic syringe cases. When possible, birds should be intubated with a noncuffed endotracheal tube (ETT). Birds do not ventilate well under anesthesia; therefore, either manual or mechanical intermittent positive pressure ventilation should be started quickly after induction.

To intubate, open the mouth with tape stirrups or a mouth speculum, and visualize the glottis at the base of the tongue. The ETT should be placed gently into the trachea and taped into place by first wrapping white tape around the ETT and then securing it to the lower beak.

It is important to monitor avian patients carefully during induction and maintenance of anesthesia. Keeping the avian patient in an appropriate plane of anesthesia is necessary, because attempts at resuscitation are usually futile. Useful visual monitoring parameters include movement in response to stimuli—wing withdrawal and toe pinch, positive palpebral and corneal reflexes, beak tone, rate and depth of respiration, venous refill time, and heart rate. Electrocardiography, capnography, and blood pressure monitoring are useful in examining trends during anesthesia. Signs of arrest include pupillary dilation, feather erection, respiratory arrest, decrease in $ETCO_2$, and sudden bradycardia or other bradyarrhythmias.

COMMON AVIAN EMERGENCIES

Blood Feathers

As new feathers grow in, they contain a vascular shaft that regresses as the feather matures. If this new blood feather breaks along the vascular shaft, then a significant amount of blood can be lost. The bleeding feather should be grasped with a hemostat and pulled out in the direction of the feather follicle to reduce the chance of skin laceration. If some bleeding occurs after the feather is pulled, then pressure can be applied to the area until the bleeding stops. Removing a broken blood feather is painful. When possible this should be done under general anesthesia and analgesia should always be administered. Pulling a broken blood feather in the wing area could result in a fracture if not done correctly.

Avian Dystocia and Egg Binding

Egg binding is a very common avian emergency, especially in small birds (e.g., Quakers, lovebirds, cockatiels, finches). Clinical signs include depression (e.g., fluffed bird on the bottom of the cage), straining (often with obvious tail bob), matted feces and urates around the cloaca, dyspnea, and occasionally paresis of the pelvic limbs.

Diagnosis is often possible by palpation of the cloacal and coelom, which may reveal a firm, rounded mass (egg) distending the area. Radiography often reveals one (and sometimes two) obvious eggs within the coelomic cavity.

Treatment depends on the condition of the patient and the size and position of the egg. Initially, attempts are made to deliver the egg medically. The patient should be treated with fluid therapy, high humidity (e.g., steam vaporizer, moist towels in a 90° F incubator), and lubrication of the cloacal area. Calcium may be administered if indicated.

If the egg is not delivered within a few hours, or if the patient's condition begins to deteriorate at any time, then the bird should be masked with isoflurane or sevoflurane and attempts to deliver the egg manually should occur. Plenty of sterile lube should be placed in the cloacal area around the egg; gentle, firm manual pressure placed behind the egg may be sufficient to expel it from the cloaca. Because these eggs are often abnormal in shape, size, and shell thickness, they may break during manipulation. Remove as much of the shell and contents as possible and return the bird to an incubator. The egg can also be imploded by placing a large-bore needle through the coelom and into the egg. The contents can be aspirated and the egg gently collapsed. This should be done under anesthesia. Once awake, the patient will often deliver the remaining contents of the egg.

Egg-bound birds can become critical very quickly, and surgical intervention may become necessary to remove the egg to prevent shock and death. If surgery is undertaken, then anesthesia must be very carefully monitored.

Toxins

Some of the most common toxins in caged birds include toxic gases, heavy metals, and toxic plants. The main key to treating toxicities in birds is to *stabilize them first.* Many toxic patients arrive at the clinic in a critical state and should be stabilized with heat, O_2, and fluids as indicated. Because no antidote exists for most of the common toxins, the patient must be treated symptomatically and with supportive care.

Ingested Toxins
Chocolate

The ingestion of even a small amount of chocolate can cause toxic effects. Chocolate contains theophylline and caffeine, which can induce hyperexcitability, cardiac arrhythmias, seizures, vomiting, diarrhea, and death. Treatment of chocolate toxicity includes supportive care and crop gavages with activated charcoal to delay continued absorption of the toxin. Cathartics such as Epsom salts (magnesium sulfate, 1 g/kg PO) or Metamucil (psyllium hydrophilic mucilloid) can be mixed with the charcoal to aid in removal of the toxins from the lower gastrointestinal (GI) tract.

Avocados and Other Plants

Although the toxicity of the avocado is still controversial, certain varieties of avocados do appear to have varying toxic potential. Simply avoiding them altogether is wise. Avocado toxicity has been described in budgerigars and canaries, with clinical signs including anorexia, fluffed feathers, respiratory dyspnea, and death. Postmortem findings often include pulmonary congestion. Treatment is primarily supportive, but activated charcoal and use of a diuretic may be indicated.

Other plants known to have toxic potential in birds include the poinsettia, rhododendron, yew, clematis, dieffenbachia, and parsley. Although studies in budgerigars have shown these and other plants to have toxic potential, wide individual and species variation to plant toxicity exists. The most common clinical signs in plant toxicoses include lethargy, diarrhea, and regurgitation.

Treatment is primarily supportive, including activated charcoal or fluid therapy if indicated.

Mycotoxins

Moldy foods such as seeds, peanuts, pelleted foods, and millet can be potential sources of mycotoxin toxicity. Treatment is symptomatic, but this toxicity can be severe and even acutely fatal.

Alcoholic Beverages

Because of such small body size, consumption of relatively small amounts of alcohol can lead to ataxia and death in birds. Treatment is supportive and symptomatic, including activated charcoal gavage.

Nicotine Ingestion

Ingestion of nicotine from chewing on cigarettes or cigarette butts can result in signs ranging from depression and cyanosis to hyperexcitability, vomiting, diarrhea, seizures, and acute death. Treatment is purely symptomatic.

Heavy Metal Ingestion (Lead and Zinc)

The two most common heavy metals causing toxicosis in birds are lead and zinc. Lead may be encountered via ingestion of costume jewelry, solder, batteries, lead-based paints, and linoleum, as well as a variety of other sources. In wild birds such as ducks and geese, lead shot is a common incidental finding on radiographs. Ingestion of lead shot is a common cause of clinical lead toxicity in waterfowl and upland game birds.

Signs of lead toxicity may be acute or chronic and include lethargy, depression, anemia, and GI signs (e.g., regurgitation, diarrhea). Neuromuscular weakness may also be present, seen as wing droop, ataxia, and leg paresis. Chronic symptoms include emaciation, blindness, seizures, and death. Radiography often reveals metallic densities in the GI tract.

Treatment includes symptomatic and supportive care such as fluid therapy, assisted feeding, antibiotics, surgical removal of the metallic foreign body if indicated, and chelation therapy. Calcium disodium ethylenediamine tetraacetate or d-penicillamine are the most common chelating agents in use. Calcium disodium ethylenediamine tetraacetate is dosed at 35 mg/kg twice a day (bid) intramuscularly (IM) for 5 days, then off for 3 to 4 days as needed until cessation of clinical signs. d-Penicillamine can be administered PO at 55 mg/kg bid for 3 to 6 weeks. Alternatively, calcium disodium ethylenediamine tetraacetate and d-penicillamine can be combined for a few days until clinical signs cease (and d-penicillamine continued for the 3 to 6 weeks). Gavage with a peanut butter or fiber-rich slurry may be used to promote passage of heavy metal from the GI tract (and continued daily until objects are gone). The passage of heavy metals should be monitored with radiography.

Zinc may be encountered in galvanized wire and wire clips, in pennies minted after 1982 (96% zinc), and in Monopoly game pieces (98% zinc). Signs of zinc toxicity include polyuria and polydipsia, weight loss, GI symptoms, weakness, anemia, seizures, and death. Treatment is similar to that for lead toxicity (discussed previously).

> *TECHNICIAN NOTE*   "Bird in a box" radiographs can be taken in critical avian patients. The technique of placing a bird in a small box and taking a single whole body radiograph does not replace traditional radiographs, but can provide a quick view of the coelom aiding in diagnosis of coelomic masses or foreign bodies such as metal.

Inhaled Toxins

Birds have a very unique respiratory system, allowing for two passes of air through the respiratory tract with each respiration. They are therefore highly sensitive to airborne chemicals, including many household cleaners.

Teflon and other nonstick cookware surfaces, including self-cleaning ovens, when overheated, can release polytetrafluoroethylene gas. Clinical signs of polytetrafluoroethylene toxicity range from depression, weakness, wheezing, and dyspnea to seizures and death. The first line of treatment is fresh air (in an O_2 cage, if possible). Stress and excitement should be avoided.

Steroids, antibiotics, diuretics for pulmonary edema, and supportive care may also be helpful.

> *TECHNICIAN NOTE*   Any odor (e.g., gasoline, fuel oil, kerosene, paint, scented candles, perfume) detected by a client is potentially harmful to a bird. Therefore the bird should be removed from the premises immediately and good ventilation ensured.

Respiratory Emergencies

Avian respiratory emergencies are some of the most difficult to treat, because patients often arrive at the clinic in such a fragile state. In addition, diagnosis can be difficult because a wide range of conditions can result in respiratory signs. Birds can present to the clinic with dyspnea for a variety of reasons including granulomas; vitamin A deficiency; bacterial, viral, and fungal infections; foreign bodies; and neoplasia.

Birds have a unique respiratory system that includes nine air sacs (four pairs and one single).

The first step to take with a dyspneic bird is to quickly assess the overall state of the patient. Because manipulation of these patients may result in death, an incubator cage with oxygen should be available. Patients that present with moderate to severe dyspnea should be placed in oxygen before any examination is performed. Any bird in severe respiratory distress should be handled with extreme care. The added stress of a simple examination can result in death. Examinations will often need to be performed systematically over a period of several minutes to hours. Patients are generally first stabilized with oxygen therapy and a heated environment. Once the patient has become more stable, fluids can be given if needed. Diagnostics are not performed until the bird has been stabilized since additional stress can result in death. Each time the patient is removed from the incubator, a brief part of the exam can be performed.

> *TECHNICIAN NOTE*   SQ fluids can be given to unstable avian patients over the back using a butterfly catheter. This technique requires less restraint and is often less stressful in very critical patients.

Lower respiratory tract signs can be the result of all of the previously mentioned causes, as well as

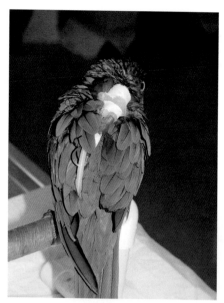

FIGURE 26-10 Air sac cannula.

immune-mediated diseases, infections, coelomic effusion, coelomic masses, and a variety of other conditions.

If a bird has an obstruction of the upper airway, an **air sac cannula** can be placed in the caudal thoracic or abdominal air sac. The patient can then breathe through the cannula instead of trying to breathe through an obstruction of the upper airways. Air sac cannulas can consist of anything from an IV catheter, endotracheal tube, or commercially made device. Aseptic technique and general anesthesia are ideal, but in a true emergency situation, the cannula may need to be placed immediately to save the patient's life (Figure 26-10). Air sac cannulas can also be used to induce and maintain inhalant anesthesia when necessary.

EXOTIC SMALL MAMMAL EMERGENCIES

Supplies
- IO catheters (22-gauge 1 1/2-inch spinal needles OR a 25 gauge, 1 1/2-inch needle used as a stylet inside a 20-gauge, 1-inch needle
- 26- to 22-gauge ¾-inch IV catheters
- 27- to 25-gauge needles
- Insulin syringes
- Fluid pump, syringe pump, or buretrol
- Syringe-case anesthesia masks
- Emeraid Diets by Lafeber

- Nutri-cal®
- Oxbow Critical Care and Carnivore Care Diet®
- 2.0- to 4.5-mm ETT
- Rabbit V-gel device
- Oral specula with light source for oral examinations
- Pediatric or infant stethoscope
- Incubator
- Oxygen cage
- Basic emergency drugs

THE EXOTIC SMALL MAMMAL PHYSICAL EXAMINATION

When possible, a complete physical examination should be performed when the animal presents to the clinic. The exotic small mammal physical examination is performed similarly to other small animals such as dogs and cats. All items are available before the exam begins. Exotic small mammals become easily stressed so it is essential to keep the "time in hand" to a minimum when necessary. A visual exam is performed before hands-on assessments. The visual examination should include information about the cage, as well as the appearance and mentation of the animal. It is important to note any toys, furniture, and bedding in the cage as well as the diet offered to the animal.

> **TECHNICIAN NOTE** Some patients may not be stable enough for a complete physical examination at the time of presentation. When this occurs, basic triage should take place and the patient treated accordingly. The physical examination may need to be performed systematically as the patient becomes more stable.

A general rule for performing a complete physical examination is to start at the head and proceed down to the tail. Heart and respiratory rates are obtained as soon as the animal is removed from the cage. If the respiratory rate seems exaggerated, recount the rate upon completion of the examination and after the animal has been placed back into the cage. Obtaining the patient's weight and temperature is a very important part of the physical examination. Since many of the mammalian patients are small, it is best to use a scale that weighs to the nearest gram. Obtaining a temperature can be challenging, but a digital thermometer is the quickest and best method (unless the patient is just too small). Normal physiologic parameters for common small mammal species are summarized in Table 26-2.

The primary deviation from the "head to tail" method of a physical examination in exotic small mammals is the oral examination. In dogs and cats the mouth is usually examined when the head is examined. The oral examination can be very stressful for exotic small mammals (ferrets are the exception) and therefore should be performed last.

Restraint

Most pet ferrets are very tractable and can easily be examined with minimal restraint. For ferrets with a tendency to bite or wiggle, a firm hold on the scruff gives good control and stimulates the relaxation reflex. Most of the examination can be performed with a little petting and treats such as a high-calorie paste like Nutrical. For SQ injections and other procedures, ferrets can be scruffed with one hand and injected with the other hand. The stretch technique, or scruffing with one hand and extending the rear legs with the other hand, is also a useful immobilization technique.

> **TECHNICIAN NOTE**   Ferrets generally yawn when they are scruffed, making it easy to obtain an oral examination (Figure 26-11).

Venipuncture

Common venipuncture sites include the cephalic, lateral saphenous, jugular, and cranial vena cava vessels. The peripheral vessels are small, which can make it difficult to obtain a full panel. Blood can be obtained from the peripheral vessels and the jugular vein using the same techniques used with dogs and cats (note that the skin is thick and the jugular vessel is more lateral than on a dog or cat). The cranial vena cava is the quickest method that yields the largest volume of blood; however, the animal

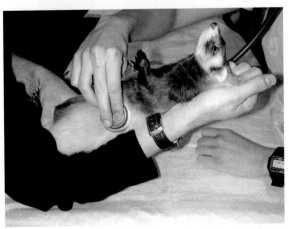

FIGURE 26-11   Ferret restraint.

TABLE 26-2	Normal Physiologic Values for Common Exotic Small Mammals*				
SPECIES	**HEART RATE (BPM)**	**RESPIRATORY RATE (breaths/min)**	**RECTAL TEMPERATURE**	**ADULT WEIGHT**	**LIFE SPAN**
Rat	250 to 450	90	35.9 to 37.5° C 96.6 to 99.5° F	250 to 520 g	2 to 4 years
Mouse	300 to 750	70 to 120	36.7 to 38.3° C 98 to 101° F	20 to 40 g	1 to 3 years
Ferret	180 to 250	10 to 30	37.8 to 40° C 100 to 104° F	Female: 600 to 950 g Male: 1 to 2 kg	5 to 8 years
Chinchilla	150 to 350	40 to 80	37 to 38° C 98.5 to 100.4° F	400 to 700 g	8 to 10 years
Guinea pig	230 to 300	70 to 130	37.2 to 39.5° C 99 to 103.1° F	700 to 1200 g	5 to 8 years
Hamster	300 to 500	60 to 220	37 to 38.6° C 98.6 to 101.4° F	85 to 150 g depending on breed	18 to 24 months
Rabbit	200 to 300	30 to 60	38.3 to 40° C 101 to 104° F	700 g to 6+ kg depending on breed	5 to 12 years depending on breed

*Information taken from Ballard B, Cheek R: *Exotic animal medicine for the veterinary technician,* ed 2, New York, 2013, Wiley; www.lafebervet.com.

must be placed under general anesthesia or heavy sedation before the sample is obtained. A 25-gauge needle attached to a 1- or 3-ml syringe is used for this venipuncture site. The patient is placed in dorsal recumbency with the front legs pulled down next to the body and the head and neck extended. The needle should be aimed toward the opposite hind limb and is then inserted at a 45-degree angle into the thoracic inlet. The landmarks used to find the insertion site include the manubrium and the first rib. Do not poke and jab this vessel trying to obtain a sample because this can lead to large hematoma formation or complete laceration. The technique described previously is the same technique used in guinea pigs (Figure 26-12).

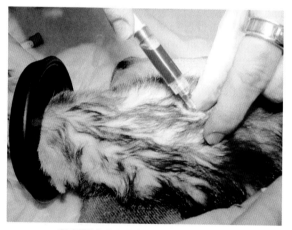

FIGURE 26-12 Ferret venipuncture.

Catheter Placement

The cephalic vein is most commonly used for placing indwelling IV catheters in ferrets. A 24-gauge ¾-inch catheter works well for most ferrets. Common IV catheterization sites for other small mammals are summarized in Table 26-3.

Ferrets are notorious for removing catheters, so adequate taping is essential. A T-port should be attached to the catheter, taped with a butterfly, and then taped around the leg. The turned up IV line should be included in another round of tape and the entire catheter wrapped in Vet-Wrap (leaving the port exposed). Close monitoring is important to prevent the ferret from becoming tangled in or kinking the IV line.

E-collars made out of a small piece of x-ray film are an effective method in preventing the ferret from chewing catheters or incisions.

IO catheterization and fluid administration is an option (often the sole option) if venous access is unsuccessful. IO catheters are most often placed in the proximal femur in ferrets (as placed in a kitten).

Fluid Therapy

Always calculate required daily fluids before administration. The daily maintenance fluid requirement for ferrets is approximately 50 to 60 ml/kg/day plus loss. The IV or IO route is preferred for very sick or dehydrated ferrets. Ferrets can be easily overhydrated because of their small body size. A syringe pump, fluid pump or Buretrol® device (Baxter Health) aids in preventing too rapid an administration of calculated fluids. When using a Buretrol,

TABLE 26-3	Common Intravenous Catheterization Sites in Exotic Small Mammals	
SPECIES	**COMMON VESSEL SITE(S)**	**CATHETER SIZE (GAUGE)**
Rabbit	Cephalic, lateral saphenous, auricular, jugular	26 to 20 IV catheter; depends on size of patient Up to an 18 for jugular Possible to place multi-lumen catheter in jugular vein
Ferret	Cephalic, lateral saphenous, and jugular	26 to 22 IV catheter 20 to 18 catheter for jugular Possible to place multi-lumen catheter in jugular vein
Guinea pig	Cephalic and lateral saphenous	26 to 22
Chinchilla	Cephalic (lateral saphenous is rarely an option due to size and anatomy)	26 to 24
Small rodents	Cephalic, lateral saphenous, lateral tail vessels (not on hamsters)	26 to 24

the total daily fluid volume can be divided into two (or optimally three) slow bolus doses. Types of IV fluids used in ferrets are similar to those used in dogs and cats.

SQ fluids can be administered in the loose dorsal scapular skin. Two or three SQ boluses can be given to meet daily fluid requirements. The use of a syringe attached to a butterfly catheter aids in easy and quick fluid administration.

Urethral Catheterization

Urethral obstruction in ferrets may arise from adrenal disease causing secondary prostatomegaly or from urethral calculi. Although relatively uncommon, urethral obstruction is a definite medical emergency. Urethral catheterization in male ferrets can be challenging because of the small size of the urethral opening and the hooked shape of the os penis. If passage of a urinary catheter in a blocked ferret is not possible, then cystocentesis or emergency cystotomy may be performed with attempts to flush the urethra normograde from the bladder.

> *TECHNICIAN NOTE*   3.5-French Slippery Sam urinary catheters generally work well for urinary catheterization in the blocked male ferret.

COMMON FERRET EMERGENCIES

Adrenal disease and insulinoma are the two most common diseases seen in ferrets in the United States. Other common problems include foreign bodies, *Helicobacter mustelae* infection, distemper, and coronaviral diarrhea (i.e., green slime disease).

Adrenal Disease

Adrenal disease is a chronic syndrome. Ferrets will frequently present on emergency with adrenal disease caused by secondary complications (including prostatomegaly) that result in urethral obstruction, weakness, anorexia, and dehydration.

A large percentage of ferrets over the age of 3 years will develop adrenal disease, most commonly in the form of benign adrenal hyperplasia and adrenal adenoma. Adrenal neoplasia occurs less commonly. Symptoms of adrenal disease usually begin with alopecia at the tip of the tail, which progresses to symmetrical truncal alopecia. Intense pruritus may accompany or precede the alopecia. Female ferrets will often present with an enlarged vulva.

A ferret with adrenal disease showing signs of debilitation should first be stabilized symptomatically. Treat with fluids, antibiotics, and/or syringe feeding if necessary. Diets such as Hill's a/d, Oxbow Carnivore Care, or meat-based baby foods can be offered or syringe-fed.

Adrenalectomy in the author's experience is the treatment of choice for most ferrets. Medical management may be more appropriate in some cases and a few options are available including, but not limited to, gonadotropin-releasing hormone analogs such as leuprolide acetate.

Insulinoma

Insulinomas are extremely common in ferrets more than 3 to 4 years old. The classic presentation is a weak, lethargic ferret, occasionally ataxic, drooling, pawing at the mouth, or in hypoglycemic seizures. Attempt to document the hypoglycemia with a blood glucose level measurement. The normal blood glucose level in ferrets is greater than 80 mg/dl. Blood glucose level below this is an indicator of possible insulinoma; blood glucose level less than 60 mg/dl is diagnostic. Ferrets that are weak, salivating, seizuring, or ataxic often have glucose levels of 20 to 40 mg/dl.

Emergency treatment of a hypoglycemic episode involves rubbing Karo or other high-sucrose syrup on the ferret's gums. Diluting Karo syrup 50:50 with tap water eases administration. For ferrets that do not respond, IV crystalloids with dextrose can be started or bolused until the ferret responds. IV fluids and corticosteroids at shock doses (dexamethasone sodium phosphate 4 to 8 mg/kg IM, IV) can be added for moribund, unresponsive ferrets. Benzodiazepines should be administered for seizure control when necessary.

Once the ferret is responsive, try to initiate frequent meals of a high-protein ferret food. Surgical therapy in patients stable enough to undergo anesthesia is considered the treatment of choice. Surgery, while not often curative, will slow the progression of the disease.

Helicobacter mustelae Gastritis and Enteritis

Clinical illness occurs in stressed young ferrets 12 to 20 weeks of age and in older ferrets exposed to newly acquired carriers that are shedding. History invariably supports this exposure.

Clinical signs include lethargy, anorexia, weight loss, and diarrhea (often with dark, tarry stools) (melena). Histopathologic lesions of clinical *H. mustelae* infection include mucous depletion, a leukocytic infiltrate in the gastric wall, gastric ulceration, and hemorrhagic gastric erosions.

Definitive diagnosis is possible by surgical or endoscopic biopsies, fecal culture, or polymerase chain reaction of combined oral, stomach, and rectal swabs.

Treatment has traditionally involved triple therapy with amoxicillin, metronidazole, and bismuth subsalicylate. Other drug therapies include the use of clarithromycin and ranitidine bismuth, or a combination of clarithromycin, metronidazole, and omeprazole or lastly clarithromycin and omeprazole.

Hydration and GI issues should always be addressed with appropriate calculated supportive care.

Coronaviral Diarrhea Syndrome

Veterinarians treating ferrets have long known of a typical diarrhea syndrome of ferrets commonly known as *green slime disease*. This syndrome has been connected with a coronaviral infection in ferrets. Clinical signs include diarrhea that becomes green and mucoid (turning to melena in severe cases), anorexia, weakness, dehydration, and emaciation. Treatment is purely supportive, with fluid therapy and feeding of slurried food via syringe if necessary. IV catheter placement and administration of IV fluids via a syringe pump, fluid pump, or buretrol is optimal. SQ fluids may be substituted if vasoconstriction makes catheter placement impossible, but this method is less effective. Antibiotics appear to expedite recovery. Syringe feeding of easily digestible foods such as Oxbow Carnivore Care may also be necessary until the ferret is eating on its own.

Foreign Bodies

Ferrets are famous for their curiosity, which includes the desire to play with and taste new objects. Rubber objects (e.g., pencil erasers and toys) are often favorite materials to chew.

Clinical signs of foreign body ingestion include anorexia, lethargy, weakness, and diarrhea. If the owner reports regurgitation, vomiting, or both, then a foreign body should be highly suspect. Foreign bodies in the small intestine may be palpable, with localized pain or discomfort on palpation. Diagnosis is based on history, clinical signs, radiography, and ultrasonography.

Treatment is usually surgical. An IV catheter is placed and the patient stabilized before surgery. Surgery should be performed as soon as possible, because these patients can become quickly debilitated. Most ferrets recover rapidly after foreign body removal and are able to eat on their own within 24 hours of surgery.

Canine Distemper Virus

Distemper is rare but can be seen in unvaccinated ferrets. This disease is highly contagious and most often fatal. Presenting signs generally include diarrhea, nasal and ocular discharge, and an orange-tinged dermatitis. Supportive care and strict isolation techniques are followed when dealing with a distemper suspect.

RABBIT AND RODENT EMERGENCIES
Restraint
Rabbits

Rabbits are built for springing with their hind legs and will often attempt to do so during restraint. The handler should always support a rabbit's back and rear legs during restraint or transport, because the act of kicking off without a firm surface to push against can result in spinal fractures.

Covering the rabbit's eyes and face with one hand can both calm the rabbit and prevent it from jumping forward during a physical examination. For transport, the rabbit's front legs may be supported and held with one hand, with a finger between the feet and its hindquarters tucked under the elbow while the other hand supports the rear legs. Alternatively, the rabbit can be placed in a football hold, with the head tucked under one elbow and the rabbit's scruff held with the other hand. To examine the abdomen or feet or for sexing, the rabbit can be cradled on its back like a baby in the technician's arm, with one hand supporting the rear legs (Figure 26-13).

Chinchillas

Most pet chinchillas are used to being handled and therefore are easy to capture and restrain. When capturing a chinchilla, it is best to place one hand under the thorax/abdomen and the other hand gently grasping the base of the tail. Once the chinchilla has been captured, it can be placed on the exam table. A chinchilla can lose patches of fur if handled roughly. This is commonly referred to as "fur slip," and because of this, a chinchilla should not be scruffed. Although not very common, "fur-slip" can happen unexpectedly during the physical examination.

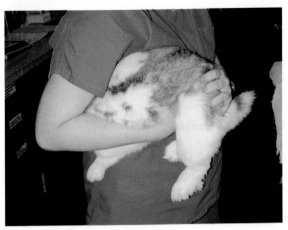

FIGURE 26-13 Rabbit restraint.

Rats

Pet rats are often used to being handled and can simply be picked up and gently supported during a physical examination. If more restraint is necessary, the rat's head can be restrained by placing your thumb on one side of the head and your index finger on the other side while still supporting the body. The rat can also be gently scruffed if necessary. For rats that are uncooperative, the base of the tail can be gently grabbed to temporarily catch the patient before restraining it. This method should only be used if the animal is not tame or not used to being handled.

Hamsters and Mice

Hamsters have a large amount of loose skin around the neck, shoulders, and back. To provide full or immobilizing restraint, the hamster's skin should be grasped between your thumb and fingertips (similar to scruffing a cat). It is important to always support the hamster's body with your other hand. Mice are restrained in a very similar manner, but can be picked up by gently grabbing the base of the tail before scruffing them.

Guinea Pigs

Most pet guinea pigs are calm and gentle animals that rarely bite; therefore they can usually be picked up out of their enclosures and placed on an exam table. Under many circumstances, guinea pigs will need only light restraint when being examined. This is usually best accomplished by supporting the hind end of the animal with one hand and cupping the other hand gently under the thorax. Scruffing a guinea pig is generally not recommended because their neck is very short and there is little skin to grip properly.

Venipuncture

Several sites are available for venipuncture in rabbits. The jugular veins yield the largest volume, but the cephalic, auricular, and lateral saphenous veins are also useful. The jugular veins can be difficult to obtain blood from in rabbits that have large dewlaps. Performing jugular venipuncture in rabbits is done in the same manner as described for chinchillas. The cephalic and auricular vessels are generally small and may not yield enough blood for a full blood panel. The lateral saphenous vein is usually the quickest and easiest vein from which to obtain a blood sample. Obtaining blood from the lateral saphenous in a rabbit is accomplished in the same manner as in a dog. A 1-ml syringe with a 27- or 25-gauge needle should be used. Proper restraint is imperative. Using a football restraint technique (done by placing the patient's head between the restrainer's side and under the restrainer's arm/armpit area while the rest of the body is supported with the restrainer's other arm) is often the easiest and safest way to obtain a quick sample. In some cases, the author will prop the patient up on a rolled-up towel so that the leg can easily be pulled away from the body.

Chinchillas

Venipuncture sites in the chinchilla include the cephalic, lateral saphenous, and jugular veins. The peripheral vessels do not usually yield enough blood for diagnostic sampling; therefore, the jugular vein is the vessel of choice when obtaining blood for a complete blood count and a biochemistry panel. Performing jugular venipuncture on a chinchilla is similar to that on a cat but technicians must be aware of "fur-slip." The chinchilla can be held in one of many different positions to gain access to the jugular vein. Choosing the position will depend on the animal as well as the preference of the phlebotomist. The chinchilla can be placed in lateral recumbency with head extended and legs pulled down toward the body. Another position involves the patient being placed in sternal recumbency at the edge of the exam table with the head extended upward and the front legs pulled down, similar to a cat. The final common position includes the chinchilla being rolled onto its back with the head extended and the legs pulled down towards the body. The vessel is held off using your thumb or index finger. The jugular vein is located in the same general area of the neck as the jugular vein in a cat. A 27- or 25-gauge needle attached to a 1-ml syringe is commonly used to obtain the blood sample. Animals that are uncooperative may need light sedation to obtain the sample.

Guinea Pigs

The peripheral vessels as well as the jugular vein can be used to obtain a blood sample from guinea pigs. The needle and syringe size as well as the positioning are the same as those for the chinchilla. Again, the peripheral vessels may not yield enough blood if a complete blood count and biochemistry are needed. Guinea pigs have very short necks; therefore, the jugular vein can be a difficult source of blood. In the author's opinion, the femoral vein is the "better" vessel to use. Obtaining blood from the femoral vein is the quickest method that yields the largest amount of blood. The patient is anesthetized to minimize the chance of lacerating the large femoral vein or artery. To obtain the blood sample, first palpate the pulse of the femoral artery in the inguinal area. The nipple can be used as a landmark to help find the pulse. Because the artery and the vein run alongside each other, the arterial pulse is used to help pinpoint the location of the vein. Once the artery is palpated, the needle (it is best to use a 1-ml tuberculin syringe with a 25- or 22-gauge needle) should be inserted at a 45-degree angle into the skin. This venipuncture site is a "blind stick." Since the vessel cannot be visualized, it is important to place slight negative pressure on the syringe as soon as the needle enters the skin. Having negative pressure on the syringe is helpful for the phlebotomist because blood will enter the syringe once the needle is properly placed into the vessel. Without negative pressure on the syringe, it is very easy to bypass the vessel and not even realize it. Once the blood sample has been obtained, the needle can be removed and the thumb or a finger placed over the insertion site to hold off the vessel.

Blood can also be obtained from the cranial vena cava (same procedure as used in a ferret), but this does not come without potential risk of traumatic bleeding into the thoracic cavity or pericardial sac. If the cranial vena cava is chosen as the venipuncture site, the animal must be under general anesthesia while obtaining the blood sample. A struggling patient will greatly increase the risk of lacerating the vena cava during the blood draw; therefore, this venipuncture site should never be used when an animal is awake.

Rats, Mice, and Hamsters

The peripheral veins as well as the jugular vein can be used, but again, these vessels are small and are difficult sample sources. In rats and mice, the lateral tail veins can be used to obtain small amounts of blood. The vessels are usually superficial and can easily be seen (unless the animal is very debilitated or obese). This can be accomplished by either using an insulin syringe or using a tuberculin syringe with a 27-gauge needle. A 27- or 25-gauge needle can also be placed into the vessel. Once there is blood in the hub of the needle, a hematocrit tube can be used to collect the blood. Generally, this site does not yield enough blood for a complete blood count and biochemistry panel. Using the femoral vein to obtain a blood sample is the quickest method that will yield the most amount of blood. The same method described for guinea pigs is also used with hamsters, mice, and rats, although a 27- or 25-gauge needle is used.

Catheter Placement

Common IV catheter sites in exotic small mammals include the cephalic, auricular (in rabbits only, also called marginal ear veins), and lateral saphenous vessels. Jugular vein catheterization is possible in ferrets and rabbits. Catheter size will vary based on the size of the patient. Commonly a 24- or 26-gauge catheter can be placed in the smaller patients, while a 22- or 20-gauge catheter can be placed in a larger patient; for example, a 4- to 6-kg rabbit. Jugular catheters will range from 22 to 18 gauge. Multi-lumen catheters can also be placed in larger patients when necessary.

The skin of some species can be thick and hard to penetrate. It is often helpful to make a skin nick incision using a 25- to 20-gauge hypodermic needle. Rabbit and chinchilla hair may be difficult to shave. A number 50 clipper blade works well to remove their fine hair.

> TECHNICIAN NOTE The skin of many exotic small mammals is often thick. Making a skin nick incision using a hypodermic needle will help an intravenous catheter advance easier.

The patient should first be placed on a nonslip surface before catheter placement. Patients should always be kept in sternal recumbency during catheter placement. Positioning the patient in lateral recumbency is often very stressful and can increase the incidence of back fractures in rabbits and stress in any species.

Unless otherwise stated in the following text, all catheterization sites follow the same basic placement and stabilization techniques. The basic technique is as follows:

The limb is shaved and aseptically prepared before catheter placement. A skin nick incision should be made using a 25- to 20-gauge needle. The catheter should be held at a 20- to 30-degree angle to the leg. Once the vessel is stabilized, the catheter can be inserted and advanced into place. An injection cap or a pediatric T-port should be placed onto the hub of the catheter. The catheter should be flushed with heparinized saline and taped into place. Taping is done in the same manner as for a dog or cat. Once the catheter has been taped into place, a sterile 2 × 2 inch gauze sponge or sterile adhesive bandage is placed over the insertion site. Roll gauze followed by an elastic wrap is used to stabilize and cover the catheter.

The cephalic vein is often small in most species, but is still the easiest to catheterize. Most patients are restrained by placing one arm around the body and gently pulling its body towards your side. The restrainer can then hold off the vessel using his or her thumb and index finger. This is very similar to the procedure for a cat.

The lateral saphenous vein is often used in ferrets, rabbits, and guinea pigs. The patient is restrained by tucking the head between the assistant's body and forearm. The patient's body is then gently restrained against the assistant's body. The assistant can place his or her hand around the hind limb and hold off the vessel. Ferrets may need to be scruffed like a cat to properly restrain them. Most ferrets like the taste of Nutri-cal, and a dollop may be placed on a tongue depressor and used to distract the ferret during catheter placement.

The auricular veins, also called the marginal ear veins, are often small, even in large rabbits. The auricular veins run along the most outer portion of the pinna. The auricular artery runs through the center of the pinna. It may be tempting to place a catheter into this vessel, but it should be avoided for the purpose of fluid therapy. Fluids and medications should not be injected into the artery.

The ear should be shaved and aseptically prepared before catheter placement. The person restraining the rabbit should also stabilize the ear by placing his or her hand around the base of the pinna. The person can then hold off the vessel with either the thumb or index finger.

A skin nick incision should be made using a 25- to 20-gauge needle. Taping at this site can be tricky because of the shape and size of the ear. Rolling the pinna around a roll of gauze or syringe case can make it easier to stabilize the catheter. Once the gauze or syringe case is in place, the catheter is taped in the same manner as the cephalic or lateral saphenous veins.

> **TECHNICIAN NOTE** When possible, ear veins should be avoided because a high chance for thrombosis, necrosis, and sloughing of ear tissue exists. Stabilizing the catheter comfortably can be difficult.

An IV catheter can be placed in the lateral tail vein of a rat. These vessels are often small; therefore, a 26- or 24-gauge catheter is used. The catheter site is aseptically prepared and a skin nick incision is made using a 25- to 22-gauge needle. The catheter should be held at a 20- to 30-degree angle to the vessel. The same technique used to place a cephalic catheter is also used for the lateral tail vein. Rats will need to be heavily sedated or anesthetized unless they are critically ill or injured (Figure 26-14).

Jugular catheters are not commonly placed in exotic small mammals, but the option is available when needed. Regular IV catheters can be placed and secured using suture. Catheter size will be dependent upon the vessel size. Multi-lumen catheters can also be placed in ferrets and rabbits. These catheters must be placed using aseptic technique. Placement is done in the same manner as that used for dogs and cats.

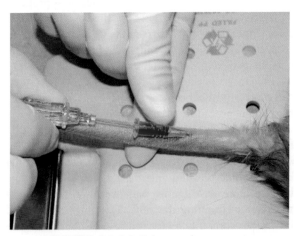

FIGURE 26-14 Tail vein catheter in a rat.

Intraosseous Catheter Placement

When placing an IO catheter into the femur, first palpate the great trochanter located on the proximal portion of the bone near the femoral head. The catheter should be placed between the greater trochanter and the femoral head. The bone is very dense and it can be difficult to advance the catheter into the bone. It is easiest to both twist the needle and push it down at the same time. This will help keep the catheter from bending as it advances into the medullary cavity. The catheter should be advanced until the entire length of the needle is in the bone. Once it is fully seated, the stylet should be removed and a 3-ml syringe with heparinized saline should be attached. The catheter should be aspirated and then flushed. If bone marrow is aspirated into the syringe, you know the catheter has been correctly placed; however, in the author's experience, bone marrow is not often aspirated. There are a few ways to check for proper catheter placement. A quick radiograph will confirm placement, but if this is not possible, the leg can be moved in a circular motion. The catheter should remain in the same plane as the femur. Once placement is confirmed, a piece of tape can be placed onto the hub of the catheter and a few simple interrupted sutures can be used to secure it. The techniques for needle advancement and checking placement are the same for all exotic animal species.

The tibial crest is the other commonly used site for IO catheter placement in exotic small mammals. In general, a 25-gauge spinal needle is used for most exotic small mammals. Placement and securing techniques are the same but the anatomy is just a little different. It is often easiest to bend the leg so that the tibial crest is palpable. The tibial crest is quite prominent in most species and in some cases placing an IO catheter here is easier even though the anatomy is smaller. Once the catheter is placed and secured, the leg is bandaged since it is more accessible to the patient compared to the femur. Bandaging is usually a better alternative than using E-collars.

Syringe Feeding Techniques

Hand or syringe feeding is an essential skill to acquire when working with exotic animals. There are several different species-specific hand feeding formulas that can be offered. Herbivorous animals such as rabbits, chinchillas, and guinea pigs can be hand- or syringe-fed formulas such as blended pellets, vegetable baby food, canned pumpkin, or the commercial diets Oxbow Critical Care for herbivores, or Emeraid Herbivore. For example, a homemade formula may consist of canned pumpkin mixed with garden vegetable baby food or blended pellets. Homemade formulas such as the one mentioned earlier are perfectly acceptable to feed as long as they are high in fiber, low in sugar, and otherwise meet the nutritional needs of the patient. Oxbow Critical Care and Emeraid Herbivore are manufactured commercially and consist of a balanced diet that can be used to provide nutritional support to convalescing herbivores. There are two techniques commonly used to syringe feed herbivorous patients. The first technique consists of loading a 60-ml catheter tip syringe and simply feeding the animal by placing the tip of the syringe into the patient's mouth. This technique works well with patients that are actively interested in eating. Some patients will actually lick the food from the syringe as it is pushed out. The other technique also consists of loading a 60-ml catheter tip syringe with the hand feeding formula but instead of feeding the patient directly with the 60-ml syringe, several 1- or 3-ml aliquots will be back-loaded from the 60-ml syringe. The smaller syringes can be placed directly into the patient's mouth with the entire amount of the food in the syringe squeezed into the mouth at one time. This seems really drawn out and tedious (and it really can be!); but for most patients, this technique works the best. If the animal is only fed one small syringe of food at a time, more food actually ends up in the patient and less on the patient, technician, or exam table. In extreme cases, the animal can be tube fed or in some species of small mammals such as rabbits, a nasogastric tube can be placed.

> **TECHNICIAN NOTE** One of the most effective ways to syringe feed an herbivorous exotic small mammal is to load several 1-ml tuberculin syringes and feed with an entire syringe at one time. This seems tedious, but more food will end up in the patient's mouth and less on the table and technical staff.

Rodents such as mice, rats, and hamsters can also be syringe-fed when needed, with a 1- or 3-ml syringe. The most common type of food used for syringe feeding includes vegetable baby food such as squash, sweet potatoes, and other various vegetable-based baby foods. If the patient is being uncooperative, a metal feeding tube (usually used in birds) can be placed into the mouth, but not down into the esophagus. The feeding tube (attached to the syringe) works well to help deliver the food by slowly dripping it into the mouth.

COMMON EMERGENCIES IN RABBITS

Dental Disease

Dental disease is a common problem in exotic small mammals such as guinea pigs, chinchillas, and rabbits (Figure 26-15). A patient that presents for drooling, anorexia, over-grooming, and/or reduced or no fecal output should be considered an emergency and treated quickly. Guinea pigs, chinchillas, and rabbits are hindgut fermenters. They need to eat continuously throughout the day and therefore defecate all the time. Not eating for 12 to 24 hours can lead to GI stasis. If this is left untreated, it can be a death sentence. The primary emergency stabilization treatments for patients presenting with dental disease (or anything causing anorexia) include pain management, fluid therapy, and force-feeding. Pain can add to the severity of GI stasis. Butorphanol is generally not an ideal drug to treat dental pain or pain caused by GI stasis. Ideally a full mu opioid such as oxymorphone is used. Buprenorphine can be used if the patient is not experiencing severe pain. Fluids such as lactated Ringer's solution (LRS) are generally given IV. If an IV is not necessary or cannot be placed, subcutaneous (SQ) fluids can be administered at a dose of 50 to 60 ml/kg/day. Using a butterfly catheter attached to a syringe makes SQ fluid administration easier. Most of these patients are small so it is hard to accurately administer fluids via a drip set and bag. If a patient is crashing and an IV cannot be placed due to poor perfusion, an IO catheter can be placed.

People often think rabbits obstruct from hairballs (trichobezoars). While this does happen, it is not very common. People talk about using pineapple juice or papaya enzymes to help break down the hairball. This is controversial and not shown to be very effective. If a rabbit or other exotic small mammal has a hairball or other GI foreign body, the animal should be treated in a similar manner to those presenting with dental disease. Basic supportive care should include pain management, fluid therapy, and force-feeding. Basic diagnostics

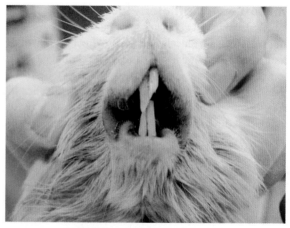

FIGURE 26-15 Dental disease.

include radiographs, abdominal ultrasound, complete blood count (CBC), and chemistry panels. Barium GI studies can be performed but GI transit time is much slower in hindgut fermenters and can therefore take 24 to 36 hours to perform a complete study. Surgery is needed if the foreign body will not pass.

Bacterial Enteritis

Enterotoxemia (caused by clostridial bacteria) and colibacillosis (caused by pathogenic *Escherichia coli*) are the two most common causes of bacterial enteritis in rabbits. Clinical signs of enteritis include soft stool to watery diarrhea containing blood or mucus, sepsis, severe dehydration, and sometimes death. Underlying causes of bacterial overgrowth include stress, lack of adequate fiber in the diet, or antibiotic therapy resulting in changes in gut flora. Diagnosis of bacterial enteritis in rabbits is based on clinical signs and fecal culture.

Treatment should be started while fecal cultures are pending. The patient should be treated empirically with enrofloxacin or metronidazole. In mild cases of enteritis, eliminating all treats and adding hay to increase dietary fiber intake may correct the problem. In cases of clostridial overgrowth, treatment consists of aggressive fluid therapy IV or IO if necessary, coupled with efforts to normalize gut flora and decrease numbers of pathogenic bacteria. Antibiotic therapy in such cases may only add to the decrease in numbers of normal bacterial flora. Metronidazole has been found to be helpful. Clearance of pathogenic bacteria may be aided by the addition of metoclopramide or cisapride, as well as the ingestion of a high-fiber diet.

Colibacillosis, on the other hand, should be treated with appropriate antibiotics based on culture and sensitivity results. Most *Escherichia coli* strains are sensitive to enrofloxacin or trimethoprim-sulfa. The clinic staff should be aggressive with fluid therapy and administer a high-fiber diet via syringe feeding if necessary. These syndromes should be treated until the rabbit is eating well on its own and producing normal feces.

Cystic Calculi and Cystitis

Cystic calculi are relatively common in rabbits and guinea pigs. Clinical signs include depression, weight loss, stranguria, hematuria, hunched stance, and depression. Discreet calculi may be palpable in the bladder. Radiography and abdominal ultrasound are useful diagnostics tests to identify calculi that may be cystic, urethral, ureteral, or renal in location.

Key Point: When performing radiography of the rabbit's bladder, do not confuse calcium sediment (radiodense sand) with cystic calculi. Calculi will appear as discreet, radiodense stones.

Key Point: Normal urinalysis in the rabbit may be characterized by calcium oxalate crystalluria and sometimes a pink or orange discoloration of the urine. A dipstick can be used to differentiate hematuria from normal pigment coloration.

Hematuria usually indicates the presence of cystic calculi. Rabbits with either calcium sludge or calcium carbonate calculi generally have excessive dietary calcium intake.

Cystitis (rare) should be treated with a 2- to 3-week course of antibiotic therapy. Trimethoprim-sulfa is usually effective.

Treatment of cystic calculi may be possible by retropulsion via repeated flushing of the bladder with saline. Usually treatment is surgical. The patient should be stabilized as indicated with IV fluids and antibiotics before cystotomy (and the calculi are submitted for quantitative analysis).

Respiratory Tract Infections and *Pasteurella*

Upper and lower respiratory tract infections are common in rabbits. *Pasteurella multocida* infection, commonly known as *snuffles,* is the most common causative agent in upper respiratory tract disease of rabbits. Other causative agents of upper respiratory tract disease include, but are not limited to *Moraxella* spp. and *Bordetella bronchiseptica.*

Clinical signs of pasteurellosis in rabbits include rhinitis and sinusitis, with nasal exudates and often excessive tearing from the eyes (i.e., epiphora), as well as conjunctivitis and often a snuffling or snoring sound audible during respiration. Sequelae of *Pasteurella* infection include otitis (when infection has spread from the nares to the middle ear), erosion of the nasal turbinates, and hematogenous spread resulting in bacteremia, fever, and acute death. *Pasteurella* pneumonia, pleuritis, and pericarditis are also possible sequelae of chronic infection.

Definitive diagnosis is by culture; however, the organism may be difficult to grow, and several culture attempts may be necessary. Treatment is based on long-term antibiotic therapy of typically 45 days or longer because of the invasive nature of the disease. Antibiotics generally effective against *Pasteurella* infection include enrofloxacin and chloramphenicol. Antibiotics should be started immediately and therapy adjusted based on the results of culture and sensitivity. The patient should be treated supportively with fluids and syringe feeding as indicated. It is imperative that a complete dental examination is performed because many of the same signs occur with both diseases.

Abscesses

Any fluctuant or firm growth on a rabbit is an abscess until proven otherwise. Pus in rabbits is solid, white, and caseous. Abscesses must be surgically excised with clean margins. When excision is not possible, such as with foot or facial abscesses, the area should be well debrided and kept open until healed. Marsupialization is the surgical procedure of choice to permit long-term flushing of the abscess pocket. Recurrence of abscesses is not uncommon.

Common pathogens causing rabbit abscesses include *Pseudomonas multocida, P. aeruginosa,* and *Staphylococcus* species. Good empiric antibiotic choices include enrofloxacin and trimethoprim-sulfa. Choice of antibiotics is optimally based on culture and sensitivity.

Uterine Adenocarcinoma

Uterine adenocarcinoma is very common in unspayed rabbits more than 4 years of age. The most common clinical sign of uterine adenocarcinoma noted by owners is hematuria, or frank blood at the end of urination. Other clinical signs include depression, anorexia, and dehydration. Metastasis to the lungs, liver, or bone may occur within the first year of the disease (or later).

Ovariohysterectomy is the treatment of choice. The rabbit should be stabilized with IV or IO fluids prior to surgery if possible. Prognosis is good if metastasis has not yet occurred.

COMMON EMERGENCIES IN RODENTS

As stated earlier, dental disease is also a common problem in exotic small mammals such as guinea pigs and chinchillas. Small rodents are treated in the same manner as rabbits.

Reproductive Emergencies

Any species of exotic small mammal can present for reproductive emergencies such as dystocia, but it is most commonly seen in guinea pigs. The pubic symphysis is fibrocartilaginous. If a female guinea pig is first bred after 6 months of age, the symphysis is less able to separate during birth, leading to dystocia. This situation often requires a cesarean section. Before surgery, radiographs, abdominal ultrasound, and (at the minimum) baseline blood work (packed cell volume [PCV], total protein [TP], blood glucose [BG] level, stick blood urea nitrogen [BUN] level) should be obtained. Painful exotic small mammals do not eat well; therefore, pain management is important as well as fluid therapy to keep the GI tract hydrated, including force-feeding when necessary.

Male chinchillas can present for penile prolapse. This is often caused by fur accumulation around the base of the penis. This is remedied by lubricating the penis and gently removing the fur ring from the penile tissue. Once the fur is removed, the penis can be placed back into the prepuce. In some cases, the patient will need to be sedated for safe removal of the fur ring. General anesthesia is not usually needed. Supportive care can be provided if necessary and include subcutaneous fluids at a dose of 50 to 60 ml/kg/day, force feeding, and pain management (Figure 26-16).

Hamsters may present for diarrhea. This is often referred to as wet tail. Wet tail is often caused by improper diet and husbandry practices. Ileitis can be caused by many different types of bacteria. Common signs include matting or wetness around the tail, diarrhea, lethargy, hunched abdomen, and in severe cases death. Supportive care includes subcutaneous fluid therapy, hand feeding when necessary, antibiotics, and a change in husbandry and dietary practices.

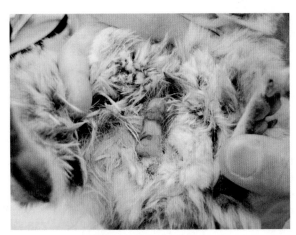

FIGURE 26-16 Chinchilla fur ring.

REPTILE EMERGENCIES

Supplies

- 25- to 20-gauge spinal needles for use as IO catheters
- Insulin syringes
- 27- to 25-gauge needles
- Basic emergency drugs
- Red rubber feeding tubes (various sizes)
- Incubator cage
- Oxbow Critical Care and Carnivore Care Diets

THE REPTILIAN PHYSICAL EXAMINATION

Performing a physical examination on reptiles is similar to performing a physical examination on most mammalian species. All items needed for the physical examination should be ready and within reach. This will help decrease the time in hand and hopefully provide a less stressful experience for both the animal and the veterinary staff. A visual pre-capture physical examination is performed to provide an assessment of the animal's attitude and mentation before it has been stressed by handling.

> *TECHNICIAN NOTE* The pupil in birds and reptiles has striated skeletal muscle. The pupillary light reflex may not be present on examination because of the voluntary control the animal has on pupil constriction.

The reptilian examination is performed in a similar manner to the mammalian species, starting with the head. A pupillary light reflex (PLR) may also be noted.

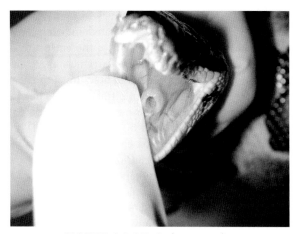

FIGURE 26-17 Oral exam, snake.

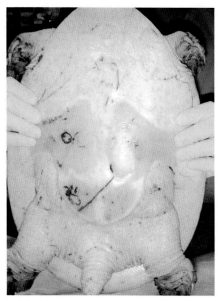

FIGURE 26-18 Systemic infection, chelonian.

Because the pupil consists of striated skeletal muscle, it is not uncommon for a PLR to be absent. The ears or tympanic membranes should also be observed. They should be clean, clear, and free of any debris.

A thorough examination of the oral cavity is an important part of performing a complete physical examination. The oral cavity can be safely opened with either porous tape stirrups or a soft plastic instrument such as a spatula (Figure 26-17). Metal speculums can be used, but caution should be taken to avoid causing trauma to the mouth. The oral cavity should be moist and pink and free of any lesions. During the oral examination, the mouth should be observed for any signs of erythema, stomatitis, or fractured teeth, and for any evidence of plaques on the mucous membranes. As you move down the body, the coelomic cavity should be thoroughly palpated. Palpation of the extremities and tail should then follow. The same techniques used to palpate dogs and cats can be used to palpate most reptiles. It is important to note any abnormalities such as soft tissue swellings, space-occupying masses (such as urinary calculi), developing eggs, neoplasia, and any current or old injuries such as fractures, burn wounds, or other types of trauma.

In snakes, usually the heart, gallbladder, and rib cage and either prey items or feces can be palpated. In lizards, it is sometimes difficult to palpate many of the organs. In some of the larger lizards, the kidneys can be palpated via a rectal examination. It is abnormal to be able to palpate the kidneys without a rectal examination. The kidneys sit in the pelvic girdle and are almost impossible to palpate unless they are enlarged or mineralized. Turtles and tortoises usually present the biggest challenge when trying to perform a complete physical examination. The shell makes it difficult to palpate most of the organs. Depending on the size of the animal, one or two fingers may be placed in the inguinal area between the hind limbs and the shell. This will enable you to palpate the coelomic cavity and look for signs of abnormalities such as cystic calculi, foreign bodies, neoplasia, or potentially eggs. It is also important to make note of the shell quality and color (or skin quality and color in lizards and snakes). If the animal has a systemic infection or is septic, petechiae and ecchymosis can often be found on the shell, especially the plastron. Petechiae and ecchymosis are also seen in other reptiles when a systemic infection or septicemia is present. In snakes, petechiae and ecchymosis are often seen on the ventral aspect of the animal, while in some lizards such as iguanas, petechiae and ecchymosis are commonly seen on the dorsal spines along the animal's back (Figure 26-18).

An accurate heart rate and respiratory rate should be noted during the physical examination. The heart rate is most easily obtained by using a Doppler. Most reptile patients cannot be auscultated with a stethoscope; therefore, the Doppler is an essential tool to have in your practice. In lizards, the Doppler probe should be placed in the same area as a stethoscope would be placed on a dog or cat. In a few species such as monitor lizards, the heart is located much more caudal in the coelomic cavity. In snakes, the Doppler probe will need to be placed on the ventral surface of the cranial proximal third of the body. In chelonians, the Doppler probe is either placed into the thoracic inlet or placed on the neck over the carotid artery (Figure 26-19).

Generally, normal physiologic values in reptiles have an extremely large range. Many reptiles can have a heart rate that ranges from approximately 10 beats per minute to about 80+ beats per minute. Heart rates and respiratory rates can vary depending on ambient temperature, age, species, and health status. The respiratory rate may range from just a few breaths per minute to 20 or more breaths per minute. The body weight will also vary depending on age, sometimes sex, nutritional status, and the species. Patients can range from as little as a few grams to several kilograms. Body condition scoring is also performed on reptiles and follows the same guidelines that are used with mammals. The scale ranges from 1 to 9 with 1 being emaciated and 9 being grossly obese. Landmarks used to score a reptile's body may include palpability of the ribs and pectoral/pelvic girdles as well as the girth of the tail.

Restraint
Snakes

Most snakes can be easily captured directly out of their carrier or cage. If the snake is aggressive, it may be necessary to use a towel along with leather gloves. In these

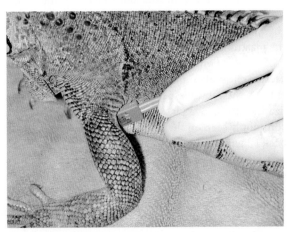

FIGURE 26-19 Doppler probe placement lizard.

cases, gently toss the towel over the snake and find the head. Once the head has been isolated and restrained, the snake can be safely taken out of the enclosure. A snake hook is used if the snake is extremely aggressive or venomous. The hook is used to hold down the head of the snake to prevent it from biting when its head is grabbed by the handler. Pressure is placed just behind the head until the head and body are restrained. Improper use of the snake hook can cause trauma to the patient; therefore, extreme caution should be used and only experienced snake handlers should be involved.

It is important to gently hold the snake directly behind the head with one hand (so it cannot turn around and bite) and support the body with the other hand.

> **TECHNICIAN NOTE** If the snake is large, more than one person may be needed to restrain it. The suggested criteria include one person per 3 feet of snake.

Lizards

Lizards can be challenging animals to both capture and restrain. Smaller lizards are easy to capture but can be difficult to restrain because they tend to squirm while they are being held. Most small lizards can simply be picked up with both hands and taken out of the enclosure. This is also true of the larger lizard species. However, some of the larger lizards can be difficult to both capture and restrain, especially if they are aggressive. If the lizard is aggressive, a towel or blanket along with leather restraint gloves should be used. It is important to remember that lizards can scratch and bite. It is therefore a good idea to wear long sleeves when possible and always keep track of the head. Long-necked lizards such as monitors can easily turn around and bite if their head is not properly restrained during capture. Keeping one hand on the neck, just behind the base of the skull, will help prevent getting bitten.

> **TECHNICIAN NOTE** It is good practice to never capture any species of lizard by the tail. Many species of lizards have a natural predatory response to voluntarily "drop" or autotomize their tail in an attempt to escape predation.

In general, lizards can be restrained by placing one hand around the neck and pectoral girdle region while the other hand can be used to support the body near the pelvis. It is important to remember that not all lizards have durable skin. Some lizards such as geckos have extremely delicate skin that can easily be damaged by capture and restraint.

Chelonians

Although chelonians (turtles and tortoises) are usually the easiest to capture, they are the hardest to restrain. Unless working with extremely large tortoises, most chelonians can just be picked up with both hands and placed on the exam table. When examining large tortoises, it is easiest to set up an exam area within the animal's enclosure or on the floor in the clinic's exam area. Since there is such a great deal of variation in size and strength, restraint techniques may vary between small and large chelonians. Once the animal's body is under control, it is imperative that the head is properly restrained. Although this is relatively easy when the animal is sick, it can be difficult on strong healthy chelonians, especially large tortoises and box turtles.

There are several ways the restrainer can gain control of the animal's head. Many turtles and tortoises are very curious. If they are placed on the table or the ground, they may start walking around to investigate. The handler will be able to grasp their head with one hand while restraining the body with the other hand. To keep control of the head, the thumb is positioned on one side of the cranial portion of the neck and the rest of fingers (or just the index finger for smaller species) on the other side of the neck just behind the base of the skull. Healthy chelonians are strong so it may take a lot of constant but gentle force to keep the turtle or tortoise's head out of the shell. If the animal is extremely active, an additional person may be necessary to help restrain the limbs and body.

Another way to gain control of the head is by trying to coax the animal out of its shell. Many chelonians will extend their head out of the shell if food is offered or if placed in a container of shallow warm water. Once the head is extended, the same techniques mentioned previously can be used to gain and keep control of the animal's head. If these techniques fail, it may be possible to slip a small blunt ear curette or spay hook under the horny portion of the upper beak, known as the rhinotheca. Once the probe has been placed, it can be gently pulled back to extend the neck to a position for the restrainer to grasp. It is important to note that this technique can be dangerous. The beak can be chipped or broken if the animal struggles or is in poor health. If a spay hook is the

tool of choice, it may be a good idea to pad the hooked portion of the instrument. Padding can simply consist of tape or an elastic wrap cut to the appropriate size.

> **TECHNICIAN NOTE** Caution should be taken when dealing with any aquatic turtle, especially snapping turtles. These species of turtles have a tendency to bite, and many of the larger turtles can cause serious bodily harm to the people working with them.

Box turtles can be the most challenging chelonians to properly restrain. Since box turtles have a hinge on their plastron, many species are able to completely tuck themselves into their shells. The easiest way to extend their head is to gently prop open the cranial portion of the carapace (upper shell) and the plastron (lower shell). Extreme care must be taken when trying to prop the shell open. It is suggested that a well-padded object be used when attempting this. This will help avoid traumatizing or fracturing the shell. Another way to extend a box turtle's head is to grasp one of the forelimbs, keeping the leg extended out of the shell until the head can be successfully pulled out and properly restrained. This method works well because once the leg is extended, the turtle will usually not close its shell down on its own leg. It is important to remember that any of these capture and restraint techniques can potentially cause a fair amount of stress to the patient. If initial attempts at capture and restraint are not successful, chemical restraint may be necessary for any reptile, especially large tortoises and box turtles (Figure 26-20).

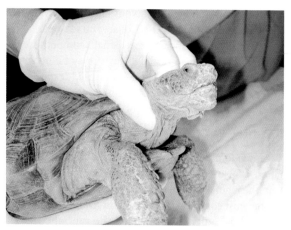

FIGURE 26-20 Chelonian restraint.

Common Venipuncture Sites in Reptiles
Snakes

The two common venipuncture sites in snakes include the caudal tail vein and the heart. Drawing blood from the tail vein is best accomplished in large snakes because it can be difficult in small snakes due to the size of the vessel. The same method used to draw blood from the ventral midline approach in lizards is used in snakes as well. Obtaining a blood sample from the heart (also called cardiocentesis) is the quickest method that will yield a large amount of blood. A 27- to 22-gauge needle attached to a 1- or 3-ml syringe is used for blood collection (size of needles and syringes will depend on the size of the snake). To obtain a blood sample, the snake should first be placed in dorsal recumbency. The heart can then be located in the cranial third of the body. The heart can move both cranially and caudally so it is best to place your thumb and index finger on either side of the heart. Look for the caudal portion of the beating heart. The needle insertion site should be two scutes (scales) below that. To obtain blood, the needle should be inserted between two scutes at a 45-degree angle. It is important to not poke around searching for the heart. Insert the needle in one fluid motion. Place slight negative pressure on the syringe and let the beating of the heart slowly fill the syringe. The palatine vessels can be used in some instances, but this technique is not suggested because it is difficult to provide hemostasis, the vessels are very small, and the mouth is filled with bacteria.

Lizards

The cephalic, jugular, and ventral abdominal vessels can be used to obtain a blood sample from various species of lizards you may encounter in your clinic; however, these vessels are not commonly used for several reasons. (1) The cephalic vein is usually extremely small, and because this is a "blind stick," a surgical cut-down may be necessary. (2) The ventral abdominal vein is not used (especially in awake animals) because of the inability to both properly restrain the animal and control hemorrhage. (3) Lastly, the jugular vein is not commonly used because in many species it is also a "blind stick" and may require a surgical cut-down to access the vessel. Lymphatic fluid contamination is also common when performing venipuncture from the jugular vein, which will skew your blood values.

The most common vessel used for lizard venipuncture is the caudal tail vein, also called the ventral coccygeal vein. There are two different techniques commonly used

to obtain blood from this vessel. These techniques include a lateral and a ventral approach. To successfully obtain a blood sample from either approach, a 1-inch or 1½-inch 27- to 20-gauge needle attached to a 1- or 3-ml syringe should be used. The size of the needle and syringe will depend on the size of your patient. Insulin syringes can be used on very small lizards, but remember to remove the needle before putting the blood into the appropriate tubes. The small needle size can cause lysis of the blood cells if pushed through the needle (the same is true for 26- or 25-gauge needles). It is important that the tail is gently restrained during the blood draw. The left hand can be used to restrain the caudal portion of the tail, while the right hand can be used to perform the blood draw. If you are left handed, just obtain your blood sample from the other side of the tail using your left hand to draw blood and your right hand to gently restrain the tail.

For a lateral approach, the needle should be inserted into the tail (between two scales) at approximately a 90-degree angle. Slowly insert the needle into the tail, keeping slight negative pressure on the syringe until either blood enters the syringe or the needle touches the vertebrae. If the needle is touching the vertebrae, slowly back the needle off the bone (still keeping slight negative pressure on the syringe) and redirect the needle into the vessel. It is important to put only slight negative pressure on the syringe while obtaining the blood sample. Too much negative pressure may collapse the vessel.

The technique for the ventral midline approach is very similar to that for the lateral approach. The needle should be inserted on midline into the tail (between two scales) at approximately a 90-degree angle. The needle should be slowly inserted into the tail, keeping slight negative pressure on the syringe until either blood enters the syringe or the needle touches the vertebrae. The blood vessel is located just ventral to the vertebrae. If you touch the vertebrae first, slowly back off of the bone until your needle is seated within the vessel (Figure 26-21).

Lizards usually struggle when they are placed on their backs, making it difficult to draw blood from them. Therefore, it is important to keep the animal in sternal recumbency while obtaining the blood sample.

Chelonians

The brachial plexus, subcarapacial venous sinus, and jugular vein are the major sites where blood can be obtained from a turtle or tortoise. The venipuncture site will depend on the size and species of the patient and the

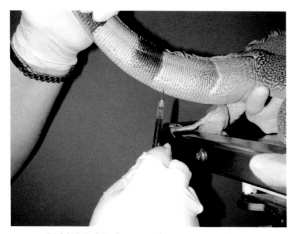

FIGURE 26-21 Lateral venipuncture, lizard.

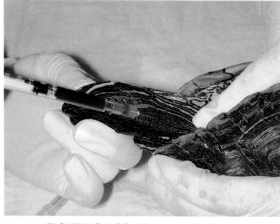

FIGURE 26-22 Chelonian venipuncture.

preference of the phlebotomist. If drawing blood from the jugular vein, the turtle/tortoise should be placed in lateral recumbency. The head and neck should be pulled away from the shell. The jugular vein can be found in the same plane as the eye and the tympanum. To obtain the sample, the phlebotomist will hold the head while the restrainer will keep the patient in lateral recumbency. A 27- to 20-gauge needle attached to a 1- to 3-ml syringe is used and will vary depending on the size of the patient. The subcarapacial venous sinus is used when jugular venipuncture is not an option. Depending on the size of the patient, a 1- to 1½-inch 27- to 20-gauge needle or a 2-inch spinal needle attached to a 1- to 3-ml syringe is used to obtain the blood sample. The needle is inserted upward at about a 60-degree angle just dorsal to the neck. Slight negative pressure should be applied on the syringe until either blood enters the syringe or bone is encountered. If bone is encountered, back away from the bone and redirect the needle. The brachial plexus, also called the ulnar venous plexus, can be used in most chelonian species. Pull the front limb away from the body and palpate the tendon near the radiohumeral joint. Generally, a 22- to 20-gauge needle attached to a 1- to 3-ml syringe is inserted at a 90-degree angle to the skin and angled towards the radiohumeral joint. The tail vein can also be used in chelonians. The same technique used in lizards can also be applied to chelonian species (Figure 26-22).

Intraosseous Catheters

It is not possible to place an IO catheter in snakes. In lizards, an IO catheter is often placed in the femur,

humerus, or tibial crest. Turtles and tortoises are difficult, but IO catheters can be attempted in the bridge of the carapace, the cranial portion of the gular scute, and the distal humerus or femur.

In reptiles, the IO catheter is placed in the distal end of the femur. This is opposite of what is done in mammalian species. The catheter is placed in the distal portion of the femur because the femoral head and greater trochanter are not easily palpated because of how they insert into the acetabulum. General placement techniques described in the mammalian section are used in reptiles as well.

IO catheterization placement in the tibial crest is done in the same manner as described in the mammalian section.

IO catheter placement in chelonian species can be difficult. There are several sites that can potentially be utilized for catheterization. The same technique described with mammals can also be used for IO catheter placement into the distal humerus and femur in turtles and tortoises.

The other two IO catheterization sites in chelonians include the cranial portion of the gular scute (bony projection found under the neck) and the cranial plastrocarapacial junction (bridge between the carapace and plastron or upper and lower shell). The shell consists of living bone and tissue under the top keratinized layer. A catheter can actually be drilled into the marrow cavity of the shell, allowing systemic access for drug and fluid delivery.

The shell is first aseptically prepared. A pilot hole is then created with a drill allowing for the spinal needle to be easily placed into the marrow cavity. Once the spinal needle is inserted, it is secured with sterile tissue glue. Placement can be verified by aspiration of bone marrow or by visualization via a dorsoventral radiograph.

IV Catheter Placement

Table 26-4 summarizes frequently used IV catheterization sites in reptiles.

Snakes

Snakes are generally difficult! The first choice for catheter placement is the tail vein. Due to the transverse processes of the vertebrae, the ventral approach is much easier than the lateral approach, but both can be done. If the ventral approach is going to be used, the snake must first be placed on its back. The skin is aseptically prepared in the same manner as with dogs and cats. The catheter should be flushed with heparinized saline and inserted between two scales at approximately a 20-degree angle. The scales are keratinized; therefore, inserting a catheter through a scale would be like inserting it through a fingernail.

The tail vein is located caudal to the "vent." If the patient is a male, the reproductive organs are housed in two diverticular sacs caudal to the "vent." The reproductive organs extend the length of about 7 to 11 scales depending on species. The catheter must be placed caudal to the reproductive organs. If the snake is a female,

the catheter can be placed more cranial to the vent. The catheter should be slowly inserted until either blood enters the hub of the catheter or bone is touched. If the catheter touches bone, it has been inserted too far and needs to be backed out slightly until it is seated into the vessel. Once blood enters the hub, the catheter should be pushed off of the stylet and seated into the vessel in the same manner as catheter placement in any other species. A T-port or intermittent infusion plug should be placed, and the catheter should be flushed with heparinized saline. The catheter is then taped into place in the same manner as you would a cephalic catheter in a dog or cat.

The same placement technique is used for the lateral approach but again placement at this site is more difficult because of the transverse processes of the vertebrae.

The second IV catheter site used in snakes is the jugular vein. The jugular vein cannot be seen without performing a surgical cut-down. The jugular vein is located between the base of the skull and the heart, in the cranial third of the body. Either the left or the right side can be used. The skin must be aseptically prepared and ideally draped. Sterile gloves should be worn while placing the catheter. Since this is a surgical procedure, a veterinarian must perform the cut-down. Once the jugular vessel is isolated, the catheter can be inserted and sutured into place. Jugular catheters are often placed for major surgical procedures and in snakes that are very ill.

Lizards

Catheters can be placed into the jugular and cephalic vessels of lizards. These vessels require a surgical cut-down for placement and in many species these veins are often quite small; therefore, they are not utilized very often. As with snakes, either the lateral or the ventral approach to the vessel can be used, but the ventral approach is generally much easier. The same techniques described for snakes are used for lizards as well.

Some people advocate IV catheter placement into the abdominal vein of lizards. This is a procedure that can be performed; however, a surgical cut-down is necessary. Catheterization at this site is hard to maintain and impractical.

Chelonians

The tail vein can potentially be used in turtles and tortoises. The same techniques described in snakes can be used for chelonians as well.

TABLE 26-4	Common Catheterization Sites in Reptiles	
REPTILE	**COMMON VESSEL SITE(S)**	**CATHETER SIZE (GAUGE)**
Snake	Jugular: must perform surgical cut-down; not common Tail: ventral aspect is most common, potentially can place from lateral aspect	26 to 20 IV catheter; depends on size of patient
Lizards	Jugular and cephalic: must perform surgical cut-down; not common Tail: ventral aspect is most common, potentially can place from lateral aspect	26 to 20 IV catheter; depends on size of patient
Chelonians	Jugular: most common Tail: placed in same manner as a lizard or snake	26 to 20 IV catheter; depends on size of patient

The jugular vein is the most commonly used vessel for IV catheterization in turtles and tortoises. The jugular vein is located within the same plane as the tympanum and the eye. Chelonians are generally placed into lateral recumbency (same manner as with venipuncture of the jugular vein) with the head and neck extended away from the body and the legs restrained alongside the body/shell. The person placing the catheter will usually restrain the head and neck. The person restraining the body can use his or her finger or a Q-tip to hold off the vessel at the thoracic inlet. The catheter site should be aseptically prepared before catheter placement. The catheter is held at approximately a 20-degree angle to the neck and jugular vessel. Once the vessel is stabilized, the catheter can be inserted and advanced once a flash is observed within the hub. This vessel is fragile and can blow once the catheter is inserted. Do not pull the catheter out if this happens because this will generally cause a larger hematoma. Keep inserting the catheter until it is seated within the vessel.

Once the catheter is properly seated within the vein, a T-port or intermittent infusion plug should be placed. The catheter should be flushed with heparinized saline and sutured into place. A "butterfly" piece of tape is placed around the hub of the catheter and tacked down to the skin using a simple interrupted suture on each side of the tape. A light wrap can then be placed around the neck.

Fluid Therapy

Fluids can be administered to reptiles by slow bolus via IV or IO catheters, or by SQ injection. Using a syringe attached to a butterfly catheter is often the quickest and easiest way to administer SQ fluids. To help avoid fluid overload, a syringe pump should be used to administer fluids via the IV or IO routes.

Tube Feeding

Hand and tube feeding is relatively simple in lizards and can be readily taught to most clients when necessary. Tube feeding in reptiles can take up to three people in the larger species. One person should be properly restraining the patient while one person opens the mouth. A proper speculum must be used to avoid trauma to the oral cavity. The feeding tube is marked by measuring from the lizard's nose to the last rib. The feeding tube is prefilled with the desired food to account for dead space. The tube is lubricated and passed gently over the glottis (located at the base of the tongue) and down the esophagus to the premarked site (done by the third person). The person administering the food should carefully watch for signs of regurgitation. Administering the food too quickly can cause it to back up into the oral cavity. Syringe feeding usually takes place one to two times a day in lizards and turtles/tortoises. Snakes may only need to be fed one time per week. Rubber feeding tubes are most often used in reptilian patients. The type of food and volume will depend on the species with which you are working and the size of the patient. Commercial hand-feeding formulas such as the Oxbow® and Emeraid® lines are commonly used. Homemade diets can be formulated as well as long as they are nutritionally sound.

Injections

Because of the renal portal system, injections should be administered cranial to the kidneys (the same is true for birds). SQ injections can be administered by tenting the skin in the dorsal scapular or femoral areas. IM injections are generally administered in the front legs.

Anesthesia

Anesthesia can be challenging in reptiles. Premedications should ideally be given before any anesthetic induction. Common premedications include butorphanol, morphine, midazolam, ketamine, telazol, and dexmedetomidine used in various combinations. Premedications are given intramuscularly in the front limbs and should be given at least 30 to 60 minutes before anesthetic induction. It is important to keep the patient warm, enabling them to properly metabolize the drugs.

While the premedications are taking effect, you, as the anesthetist, should prepare for the anesthetic procedure. All instrumentation should be organized and ready to place once the patient has been anesthetized. Common monitoring techniques used for reptiles during anesthesia include heart rate (HR), respiratory rate (RR), mucous membrane (MM) color, ECG, Doppler, sphygmomanometer, blood pressure (BP) cuff, ETCO$_2$, and a temperature probe. The ECG is placed in the same manner as in mammals if you are going to use ECG pads. In some cases, these do not work well because of the scales; therefore, alligator clips can also be used, but the teeth should be flattened when possible. Sometimes these techniques do not work or the patient's skin may be too delicate. If this is the case, needles can be pushed through the skin with the alligator clips attached to the needles.

An IV or IO catheter should be placed when possible. Ideally the IV or IO catheter is placed before anesthetic induction, although this is nearly impossible in most reptile species. Having an IV or IO catheter in place will provide systemic access if an emergency occurs during induction and it also provides easy access for anesthetic induction. Injectable anesthetics are generally preferred over inhalant inductions because reptiles can hold their breath for long periods of time.

Propofol is the most common injectable anesthetic drug used in reptiles. If a catheter is not possible, propofol can be given using a butterfly catheter or a normal syringe and needle. Propofol is given slowly over a few minutes. Once the patient has been induced, it should be intubated and placed on isoflurane at an appropriate percentage. Sevoflurane can be used, but does not seem to work as well in many reptile species. The patient should be placed on a ventilator or bagged by hand to provide intermittent positive pressure ventilation (IPPV) throughout the procedure since reptiles do not breathe well on their own while under anesthesia. It is very important to keep the patient at an appropriate temperature during the surgical procedure. For most species of reptiles, core body temperature should be kept between about 85° and 90° F. If the patient is kept too cold, the drugs may take hours to metabolize and the patient will likely have a prolonged recovery time. Lactated Ringer's solution is commonly used at a rate of 5 ml/kg/hr.

COMMON SNAKE EMERGENCIES

Predator/prey syndrome is seen in snakes that are fed live prey (e.g., rats, mice). This occurs because the owner leaves the prey item in the cage unsupervised and if the snake does not eat it (due to anorexia, stress, poor husbandry, for example), the prey item becomes hungry and starts chewing on the snake. Management includes wound care (cleaning and débriding), radiographs, complete blood count (CBC) and chemistry panels, antibiotics, and fluid therapy. Subcutaneous crystalloid fluids are administered, but can also be given intracoelomically at 10 to 30 ml/kg/day. The patient often needs wet to dry bandaging until the wounds are healed. Wounds in snakes can take several weeks to months to fully heal. Patients need to be heavily sedated or anesthetized for wound care (Figure 26-23).

Anorexia can be seen in any snake, but it is very common in species such as ball pythons. It is not un-

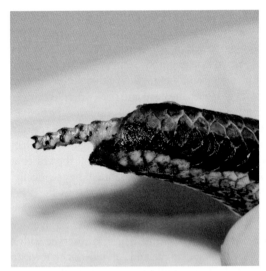

FIGURE 26-23 Wound in snake.

common for some species of snake to go for 6 months or more without eating. Common causes of anorexia include improper husbandry and environmental conditions, wrong prey being offered, stomatitis, and general disease. Supportive care with subcutaneous or intracoelomic fluids should be given at 10 to 30 ml/kg/day as well as soaking for 15 to 30 minutes, one to two times daily in warm water. Tube feeding should start off slow with either just water or a very diluted carnivore liquid formula. As the snake becomes more stable, the caloric value can be increased each week. In many cases, snakes are only tube fed about one time per week until they are healthy again and eating on their own.

COMMON REPTILIAN EMERGENCIES
Metabolic Bone Disease

Metabolic bone disease (MBD) is common in lizards such as iguanas, chameleons, and geckos. MBD is an umbrella term used to cover a variety of disease processes caused by poor husbandry and diet. Dietary imbalances (either too little or too much) of vitamin D_3, calcium, and phosphorus can lead to MBD as well as improper lighting and temperature gradients. Signs of MBD include slow growth, kyphosis of the spine, seizures, tremors, twitching, anorexia, thickening or softening of the bone, and fractures. Damage to the bones is generally not reversible. Patients presenting with MBD need supportive care including proper temperature support for the specific species, fluid therapy (can be IV, IO, SQ, ICe

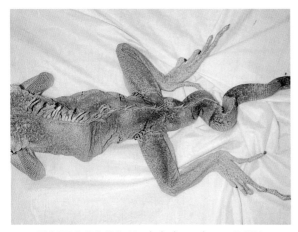

FIGURE 26-24 Metabolic bone disease (MBD).

[intracoelomic], or soaking in warm water bath), force feeding species appropriate diet, and if needed calcium supplementation. Basic diagnostics include radiographs, CBC, ionized calcium, and chemistry panels. Long-term treatment and husbandry changes are required to properly treat this disease (Figure 26-24).

Reptile Dystocia and Egg Binding

A very gravid lizard will often go off feed and therefore needs to be on an adequate plane of nutrition, including adequate calcium intake, before laying her clutch. Appropriate environmental conditions also need to be met, with a species-appropriate ambient temperature and provision of an appropriate nesting area. The nest box should be large enough for the lizard to enter and turn around in and contain moist bedding at least 2 inches deep. If any of the previously mentioned conditions are not met, then the lizard may become egg-bound (i.e., unable to lay her eggs).

Hypocalcemia may precede and be an underlying cause of egg binding, or the egg-bound condition itself can result in a hypocalcemic state. The typical egg-bound lizard initially arrives at the clinic anorectic and lethargic. In the later stages, egg-bound lizards may demonstrate profound weakness, dehydration, muscular twitching, and sometimes overt seizures due to hypocalcemia.

Diagnosis is based on history, clinical signs, and usually radiography. Although reptiles have eggs that appear similar to avian eggs on a radiograph, reptiles often have soft-shelled eggs with almost a soft tissue density (often described as leathery).

Critical patients should first receive medical treatment. Start with providing an appropriate environment, warm-water soaks, rehydration, and calcium supplementation. Critical or very ill patients will likely require surgical salpingectomy. The patient should be stabilized before surgery with SQ, ICe, IV, or IO fluids; warmth; and calcium supplementation.

Abscesses

Reptiles form caseous abscesses that often appear as firm, raised swellings. These abscesses are usually traumatic in origin and can be found anywhere on the body.

Treatment consists of aggressive surgical excision of the abscess, followed by copious flushing with antibacterial solution such as chlorhexidine (Nolvasan). The abscess should be left open to heal by second intention.

Foreign Bodies

Foreign body ingestion is not uncommon in lizards and chelonians that are allowed to roam freely around the home or outside. Wood chips and other indigestible bedding material can also cause potential GI blockage.

Foreign bodies should be on the "rule out list" for any anorectic lizard. Anorexia and lack of fecal production may be the only clinical signs of blockage early in the condition. Progressive dehydration, emaciation, and profound weakness will develop in later stages.

Radiography is often diagnostic; treatment of obstructive foreign bodies is surgical. IV or IO catheterization for fluid support is advisable in more advanced cases. Antibiotics such as amikacin may be indicated in cases in which abdominal contamination from GI leakage is suspected (Figure 26-25).

Renal Failure

Renal failure in reptiles mimics the clinical picture of MBD. Symptoms include dehydration, lethargy, anorexia, and often secondary osteomalacia. Diagnosis is possible with radiography and evaluation of blood calcium, phosphorous, and uric acid levels. On radiographs, the renal silhouette will often be enlarged and radiodense, and dystrophic mineralization of tissues may be visualized.

Treatment includes IV or IO fluids, supplementation of calcium if loss has occurred, and oral phosphate binders if hyperphosphatemia is present. Husbandry changes are usually necessary as dehydration is often a key factor in renal failure.

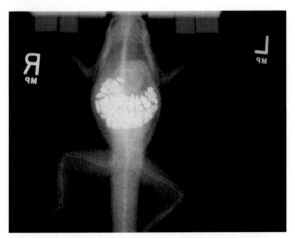

FIGURE 26-25 Radiograph foreign body, lizard.

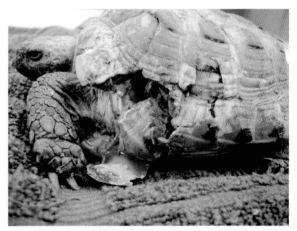

FIGURE 26-26 Shell fracture.

COMMON CHELONIAN EMERGENCIES

Chelonians can present for pneumonia any time of the year, but it is most commonly seen after awaking from hibernation. Signs include lethargy, anorexia, dyspnea, nasal discharge, and buoyancy issues in aquatic turtles. Diagnostics include radiographs and/or computed tomography, CBC, and blood chemistry panels. Supportive care and treatment involve fluid therapy, force-feeding, proper heating in enclosure, and antimicrobial therapy. Fluids are given subcutaneously or intracoelomically (soaking, IV, and IO are also potential options).

Hypovitaminosis A is most commonly seen in aquatic turtles. As with most reptile emergencies or diseases in general, it is caused by poor husbandry—specifically a diet lacking in vitamin A. Patients present with conjunctivitis, blepharitis, nasal discharge, swollen eyelids, aural abscesses, and dyspnea. Supportive care includes fluid therapy and tube feeding if needed, treatment with parenteral vitamin A, and husbandry corrections. Ear abscesses often need to be lanced and cleaned.

Being hit by a car can happen to any reptile, but it is most commonly seen in wild turtles and tortoises (at least those that survive long enough to make it to the hospital). Shell cracks and fractures are most commonly seen after being hit by a car. Basic supportive care should be administered starting with pain management, fluid therapy, heat support, and wound care. Fluids can be administered SQ, IV, IO, or ICe although subcutaneous is the most common route. Subcutaneous fluids are usually administered into the inguinal or axillary regions. You should always aspirate before injection to make sure your needle is not in the bladder or lung. Soaking is not recommended for patients with shell fractures. Once the patient has been stabilized, the shell fractures can be managed. The extent of the crack or fracture will dictate treatment. Superficial cracks can be treated by applying quick-drying epoxy with or without sterile fiberglass attached to the shell. Full-thickness fractures will likely need surgical intervention before the shell is sealed (Figure 26-26).

The avians, reptiles, and **exotic small animals** patient bring another set of challenges, especially when they arrive in an emergent state. The veterinary technician can develop lifesaving skill sets to assist in caring for these unique patients by attending continuing education seminars and volunteering in wildlife centers. Many veterinarians who specialize in this area welcome other veterinary professionals to visit and observe. All involved in emergency medicine are encouraged to be open to learning about all species since being prepared for anything to enter the hospital is the first step in saving lives.

SUGGESTED READINGS

Ballard BM, Cheek R: *Exotic animal medicine for the veterinary technician*, ed 2, New York, 2010, Wiley-Blackwell.

Bryant S: *Anesthesia for veterinary technicians*, New York, 2010, Wiley-Blackwell.

Carpenter JW, et al.: *Exotic animal formulary*, ed 4, St Louis, 2013, Elsevier.

Harrison GJ, Bightfoot TL: *Clinical avian medicine, Volumes 1 and 2.* Palm Beach, FL, 2006, Spix Publishing.

Longley LA: *Anaesthesia of exotic pets*, St Louis, 2008, Saunders.
Mader DR: *Reptile medicine and surgery*, St Louis, 2006, Saunders.
Mader DR, Divers SJ: *Current therapy in reptile medicine and surgery*, St Louis, 2014, Saunders.
Mitchell M, Tully T Jr: *Manual of exotic pet practice*, St Louis, 2008, Elsevier Health.

Quesenberry KE, Carpenter JW: *Ferrets, rabbits, and rodents: clinical medicine and surgery*, ed 3, St Louis, 2012, Saunders.
Ritchie BW, et al.: *Avian medicine: principals and application*, Lake Worth, FL, 1994, Wingers Publishing.
www.lafebervet.com.

SCENARIO

Scenario

A 5-year-old, female spayed Netherland Dwarf rabbit presents to the clinic for a 36-hour history of lethargy, anorexia, bruxism, and drooling. On physical examination, you find crusting on the forelimbs and a lack of gut sounds in all four quadrants. The vital signs are as follows: heart rate 300 beats/min, respiratory rate 100/min, pulse weak, mucous membranes pink, capillary refill time 3 seconds. The patient is quiet, alert, and responsive and is slightly dehydrated based on skin turgor and capillary refill time.

Questions

- Would you consider the initial assessment normal?
- How would you categorize the level of severity of this patient?
- Are there any other diagnostics to consider?
- How would you proceed with stabilization?
- Would this patient require hospitalization?

Discussion

Based on the presentation, this patient likely has GI stasis secondary to dental disease. This is an emergency. Dental disease is common in exotic small mammals such as rabbits. Rabbits are hindgut fermenters. Anorexia for as little as 12 to 24 hours can lead to GI stasis and death if not quickly treated. Dental disease is also very painful. Pain often leads to inappetence and anorexia in most exotic small mammals.

To properly work-up this patient, a complete blood count and biochemistry panel should be performed. This will help assess overall organ function. A thorough oral examination should be performed. This is done using an oral specula with a light source. The entire mouth, including the molars and premolars should be visualized. Thorough oral exams generally need to be performed under heavy sedation or anesthesia. If further assessment of the oral cavity is deemed necessary, skull radiographs and a CT can be performed.

This patient needs to be stabilized. While most of the vital signs are within normal limits, the patient is dehydrated and would benefit from fluid therapy. Common fluid routes include intravenous, subcutaneous, and intraosseous (only when IV access is not an option). Routes are chosen based on the patient's status.

Pain management is extremely important. Opioids should be chosen based on the type of pain being experienced. Most dental pain is moderate to severe. Buprenorphine is acceptable for mild to moderate pain, but full mu opioids should be used for patients experiencing severe pain.

Lastly, this patient should be syringe-fed. Rabbits need to eat frequently throughout the day to keep the GI tract moving properly. A commercial critical care diet made for herbivores should be administered in multiple small meals throughout the day.

MEDICAL MATH EXERCISE

Calculate the hourly fluid rate in milliliters required for a 3-kg rabbit, using a rate of 60 ml/kg/day.

## 27

Disaster Medicine

Amy N. Breton

KEY TERMS

Decontamination
Posttraumatic stress
 disorder
Search and rescue
Triage

CHAPTER OUTLINE

Legal Issues
Types of Disasters
Triaging
 START Method
 SAVE Method
Owner in the Disaster
Self-Protection
Common Emergencies
 Shock
 Orthopedic and Soft Tissue Injuries
 Wounds
 Neurologic Injuries
 Hyperthermia and Hypothermia
 Smoke and Burn Injuries
 Near Drowning

Search and Rescue Canines
 Stray Animals
 Decontamination
Surgery
Record Keeping
Rechecking Appointments
**Helping the Local Veterinary
 Infrastructure**
Personal Recovery after the Disaster
Structure of a Disaster
Becoming Involved
Joining a Team
Disaster Training
Conclusion

LEARNING OBJECTIVES

After studying this chapter, you will be able to:

- Understand what a disaster is and how the veterinary community is affected.
- Understand the various methods of mass triaging.
- Understand the environmental and mental hazards of working in a disaster.
- Understand how to set up and create a clinic disaster plan.
- Understand the legal issues of volunteering in a disaster team.
- Understand how to join a disaster team.

Disaster medicine has been a topic in veterinary medicine for the past 25 years. However, after the terrorist attacks in the United States on September 11, 2001 (often referred to as *9/11*), disaster medicine was a topic that was pushed to the forefront. Before that event, most of veterinary disaster medicine was focused on natural disasters. The veterinary community trained and planned their response in the event of a hurricane, tornado, flood, or earthquake. After 9/11, the focus shifted to how the industry should deal with artificially created disasters. However, Hurricane Katrina showed the veterinary community the horrific devastation that can occur from a natural disaster. As a result of the poor response to Hurricane Katrina, many veterinarians, animal organizations, and state and local officials worked together to help

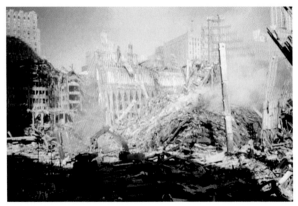

FIGURE 27-1 Scene from New York City World Trade Center after the terrorist attack of September 11, 2001.

create the PETS Act, which was signed into law by President George W. Bush on October 6, 2006 (Government Tracking of Bills, 2013). The PETS Act requires local and state emergency preparedness authorities to include in their evacuation plans how they will accommodate household pets and service animals in case of a disaster (Government Tracking of Bills, 2013). Local and state authorities must submit these plans in order to qualify for grants from the Federal Emergency Management Agency (FEMA) (Government Tracking of Bills, 2013).

Approximately 46% of Americans own a pet; therefore when a disaster strikes, animals usually are involved (Humane Society of the United States, 2013).

> *TECHNICIAN NOTE* Today veterinarians and technicians are considered first responders (Figure 27-1). When pets are injured the public will seek the help of the local veterinary community. The recent disasters such as Hurricane Sandy, tornadoes in the Midwest, and wild fires in Colorado and California have shown that veterinary professionals are not prepared for care of the animals in their communities.

Disaster medicine can appear vastly different from the medicine that veterinary professionals practice every day. Even during the busiest times, such as when working in an emergency department, some control of the situation is possible. During a disaster, the situation can quickly become out of control at any moment. Technicians should understand what types of disasters they might experience and how to handle different disaster

situations. In addition, all veterinary hospitals should have an established disaster plan. Being prepared before a disaster will help prevent the veterinary hospital from becoming a victim during a disaster.

Disaster medicine is vastly different from other disciplines of veterinary medicine. A disaster occurs when community resources become overwhelmed, causing the inability to function normally (Heath, 1999). This type of situation is unpredictable, whether it is artificially or naturally created. Artificially created disasters include terrorism events, fires, and hazardous material spills. Examples of natural disasters include fires, hurricanes, tornados, tsunamis, earthquakes, and droughts.

Working as a technician during a disaster is vastly different from working as a technician in a clinic setting. Stress, working conditions, types and numbers of animals involved, and the legal issues of working during a disaster all contribute to making it a unique and challenging situation.

Stress is a common feature in the daily life of an emergency critical care veterinary technician. Multiple traumas, a fast-paced environment, and the inability to take breaks are all considered routine, and the stress experienced is multifaceted. Most technicians who become involved in a disaster situation reside near or in the town where the disaster has occurred. The local veterinary hospital may be the only functioning veterinary hospital in town; therefore the amount of responsibility for those who work at the hospital can become enormous during a disaster, and the clinic may become overwhelmed with people and their pets.

> *TECHNICIAN NOTE* Individuals assisting during the crisis should care for their family members and themselves first—only then will they be able to remain truly focused on the needs of others.

The conditions (Figure 27-2) encountered during a disaster are different from those found in a regular clinic setting and can contribute to an already stressful situation. Working outdoors, with limited supplies, unfamiliar people, and different organizations, is considered common. Mosquitoes, gnats, flies, and other insects may be numerous. Keeping patients clean and dry may be very difficult, and surgery may not be possible.

Even the smallest things that are taken for granted may become luxuries. For example, electricity and

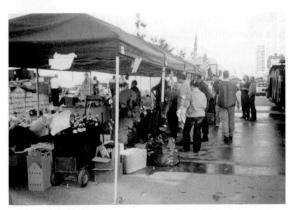

FIGURE 27-2 Outside veterinary field hospital.

running water may not be available. A clinic that is affected by a disaster must look at its capabilities in the aftermath of the disaster. Members of the clinic should fully assess what they *can* offer versus what they *cannot* offer to the public. Looking at the entire situation and assessing what would be most beneficial for the clinic and the clients are important.

Locating a fully functioning veterinary hospital (outside of the devastated area) to which clients can be referred is critical. Hospitals that are not fully functioning may be used as boarding facilities. The staff needed for boarding animals is minimal in comparison to a staff needed to medically treat animals and will therefore allow staff members to have more time to deal with personal problems caused by the disaster. Creating an individual and community veterinary hospital disaster plan will help alleviate some of the stress associated with assisting in an artificially created or natural disaster (Box 27-1).

The types of animals needing assistance during a disaster may be numerous. The area veterinary hospitals involved must know their limitations. A protocol should be created for employees to follow. Local farmers, wildlife rehabilitators, park rangers, game wardens, zookeepers, and members from the United States Fish and Wildlife Service can be used as a resource; they can assist in developing the protocols and training the support staff on handling different species.

LEGAL ISSUES

Veterinary professionals who help in a disaster must comprehend the legal issues involved in the situation. Injuries to the support staff, animals, and owners must be understood and addressed. Before joining a disaster team, you should be sure to ask yourself the following questions:

- Do you have health insurance?
- What will happen if you become injured and cannot work?
- Will your job allow you to take time off to help with disaster relief?

Workers' compensation does not apply when someone is injured outside of his or her job. An employer is not required to keep a staff person's position available if the person volunteers and is injured during a disaster. Addressing these concerns and talking to the employer before accepting to volunteer are important.

Most responders fall under the protection of the Good Samaritan laws. In each state the Good Samaritan laws regarding animals may vary. The clinic staff should know if the state in which they are working has a written Good Samaritan animal law that protects individuals who volunteer to help during a disaster.

The American Animal Hospital Association took a stand regarding veterinarians and technicians when they published the following position statement:

> *"Any veterinarian or veterinary technician who, in good faith, renders emergency care, without remuneration or expectation of remuneration, to a sick or injured animal shall not be liable for any civil damages resulting from his or her acts or omission, except for such damages as may result from acts of gross negligence or wanton acts or omissions."*

This type of law would serve to encourage veterinarians and veterinary technicians to assist with emergency veterinary care (American Animal Hospital Association Board of Directors, 1994).

TYPES OF DISASTERS

- **Terrorism: Search and rescue** (S&R) dogs with burned or lacerated feet are common. Smoke or other toxic gas inhalation may cause the dogs to become very sick. Dehydration from overwork and heat is common. Stress diarrhea may also occur. Animals may be trapped inside nearby buildings and arrive at the clinic stressed, dehydrated, and emaciated.
- **Foreign animal disease:** Veterinarians working with large animals are usually the first to diagnose foreign animal disease. Veterinarians should carry with

BOX 27-1	Veterinary Clinic Disaster Plan Details

- Basic responsibilities
  Establish an incident command system (ICS) for the clinic.
  Keep current contact information for all employees.
- Information to be kept offsite
  Insurance papers
  Inventory of everything (with cost)
  Written business plan
  Copy of computer records (updated and replaced every week)
  Pictures of and receipts for items used in the clinic
  Pictures of the clinic (interior and exterior)
  List of suppliers, contact numbers, and delivery schedule
- Explanation of the clinic's role during a disaster
- Policies created before the disaster
  Will the clinic accept wildlife?
  Will the clinic accept farm animals?
  Will the clinic function as a kennel for strays?
- Charging clients during disasters
  Will the clinic work for free, at a discount, or remain closed?
  Will the clinic donate goods and services to those in need?
- Establishing a community veterinary disaster plan
  Talk to colleagues and get phone numbers.
  Develop an agreement before the disaster occurs.
  Decide if profits are shared.
  Decide to use another clinic for a certain percentage of patients.
  Determine what equipment is available for use at other clinics.
  Decide if personnel can be exchanged to help at other clinics.
  Find a clinic outside an affected area that may be able to help. If all clinics are out of service, find out if a larger facility exists out of the area.
  Find an off-site location where clinics can pool resources.
  Compile a verbal stockpile system for pharmaceuticals.
  Discover if a facility is available for isolating animals.
  Animals with bite wounds (possible rabies)
  Animals with the same disease (if in large numbers)
- Maintaining accurate records of animals seen
  Have a form in duplicate ready to use.
  Take a photograph to document the animal.
  Place identification bands on all animals.

- Supplies for the clinic (to be kept in a secure and separate area)
  Generators
  Tarps
  Rope
  Wet-dry vacuum
  Leashes
  Cardboard cat carriers
  Disposable isolation gowns
  Disposable medical gloves
  Masks
  Set of muzzles
  Set of wildlife gloves
  Caution tape
  Orange cones or flags
  Polaroid camera and film
  Duct tape or other heavy-duty tape
  Portable floodlights
  Flashlights
- Training for the clinic disaster team
  Hazardous materials (two people should take level-one course)
  ICS system (two people should take level-one course)
  Online training (provided by Federal Emergency Management Agency [FEMA])
  On-site training (provided by Humane Society of the United States [HSUS] throughout the year [includes hands-on training])
  Have someone become familiar with posttraumatic stress disorder (PTSD), and have contact numbers on hand for organizations that provide help for PTSD.
- Additional considerations
  Have everyone trained on how to triage mass casualties.
  - Agree on a triage method.
  - Use role-playing techniques.
  Have everyone familiar with the medical forms used during a disaster.
  Gather all important contact numbers, including the following:
  - Wildlife experts
  - PTSD help numbers
  - Grief-counseling numbers
  - Poison control
  - Local/state/federal official numbers

them a list of whom to contact if a foreign animal disease is suspected. Typically the United States Department of Agriculture is notified immediately. The clinician should research the disease to better explain the illness to owners. He or she should also expect to handle questions such as, "Can my dog get mad cow disease?" Volunteers from the veterinary community may be needed to help perform physicals on animals or to deal with questions from the general public in a large-scale epidemic.

- **Fire:** During a wild fire, animals often run scared and relocate themselves in yards and barns where they do not belong. House pets may be abandoned and brought in by local rescue groups. Dehydration, stress, and anorexia can be common. The proper authorities, such as the United States Fish and Wildlife Service or local wildlife rehabilitators, should ideally handle wildlife. Clients may bring burned or injured birds and squirrels to the veterinary hospital in the area. The clinic should post a list of contact numbers of those individuals equipped to deal with wildlife before the disaster.

- **Hurricanes and tornadoes:** Wildlife may be relocated to unexpected places. Snakes, spiders, and birds may end up in places that are not desirable. Often times, house pets are abandoned. Dehydration, stress, and anorexia can be common. Clients may be calling with questions on how to get snakes or birds out of their homes. The clinic should have telephone numbers of wildlife removal companies that can deal with such questions.

- **Floods:** Often house pets are abandoned during floods. Dehydration, stress, anorexia, and near drowning can be common. Pets may end up in towns far away from their homes. Owners may not realize that they should contact veterinary hospitals to help find their pets.

TRIAGING

The term **triage** comes from the French word that means *to sort*. During a disaster, patients must be triaged in a way that will benefit the most animals. You may have to triage mass casualties and many different species at once.

When triaging animals during a disaster, thinking "outside" of the disaster is important. Several scenarios may give a false sense of the patient's condition.

Preexisting illnesses may be present in several patients. Animals may start to acquire new illnesses that are not related to the disaster. For example, the dog that initially arrived at the clinic with a large laceration comes back because of pancreatitis, or the cat that came in for hypothermia develops pyelonephritis. Deciding if you are just dealing with emergencies or long-term hospitalized care is important if you are involved in the hospital issuing care. Attempting to function as a "regular" emergency hospital *and* a "disaster" hospital often does not work well for the staff or for the pets. If the hospital chooses to deal with disaster animals only, then clients should be informed that the hospital's focus is on helping only those animals. Most clients will understand this policy, and their devotion to the clinic will only grow stronger because of the dedication shown by staff members in helping those animals affected by the disaster.

Having an organized approach will help ensure that the most patients possible are triaged appropriately. A method must be designed for dealing with numerous patients at once.

> **TECHNICIAN NOTE**   Two methods can be used to efficiently triage during a disaster: (1) START (**S**imple **T**riage **A**nd **R**apid **T**reatment) and (2) SAVE (**S**econdary **A**ssessment of **V**ictim **E**ndpoint) (Wingfield and Raffe, 2002). Both methods were developed for triaging human casualties during war and disasters. To date, no similar method has been specifically designed for triaging animals; however, both START and SAVE are widely accepted in the veterinary community as efficient triage methods for dealing with nonhuman patients.

START METHOD

With the START method, each animal is quickly assessed for respiration, alertness, and perfusion status. This is also known as their *RAP status*. Using this system, animals are color-coded and moved to their color-coded areas. Animals should be marked with the appropriate color. Owners can be given cards for their animals, and unowned animals can be marked with identification bands. The date, the time, the initials of the person who triaged, the initial problem, and the color should all be listed. As a base, animals that are walking are considered *green*. These are animals that have minimal injuries and are considered stable enough to wait for medical treatment. Having every

TABLE 27-1	Start Color Code System
COLOR	**TYPE OF INJURY**
Red	Critical—The patient must receive simple life-saving procedures to ensure survival.
Yellow	The patient should survive as long as simple care is given within a few hours.
Green	Minor injuries—The patient can wait for treatment and still survive.
Black	Dead or dying—The patient's injuries are very severe, and the patient is unlikely to survive regardless of the treatment received.

staff member in the clinic become familiar with the color-coded system will help decrease confusion if and when disaster strikes. Using the START method, animals can be quickly assessed and brought to appropriate treatment areas to receive the treatment needed. Areas should be established and staffed to deal with that particular color animal. Animals may need to be reassessed as time passes. Reassessment times should be agreed upon so that animals will not be forgotten. An animal's status may change, and it may be given a different color depending on the current condition (Table 27-1).

SAVE METHOD

The SAVE method is much faster than the START method and works well when resources and personnel are limited. It will help to conserve the resources and personnel by focusing them on patients who have the best chance of survival. Using the SAVE method, patients are divided into the following three categories:

1. Those who will die regardless of the treatment
2. Those who will survive regardless if treated or not
3. Those who will benefit if medical intervention occurs immediately

Only those that fall in groups two and three are given care. Group number two is put on "hold" while group number three is treated. After group number three has been dealt with, group number two can be reassessed and treated. Placing an animal in one of the groups is a judgment call and can be difficult at times. Decisions must be made quickly to save the most patients possible.

OWNER IN THE DISASTER

Dealing with pet owners can be very stressful during a disaster. Their houses may have been destroyed, family members may be missing or injured, and all of their personal belongings may be gone. As in the case of many natural disasters, their pets may be all they have left. Finding assistance for clients often will be as important as helping their pets. These clients may not be equipped to deal with their pets' conditions, and their decisions may not be rational.

> **TECHNICIAN NOTE** Understanding **posttraumatic stress disorder (PTSD)** will assist everyone in this situation. The clinic should have contact numbers available for owners of local specialists who deal with PTSD. Grief counseling can also be suggested.

Owners, kennel owners, breeders, zookeepers, and farmers all know how to handle their animals well. In most disasters, *the more hands the better* method holds true. Certainly not every owner can help during a disaster. Many of these owners may be distraught and unable to deal with the current situation. Every situation is unique and must be considered on an individual basis.

SELF-PROTECTION

Self-protection during a disaster is important. The rate and severity of bites and scratches increase during a disaster. Preventing injury to the handlers and medical support staff is a priority (Box 27-2).

Location and surroundings in and around a disaster area are often unpredictable and dangerous.

> **TECHNICIAN NOTE** Any disaster is considered a *hazardous working environment*. During an average day in an emergency clinic, bumping into a cabinet or tripping over a rolled up piece of carpet is something we attempt to avoid. However, during a disaster, walking into a puddle of water where a live wire fell or reaching into the bottom of a drawer to find a rattlesnake could be a deadly mistake; therefore veterinary professionals must remain alert during a disaster.

Marking dangerous areas with cones or caution tape will help decrease the amount of injuries. A safety officer should be appointed to help make staff aware of the dangers. A briefing should occur before each new shift, and a safety officer should speak to the group about concerns. During a disaster, a safety officer should always be on duty to monitor the situation.

COMMON EMERGENCIES

Even though a disaster is occurring, animals that arrive at the clinic as emergencies should still be considered just emergencies. One of the biggest differences seen during an emergency is that animals may come without owners and no identification—this is when the Good Samaritan laws apply.

The clinic should not overtreat the patient. Ear mites and matted fur can be uncomfortable but certainly are not an emergency. During a disaster, treating animals should be done using appropriate judgment, understanding that time and resources are limited.

Disasters create many types of conditions and emergencies. The topics discussed have ranged from radiation exposure, weapons of mass destruction, biologic warfare, chemical warfare, explosives, and foot and mouth disease. The following lists are emergencies that have occurred during disaster situations in the United States.

SHOCK

Shock is a very common emergency during a disaster. Most of the time an injury has caused the shock, but certainly some animals can go into shock because of stress. Before treating the shock in the animal, the clinician should assess the animal's overall condition and decide whether reversing the shock will give the animal a good chance for survival.

ORTHOPEDIC AND SOFT TISSUE INJURIES

Orthopedic and soft tissue injuries are common during a disaster. Not all orthopedic and soft tissue injuries are

emergencies. Being able to refer nonemergency patients to a clinic that is not affected by the disaster may be the best option. Most orthopedic and soft tissue injuries are not life threatening, but they certainly can be painful. Providing pain relief by administration of an analgesic and stabilizing the affected area by application of a bandage (if appropriate) can be done quickly before referring the patient elsewhere.

WOUNDS

Wounds of all types are common during a disaster. Certainly a dog can live with a minor laceration to its pad. It may be painful, but it will live. However, a stick impaled through the abdomen is a wound that is an emergency. Being able to stabilize the patient may be a possibility, but surgery may not be an option. Euthanasia may be the only option, unless the patient can be transferred to a fully functional hospital.

NEUROLOGIC INJURIES

Neurologic injuries can occur for varying reasons during a disaster. Smoke inhalation may cause an animal to arrive in an altered state. Another scenario is being thrown around the yard during a tornado and suffering spinal trauma. Performing a complete neurologic assessment of the patient is necessary. Some patients that suffer head trauma or other neurologic disorders may take a long time to recover. Most neurologic patients require constant monitoring. During a disaster, cage space and staff may be limited. Waiting a week or more to see if the patient recovers from head trauma may not be an option.

HYPERTHERMIA AND HYPOTHERMIA

Hyperthermia and hypothermia are very common during a disaster. Knowing where and how the patient was rescued is important. Rushing to warm the patient may not be beneficial. Although hyperthermia or hypothermia always has a cause, the clinician may not discover it during the time of the disaster. However, considering all possibilities and determining what the overall prognosis is for that patient are important.

SMOKE AND BURN INJURIES

Animals that have been involved in a fire or have been burned smell like smoke, have whiskers or hair that has been singed, are covered in soot, or have visible burns. Oxygen should be immediately given to these patients even if respiratory signs are not apparent. Providing oxygen will help with carbon monoxide elimination and tissue hypoxia. Clinical signs will often worsen for up to 48 hours after exposure. Once admitted, the animal's condition can become life threatening.

NEAR DROWNING

The true definition of a near-drowning victim is "survival for at least 24 hours after underwater submersion." If the patient dies before 24 hours, then the animal is considered a drowning victim. During a flood or hurricane, near-drowning victims are common. Symptoms of near drowning may include respiratory signs, hypothermia, pulmonary edema, and vomiting. Respiratory changes may be delayed by up to 48 hours after the incident because of infection from contaminated water. Neurologic signs may include lethargy, stupor, coma, or seizures as a result of the cerebral acidosis, electrolyte changes, and increased intracranial pressure. Providing oxygen, antibiotics, intravenous fluids, and heat therapy may be indicated. Long-term prognosis varies based on how much water was aspirated, how long the patient was submerged, the patient's age, and any other preexisting conditions. It may also be possible for a patient to fall into water contaminated with a toxic substance such as bleach.

SEARCH AND RESCUE CANINES

TECHNICIAN NOTE Any medical condition in an S&R dog is an emergency. S&R teams vary and can be state, private, or federally formed. The federally recognized teams are categorized as task forces, with most states having one or more. State and federal laws protect many of these dogs. During a disaster, S&R dogs must get back to working status as quickly as possible.

In most cases the handler of an S&R dog will want to be present for any treatment performed on the dog. Sometimes it may be mandatory that the handler is present. Canine police dogs are better handled with their owners present to provide commands. Some police dogs are dual trained for both police work and S&R work. Understanding that the dog is the handler's partner and team member is important; the person cannot help with disaster relief if he or she does not have a working dog.

Occasionally S&R dogs encounter unique hazards that cause them harm. In the aftermath of the 1995 Oklahoma City bombing, the 9/11 attack in New York, and the tornadoes in Oklahoma, dogs used to search the rubble for survivors were exposed to inhalant toxins while working. Several routes of exposure exist:

- **Respiratory exposure:** Dogs cannot wear gas masks. Substances such as fiberglass or halogenated gases may cause symptoms of pulmonary edema or respiratory tract irritation.
- **Dermal exposure:** Corrosive agents may burn or injure the skin.
- **Oral exposure:** Ingestion of materials is a potential hazard for any dog. Detergents, acidic toxins, and other materials may be licked or ingested on purpose or by accident.
- **Ocular exposure:** During 9/11, many dogs arrived at the field hospital with red, injected sclera. Liquids splashing into eyes or even debris blowing onto the eyes can cause serious eye injuries.

If a toxin is suspected, the clinician should call an animal poison control center for advice. Remember also that you may not be able to make telephone calls and having book references on hand is an important backup plan. After 9/11, veterinarians wrote many toxicology reports regarding S&R dogs, and the national poison centers have all that information. Injuries will be different for every disaster.

The 9/11 terrorist attacks inspired one of the largest showings of S&R dogs in the history of the United States (Figures 27-3 and 27-4). Hundreds of S&R dogs were called into action. Experiences gained from working with so many S&R dogs provided a wealth of knowledge for future disasters involving working dogs.

Several medical conditions were common for S&R dogs during 9/11. S&R dogs were more susceptible to dehydration because they worked long shifts in the heat. During a disaster, a clinic may become the "checkpoint" for the medical evaluation of S&R dogs before and after each shift. Offering this service to S&R teams is a great way to provide help during a disaster, because most S&R teams do not have staff veterinarians. During 9/11, most S&R dogs were given subcutaneous fluids after each shift to help combat dehydration. Handlers who had fluids given to their dogs noticed a dramatic improvement in energy level and attitude. Because S&R dogs love to work and are driven to perform, the handler may never see any signs of dehydration until the animal is too ill to

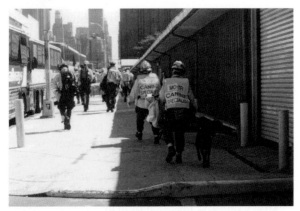

FIGURE 27-3 Missouri Task Force One going to work during 9/11.

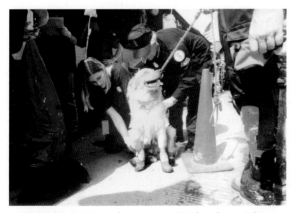

FIGURE 27-4 Author assesses S&R dog during 9/11.

recover (Otto et al, 2003). Severe dehydration can lead to hypovolemia. These dogs must then be hospitalized until they are stable. Handlers should be instructed on ways to prevent dehydration. Taking more frequent and longer breaks and ensuring dogs drink an appropriate amount of water are keys to preventing dehydration.

Stress diarrhea was found to be common in dogs that worked for long hours under stressful conditions. If diarrhea is severe enough, then it can lead to dehydration. In severe cases the diarrhea became hemorrhagic. Keeping a close eye on S&R dogs and addressing diarrhea as soon as it begins are both important factors in keeping these dogs working.

During 9/11, several dogs had hemorrhagic cystitis (Otto et al, 2003). All dogs responded to supportive care, and no evidence of toxicosis or infectious disease was

ever found (Otto et al, 2003). Minor skin infections also occurred. Bathing the dogs and administering antibiotics helped with most skin infections. Other issues of S&R dogs included minor lameness, minor lacerations, ear infections, and eye infections.

Most S&R dogs did not wear booties while working during the crisis, because booties tended to decrease traction and inhibit their ability to walk. Despite their feet being unprotected, a remarkably low occurrence of injuries to the pads was reported. Thousands of booties for dogs were donated and initially given out to handlers, but after weeks passed with limited injuries, the handlers found it best to work their dogs without the booties.

STRAY ANIMALS

Ideally stray animals should be handled by the local shelter or humane society. It is important to remember that during a disaster everyone should welcome working with new groups and people. An individual organization cannot effectively manage a disaster situation by itself. This point was exhibited during Hurricane Katrina.

More than 6000 stray animals were transported for care at the Lamar-Dixon Exposition Center (the largest created sheltering facility). The large number of stray animals during Hurricane Katrina could not have been predicted by anyone. One thing became quite obvious. The situation quickly spiraled out of control and despite many organizations already being involved, many more were brought in to help.

Veterinarians should not act as shelters without the supervision of another organization, but they can certainly care medically for the sheltering of animals. It is important that the veterinary team and shelter work together to help each other during a disaster. Groups like the Humane Society of the United States, the American Society for the Prevention of Cruelty of Animals, and other local shelter organizations should be recruited to help with the sheltering and placement of animals during a disaster. These groups understand the legal issues with taking in stray animals and usually boast large databases necessary for finding the owners. That being said, large veterinary schools and facilities have been turned into overflow shelters if their community cannot meet the demand. During the 2012 fires in Colorado the veterinary school saw more than 100 animals brought in to board in a temporary shelter in the school. This required more than 100 around-the-clock volunteers. Although not ideal, it was an important function that the school played in the community at the time of a major disaster. Ultimately, the school had to decide if it could afford to give this resource to the community.

There are many issues of awareness that must be known for shelter animals of veterinarians and technicians. These animals are under a lot of stress. They may exhibit behaviors during a disaster that they would not normally show under normal circumstances. There is an increase of aggression during times of disasters and it is important to be careful when dealing with these animals. Nothing is more stressful than losing your owner, swimming in flood waters, and being pulled out by a stranger, locked in a crate, placed next to 60 other barking dogs, and transported to a strange facility where a stranger wants to perform a physical on you.

In one 6-hour period one night, more than 300 animals were triaged by a veterinary staff of 10 mainly using the SAVE method—this is a little less than 1 minute for an animal needing to be triaged. Being able to perform individual physical exam on each animal became impossible, so animals were assessed on "who will die, who will live and who needs medical attention right now" basis. Emergency and critical care technicians have a great ability to think and act quickly. Having such skills was important in that situation. Eventually veterinarians and technicians went back and performed physicals on every animal. It is important to note that although it would have been ideal to have a veterinarian perform a physical on every animal, that quickly became impossible. Technicians needed to be able to auscult animals well, identify any abnormal heart and lung sounds, and notify the veterinarian. They needed to perform complete physical exams, just like they would in a clinic setting. Starting with the head, looking at the eyes, feeling and looking at all limbs, palpating the abdomen, and checking under the tail are all important to a complete physical examination. Though the situation of Lamar-Dixon was extreme (and hopefully will never occur again), technicians in this situation played a vital role in the care of the animals.

Many stray animals arrive without any identification. Ideally, the local shelter agency on the scene should be responsible for identifying and keeping track of the animals. Using ID bands, taking pictures, and noting unique markings are all important to ensuring the animal is not lost in the system. Remember, the goal of these animals is to find their owners.

No matter how many stray animals present, they should never be euthanized because there are "too many." Remember that people may have nothing and looking for their pet may be the only thing that keeps them motivated. Even at Lamar-Dixon, animals were never casually euthanized. Highly aggressive animals were kept alive in hopes their owners would find them.

> **TECHNICIAN NOTE** Technicians are wonderfully compassionate. It is important to remember to bring that compassion with you to a disaster.

Lashing out at owners for deserting their pets benefits no one. During Hurricane Katrina some individuals who rescued animals from homes left spray-painted derogatory messages on the owners' doors. As a technician, we must remember that we were not in that person's position. When owners arrive looking for their pet, compassion and understanding are vital.

All stray animals should be handled with gloves. Vaccine and disease history is unknown. Many stray animals during Hurricane Katrina were covered in dirt and oil. Skin problems were a big issue following Hurricane Katrina. Many of the animals had rashes, bites from fire ants, and hair loss.

Any animal with signs of a possible contagious disease should be isolated immediately. This became a big problem at Lamar-Dixon because it was an open-air barn. Best efforts were made to keep contagious animals separated by isolating a few barn stalls. Only designated people were allowed to treat those animals to help reduce dissemination. Overall, there were very few animals that got sick.

Because of the shear magnitude of the amount of animals being sheltered in one facility, there have been many lectures and articles written about the disaster within the disaster of Hurricane Katrina. It is obvious that much went wrong on both the human and the animal disaster side. One thing Hurricane Katrina has provided the animal community is an opportunity to talk and find solutions so that a better response can be initiated the next time such a catastrophe occurs.

DECONTAMINATION

Decontamination of animals became critical during 9/11 and Hurricane Katrina (Figure 27-5). S&R dogs during 9/11 were arriving at the field hospitals covered

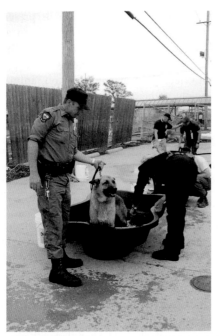

FIGURE 27-5 Search and rescue (SAR) dog is hosed down for decontamination.

in dirt and grime. Katrina dogs had waded in flood waters with oil and debris floating in it.

One of the biggest treatments administered during 9/11 and Katrina was decontamination of the S&R dogs and other pets. Washing them down and trying to remove any hazardous materials after they were done searching was extremely important. Most information compiled on decontamination of animals has been adapted from human medical research.

> **TECHNICIAN NOTE** First and foremost, veterinary staff must protect themselves. Vomit, urine, and feces of pets may contain hazardous materials. Wearing gloves, disposable gowns, and even eye protection is a required.

Pets should be assessed for any life-threatening ailments first. The clinician should remember that symptoms from a toxic substance may not appear until long after exposure. Keeping track of pets' symptoms is key to helping with a diagnosis. For example, if a few of the pets brought to a clinic begin to cough and the clinician suspects that the coughing is the result of exposure to an airborne toxic substance, then all S&R dog handlers and pet owners should be notified so that precautions can be taken to prevent further toxicosis.

Bathing with a detergent soap (e.g., Dawn, GOJO) and water became routine when dogs were searching the World Trade Center areas. This helped to remove any oil-based contaminants that the dogs may have encountered. Flushing of the eyes and nostrils with saline can help remove any irritants. Changing gloves and gowns between patients is ideal. Animals brought to Lamar-Dixon and other facilities were hosed down and washed with Dawn liquid dish soap. All people washing the animals needed to wear gloves, aprons, and boots.

Using extra precautions when dealing with animals during a disaster is important, because they have the potential to be covered in corrosive materials that can be damaging to the veterinary staff. Protecting oneself first and then treating the patient is the safest way to handle a potential exposure to a toxic substance.

SURGERY

Taking a patient to surgery during a disaster should only occur in an emergency, if the patient's prognosis will benefit from it, and if the clinic has the resources to safely perform the procedure. Appropriate precautions must still be taken to ensure the patient's safety.

Patients that are stable should be referred to another clinic that is fully functioning. Fractures, major lacerations, most ocular injuries, and some hemoabdomens are surgeries that are not emergencies and should be done only under pristine conditions.

Performing surgery requires more staff, uses more resources, and restricts cage space for an extended period of time. Taking a patient to surgery may decrease the number of other patients that can be seen and treated at the hospital. It is important to consider the overall effects that taking a patient to surgery during a disaster will have to the entire clinic, staff, and other patients.

RECORD KEEPING

One of the most important tasks in emergency medicine is the ability to keep accurate records.

> **TECHNICIAN NOTE** During a disaster, having premade forms ready for use to keep accurate records is important.

Many times disaster teams "hit the ground running." They usually set up a working area and start seeing patients immediately. Throughout many disasters one of the realities is that medical records were poorly, if ever, kept. Owners and handlers that returned to the veterinary field hospital a few days later had to communicate what had been done to their dogs during the previous visit. No computers were available and electricity was limited at the field hospital. Physical exam forms should be preprinted in duplicate carbon copy. This way a record can be kept at the working field hospital and one can be given to the owner.

Even during a disaster, maintaining accurate records is important. This is especially true if no owner is present. If an animal's owner is eventually found, then he or she will want to know how the pet was treated during the separation period—hence accurate records are needed. A medical record is a legal document. For example, if it was deemed that a pet should be euthanized and an owner is later found, being able to provide a record describing why the pet was euthanized is important. All veterinary clinics should have printed forms (created in duplicate) for use in disasters. Multiple copies should be made in advance and stored in the event they are needed. Forms should be fast and easy to use; checking boxes and circling answers is the easiest way to record basic information. If your clinic works on a paperless system, it is important you have the ability to write records in the event you have no computers.

Having an instant camera ready is very useful to take pictures of unowned animals. Although you may not have computer power to store them, it can be something you can do later once power is restored. If an animal must be euthanized and an owner comes to identify the animal, then a photograph is important. Stapling the pictures to the patient's record will provide quick access to the picture if an owner is trying to locate his or her pet.

The Humane Society of the United States (HSUS), Petfinder.com, and other rescue organizations have computer systems that form a list of animals that have no owners. Since Hurricane Katrina, even more emphasis has been placed on record keeping. When taking in and treating an unknown animal, the clinic staff should find the local group that is handling rescue and placement of animals so that the animal can be added to the database. Owners may not think to look for their pets at veterinary clinics and may only go to the rescue organization for assistance.

RECHECKING APPOINTMENTS

Plans should be made for postdisaster care of each animal that enters the hospital. The client should be encouraged to return to the regular veterinarian for follow-up care. However, if the client's hospital is closed for an extended time, then a recheck appointment at the nearest facility should be scheduled.

Providing owners with enough medication is also another consideration. The clinician should limit the amount dispensed to avoid depletion of stock supplies. Clients should be instructed to follow up with their regular veterinarians once they are open for business. Local veterinary hospitals should assemble a verbal and written "stockpile" system before the disaster strikes. Accurate records should be maintained so that hospitals can be reimbursed after the disaster subsides.

HELPING THE LOCAL VETERINARY INFRASTRUCTURE

Talking to other local clinics before a disaster occurs and creating a support team will help the clinician's facility and the local community. Being able to share equipment and even personnel can be a huge benefit to multiple clinics during a disaster. Talking to local shelter groups and letting them know what services you can provide them can be a huge benefit. Making contact before a disaster always helps during a disaster.

Communication before a disaster will help to expedite things during a disaster. If all local veterinarians had each other's contact numbers, then when a disaster struck they could easily communicate with each other to assess damage, determine what clinics could function, and decide who needed help. Ultimately the goal of any disaster is to get the local community functioning by itself again. Once that occurs, the situation stops being a current disaster (Box 27-3).

PERSONAL RECOVERY AFTER THE DISASTER

Being aware of PTSD is very important. All responders, no matter what the magnitude of the disaster, have the potential to suffer PTSD. A "debriefing" should be done at the end of each day that someone has worked in a disaster. This should include asking how tired the person is, what bothered the person the most, how he or she

BOX 27-3	Personnel Disaster Kit for Disaster Responders

- Flashlight
- Batteries for flashlight and all electronics
- Small battery-operated radio
- Medications
  - Personal prescription drugs
  - Over-the-counter drugs
- One week of clothing
- Garment bag
- Immunization record
- Medical record
- Important documents
  - Homeowner's policy
  - Health insurance policy and identification cards
  - Credit card numbers
  - Bank numbers
- Current contact number list of family members and friends
- Laundry detergent
- First aid kit
- Travel size shampoo/conditioner/soap/toothpaste
- Extra toothbrush
- Extra towel
- Duct tape
- Trash bags (multiple sizes)
- Sunscreen
- Bug repellent
- Candles
- Toilet paper
- Water bottles

is dealing with the disaster, and if the person wants to return to help the next day. Realizing that each person deals with stress differently is important. Creating opportunities for each person to talk and share feelings is equally important. Ideally a couple of people in the clinic should not be directly involved in dealing with veterinary medicine during the disaster. These individuals can include administrators or receptionists. Sometimes just having someone who will listen will make all the difference when dealing with the stress of the disaster. If someone appears to be suffering from PTSD, then seeking appropriate help is important.

People who were involved in rescue efforts or who were victims of a disaster may suffer from PTSD. This syndrome was initially diagnosed in people who served in the military during war times. It has now been recognized in anyone who has been involved with a disaster or traumatic event. The National Center for Post-Traumatic Stress Disorder (www.ptsd.va.gov/index.asp) has a wide variety of information for anyone affected by a disaster (United States Department of Veterans Affairs, 2013). The National Center for PTSD states that 8% of men and 20% of women will experience PTSD symptoms (United States Department of Veterans Affairs, 2013). About 30% of those afflicted will suffer from a chronic form for the rest of their lives (United States Department of Veterans Affairs, 2013). The National Center for Post-Traumatic Stress Disorder's website contains some valuable links to other websites that provide help for those suffering from PTSD.

Relaxing after a disaster can be very difficult. Usually people push themselves to their limits by working 16- to 18-hour days. They never stop to think of themselves and feel that more needs to be done, at the clinic or at home. After the disaster is over and life starts to return to normal, it can become very difficult to relax, because the body and mind have a difficult time slowing down.

Continuing to eat well, taking regular breaks, and having periods of scheduled "down time" to avoid burnout are vital. Everyone must care for himself or herself before offering care to others.

STRUCTURE OF A DISASTER

All disasters start at a local level. This is true with every tornado, flood, or terrorist event. The local community government usually contracts with a single primary group, which agrees to oversee and coordinate other individuals/agencies to manage the functions of a disaster. As a veterinary technician, your clinic may be contacted to see if they are able to provide medical care to the pets of the community. There may be an established local disaster team that has a medical component ready for the local town government.

If the local infrastructure is overwhelmed, they will then reach out to the regional or state resources. All states in the United States have a state emergency management agency (EMA). The local town will contact their EMA and request specific assistance. For example, they may need veterinary care for a large number of animals or temporary housing for displaced residents. States and local towns rely heavily on nonprofit organizations and groups of volunteers to provide specialty services they cannot fulfill. Although there are a lot of disaster teams in the United States, not every state has a State Animal Response Team (SART). While the term "state" animal response team is used readily, it is important to note that almost all SART teams are not part of the state government. They are usually independent nonprofit organizations. Most SART teams have memorandums of understanding (MOU) or contracts with the state in which they reside. Getting involved on a local level is a great way to start learning about disaster medicine, but it is important to check to see what they have in place for medical and liability insurance to cover you if you are injured. It is important to note that many SART teams focus solely on rescue and housing of animals in a disaster and often still rely on the local veterinary clinic to provide medical support.

If the disaster overwhelms the state resources, then the state must ask for federal help. The governor of that state must declare a state of emergency and then ask for federal help. The federal government then may elect to use the only federal veterinary team, National Veterinary Response Team (NVRT), if a state team cannot adequately meet the demands. Calling in the NVRT team is expensive and is something usually done as a last resort.

It is important to recognize that as more people are called in to help, the chain of command usually (not always) passes onto the next group that was contacted. First, it is the local authorities who are in control of the scene. When the local authority calls in the state, it is typically the state authority that is in charge. If the state calls in the federal authorities, it is typically the federal authority that is in charge. Any disasters of national security (terrorism) fall under the jurisdiction of the federal government and they are automatically in charge of the scene.

BECOMING INVOLVED

Often disasters strike without warning. One of the largest issues during Hurricane Katrina was the number of people who came in to help with the 6000 animals at the Lamar-Dixon Exposition Center. Managing and dealing with the thousands of people who showed up became very difficult and hindered the relief efforts of many teams. It is important to realize that although you may want to help, you may not be allowed to. Many states will not allow out of state veterinarians and technicians to practice in their state. An organization that is already on the scene operates with a set of rules and regulations with which you may not be familiar.

BOX 27-4	Pet Disaster Kit for Pet Owners

Items to be packed up and stored away in bag:
- Current medical records including vaccinations
- Extra leash and collar
- Identification tags for all collars or harnesses
- Current photographs and written descriptions of pets
- Extra bowls
- Small bag of cat litter and small cat litter box
- Can opener
- Phone number of veterinarian
- Extra towels

Items on checklist that must be brought if disaster occurs:
- Two-week supply of any medications needed (should always be kept in the house)
- Carrier
- Two-week supply of food (should always be kept in the house)
- Pet beds
- Pet toys
- Three-day supply of water

Disasters occur all the time. Whether it be a small local disaster or a large federal disaster, you may be asked to be involved. Unless you are part of the organization already on the scene, you must remember to follow their rules and guidelines or you may be asked to leave. Even though you may have exemplary skills as a veterinary technician in a clinic, you may end up hindering the relief efforts if you do not understand the system in place. Getting involved in a disaster team or taking some online training can make you a much better asset during a disaster.

First and foremost, you must be able to help yourself. If you are not prepared for yourself, your family, and your own pets, then you are acting against the relief efforts. A small disaster pack of personal items and a disaster pack for pets located in a designated area can be prepared before a disaster strikes (see Boxes 27-3 and 27-4).

JOINING A TEAM

TECHNICIAN NOTE Joining an animal disaster team is another great way to become involved. It takes time and commitment to join one of the teams. Speaking to team members and visiting their websites will help provide more in-depth information. This will also allow you to see if a team is the right choice for you.

Joining a team will help keep you protected when working in a disaster. National and federal teams offer liability insurance and health insurance, should you become injured while working in a disaster. Some state and local teams offer insurance as well, but it is best to check to see if you are covered in case of a disaster.

With the exception of NVRT, when you decide to join a disaster team it is important to recognize your employer is not required to hold your job. The NVRT team members fall under the USERRA Act, which means their employer must let them deploy and must retain their position when they return. If you are not part of this team, it is imperative that you get permission to be on the team and to take a leave of absence to work in the disaster. It is important to note there are local, state, national, and federal disaster teams.

Local teams are generally smaller and are nonprofit organizations. The members involved may have extensive training or none. Their focus is on their community. These teams are usually termed "regional animal response teams" or "community animal response teams." Many times the focus of these groups is sheltering and rescue. Obtaining the advice of a veterinary professional is important to these teams. Unfortunately, they often do not offer insurance or payment should the person become injured.

State teams are often nonprofit organizations whose focus is anything state related. These teams have members from across the state and are often larger than the local groups. These are generally termed "state animal response teams." Although they are termed "state" they generally have no official position within the government of the state. They often seek out an MOU with the state and offer their resources in times of a disaster, much like the American Red Cross. Usually members have more training than the local team, but not always. Insurance may be offered to members, but it is important to check if this is available.

National teams are nonprofits whose focus is anything in the United States. Some teams offer assistance to the territories (e.g., Puerto Rico) of the United States. These teams have members across the country and resources in numerous states. Some of the largest include the following:

- Veterinary Medical Assistance Teams (operated by the American Veterinary Medical Association)
- National Disaster Animal Response Team (operated by the Humane Society of the United States)

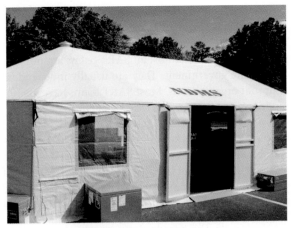

FIGURE 27-6 VMAT field tents.

- ASPCA's Field Investigations and Response Team
- Emergency Relief Team (operated by the International Fund for Animal Welfare)
- Red Rover

National teams often, but not always, offer insurance to volunteers. Some of these teams you can join on a per diem basis and be paid, although positions are hard to obtain generally. Because of their size they have the ability to ship supplies and people around the country. They also have a significantly larger number of members than state or local teams. National teams often require training in order to be deployed as a member.

Federal teams must be operated by a federal government agency. The NVRT teams are part of the National Disaster Management System that falls under the U.S. Department of Health and Human Services. When called into action, these highly trained veterinarians and technicians are considered to be part-time employees of FEMA. FEMA will activate the team, giving them as little as 12-hours' notice that they are going to be deployed. Members can be deployed up to 14 days. The team is self-sufficient and can establish a fully functioning (including minor surgery) veterinary hospital (where technicians can use their medical skills during a disaster). Members are required to fulfill training requirements before they are considered deployable. If activated, then the team members are paid a salary and are covered by federal workers' compensation. They are also protected under the Federal Tort Claims Act against any personal liability during deployment and are exempt from licensure, certification, and registration requirements outside of the state in which they are registered (Figure 27-6).

Graph 1.0

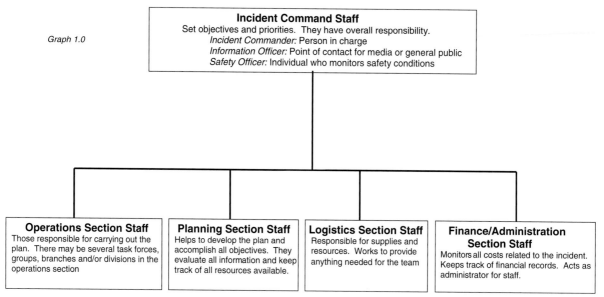

FIGURE 27-7 Incident command staff graph.

DISASTER TRAINING

Training is needed in any disaster situation. The two main requirements are (1) training for personal protection and (2) training for the actual disaster.

Becoming certified in a level I hazardous materials (i.e., hazmat) course is a must for at least one member of the clinic's disaster team. Most animal disaster teams require a level I hazmat course. Local fire departments often offer such courses throughout the year. Online training is available through FEMA (www.fema.gov/about/training). In most cases these courses are free. Courses focus on how to read hazardous materials signs and the basics of what to look for when entering a disaster scene. Certain websites (e.g., www.saferesponse.com) also offer a free online hazmat course. Taking a hazmat course will assist any disaster responder.

The incident command system (ICS) has become a universal system for those dealing with any type of disaster. It was developed by a California fire department in the 1970s. Since then, local, state, and federal branches all use the ICS system. The ICS is designed to have certain key people fill specific duties and establish a chain of command. Many local fire departments, as well as FEMA, offer ICS courses for free.

One person in the veterinary hospital should familiarize himself or herself with the ICS system to make

it easier to communicate with local, state, and federal responders during a disaster. The ICS system can be applied to the smallest of veterinary hospitals. If each clinic appoints key members using ICS before the disaster happens, then it will be easier to function if one does occur. Using the ICS system, a person would be designated as the *Incident Commander* or *Administrative Officer* (Figure 27-7).

Training for individual disasters can vary. The myriad of disasters that can occur require flexible skills. Thinking "outside of the box" when dealing with certain situations is common. For example, having a clean, sterile environment to repair a laceration may not be feasible. Placing a large sterile drape under the patient may be the best solution. Lack of intravenous poles may require innovative ideas on how to hang fluid bags.

Many veterinary conferences have started to include disaster medicine as a topic. The International Veterinary Emergency and Critical Care Conference, held once a year, has had disaster medicine as a topic since 1998. The National Disaster Medical System (NDMS) offers a conference once a year (Integrated Training Summit) specifically geared toward the NDMS teams, which include topics in veterinary disaster medicine presented by members of the National Veterinary Response Teams (NVRT). There are also national and international disasters occurring yearly that work to bring first responders and disaster professionals together.

BOX 27-5 | Sites That Contain Information on Disaster Training

National Disaster Medical System: www.ndms.dhhs.gov
Federal Emergency Management Agency (FEMA): www.fema.gov
Department of Homeland Security: www.dhs.gov
American Veterinary Medical Association: www.avma.org
American Animal Hospital Association: www.aahanet.org
American Veterinary Medical Foundation: www.avmf.org

Many organizations (government and private) are devoted to disaster medicine (Box 27-5). Organizations like the FEMA offer online disaster training. For example, FEMA offers free courses on the ICS and livestock in disasters through their Emergency Management Institute. Many of the organizations listed in Box 27-5 also will provide brochures and other written materials on disaster medicine. The American Veterinary Medical Association offers a great guide to pet owners on how to prepare for a disaster. The HSUS provides a free online manual for the general public and animal care providers on preparing for and dealing with animals in disasters. Many of the courses and literature offered by these organizations are provided at little or no cost.

Very few books have been published on veterinary disaster medicine, and most published before 9/11 contain outdated material. Several veterinary emergency books have started to include chapters on disaster medicine. Since 9/11 a couple of books specific to veterinary medicine in disaster have been printed.

Technicians and veterinarians should realize that some of the best information is obtained through personal experience.

CONCLUSION

Disaster medicine is an evolving field of veterinary medicine. Becoming involved may not be a choice; therefore being prepared before a disaster is important. Veterinary hospitals can create a plan to expedite patient care during a disaster. In addition, veterinary professionals should become educated and know what resources are available during a disaster so that they can provide the best care possible.

REFERENCES

American Animal Hospital Association Board of Directors. Last revised March 2010. Accessed online at. www.aahanet.org/Library/GoodSamaritan.aspx, June 1994. Oct 8, 2013.

Government Tracking of Bills. Accessed bill online at. www.govtrack.us/congress/bills/109/hr3858, Oct 8, 2013.

Heath S: *Animal management in disasters,* St Louis, 1999, Mosby.

Humane Society of the United States. Accessed online at. www.humanesociety.org/issues/pet_overpopulation/facts/pet_ownership_statistics.html, Oct 8, 2013.

Otto C, Franz M, Kellogg B, et al.: *Field treatment of search dogs: lessons learned from the World Trade Center disaster,* Proceedings of the Long Island Veterinary Medical Association Toxicology and Search and Rescue Dogs 43–52, 2003.

United States Department of Veterans Affairs. Accessed online at www.ptsd.va.gov, Oct 8, 2013.

Wingfield W, Raffe W: *The veterinary ICU book,* Jackson, WY, 2002, Teton NewMedia.

SCENARIO

Purpose: To provide the veterinary technician with the ability to think about how he or she would design a disaster plan for the clinic.

Stage: Emergency clinic is a 24-hour facility with at least two technicians, one receptionist, and one doctor present at all times.

Scenario
A category 4 hurricane is likely to hit 30 miles south of your veterinary clinic/boarding facility in the next 36 hours. Town officials have called for an evacuation. It is Labor Day weekend and you have 15 dogs and 20 cats boarding. You also have 10 hospitalized patients. Most of the pets' owners are more than 50 miles out of town and at least 4 are out of the country.

Delivery
- Staff reviews, divides into groups, and has **10 minutes** to discuss the situation.
- Discussion should continue without goal being to find the right answer.

Questions
- What steps should you have in place before the hurricane hits?
- List some ideas of how and when you plan to evacuate.

SCENARIO—cont'd

- List some ideas of where you plan to evacuate the animals.

Key Teaching Points
- Provides veterinary technicians the opportunity to discuss how they would deal with evacuating hospitalized patients.

References
- Box 27-1 should be used as a reference on preparing a veterinary clinic for a disaster.

Discussion
Please note: There is no right answer in disaster medicine.

Before the Hurricane, Consider:
- Setting up an MOU with a clinic or clinics in a "safe" area to transport the pets.
- Consider an MOU that includes using your equipment and/or personnel.
- Should have all owners' contact information, including email, hotel phone numbers, cell phone numbers, and in case of emergency numbers.
- Should have a policy in place about procedures your clinic/facility will follow in case of a disaster (e.g., all pet owners must arrange for their animal to be picked up 48 hours before landfall; all owners recognize that if the facility must evacuate their animal, they will be charged an additional charge per week for transportation and care of their pet, for example).
- Should provide the owners (either via contact info or ahead of time in initial paperwork with every visit) clinic emergency contact information in case they have to reach the clinic. Alternative is to have an answering service take your calls.

How/When/Where to Evacuate:
- Contact owners as soon as you get the evacuation order so that they have as much time as possible to get their pets or arrange for someone else to retrieve their pets.
- Pets should have waterproof ID on them: ID bands, ID cards, ID on leashes/carriers along with photo IDs.

- Medical records must be copied and placed in a waterproof sleeve and be kept with each pet. A duplicate of this record should be backed up electronically **or** transported away from the area in a hard copy file with vet staff.
- All medications that may be needed for hospitalized patients should be taken with you to help offset other clinics' costs (e.g., IV fluids, antibiotics).
- If the hospitalized patients cannot be moved a long distance, a facility in your area should be designated where all hospitalized pets are kept and a reserve staff is selected to ride out the storm with the animals. The facility must have a generator and food/water supply for humans/pets, and be in a secure building that is unlikely to flood. The alternative is to get permission from the owners to move patients at risk or to humanely euthanize pets.
- Pack emergency medical kits in case an animal has an emergency medical complication while being transported.
- Town officials should be notified and media should be contacted in case owners are looking for their pets before you can contact them.
- Evacuation should start occurring at least 24 hours before the hurricane.
- Town officials should be notified about the evacuation location. Usually the state requires facilities to file plans at the beginning of every season.
- Watch the local news to find out what areas are expected to be affected and then evacuate to "safe" area.
- All owners should ideally be notified. It is preferable if they can come and transport their own pet so that the liability does not fall on the clinic.
- Post updates on your clinic's phone line and on your website regarding the status of your evacuation and the process by which owners can claim pets.
- All animals should be restrained and secured appropriately during transport. No loose dogs or cats in cars!
- If roads are backed up, contact local officials and see if they can provide an escort.

Maintaining a 24-hour emergency critical care team is very challenging, but it can be done successfully using proper scheduling techniques. Proper scheduling includes considering how changing schedules or rotating workers will affect their lives personally and physically.

This section describes how using different rotations and maintaining a routine to optimize sleep can help alleviate the stress of working overnights or rotations.

Veterinary personnel need to understand the liability risks that they take when assuming responsibility for the medical care of critically ill or injured patients. Many times the owners are extremely distraught and may be unable to make a decision that will be beneficial for all individuals involved.

Veterinary personnel need to be able to identify and minimize risks to themselves while still being able to provide the immediate care for patients. The importance of informed consent, documentation, and communication are discussed.

## 28

The Art of Scheduling

Andrea M. Battaglia

CHAPTER OUTLINE

Sleep Deprivation
Creating the Optimal Shift for Employees
  Length of Shifts

Helpful Hints for Day Sleeping
Working the Night Shift
  After the Shift
Conclusion

LEARNING OBJECTIVES

After studying this chapter, you will be able to:

- Define shift work and how it can impact a person.
- Understand how to create a shift structure to optimize health and wellness.
- Provide the veterinary technician with ideas on how to be a healthy shift worker.

KEY TERMS

Circadian dysrhythmia
Rotations
Shift work
Shift work maladaptive syndrome (SMS)
Sleep deprivation

One common reason why technicians leave a position in emergency or critical care is because of the inconsistency of a schedule or the inability to continue shift work. **Shift work** is defined as being a process that is designed to accommodate a 24/7 operation. The hours worked are outside a normal business day and include evening, nights, and early morning hours. Some shift structures may include **rotations**. In 1952 researchers from the University of Minnesota began looking at how biologic rhythms dictate human desires, moods, and abilities. They began to study every feature of metabolism, growth, injury, and illness. Chronobiology was developed, and the advances in this area have been very helpful in determining how to support people involved with shift work.

Managers responsible for scheduling a team of 24-hour emergency or critical care veterinary technicians must consider many factors: how changing a specific person's shift may affect his or her personal, physical, and emotional well-being; whether rotations are necessary; and what schedule best fits the needs of the hospital. The manager of the schedule should communicate and reevaluate each veterinary technician's progress during training periods and when a change in shifts is necessary. Surveying the team assists in obtaining information needed to properly assess how an individual is adapting and provides the individual shift worker with an opportunity to share his or her thoughts (Figure 28-1).

Shift work maladaptive syndrome (SMS) and **circadian dysrhythmia** are terms used for conditions now recognized by the medical community to diagnose the negative effects of shift work.

Evaluation of the Shift Structure and Schedule

Refer to the following shift structure when answering questions.

1st shift- 7:am-5:pm   2nd shift-4:pm-2:am   3rd shift-11:pm-9:am

Name: _____   **Date:** _____

	1-Strongly Agree	2-Somewhat Agree	3-Neutral	4-Somewhat Disagree	5-Strongly Disagree
I would prefer a shift rotation.	☐	☐	☐	☐	☐
I would prefer having a set schedule on a specific shift.	☐	☐	☐	☐	☐
I would prefer rotating every 2 weeks.	☐	☐	☐	☐	☐
I would prefer rotating every 4 weeks.	☐	☐	☐	☐	☐
I would prefer rotating every 3 months.	☐	☐	☐	☐	☐
I would prefer rotating every ___ (day/week/months).	☐	☐	☐	☐	☐
I would prefer rotating through all shifts.	☐	☐	☐	☐	☐
I would prefer rotating through 1st and 2nd shifts.	☐	☐	☐	☐	☐
I would prefer rotating through 2nd and 3rd shifts.	☐	☐	☐	☐	☐
I would prefer working the 1st shift.	☐	☐	☐	☐	☐
I would prefer working the 2nd shift.	☐	☐	☐	☐	☐
I would prefer working the 3rd shift.	☐	☐	☐	☐	☐
I would prefer working _____ shift.	☐	☐	☐	☐	☐
I would prefer working 3-12 hour shifts/week.	☐	☐	☐	☐	☐
I would prefer working 4-10 hour shifts/week.	☐	☐	☐	☐	☐
I would prefer working 5-8 hour shifts/week.	☐	☐	☐	☐	☐
I would prefer working all days in a row.	☐	☐	☐	☐	☐
I would prefer a split week. (ie. 2 days on/2 days off)	☐	☐	☐	☐	☐
I would like the opportunity to work overtime.	☐	☐	☐	☐	☐
The present shift structure has improved my ability to maintain my health and wellness.	☐	☐	☐	☐	☐
The present shift structure has allowed me to maintain work life balance.	☐	☐	☐	☐	☐
The present shift structure has improved my ability to provide excellent patient care.	☐	☐	☐	☐	☐

FIGURE 28-1 Schedule survey.

> **TECHNICIAN NOTE** The primary cause of SMS is **sleep deprivation** due to the disruption of the circadian rhythms. Manifestations of these effects can be emotional and physical.

Managers may receive complaints that one of the veterinary technicians has been very moody and irritable lately. The ability to be empathetic may decrease. These behaviors may be out of character for the individual, and when approached with the concern, the person may become very emotional and upset. SMS may be the problem and should be considered.

Reports of an increase in errors including making medical math miscalculations, administering incorrect medications, or forgetting assigned treatments during a shift can manifest. Other problems include sleep-awake disorders, gastrointestinal disorders, and cardiovascular disorders.

SLEEP DEPRIVATION

The light of the sun and the darkness of the night reset the internal biological clock, or circadian rhythm, each day. Those who work the late shift (also called the *graveyard shift* or *night shift* [e.g., 11 PM to 6 AM]) are at the greatest risk, because around 3 am the body is at its lowest ebb and the daily biological clock is reset. This conflict is called *circadian dysrhythmia.* Those who work evenings and nights are continually readjusting this clock. The majority of people soon revert to a daytime schedule. Some individuals work very well at night and have been labeled as "night owls." These people are able to sleep well during the day and adjust hours of sleep without any problem. It is genetically determined whether or not a person will be able to sleep during the day, and aging will decrease the speed of circadian adaptation to night shifts.

The most common complaint of people working various shifts is sleep deprivation. The average person needs 7.5 to 8.5 hours of sleep each day. The veterinary technician who works the night shift averages 5 to 7 hours less sleep per week than the person who works the day shift. Over time this leads to serious physical problems.

Sleep-deprived people are more susceptible to colds, flu, and gastrointestinal problems. People who work nights are more prone to heart disease, accidents, and obesity.

Women who work rotating shifts may have more difficulty conceiving. Two European surveys found that women working irregular shifts were twice as likely to experience delays in conceiving. The numbers of miscarriages and low birth weights also were higher in women with unstable work schedules.

Depression and chronic fatigue also are common among night workers. If poor morale is affecting the staff, then fatigue may be the cause.

Weight gain commonly affects shift workers because of the tendency to snack on unhealthful foods. Attaining a standard mealtime is difficult during these hours. Research has also suggested that sleep-deprived people have larger appetites. Boredom also can increase snacking during these hours.

Many studies have been done over the years to determine how to help people adapt to shift work. About 25% of our workforce is involved in shift work; the Centers for Disease Control and Prevention (CDC) has cited that an average of 15.5 million people are involved in shift work. Law enforcement, news publishing, emergency services, hospitals, food services, printing, military, airlines, paper production, and railroads are just some of the industries affected. It is clear that many lives depend on people who are fully functional while the majority of the population is sleeping.

CREATING THE OPTIMAL SHIFT FOR EMPLOYEES

Scheduling is one of the greatest challenges a manager faces. What works for one person may not work for the others—a schedule that meets the needs of the employees may not meet the needs of the hospital.

The conversations regarding the expectations for the employee to be involved with shift work begin during the recruitment and interview process. To create a successful schedule, the manager should begin by determining the best shift for each person. Each veterinary technician should be interviewed to determine what would work best for him or her. The staff should be allowed to submit their own ideas. They should know that their preferences may not be possible, but the manager is willing to consider all possibilities. Open and frequent communication promotes teamwork.

The manager should discuss possible scenarios that may occur on different shifts to determine which veterinary technicians may be able to handle specific shift expectations. Allowing the applicants to shadow during different shifts will allow them to interact with veterinary technicians who work nights and ask questions they may have about working the different hours.

Most procedures and activities will occur during the day. The person who works during the day is someone who enjoys the busy pace, as well as working with many people (and occasionally different services).

The person scheduled to work the second shift assists in bridging the gap between the two shifts. This person also enjoys the busy pace and communicates well with coworkers. The hours tend to be very busy for emergency clients.

The overnight shift requires someone who is experienced and works well independently. His or her ability to observe and interpret observations should be excellent. Many times the overnight veterinary technician is the primary caregiver and needs to be able to relay important information over the phone to the doctor. The person should be able to communicate well not only to the professional staff but also to the clients.

> *TECHNICIAN NOTE* The overnight shift is a time when communication is necessary, and it must be very clearly stated and as detailed as possible. Most people this individual will be communicating with are people whose sleep cycle has been disrupted.

The manager should overlap staff schedules for at least 1 to 2 hours. The combined team from the two different shifts is able to work closely together to complete procedures or treatments before the previous shift leaves. Overlapping shifts promote a team effort to accomplish the same goal; it also gives the team time to complete thorough case reviews and updates and answer any questions that arise once the relief shift begins to assess patients' conditions. The overlap also gives the combined team time to interact with coworkers and help eliminate the feeling of isolation that sometimes occurs among veterinary technicians who work nights.

Consistency is extremely important. The ideal situation would be to eliminate shift rotation schedules (because it sometimes takes days for the body to adjust to a new schedule). The clinic should have a pool of part-time people to cover for vacations, holidays, personal days, and sick leave. This reduces the number of times regular staff people must rotate shifts and increases the consistency of the schedule.

Finding people who are interested in working only nights is difficult, so rotations have become part of the system.

A variety of rotations have been developed. Some rotations are more beneficial to the normal body rhythms; others are detrimental. Optimized shift rotation schedules are schedules designed specifically to meet the normal daily rhythms or circadian cycles of human physiology.

The most beneficial rotations are slow rotations in which each person stays on a specific shift 5 to 14 days. Two weeks on a specific shift is best. Slow rotation by phase advance is the rotation from night to afternoon to morning; this rotation method is considered to be physiologically and emotionally harmful.

Slow rotation by phase delay is the rotation from morning to afternoon to night and is considered to be the ideal shift rotation. When the veterinary technician rotates through this shift structure, he or she gains 8 hours of sleep.

Rapid rotations also occur, which are shifts that rotate the veterinary technician through several shifts during 1 week. Rapid rotations are considered the worst type of schedule. The daily rotation disrupts the body rhythms, making it very difficult for the veterinary technician to be productive.

The next category is the dedicated shift, in which the veterinary technician is assigned to a single shift during his or her stay with the practice. This is preferred to any rotation but in many cases is not an option.

LENGTH OF SHIFTS

Extended shifts began to increase in human nursing in the 1980s. An increase of needle stick injuries, patient-care errors, and other work-related accidents has been well documented in nurses who work the extended shifts. It has been shown through sleep and neurobehavioral tests that people who work beyond 8 hours begin having decreased cognitive function and ability. European nurses typically work 37-hour work weeks and are often prohibited from working 12-hour shifts; 12-hour shifts are highly discouraged because of the risk involved but continue to be very popular as a result of the limited number of days the employee needs to work.

TECHNICIAN NOTE   Shift schedules should be evaluated routinely. Employees working night shifts should be monitored for productivity and for the physical and emotional effects of the schedule. This will help prevent employee turnover and accidents caused by fatigue.

In addition, sleep schedules should be posted so that the staff can avoid calling sleeping employees, if possible. The supervisor of the veterinary technician working nights should avoid encroaching on employees' sleep time when scheduling mandatory meetings or performance reviews.

The manager responsible for the schedule should remember that not every schedule will work for every team, and what is currently working may need to be adjusted depending on the needs of the hospital. Many options are available; involving those individuals who will be directly affected by the shift structure is important.

HELPFUL HINTS FOR DAY SLEEPING

TECHNICIAN NOTE   Emergency and critical care veterinary technicians must make an extra effort to take care of themselves to be efficient and productive workers during all hours. Applicants for positions in a 24-hour unit must understand that they may be expected to work different shifts.

Many people agree to these arrangements without understanding how such schedules can impact their personal and professional lives.

A new veterinary technician working nights can try taking a 3-hour nap before the shift begins and sleeping right after the shift is over. The goal is to increase the sleep time after the shift and decrease it before the shift. This gradual change has worked for many.

The veterinary technician working nights can become a successful day sleeper; he or she should keep the routine as consistent as possible. When trying to establish a healthy sleep pattern, the technician also should do the following:

- Go to bed immediately after work—Resist the temptation to do anything because this stimulates the body clock to go into the day mode. Exercise should be planned after sleep.

- Exercise at least five times a week for emotional and physical well-being.
- Seek total darkness—This can be accomplished by using dark, heavy drapes or black plastic garbage bags over the windows to block any sunlight. A blindfold may be a good investment.
- Be vocal about the need for peace during these hours—Inform friends about sleep schedules, put a "Do Not Disturb" sign on the door, and wear earplugs if necessary.
- Use white noise—White noise has been used as a sleep inducer and has been found to be very successful for some people. White noise is acoustic or electrical noise in which the intensity is the same at all frequencies. Fans and bubbling fish filters are two examples. Tapes and machines made specifically for white noise also are available.
- Keep the environment cool—Many people sleep better in a cooler environment. Adjust the thermostat to a comfortable temperature.
- Take a bath—Having a hot bath 1 to 2 hours before sleep will raise your body temperature. You begin to feel sleepy as your body temperature decreases after the bath.
- Avoid using sleep inducers—Melatonin supplements are commonly used to help travelers avoid jet lag, get some sleep, and reset their body clocks. Melatonin is the sleep-inducing chemical released in the brain during the hours of darkness. The synthetic form may be helpful in assisting the body to adjust to the first few days of night shift work, but no studies have been done to evaluate the safety of chronic use.
- Do not use sleeping pills—Sleeping pills are not recommended because of the psychologic addiction that may occur. Any such drugs should be used in moderation. It may be best to use them only on the first day after the first night back on the night shift.

It takes extra effort for the night worker to arrange a sleep schedule, but doing so is worth it. In the book *Restful Sleep*, Deepak Chopra writes, "The purpose of sleep is to allow the body to repair and rejuvenate itself. The deep rest provided during sleep allows the body to recover from fatigue and stress and enlivens the body's own self repair and homeostatic, or balancing, mechanisms."*

---

*From Chopra D: *Restful sleep*, New York, 1994, Harmony Books.

WORKING THE NIGHT SHIFT

To become as productive, efficient, and healthy as possible when working the night shift, emergency and critical care veterinary technicians should do the following:

- Drink plenty of water—Dehydration was noted to be very common among people who work at night.
- Avoid caffeinated beverages after midnight during the shift—Caffeine remains in the body for an average of 6 hours and can interfere with sleep and cause indigestion. One should reduce the consumption of caffeine slowly if accustomed to consuming large quantities. Withdrawal symptoms include headaches and nausea.
- Plan to eat the biggest meal of the day during the lunch break on the night shift—Doing this will help limit snacking throughout the shift.
- Bring plenty of healthful snacks for late-night cravings.
- Exercise during the night shift—Exercising during the night shift has been proven to increase alertness and ability to sleep during the day. Take at least 20 minutes to do some aerobic exercise. Walking the animals during the shift may not be enough unless the caseload of ambulatory animals is high. Walking up stairs or around the hospital may be necessary.

Veterinary technicians should also remember that bright light therapy for night workers is becoming very popular. It helps the body clock shift to an active mode by suppressing the secretion of the nighttime hormone melatonin. Bright lights also may enhance the effectiveness of serotonin and other neurotransmitters, which shift the circadian rhythm (10,000 lux therapy is the intensity suggested, which is 20 times the intensity of average indoor light). Spending 3 to 6 or more hours under bright lights increases alertness during the night shift and the ability to sleep during the day. Practices can install these light sources, or light boxes can be purchased individually.

AFTER THE SHIFT

After a shift, limiting exposure to sunlight and avoiding eating a breakfast-type meal are good practices. Dark sunglasses can be used on the ride home.

If a person cannot adjust to the night shift, the only other solution may be a day shift. People in their middle forties to early fifties have greater difficulty adjusting to these shifts.

CONCLUSION

The veterinary technician who chooses to work in an emergency and critical care unit may be asked to work a variety of shifts during his or her employment. The shift worker and the employer must understand the physical and psychological strain this type of work can cause. Once this is understood and accepted, the people involved with shift work can take the necessary steps to decrease the negative impact of shift work. The person responsible for scheduling and the shift workers must act as a team. The veterinary technician must be committed to making an extra effort to obtain a restful sleep and the person responsible for scheduling the shift workers must be committed to providing optimal rotations to prevent disruption to the workers' normal body rhythms. Patient and personnel safety and well-being will improve when all are committed to providing a healthy environment for the shift worker.

SUGGESTED READINGS

Campbell S: Effects of timed bright-light exposure on shift work adaptation in middle-aged subjects, *Sleep* 18(6):408–416, 1995.

Caruso C: Negative impacts of shiftwork and long work hours, *Rehabil Nurs* 0:1–9, 2013.

Chopra D: *Restful sleep*, New York, 1994, Harmony Books.

Czeisler CA: Rotating shift work schedules that disrupt sleep are improved by applying circadian principles, *Science* 217:460, 1982.

Dearholt SL, Feathers CA: Self-scheduling can work, *Nurs Manage* 28(8):47, 1997.

DeMoss C, McGrail M, Haus E, et al.: Health and performance factors in health care shift workers, *J Occup Environ Med* 46:1278–1281, 2004.

Geiger-Brown J, Lee CJ, Trinkoff AM: The role of work schedules in occupational health and safety. In *Handbook of occupational health and wellness*, New York, 2012, Springer Science + Business Media, pp 207–322.

Geiger-Brown J, Roger VE, Trinkoff AM, et al.: Sleep, sleepiness, fatigue and performance of 12-hour-shift nurses, *Chronobiol Int* 29(2):211–219, 2012.

Goodkind M: Night shifts can be easier, Stanford University Medical Center News Bureau, *Health Tips*, Jan 1996.

Gumenyuk V, Roth T, Drake CL: Circadian phase, sleepiness, and light exposure assessment in night workers with and without shift work disorder, *Chronobiol Int* 29(7):928–936, 2012.

Han K, Trinkoff AM, Storr C, et al.: Comparison of job stress and obesity in nurses with favorable and unfavorable work schedules, *JOEM* 54(8):928–983, 2012.

Keller S: Effects of extended work shifts and shift work on patient safety, productivity, and employee health, *AAOHN J* 57(12): 497–502, 2009.

Lewy AJ: Treating chronobiologic sleep and mood disorders with bright light, *Psychiatr Ann* 17(9):664, 1997.

Scott A: Shift work and health, *Primary Care* 27(4):1057–1079, 2000.

Slon S: Night moves, *Prevention* 49(6):106, 1997.

Trinkoff A, Geiger-Brown J: Sleep-deprived nurses. In Koppel R, Gordon S, *First, do less harm*, Ithaca and London, 2012, Cornell University Press, pp 168–178.

Other Resources

Healthcare Tips for the Shift Worker: www.mayoclinic.com.

Lark and Owl Self-Test: www.sph.uth.edu.

Plain Language About Shift Work: DHHS (NIOSH) Pub No. 2004-143. www.cdc.gov.

Sleep Hygiene Poster: www.cci.health.wa.gov.au.

29 Client Communication in an Emergency

Jim Clark

CHAPTER OUTLINE

Why Communication Matters
Fielding Telephone Calls
Initial Greeting of Clients
Expressing Empathy
Communicating Effectively with
  Emergency Clients
Presenting Critical Care Estimates

Exam Room Communication
Presenting Estimates
Discussing Euthanasia
Communicating with Challenging
  Clients
Communicating with Referral
  Practices

KEY TERMS

Critical care estimate
Empathy
End-of-life
  decision-making
Mixed signals
Nonverbal
  communication
Open-ended questions
Open posture
Paraverbal
  communication
Perceived wait time
Reflective listening
Validation

LEARNING OBJECTIVES

After studying this chapter, you will be able to:

- Understand why communication is more challenging in emergency practice.
- Identify the three key communication needs of veterinary emergency clients.
- Handle emergency telephone calls professionally and efficiently.
- Demonstrate how to express empathy, both verbally and nonverbally.
- Use open-ended questions and reflective listening when collecting a history.
- Apply principles of nonverbal communication, including use of an open posture.
- Tailor the communication approach to the situation and client preference.
- Improve the approval rate for cost estimates by using proven communication skills.
- Provide communication support to clients facing end-of-life decisions.
- Utilize appropriate tools to defuse angry clients.
- Demonstrate warm and professional communication with referral practices.

WHY COMMUNICATION MATTERS

One of the most important tasks in veterinary general practice is communicating effectively with clients. Effective communication is even more essential in emergency practice because: (1) medical conditions are, on average, more severe and more acute; (2) clients typically lack a trusting relationship with the emergency doctor and other medical staff; (3) discussion of diagnostic and management options may be more complex; (4) clients are more likely to be affected by strong emotions; and (5) the cost of care is likely to be higher.

> **TECHNICIAN NOTE** Experienced emergency technicians know that just one communication misstep can create a disastrous situation, *even when excellent medical care was provided by a highly competent healthcare team!* A breakdown in client communication by *any* member of the healthcare team weakens the entire chain of communication.

In this chapter, we will review some of the key principles and most recent information regarding effective communication in a medical setting. Our focus will be on communicating with clients, but many of the principles also apply to communicating well with fellow team members. If you are like most people, you already assume you are a good communicator. Although that may be the case, I encourage you to consider how you can further improve your communication skills in emergency practice, inspiring others to follow your example.

> **TECHNICIAN NOTE** Communication is a core clinical skill that every member of the emergency healthcare team should strive to further develop.

FIELDING TELEPHONE CALLS

Client communication in emergency practice typically begins with a telephone call handled by a technician or client service representative (CSR). Depending on their level of medical knowledge, CSRs often consult with technicians or doctors to ensure clients receive accurate advice and recommendations. It is important to recognize that each phone call from a potential client creates a *first impression* of the practice. Try to answer the call in three rings or less and strive to convey warmth, caring, and competency. Our goal should be to understand the client's concern(s), provide support, and offer helpful advice. The most skilled technicians achieve these goals while also handling calls efficiently.

Figure 29-1 shows one approach to handling calls professionally and efficiently. Notice that step 2 (very early in the call) suggests asking if the client would like to come to your hospital. Because many clients have already decided to seek an exam (calling just to verify you are open or find out costs or directions), asking this question is far more efficient than obtaining a detailed description of the pet's situation on every call. Other clients, however, are uncertain if their pet needs to be seen.

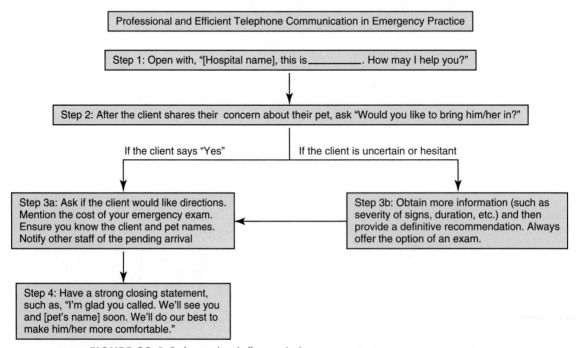

FIGURE 29-1 Professional and efficient telephone communication in emergency practice.

In this case, it is important to ask enough questions to understand the pet's situation.

If you feel the pet should be seen, state that definitively. For example, "Based on what you've described, I think Max should *definitely* be examined tonight." This is more compelling than saying, "I *think* it *might* be a good idea to bring Max in." Even if we feel the situation is *not* emergent, it is still wise to offer the client the option of an exam. For example, by saying, "From what you've shared, I'm uncertain if this is an emergency. We'd be happy to see Max, if only for all of our peace of mind." Always err on the side of patient safety and never make a diagnosis or rule out an emergency over the phone.

INITIAL GREETING OF CLIENTS

When a client arrives with his or her pet at your emergency hospital (or, in large animal mobile practice, you arrive on site), it is essential to greet the client and assess the patient quickly. Because of the repetitive nature of our work, *it is easy to forget what a stressful situation this is for our clients and patients!* According to a comprehensive survey, 85% of pet owners view their pet as a family member (Brown and Silverman, 1999). Witnessing an event such as a seizure or hit-by-car is very traumatic for most pet owners, whereas these may be everyday occurrences for technicians in emergency practice.

> *TECHNICIAN NOTE* In addition to attending to the immediate medical needs of patients upon arrival, we must also recognize when clients are in distress and provide support.

EXPRESSING EMPATHY

One of the best ways to help clients feel more comfortable on arrival is to express **empathy**.

> *TECHNICIAN NOTE* Empathy has been defined in many ways. In essence, it is the ability to recognize, experience, and express the feelings of another person. Whereas sympathy is the intellectual exercise of putting oneself in another's shoes, empathy incorporates an emotional aspect as well.

In a review of 20 years of patient-satisfaction research in the human emergency room (ER), empathy/attitude was identified as one of five key correlates with satisfaction (Welch, 2010). Research in the veterinary field has shown that veterinarians underutilize empathy statements, using them in only 7% of appointments in one study (Shaw et al, 2004). Table 29-1 provides practical suggestions for expressing empathy both verbally and nonverbally.

COMMUNICATING EFFECTIVELY WITH EMERGENCY CLIENTS

There are several important principles to keep in mind when communicating with clients.

> *TECHNICIAN NOTE* I believe veterinary emergency clients have three key desires: (1) to understand their pet's medical condition; (2) to feel in control; and, (3) to feel understood.

Achieving these objectives is the job of EVERY member of the healthcare team. When communicating a recommended test or treatment, we should convey both *what* it is and *why* it will benefit the patient. Whenever we have the opportunity, we should help our clients feel in control of their pet's care. Clients who feel in control are more likely to approve the medical care we recommend. In order for clients to feel understood, we need to express genuine concern, using both verbal and nonverbal expressions of empathy.

Good communicators recognize that the majority of communication during in-person interactions occurs

TABLE 29-1	Expressing Empathy Verbally and Nonverbally	
VERBAL EXPRESSIONS OF EMPATHY	**NONVERBAL AND PARAVERBAL EXPRESSIONS OF EMPATHY**
"I can see you're very concerned about Max."	Facial expression of concern with caring tone of voice
"I'm sorry you had to come in at this hour."	Good eye contact
"I'm sure you're worried about Max's vomiting"	Open body posture with arms at sides (vs. arms crossed)
"I'm so sorry that Max isn't feeling well tonight."	Leaning or kneeling to match height with client and/or pet

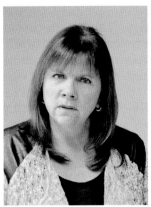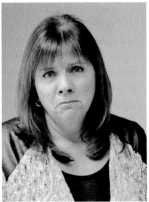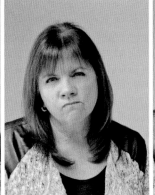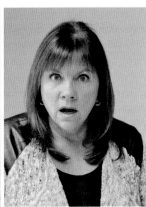

FIGURE 29-2 Can you correctly identify this client's emotions? From left to right: (1) skeptical; (2) sad; (3) angry; (4) surprised.

*non*verbally and *para*verbally. **Nonverbal communication** includes facial expressions, body posture, body movements, and body position relative to our client. **Paraverbal communication** is *how* we say things, including our tone, rate, volume, and rhythm. When communicating with clients, pay close attention to the nonverbal signals you are sending and to those displayed by the client. Adopt an open posture, with legs uncrossed and arms hanging at your sides or resting with palms open in front of you. According to communication expert Carol Goman, PhD, individuals with open body positions are perceived more positively and are more persuasive (Goman, 2008).

When clients experience "**mixed signals**" (for example, they hear us say we are concerned about their pet but our tone and posture suggest otherwise), clients will trust the nonverbal signals over the verbal message. If you are presenting an estimate and the client says "yes" but their nonverbal communication appears inconsistent, pay attention to that! It may be helpful to say, "I'm sensing that you have some concerns about these costs. Can I be of help?" Figure 29-2 shows a variety of facial expressions. Can you correctly identify this client's emotions?

PRESENTING CRITICAL CARE ESTIMATES

If upon arrival a pet is determined to need immediate care, many emergency practices present their clients with a "**critical care estimate**" (often ranging from $200 to $600) to cover the cost of just the initial diagnostic tests and treatments. If communicated poorly, clients may develop the perception that we care more about money

than helping animals. As discussed earlier, we should pay attention to both *what* we say and *how* we say it!

Here is one approach: "I know you must be worried about Max [empathy statement]. Dr. Jones is concerned about Max's condition ["warning shot"] and we've made caring for Max a top priority right now [reassurance]. Dr. Jones wants to meet with you, share her findings, and answer your questions [signaling the client will have some control], but right now she needs to be with Max [personalizing the message by repeating the pet's name]. May I share her recommendations? [allowing a pause for the client to think and using a question to signal client control] She would like to give Max an injection to make him more comfortable [*what* and *why*], place a line in a blood vessel to give Max some fluids to support his blood pressure, and run some basic blood tests to see how his main organ systems are functioning. We'd like your authorization [client control] to provide this care and want you to know the costs in advance [reassurance]. The cost of these initial steps will be approximately $500. Are you comfortable placing a deposit in that amount? [signaling client control by presenting a question rather than a demand]"

Notice the effort to help Max's owner understand the situation, feel in control, and "feel felt." This increases the likelihood of effective communication and approval of our recommendations, though there will obviously still be clients who decline care or misinterpret our efforts. When breaking bad news to clients, for example, that their pet has a life-threatening problem, be especially aware of how you communicate the information. Table 29-2 shares some "Do's and Don'ts" for breaking bad news.

TABLE 29-2	Do's and Don'ts for Breaking Bad News	
DO	**DON'T**
Provide a "warning shot."	Immediately "drop the bomb."
Proceed slowly and include pauses.	Rush to explain everything.
Express empathy.	Focus on just the facts.
Use concise "talking points."	Provide lengthy explanations.
Check in frequently for understanding.	Discourage questions.
Ask if the client has family or friends for support.	Assume the client has adequate support.

Because of the unscheduled nature of emergency work, clients will sometimes be kept waiting. Human patients tend to overestimate wait times and the urgency of their medical situation (Welch, 2010). Research by Burch and colleagues suggests that perceived (vs. actual) wait time was the most important factor in human emergency room satisfaction and that unoccupied time is perceived as longer than occupied time (Burch et al, 1993). When clients are kept waiting, keep them occupied by providing frequent updates, both on the status of their pet and on the expected wait time. Providing video presentations, a variety of current magazines, and self-served amenities such as coffee and tea may also be helpful.

EXAM ROOM COMMUNICATION

In small animal emergency practice, clients are typically moved from a reception area into an exam room to meet with a doctor. The role of veterinary technicians in the exam room varies: technicians may collect initial baseline medical data and obtain detailed histories or instead obtain very minimal information. Upon entering the room, introduce yourself and your role. For example, "Hi, Ms. Davis. My name is Karen and I'm a veterinary technician. I'll be getting some initial information on Max and then you'll be meeting with Dr. Jones. She's a very experienced emergency doctor and loves Labs. I think you'll like her."

Notice in the preceding example that the technician Karen gave a brief positive "testimonial" about Dr. Jones. This can be very helpful in reassuring the client and improving the client's first impression of the doctor. If you are collecting the history, begin by asking the client an open-ended question such as, "So what brings you in tonight with Lady?" Even if you already know the client is concerned about a specific problem (such as vomiting), it is still helpful to use an open-ended question such as, "What are your concerns about Lady?" This provides clients with a chance to *tell their story*, often revealing more information than you would have obtained using just closed-ended questions (which can be answered with a single word). Research has shown that veterinarians underutilize **open-ended questions** (Shaw et al, 2004). As clients share their story, avoid interrupting them.

Effective communication requires effective listening skills. Because our animal patients cannot speak for themselves, it is critical that we glean as much historical information as possible from their owners. Reflective listening requires you to listen with attention and then share a brief synopsis of what you have heard. For example, "So what I'm hearing is that Lady has vomited 6 times in the past 12 hours and that you noticed some blood when she last vomited 1 hour ago. Is that right?" Reflective listening shows clients you are interested and paying attention. It also helps ensure the information is correct, potentially improving diagnostic accuracy (Kurtz et al, 2004).

Technicians are often required to share medical information with clients, including diagnostic test results, and to explain medical procedures. In a 2013 *Consumer Reports* survey of 1000 Americans, the number one complaint about human physicians was their "unclear explanations of problems." When conveying information, remember that clients only retain a small percentage of what we tell them. Keep your explanations organized and brief while avoiding use of medical jargon. Check in frequently with clients, for example by asking, "Am I explaining this clearly? What questions do you have?" The best communicators adapt to their clients; for example, some clients want only the "big picture," whereas other clients are very detail oriented. Many clients care most about their pet's comfort and likelihood of recovery, so it is important to discuss these issues.

> **TECHNICIAN NOTE** When possible, provide key information in both verbal and written form. Many clients will learn best when you draw a picture, demonstrate a technique, or assist clients themselves in performing a procedure (such as instilling an eye medication).

PRESENTING ESTIMATES

Technicians also commonly review cost estimates with clients. Table 29-3 lists do's and don'ts when discussing finances with clients. These conversations can at times be challenging because money is at the root of many client conflicts. In our efforts to be patient advocates, we can unconsciously cause clients to feel pressured to approve care they do not understand or cannot afford.

TABLE 29-3	Do's and Don'ts When Discussing Finances with Clients	
DO	**DON'T**	
Avoid surprises—share costs in advance.	Expect clients to pay for care they did not approve.	
Present estimates with confidence.	Verbally or nonverbally project hesitancy.	
Sit or stand *next to* the client.	Sit or stand directly *across from* the client.	
Be empathetic about the costs of care.	Judge clients who cannot afford recommended care.	
Explain how each item benefits the pet.	Present a list of items without any explanation.	
Provide a breakdown of included items before the total.	Give clients just the total cost.	
Be very clear about the time frame covered.	Expect clients to understand future expected costs.	
Remind clients they are in control.	Pressure clients to approve care.	
Update clients when additional costs arise.	Hit clients with unexpected charges at discharge.	

Counter-intuitively, when clients feel *less* pressured they are more likely to approve care. Help clients feel in control (because, after all, they do have the final say in what care will be provided) by using statements such as, "you're in the driver's seat," or "we want to work within your budget." When presenting estimates to clients, be sure to explain how recommended tests and treatments will *benefit* the pet. Rather than presenting an estimate across a counter, try sitting down next to your client. As shown in Figure 29-3, this conveys a more collaborative approach and is likely to be more successful.

DISCUSSING EUTHANASIA

Another communication challenge for technicians is discussing end-of-life decisions and euthanasia ("good death" in ancient Greek). Unfortunately, we find ourselves in these situations more often in emergency practice than in general practice. We have the added challenges of lacking a prior trusting relationship with our clients and facing time pressures on busy shifts. A thorough discussion of this important topic is beyond the scope of this chapter, but several key principles are to provide privacy, respond to emotions with empathy, slow down, avoid medical jargon, be honest but compassionate, and explore the client's thoughts and feelings. If clients choose to be present when their pet is euthanized, it is important to discuss the process in order to avoid alarming surprises.

According to a Canadian survey of pet owners who had recently euthanized a pet, approximately 27% experienced severe grief and 50% questioned if they had made the right decision or felt guilty about the decision

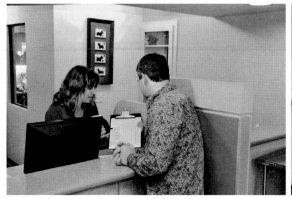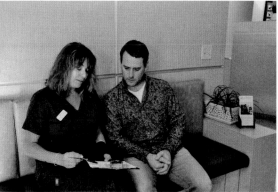

FIGURE 29-3 Nonverbal communication during estimate presentation.

(Adams et al, 2000). Once our client has made the decision to euthanize his or her pet, it is essential that we *respect and validate* the decision. For example, we might say, "Based on Pepper's condition, I think your decision is a compassionate one that will prevent further discomfort."

An analysis of euthanasia discussions in veterinary practice suggested that some veterinarians fail to adequately explore key areas, such as client feelings, ideas, and expectations (Borden et al, 2010). We may also err in end-of-life communication by talking too much, neglecting to explore our client's goals, skirting open discussion of feelings, and failing to validate our client's decisions and feelings.

COMMUNICATING WITH CHALLENGING CLIENTS

The reality is that communicating with some emergency clients is difficult. I prefer to view these individuals as "challenging clients" rather than "difficult clients." Although you cannot control the behavior of another person, you can control your own perspective and behavior. We should view these situations as professional challenges where we have a chance to test our best communication skills! Begin by asking yourself if the client (1) understands; (2) feels in control; and (3) feels understood. Odds are good that there is a disconnect in one or more of these areas. Avoid taking comments personally. We often just need to respectfully listen, ask questions for clarification, and seek mutual understanding. Communication rookies will instead respond by quoting policy, "digging in" to their positions, and emphasizing differences rather than seeking common ground.

If you ever feel your personal safety is at risk when communicating with an angry client, pay attention to that "gut feeling" and immediately take steps to protect yourself. According to VIN consultant Michele Gaspar, patients in human hospitals appear to be becoming more reactive and aggressive (Gaspar, 2012).

TECHNICIAN NOTE Many angry clients are reacting to underlying feelings of vulnerability, loss of control, fear, and/or anticipatory grief. Thankfully, most of these clients will respond to effective communication.

Adopt an open body posture, listen without interruption, respond in a calm and professional tone, express empathy, offer an apology, talk about common goals, and seek a mutually satisfactory solution. This is an excellent time to use **reflective listening**. Note that, when necessary, you can express empathy and apologize without assuming responsibility. For example, "Mr. Cornell, I can see you are very upset and I'm so sorry about that." I have also found it helpful to sit down, let the client vent, ask questions before offering any solutions, and take notes (signaling the importance of the information). Use of these tools will improve your success in these challenging situations.

COMMUNICATING WITH REFERRAL PRACTICES

In addition to communicating with clients, emergency technicians often interface by phone with doctors and staff at surrounding referral practices. When doing so, always keep in mind the importance of the referral relationship; these practices are our MOST important clients! We should handle these calls with warmth and professionalism, seeking to provide support and expressing our thanks for their trust and referrals. At times, clients will make derogatory remarks about their family veterinarian. Experience suggests we should always take these comments with a large grain of salt. Similarly, we hope that our referring veterinarians will not believe some of the things they hear about our emergency practices! Our relationship and communication with our referral hospitals should be based on mutual respect and the shared goal of providing excellent patient care and client service.

Use of the communication tools discussed in this chapter has the potential to improve client satisfaction and diagnostic accuracy while reducing complaints and litigation (Levinson et al, 1997). Effective communication also makes our work more fun and allows us to provide better care to our animal patients and their owners.

REFERENCES

Adams CL, Bonnett BN, Meek AH: Predictors of owner response to companion animal death in 177 clients from 14 practices in Ontario, *J Am Vet Med Assoc* 217:1303–1309, 2000.

Borden LJ, Adams CL, Bonnett BN, et al.: Use of the measure of patient-centered communication to analyze euthanasia discussions in companion animal practice, *J Am Vet Med Assoc* 237:1275–1287, 2010.

Brown JP, Silverman JD: The current and future market for veterinarians and veterinary medical services in the United States, *J Am Vet Med Assoc* 215:161–183, 1999.

Burch B, Beezy J, Shaw R: Emergency department satisfaction: what matters most? *Ann Emerg Med* 22:586–591, 1993.

Consumer Reports Magazine, June 2013.

Gaspar M: Veterinary Information Network Web site: *Electronic rounds: working with reactive clients: de-escalation techniques for volatile situations*, Published Oct 28, 2012 at www.vin.com/members/cms/document/default.aspx?id=5579718&;pid=6257&catid=&said=1.

Goman CK: *The nonverbal advantage: secrets and science of body language at work*, San Francisco, 2008, Berrett-Koehler.

Kurtz SM, Silverman J, Draper J: *Teaching and learning communication skills in medicine*, Arbingdon, U.K. 2004, Radcliffe Medical Press.

Levinson W, Roter DL, Mullooly JP, et al.: Physician-patient communication. The relationship with malpractice claims among primary care physicians and surgeons, *J Am Med Assoc* 277:553–559, 1997.

Shaw JR, Adams CL, Bonnett BN, et al.: A description of veterinarian-client-patient communication using the Roter Method of Interaction Analysis, *J Am Vet Med Assoc* 225:222–229, 2004.

Welch SJ: A review of human patient satisfaction literature over the past 20 years, *Am J Med Qual* 25(1):64–72, 2010.

SCENARIO

Telephone Role-Playing Exercise

Purpose: To provide an engaging interactive experience where technicians can actively practice and evaluate the professional and efficient handling of common situations encountered during telephone conversations in emergency practice.

Delivery: Have team members pair up. Give each team member a memo card with one of the scenarios described below. Each team member will role-play as the client described on the memo card while their partner role-plays receiving the call at the hospital.

Scenario A

Your 7-year-old domestic shorthair cat has been vomiting repeatedly over the past 2 days and you are both concerned and fed up with the mess. You have already made the decision to come in, so are just calling to check on availability of care and cost of the exam.

Scenario B

Your 7-week-old Rottweiler puppy is lethargic and has bloody diarrhea. You are unsure if an exam is really warranted.

Scenario C

Your 7-month-old unspayed female cat is suddenly behaving very strangely. She is vocalizing a lot and rubbing up against you. She is a solo indoor-only cat with no other signs of concern.

Scenario D

Your 7-year-old German shepherd's stomach suddenly seems distended and he has been retching for the past hour.

Discussion

Upon completion of the role-play, have each team member share what went well and what could have been "even better yet." Using the skills discussed in this chapter, discuss these scenarios and describe how to handle the calls both professionally and efficiently, while erring on the side of protecting patient safety.

Key Teaching Points

- Provides technicians with the opportunity to tailor their communication approach to the situation, improving efficiency.
- Provides technicians with the opportunity to demonstrate appropriate professional verbal and paraverbal communication with simulated clients.
- Provides technicians with the opportunity to learn from their peers as well as the instructor.

Index

A

Abdomen, injury to, 266
  assessment of, 266
  management of, 266
  monitoring of, 266
Abdominal distention, anesthesia and, 167
Abscesses
  meibomian gland, 409
  prostatic, 400, 400f
  rabbit and rodent emergencies and, 475
  in reptile emergencies, 485
Accelerated idioventricular rhythm, 310, 310f
Acepromazine, 174
Acetaminophen, in toxicologic emergencies,
  447–448
Acetylcysteine, 410
Achlorhydria, 441
Acid citrate dextrose (ACD), 91t
Acid-base status, 22
Acidosis
  in diabetic ketoacidosis, 355
  trauma and, 256
Acquired coagulopathies, 274–275
  dilutional coagulopathies in, 275
  dysfunctional synthesis in, 274–275
  factor activation defect in, 274
  factor consumption in, 275
Acquired myasthenia gravis, 426
  diagnostic confirmation of, 427
ACT. *see* Activated clotting time
ACTH. *see* Adrenocorticotropic hormone
  (ACTH)
Activated charcoal (AC), for toxicologic
  emergencies, 436
Activated clotting time (ACT), 279–280, 323
Activated partial thromboplastin time, 279
Acuity, of patient, 212
Acute Addisonian crisis. *see*
  Hypoadrenocorticism
Acute bacterial prostatitis, 401
Acute hemolytic transfusion reactions
  (AHTRs), 101
Acute kidney injury (AKI), 383
  causes of, 384, 384b
  clinical presentation of, 384
  diagnosis of, 385
  drug therapy for, 386
  fluid therapy for, 385–386
  nutritional support for, 386
  response to treatment for, 386
  treatment of, 385–386
Acute nucleus pulposus extrusion, 424, 424f

Acute pain scales, 13b
Acute renal failure, fluids for, 72t
Addison's disease. *see* Hypoadrenocorticism
Adenoma, in cornea, 409
Adenosine triphosphate, 280–281
Adhesives, in toxicologic emergencies, 447
Adjunctive/adjuvant analgesics, 157–160
  dose for, 160
Admission form, 216, 219f
Adrenal disease, in ferret emergencies, 468
Adrenocortical insufficiency, fluids for, 72t
Adrenocorticotropic hormone (ACTH), 356,
  361
Adulticide therapy, complications of, 314
Advanced life support, 240
  atropine in, 240
  calcium therapy for, 241
  drug administration route for, 241–242,
    242b
  drug delivery methods for, 241b
  drugs for, 240–242
  epinephrine in, 240
  fluids for, 241
  lidocaine in, 240–241
  reversal agents in, 241
  sodium bicarbonate in, 241
  vasopressin in, 240
Afterload, 302
Agenesis, eyelid, 409, 409f
Agglutination test, 19f
Agonal breaths, 236–237
AHTRs. *see* Acute hemolytic transfusion
  reactions (AHTRs)
Air embolism, 53–54
  anesthesia and, 184t–188t
Air sac cannula, 465, 465f
Airborne transmission, of disease, 193
Airflow system, in isolation unit, 203
Airway
  basic life support and, 237b
  obstruction of, 328
Airway access, emergency supplies and, 236b
Airway disruption, intubation and, 178
Airway humidity, mechanical ventilation and,
  141–142
Airway management, rabbit V-gel device for,
  453–454
Airway obstruction, intubation and, 178,
  178b
Airway swelling, intubation and, 178, 178b
Albumin, 82
  measurement of, 167–168

Alcoholic beverages, in avian emergencies,
  463
Alcohols, as disinfectant, 199t–200t
Alfaxalone, 175
Allergic reactions, in transfusion therapy,
  100–101, 100f
Allium species, 439–440
Alloantibodies, problems from, 90
Alpha$_2$ (α_2) agonists, 155–156
  reversal of, 156
American Philosophical Association (APA), 3
American Veterinary Medical Association
  in disaster medicine, 504
  field tents, 502f
Amikacin, 485
Amino acids, preparations of, 118
Ammonium urate uroliths, 382–383
AMPLE mnemonic, 254–255
Analgesia, 171–172
  for spinal cord injury, 425
  topical, 154
  in traumatic emergencies, 259, 259b
Analgesia injection
  in joint space, 155
  in peritoneal space, 155
  in pleural space, 155
Analgesics, 171–176
  adjunctive and adjuvant, 157–160
    dose for, 160
  CRI of, 156–160
  for pain, 150–152, 151b
Anaphylaxis, 100–101
  anesthesia and, 184t–188t
  distributive shock from, 225
Anemia, 17, 280–289
  abdominal palpation in, 287
  aplastic, 285
  blood smear in, 287–288
  blood transfusion for, 99
  chemistry profile in, 288
  of chronic disease, 284
  clinical assessment of, 285–288
  Coombs' test for, 288
  dysfunctional hemoglobin species in, 285
  erythropoiesis, reduced or ineffective,
    284–285
  hemogram in, 287–288
  hemolytic, 282
  history of, 285–286, 286b
  hypochromic, 287–288
  laboratory tests of, 287–288
  macrocytic, 287–288

Note: Page numbers followed by "b", "f" and "t" indicate boxes, figures and tables respectively.

Anemia (Continued)
  miscellaneous information in, 288
  nonregenerative, 285
  physical examination in, 286–287
  platelet count, 288
  red blood cells
    destruction of, 282–284
    loss of, 281–282
  from reduced or ineffective erythropoiesis, 284
  saline agglutination test for, 288
  tick titers in, 288
  treatment and management of, 289, 289b
  urinalysis in, 288
Anesthesia
  abdominal distention and, 167
  air embolism and, 184t–188t
  anaphylaxis and, 184t–188t
  atrioventricular block and, 184t–188t
  for avian emergencies, 462
  balanced, 171
  bradycardia and, 184t–188t
  controlled ventilation and, 179, 179f
  in critically ill or injured patient, 165–190
  cyanosis and, 184t–188t
  definition of, 166
  drugs for, 170–171, 170b
  in E tube placement, 112
  emergencies and complications during, 184–188, 184t–188t
  epidural analgesia and, 172–173
  ETCO$_2$ decrease and, 184t–188t
  ETCO$_2$ increase and, 184t–188t
  fluid therapy for, 183
  goals of, 171
  hypertension and, 184t–188t
  hypotension and, 184t–188t
  hypothermia prevention during, 183
  hypoventilation and, 184t–188t
  induction of, 170b, 174–175, 174b
  lack of thoracic expansion and, 184t–188t
  local/regional, 172
  malignant hyperthermia and, 184t–188t
  miscellaneous supplies for, 170b
  monitoring equipment for, 170b
  monitoring of, 179–181, 180b
  multifocal ventricular premature contractions and, 184t–188t
  oxygen saturation decrease and, 184t–188t
  patient maintenance under, 178–179
  patient recovery from, 188–189, 188b
  perivascular injection and, 184t–188t
  premedication and, 173–174
  preparedness for, 169–170
  principles of safe, 171b
  regurgitation/vomiting and, 184t–188t
  respiratory rate and, 167
  setting up for, 170b
  sinus arrest and, 184t–188t
  stabilization before, 168–169, 168b
  success goals of, 166–168, 166b
  supportive measures needed during, 183–184

Anesthesia (Continued)
  supraventricular tachycardia and, 184t–188t
  surgery set up and, 170, 170b
  tachycardia and, 184t–188t
  temperature conservation and, 183, 183f
  temperature monitoring and, 180–181
  weight evaluation and, 167
Anesthetic machine, preparation of, 170b
Anesthetic sheet, 169–170
Anesthetics, 173t–174t
  local and regional, 154
Anestrus, 392
Animal disaster team, 501b
Ant traps, in toxicologic emergencies, 443
Antagonist opioids, mixed agonist and, 153–154
Antagonists, 154
Anterior chamber, ocular emergencies of, 411
Antibiotics
  for diabetic ketoacidosis, 356
  for ocular emergencies, 406t–407t
  for otitis media/interna, 422
Anticholinergics, for gastrointestinal emergencies, 337–338
Anticoagulant-preservative solutions, 90, 91t
Anticoagulant rodenticide toxicity, 274
Anticoagulant rodenticides, 443–444
Anticoagulation, disorders in, 275–276
Antidotes, for toxicologic emergencies, 436, 436t
Antiemetics, for gastrointestinal emergencies, 337–338
Antihemophilic, 270t
Antiinflammatories, for ocular emergencies, 406t–407t
Antimicrobial impregnated central venous catheters, 44
Antimicrobial stewardship, 204
Antiparasitics, in toxicologic emergencies, 441–443
Antiprostaglandins, 152
Anti-proteinases/anti-collagenases drugs, 406t–407t
Antithrombin, deficiency of, 275
Antiviral drugs, for ocular emergencies, 406t–407t
Aortic stenosis, emergencies associated with, 295t
APA. see American Philosophical Association (APA)
Aplastic anemia, 285
Apomorphine, 435
Appendicular skeletal injuries, 425
Appetite, stimulants, 111
Approach, for patient, in emergency receiving, 214–216
Appropriate staff, 4
aPTT. see Activated partial thromboplastin time
Art of scheduling, 507–514
  day sleeping and, 512, 512b
  night shift and, 513

Art of scheduling (Continued)
  optimal shift for employees and, 510–512
  sleep deprivation and, 510, 510b
  survey of, 509f
Arterial blood gases (ABGs), 124–126
Arterial blood pressure, shock and, 231
Arterial catheter, 24
Arterial oxyhemoglobin saturation (SaO$_2$), 281
Arterial pH, shock and, 232
Arterial sampling, 23–24
ASPCA Animal Poison Control Center, 432b
Aspiration pneumonia, 330–331
  risk of, 427
Assisted feedings, 111
Association of Veterinary Hematology and Transfusion Medicine, 79
Asystole, 243, 243b, 244f
Atracurium, 177, 177b
Atrial fibrillation, treatment of, 310
Atrial septal defect, emergencies associated with, 295t
Atrioventricular block, anesthesia and, 184t–188t
Atrioventricular valve dysplasia, emergencies associated with, 295t
Atropine, 173–174, 173t–174t
  in advanced life support, 240
  for emergency situations, 454
Attire, for infection control, 195, 195b
Auscultation, 14, 14b
  of heart, 295, 295b
Autoagglutination, 18f
Autoimmune hemolytic anemia, 282
Autotransfusion, 103, 103b
  for traumatic emergencies, 250, 250f
Autumn crocus, in toxicologic emergencies, 438
Avian daily fluid requirement, 462b
Avian emergencies, 454–465
  alcoholic beverages in, 463
  anesthesia for, 462
  avocados in, 463
  of blood feathers, 462
  chocolate in, 463
  common, 462–465
  dehydration in, 461
  dystocia and, 462–463
  egg binding in, 462–463
  fluid administration in, 461–462, 461f, 461b–462b
  from ingested toxins, 463–464
  inhaled toxins in, 464, 464b
  intraosseous bolus volumes in, 460b
  intravenous bolus volumes in, 460b
  IV catheter placement in, 459–460, 459f, 459t, 460b
  lead ingestion in, 463–464
  metal ingestion in, 463–464, 464b
  mycotoxins in, 463
  nicotine ingestion in, 463
  physical examination for, 455–462, 455f–456f, 455b

Avian emergencies *(Continued)*
  respiratory, 464–465, 464b
  restraint for, 455–458, 455b, 457f
  supplies for, 454
  toxins in, 463
  tube feeding for, 460–461, 460b, 461f
  venipuncture for, 457–459, 458f, 458b
  zinc ingestion in, 463–464
Azotemia, 21, 360

B

Babesia canis, 86b
Backward failure, of heart, 304
Bacterial enteritis, in rabbit and rodent
    emergencies, 474–475
Bacterial pneumonia, 329–330
Balanced anesthesia, 171
Bandages, in traumatic emergencies, 259–260
Basic life support
  blood flow and, 237
  cardiopulmonary resuscitation and,
      237–243, 237b
  chest compressions and, 237–239
  ventilation and, 239, 239b
BCM. *see* Blood crossmatch (BCM)
BCS. *see* Body condition score (BCS)
Benign prostatic hypertrophy (BPH), 401
Benzodiazepines, 175–176
Beta oxidation, in diabetic ketoacidosis, 352
Bicarbonate ion (HCO_3-), 25
Bilirubin, anemia and, 286, 288
Biosecurity, 193–194
Bisphosphonates, for hypercalcemia, 364
Blanket warmer, for traumatic emergencies,
    252
Blastomycosis, 330
Bleach, in toxicologic emergencies, 447
Bleeding time test, 278–279, 278f, 278b
Blocked cat, 374–379
  catheterization for, 376–377, 376f,
      377b–378b
    managing indwelling urinary catheters,
        377–379, 378f, 378b
    response to treatment, 379
  clinical presentation of, 375
  diagnosis of, 375–376
  treatment for, 376
Blocked dog, 379–383, 380f
  catheterization for, 381, 381b–382b, 382f
  clinical presentation of, 380
  diagnosis of, 380, 380f
  response to treatment for, 382–383
  treatment of, 381
  urohydropropulsion and, 381–382
Blood, portions of, 79
Blood administration, 96–100
Blood banks, 79
Blood collection, 90–96
  leukoreduction in, 96
  processing of, 94–95
  storage lesions in, 96, 96b
  storage of, 94–95

Blood collection *(Continued)*
  systems of, 14f, 90–92, 92f
  techniques of, 92–94
    canine, 92–94, 92b–93b, 93f
    feline, 94, 94b
Blood compatibility, 96–97
Blood component, preparation of, 98–99, 98b
Blood component therapy, for vWD, 273
Blood crossmatch (BCM), 97
  parts of, 97
  procedure for, 98b
Blood donor
  canine, 86, 86b
  feline, 89, 89b
Blood feathers, in avian emergencies, 462
Blood filters, 100
Blood flow, in basic life support, 237
Blood gas analysis, 22–25, 22f
  definitions of, 24–25
  equipment for, 23
  indications for, 23
  interpretation for, 24–25
  manufacturers of equipment, 41
  normal values of, 25t
  simple, 25
  technique for, 23–24
  troubleshooting for, 24, 24b
Blood gases, 323
  shock and, 232
Blood glucose, in diabetic ketoacidosis, 356
Blood pressure
  fluid therapy and, 66
  gastrointestinal emergencies and, 335
  preanesthetic, 167
  in traumatic emergencies, 254
Blood pressure monitoring, 32–35
  anesthesia and, 181, 181b
  direct arterial pressure monitoring and, 33
  Doppler ultrasound flow detectors and,
      34–35, 34f
  equipment for, 32–33
    manufacturers of, 41
  indications for, 32
  indirect, 33–35, 34b
  interpretation for, 35
  technique for, 33–35
  troubleshooting for, 35
Blood smear, 287–288
Blood sources, 83–90, 86b–88b, 88f, 90
Blood tests, interpretation, 21
Blood types, 86–87, 96–97
  in canines, 87, 88t
Blunt trauma, 263
Body condition score (BCS), 107, 119–120
Body water, 62–63, 62f
Body weight
  fluid therapy and, 66–67, 66b, 67f
  monitoring of, 119–120
  reassessment of, 119–120
  restoration of healthy, 107–110
Bone marrow, dysfunction of, 284
Bone resorption inhibitors, for
    hypercalcemia, 364

Bordetella bronchiseptica, 329–330
  in rabbit and rodent emergencies, 475
Botulism, 426
Brachycephalic airway syndrome (BAS), 328,
    329f
Bradyarrhythmias, treatment of, 311, 311f,
    312t, 313f
Bradycardia, anesthesia and, 184t–188t
Breathing, basic life support and, 237b
Broad-spectrum antibiotics, for
    gastrointestinal emergencies, 337
Bromethalin, in toxicologic emergencies,
    444–445
Buccal mucosal bleeding time (BMBT), 28,
    29b, 278, 278f, 278b
Bulldogs, dystocia in, 393
Buphthalmia, cat with, 408
Bupivacaine, 172
Buprenorphine, 154, 172
  for gastrointestinal emergencies, 338
Buretrols, 73, 76f
Burn injuries, in disaster medicine, 494–495
Butorphanol, 172
  CRI dosage for
    in cats, 158t
    in dogs, 159t
  for gastrointestinal emergencies, 337–338
Butorphanol tartrate, 154

C

Caffeine, in toxicologic emergencies, 440
Calcitriol, for hypocalcemia, 367t
Calcium, 270t
Calcium carbonate, for hypocalcemia, 367t
Calcium chloride, for hypocalcemia, 367t
Calcium gluconate, for hypocalcemia, 367t
Calcium lactate, for hypocalcemia, 367t
Calcium oxalate uroliths, 383
Calcium sludge, in rabbit, 475
Calcium therapy, for advanced life support,
    241
Calcium-containing fluids (lactated Ringer's),
    355b
Calciuretic diuretics, for hypercalcemia, 364
Canine
  blood collection in, 92–94, 92b–93b, 93f
  blood donor, 86, 86b
  blood type frequencies in, 88t
  cantankerous, 57–58
  infectious disease screening, 87t
  RBC dosing formula for, 99b
Canine distemper virus, 469
Canine flu, 330
Canine-specific albumin, 82
Cantankerous canine, intravenous catheter
    and, 57–58
Capillary refill time (CRT)
  mucous membrane color and, 64
  shock and, 226, 226t
Capnography, 37
Capnometry, 37, 182–183, 182f
Carbamates, 442

Carbon monoxide, 285
Carboxyhemoglobin, 285
Cardiac arrhythmias, 305, 308–312, 308b
    client complaints in, 308
    diagnostic imaging and electrocardiogram
        of, 308
    medical treatment of, 308–309
    monitoring of, 311
    pacemaker therapy for, 311–312, 313f
    physical findings in, 308
    precordial thumps in treatment of, 312
Cardiac glycosides, in toxicologic
        emergencies, 438
Cardiac output
    anesthesia and, 166
    oxygen delivery and, 224
Cardiac physiology/pathophysiology,
        overview of, 302–303
Cardiac pump theory, of blood flow, 237
Cardiac rhythms, 243
Cardiac tamponade
    client complaints in, 314–315
    clinical signs of, 315
    diagnostic imaging and electrocardiogram
        of, 315
    monitoring of, 315
    pericardial effusion and, 314–315
    treatment of, 315
Cardiac ultrasound, for heart disease, 293
Cardiogenic shock, 224, 303–304
    pathophysiology of, 224–225
Cardiomegaly, 296
Cardiomyopathy, 294
    secondary to hyperthyroidism,
        emergencies associated with, 295t
Cardiopulmonary arrest (CPA), 234
    care after, 244–245
    recognition of, 236–237, 237b
Cardiopulmonary resuscitation (CPR), 56
    assessing effectiveness of, 239–240, 240f
    for avian, reptilian, and small animal exotic
        patient, 453–454, 453b
    basic life support and, 237–243, 237b
    blood flow mechanism of, 237
    code, 216
    current practice in, 234–246
    equipment for, 236, 236b
    facilities for, 235–236, 236b
    preparation for, 235–236
    recognizing need for, 236–237, 237b
    responsibilities of, 235t
    staff and, 235, 235b
    tasks of, 235t
Cardiovascular emergencies, 292–318
    common signs in, 294b
Cardiovascular status, anesthesia and,
        180–181
Cast padding, 55
Castor beans, in toxicologic emergencies, 439
Cataracts, 412, 412f
Cathartic
    sodium sulfate as, 449–450
    for toxicologic emergencies, 436

Catheter(s)
    for parenteral nutrition, 117–118
    peripheral, 54–55
    placement of
        in ferret emergencies, 467, 467t
        for rabbit and rodent emergencies,
            471–472, 471b–472b, 472f
Catheterization
    for blocked cat, 376–377, 376f, 377b–378b
    for blocked dog, 381, 381b–382b, 382f
    intraosseous, 56
Caval syndrome, 312–313
    client complaints in, 313
    diagnostic imaging and electrocardiogram
        of, 313–314
    monitoring of, 314
    physical findings in, 313
    surgical treatment of, 314
Celiotomy, 341
Centers for Disease Control and Prevention, 59
Central line, 46
Central venous pressure (CVP), 39–40, 39b,
        40f, 302
    equipment for, 39–40
    fluid therapy and, 67, 67f
    indications for, 39
    interpretation for, 40
    shock and, 231–232
    technique for, 40
Central vestibular disorders, peripheral
        vestibular disorders and, 421t
Cerebral spinal fluid (CSF), 62
Cervical soft tissue, injury to, 264–265
    assessment of, 264–265
    management of, 265
    monitoring of, 265
Cesarean section, 393–394
    goal of, 395
Challenging clients, communication with,
        521, 521b
Chelonian emergencies, 486, 486f
Chelonians
    catheterization site in, 482t
    IV catheter placement in, 482–483
    restraint for, 478f, 479, 479b
    venipuncture for, 480–481, 481f
Chemistry, manufacturers of equipment, 41
Chemosis, 15f
Cherry eye, 409
Chest compressions, 237–239
Chest injury, 265–266
    assessment of, 265
    management of, 265
    monitoring of, 265–266
Chest wall, deformities of, 327
Chinchilla(s)
    intravenous catheterization site in, 467t
    physiologic values of, 466t
    restraint for, 469
    venipuncture for, 470–471
Chinchilla fur ring, 476f
Chlorhexidine gluconate, as disinfectants,
        199t–200t

Chlorhexidine patches, 59
Chocolate
    in avian emergencies, 463
    in toxicologic emergencies, 440
Cholecalciferol, toxicologic emergencies
        with, 445
Christmas factor, 270t
Chronic kidney disease, 284
Chronic kidney failure (CKF), 383
    alternative treatments for, 387
    causes of, 384
    clinical presentation of, 384
    diagnosis of, 385
    drug therapy for, 387
    fluid therapy for, 387
    hemodialysis for, 388, 388f
    nutritional support for, 387
    peritoneal dialysis for, 387–388
    renal transplantation for, 388, 389f
    response to treatment for, 387
    treatment for, 387–388
Chronic renal failure, fluids for, 72t
Chronic valvular disease, emergencies
        associated with, 295t
Chronobiology, 508
Circadian dysrhythmia, 508, 510
Circulation, basic life support and, 237b
Citrate intoxication, 102
Citrate phosphate 2 dextrose (CP2D), 91t
Citrate phosphate dextrose (CPD), 91t
Citrate phosphate dextrose adenine 1
        (CPDA-1), 91t
Cleaning, for infection control, 198, 198b, 201
Client
    communication, in emergency, 515–522,
        517b
    in emergency receiving, 211–212, 213f
    greeting of, in emergency receiving, 214,
        214b
    initial greeting of, 517, 517b
Client service representative (CSR), 516
Closed-ended questions, 519
Closed-suction drainage, for peritonitis, 348
Coagulation, 270
    amplification phase of, 271
    cell-based model of, 271f
    initiation phase of, 271
    propagation phase of, 271
Coagulation cascade, 270, 270f
Coagulation factors, 270, 270t
    replacement of, 275
Coagulation parameters, in preanesthetic
        exam, 168
Coagulation tests, 28–30, 28b
    equipment for, 28
        manufacturers of, 41
    indications for, 28
    interpretation for, 29–30
    technique for, 28–29
    troubleshooting for, 29
Coagulopathies
    hereditary, 272t
    trauma and, 256

Coccidiodomycosis, 330
Collagen, 270
Collagenase ulcers, of cornea, 410
Collapsed vascular system, 58
Collection system, closed, 21f, 22
Colloid osmometer measures, of COP, 26
Colloid osmotic pressure, 25–27, 26b
  equipment of, 26
  indications for, 26
  interpretation for, 27
  shock and, 232
  technique for, 26
  troubleshooting for, 27
Colloids, 69–73, 230
  natural, 26
Common vehicle transmission, of disease, 193
Communication, 4
  with challenging clients, 521, 521b
  client, in emergency, 515–522
  critical care estimate, 518–519, 519t
  discussing euthanasia, 520–521
  in emergency receiving, 216, 216
  estimates and, 520, 520f, 520t
  exam room, 519–520, 519b
  importance of, 515–516, 516b
  with owner, in traumatic emergencies,
    263, 263b
  with referral practices, 521
  telephone calls and, 516–517, 516f
Compassion fatigue, 6
Compensated shock, 227–228
Component therapy, 79
Concept mapping, 4–5
Congestive heart failure, 304
  emergency treatment of, 305–306, 306t
  fluids for, 72t
Constant rate infusion (CRI), of analgesia,
    156–160
  calculation of, 151b
  in cats, 158t
  in dogs, 159t
Constant rate infusions, calculation of, 231f
Contact transmission, of disease, 193
Continuous chest suction device, 327f
Continuous renal replacement therapy
    (CRRT), 388, 388f
Contractility, of heart, 302–303
Contraindications, colloids, 72–73
Controlled ventilation, anesthesia and, 179,
    179f
Convulsion or (epileptic) fit, 416
Coombs' test, for anemia, 288
"Coonhound Paralysis," 426
Corneal sequestrum, 411
Corneal ulcers, 409–410, 410f
Coronaviral diarrhea syndrome, in ferret
    emergencies, 469
Corticosteroids, for spinal cord injury,
    425–426
Cortisol, hypovolemic shock and, 225
CPA. see Cardiopulmonary arrest (CPA)
CPR. see Cardiopulmonary resuscitation
    (CPR)

Crash cart
  emergency kit and, 236, 236f
  for traumatic emergencies, 248–249, 249f
CRI. see Constant rate infusion (CRI)
Critical care estimate, 518–519, 519t
Critical thinking, 1–8
  defining, 3, 3f–4f
  delivering information received, 5–6
  developing, 4–5
  impacts in decision making, 3
  sustaining the development and use of,
    6–7, 7b
Critically ill patient
  monitoring of, 9–42, 13b
    clinical pathologic, 14–16, 15b
    physical examination, 13–14
  nutritional support for, 106–122
  record for, 10f–12f
Cryoprecipitate, 81–82, 84t–85t, 273
Cryosupernatant, 81–82, 84t–85t
Cryptococcosis, 330
Crystalloids, 25–26, 69, 69f, 229–230, 230b
Currants, in toxicologic emergencies, 439
Cyanosis, 254, 320–321
  anesthesia and, 184t–188t
Cycad (sago) palm, in toxicologic
    emergencies, 438–439
Cycasin, 438
  poisoning of, 438
Cyclophotoablation, 408
Cystic calculi
  in guinea pig, 475
  in rabbit and rodent emergencies, 475
Cystitis, in rabbit and rodent emergencies, 475
Cystocentesis, 373
Cysts, prostatic, 400

D
DAMNIT V scheme, 418f
Day sleeping, art of scheduling and, 512, 512b
DDAVP. see Desmopressin
DEA. see Dog erythrocyte antigen (DEA)
Debriefing, 218–220, 220b
Decompensated shock, 227–228
Decontamination, 433–435
  during hurricane Katrina, 497–498
  of search and rescue canines, 497–498,
    498f, 498b
Defibrillation, 242–243, 242b
Dehydration, 17
  anemia and, 287, 287b
  in avian emergencies, 461
  fluid therapy and, 64, 65t
  fluids for, 72t
Delivery systems, of fluid therapy, 73–74,
    73f, 76f
Dental disease, rabbit and rodent
    emergencies and, 474–476, 474f
Dental nerve blocks, 155
Deoxyhemoglobin, 125b
Depolarizing muscle blocking agents,
    176–177

Dermal exposure, 495
  in toxicologic emergencies, 434
Descemetocele, 410, 410f
Desmopressin (DDAVP), 273–274
Desoxycorticosterone pivalate (DOCP), 360,
    360t
Device-based monitoring, 30
Dexamethasone sodium phosphate, 359–360,
    360t
Dexmedetomidine, 157–160, 175
  dose for, 157
Dextrans, 71
Dextrose supplementation, anesthesia and,
    183–184
Diabetic ketoacidosis (DKA), 352–356
  clinical signs of, 352b
  clinicopathologic values of, 353t
  definition of, 352
  fluids for, 72t
  monitoring for, 356, 356b
  nursing care for, 356
  potassium supplementation
    recommendations for, 354, 355t
  presentation of, 352
  stabilization supplies for, 354b
  treatment of, 352–356
Diaphragmatic hernia, 326–327
Diarrhea, 333
  assessment of, 334b
  fluids for, 72t
Diastolic dysfunction, causes of, 225
Diastolic function, of heart, 303
Diastolic murmurs, 296
Diazepam, 175, 417–418
Diestrus, 392
Diet
  "blenderized," 112–116
  enteral, 117
  feeding tube and, 116–117
  liquid, 111–112
Dihydrotachysterol, for hypocalcemia, 367t
Dilated cardiomyopathy, emergencies
    associated with, 295t
Dilutional coagulopathies, 275
Direct arterial pressure monitoring, blood
    pressure monitoring and, 33
Disaster kit
  for disaster responders, 500b
  for pet owners, 501b
Disaster medicine, 488–506, 489b
  American Veterinary Medical Association
    in, 504
  burn injuries in, 494–495
  common emergencies in, 494–495
  disaster
    structure and, 500–501
    types and, 490–492
  hurricane Katrina and, 488–489
  hyperthermia and hypothermia in, 494
  incident command system in, 503
  injury prevention in, 493, 494b
  involvement in, 501
  legal issues with, 490

Disaster medicine (Continued)
    local veterinary infrastructure in, 499, 500b
    near drowning in, 495
    neurologic injuries in, 494
    orthopedic injuries in, 494
    owner in, 493, 493b
    personal recovery after disaster in, 499–500
    rechecking appointments in, 499
    record keeping in, 498–499, 498b
    search and rescue canines in, 495–498,
        495b, 496f
    self-protection in, 493–494, 493b
    shock in, 494
    smoke in, 494–495
    soft tissue injuries in, 494
    surgery in, 498
    triaging in, 492–493, 492b
    wounds in, 494
Disaster plan details, for veterinary clinic,
    490, 491b
Disaster responders, disaster kit for, 500b
Disaster training, 503–504
    sites of, 504b
Disease transmission, infection control and,
    193
Disinfectants, for infection control, 192,
    199t–200t
    bottles of, 200–201, 201f, 201b
    dilution of, 200–201
Disinfection, for infection control, 198–201,
    199t–200t, 200b
Disseminated intravascular coagulation, 271,
    276
Distended superficial epigastric veins,
    anesthesia and, 167, 167f
Distributive shock, 224
Diuretic therapy, for heart failure, 306
    monitoring of, 308
DKA. see Diabetic ketoacidosis (DKA)
Dobutamine, 230
DOCP. see Desoxycorticosterone pivalate
    (DOCP)
Dog. see Canine
Dog erythrocyte antigen (DEA), 86–87, 87b
Dopamine, 230
Doppler echocardiography, for heart disease,
    300
Doppler imaging, for gastrointestinal
    emergencies, 335
Doppler ultrasound flow detectors, blood
    pressure monitoring and, 34–35, 34f
Droplet transmission, of disease, 193
Drug(s)
    for advanced life support, 240–242
    for anesthesia, 170–171, 170b
    ophthalmic, 406t–407t
    for pain, 152–153
Drug administration route, for advanced life
    support, 241–242, 242b
Drug delivery methods, for advanced life
    support, 241b
Drug interactions, in antiarrhythmic therapy,
    309

Dyspnea, 319
    in pulmonary edema, 326
Dystocia, 392–397, 393b, 397f
    avian, 462–463
    in bulldogs, 393b
    causes of, 393
    diagnosis of, 394, 394f
    in reptile emergencies, 485
    screening for, 394b
    signs of, 393b
    treatment for, 394

E

E-collar oxygen hood, 127t
E tube. see Esophagostomy (E) tube
Ecchymoses, 18f, 335, 335f
Echocardiography, for heart disease,
    299–302, 302b
Eclampsia, 400
Ectropion, 409
EDTA (ethylenediaminetetraacetic acid)
    tube, 16, 19b
Egg binding
    in avian emergencies, 462–463
    in reptile emergencies, 485
Ehrlichia canis, 86b
Electrocardiogram
    of cardiac arrhythmias, 308
    of cardiac tamponade, 315
    of Caval syndrome, 313–314
    of feline aortic thromboembolism, 316
    for heart disease, 293, 296, 297t
        cardiac rhythm disorders, determination
            with, 298t
    for heart failure, 304–305
    methods for measuring, 305f
    of pericardial effusion, 315
    in preanesthetic exam, 168, 168f
    shock and, 231
Electrocardiogram monitoring, 35–37
    equipment for, 36
    indications for, 35–36
    interpretation for, 37
    technique for, 36–37
    troubleshooting for, 37, 37b
Electrocardiography, 181
Electrocautery device, in surgery set up,
    170
Electrolyte and chemistry analyzers, 19–21
    equipment for, 20, 20f
    indications for, 19–20
    interpretation for, 21, 21b
    technique for, 20
    troubleshooting for, 20–21
Electrolytes
    anesthesia and, 167
    in antiarrhythmic therapy, 309
    in diabetic ketoacidosis, 356
    shock and, 232
Embolism, air, 53–54
Emergency, client communication in, 515–522
Emergency kit, crash cart and, 236, 236f

Emergency receiving, 207–222, 209b, 212f
    assessment of patient, 212
    communication in, 216
    entrance of, 210
    facility for, 210–212
    preparation for, 209–210
    re-energizing in, 216–220, 220f
    treatment area of, 210–211, 211f–212f
    waiting room of, 210
Emergency Severity Index (ESI), 214
Emergency supplies, 236b
Emergent, approach for, in emergency
    receiving, 214
Emesis, for toxicologic emergencies, 434
Empathy, expressing, 517, 517t, 517b
End-of-life decisions, 520
End-stage liver disease, fluids for, 72t
End-tidal carbon dioxide ($ETCO_2$)
    anesthesia and, 184t–188t
    monitoring, 37–39
        equipment and technique for, 38, 38f
        indications for, 37–38
        interpretation for, 38–39, 39b
        troubleshooting for, 38
Endocarditis, 294
Endotracheal intubation, 323
Endotracheal tubes
    clear, 169, 169b
    cuffed, 178
Enhanced elimination techniques, 436
Enophthalmos, 409
Enteral nutrition, 110–117, 111t, 112b–116b,
    116f
    complications of, 119–120
    for trauma patients, 262–263
    worksheet calculation for, 117b
Enteritis, in ferret emergencies, 468–469
Enteroplication, 345
Enterotoxemia, 441
Entrance, of emergency receiving, 210
Environmental toxins, in toxicologic
    emergencies, 446–447
Epidural analgesia, anesthesia and, 172–173
    for pain, 160, 160f
Epigastric veins, distended superficial,
    anesthesia and, 167, 167f
Epilepsy, 415–416
    classification of, 415–416
    types of, 416
Epinephrine
    in advanced life support, 240
    hypovolemic shock and, 225
Episodic disorders, seizures and, 416
Ergocalciferol, for hypocalcemia, 367t
Erythropoiesis, reduced or ineffective, 284–285
Erythropoietin, 284
    suppression of response to, 284
Esmolol, 309–310
Esophageal foreign bodies, 342
    clinical signs of, 342
    diagnosis for, 342
    history of, 342
    treatment of, 342

Esophageal stethoscopes, 13f
Esophagostomy (E) tube, 111t, 112
   placement of, 112b–116b
   volume for, 117
Estimates, communication and, 520, 520f, 520t
Estrus, 392
Ethylene glycol, in toxicologic emergencies, 446–447
Etomidate, 175
Euthanasia, discussing of, 520–521
Exam room communication, 519–520, 519b
Exophthalmos, 407
Exotic small mammal emergencies, 465–474
   physical examination for, 465–468, 465b, 466t
   supplies for, 465
Extended shifts, 511
External cardiac compression, 237–238, 238f, 238b
Extracellular fluid, 68, 76t
Extracellular fluid volume depletion and overload, clinical signs of, 76t
Extremity temperature, shock and, 226t, 227–228
Eye
   diagram of, 407f
   position, fluid therapy and, 64
Eyelid, ocular emergencies of, 409
EZ-IO catheters, 56

F

Febrile nonhemolytic transfusion reactions (FNHTRs), 101
Federal Emergency Management Agency (FEMA), 502
Feeding tube
   complications of, 110–111
   selection of, 111, 111t
Feline
   blood collection in, 94, 94b
   blood donor, 89, 89b
   with buphthalmia, 408
   infectious disease screen for, 89t
   male, catheterization for, 376–377, 376f, 377b–378b
Feline aortic thromboembolism, 315–316
   client complaints in, 315
   clinical signs of, 316
   diagnostic imaging and electrocardiogram of, 316
   goals of therapy in, 316b
   treatment of, 316
Feline asthma, 329
Feline idiopathic vestibular syndrome, 421
Feline seizures, 417
FEMA. see Federal Emergency Management Agency (FEMA)
Fentanyl, 156–157
   CRI dosage for
      in cats, 158t
      in dogs, 159t
   dose for, 157

Fentanyl citrate, 153
Ferret, physiologic values of, 466t
Ferret emergencies
   adrenal disease in, 468
   catheter placement in, 467, 467t
   common, 468–469
   coronaviral diarrhea syndrome in, 469
   enteritis in, 468–469
   from foreign bodies, 469
   gastritis in, 468–469
   Helicobacter mustelae in, 468–469
   insulinoma in, 468
   restraint for, 466, 466f, 466b
   venipuncture for, 466–467, 467f
FFP. see Fresh frozen plasma (FFP)
Fibrin degradation products (FDPs), 271
Fibrin split products (FSPs), 271
Fibrin-stabilizing factor, 270t
Fibrinogen, 270t
Fibrinolysis, 271
Fibrocartilaginous embolic myelopathy (FCEM), 425
Fight or flight response, 218
FiO_2, 124, 137
Fire, disaster medicine and, 492
First aid, for traumatic emergencies, 252–253
Flail segment, 327
Floods, disaster medicine and, 492
Flow rate, of oxygen, 126
Flow-by oxygen, 126, 127f, 127t, 321–322
   in gastrointestinal emergencies, 336
Fludrocortisone acetate (Florinef), 360, 360t
Fluid administration
   in avian emergencies, 461–462, 461f, 461b–462b
   via intraosseous catheter, 229f
Fluid flow rates, 229t
Fluid resuscitation, 226, 229–230, 229b, 335–336
Fluid support, anesthesia and, 183–184
Fluid therapy, 61–77
   for acute kidney injury, 385–386
   administration and, 64–65
   blood pressure and, 66
   body water and, 62–63, 62f
   body weight and, 66–67, 66b, 67f
   central venous pressure and, 67, 67f
   for certain diseases, 72t
   for chronic kidney failure, 387
   complications of, 74–77
   delivery systems of, 73–74, 73f, 76f
   emergency admission and, 65–66, 66f
   eye position and, 64
   in ferret emergencies, 467–468
   for gastrointestinal emergencies, 337
   history and, 63–64, 64f
   in-hospital monitoring of, 66–68
   osmolality and, 68
   for pancreatitis, 347
   patient assessment of, 63–66
   physical exam of, 63–64, 64f
      mentation and, 67–68, 68b
   pulse rate and, 64
   regulating, 75b

Fluid therapy *(Continued)*
   for reptile emergencies, 483
   routes of administration, 63t
   skin tent and, 64
   skin turgor and, 64
   temperature and, 64
   urine production and, 66
   volume overload and, 74–77
Fluid types, 69
Fluids
   administration of, in traumatic emergencies, 257–258
   for advanced life support, 241
FNHTRs. see Febrile nonhemolytic transfusion reactions (FNHTRs)
Focal seizures, 416
Foods, in toxicologic emergencies, 439–441
Footbaths, 203
Footmats, 203
Footwear, for infection control, 197
Foreign animal disease, 490–492
Foreign bodies
   esophageal, 342
   in ferret emergencies, 469
   gastrointestinal, 342–343
   in gastrointestinal emergencies, 334, 342
   in reptile emergencies, 485, 486f
Forward failure, of heart, 303–304
FP. see Frozen plasma (FP)
Fractional shortening, 300
Fractious feline, intravenous catheter and, 57–58
Frequency (F), 136–137
Fresh frozen plasma (FFP), 81, 84t–85t
Fresh whole blood (FWB), 79, 84t–85t
Frozen plasma (FP), 81, 84t–85t
Fungal pneumonia, 330
Furosemide, 306, 428
FWB. see Fresh whole blood (FWB)

G

G tube. see Gastrostomy (G) tube
Gallop sounds, 296
Garbage toxicity, in toxicologic emergencies, 441
Gastric dilation and volvulus, 343–345
   clinical signs of, 343
   diagnosis of, 344, 344f
   history of, 343
   pathophysiology of, 343
   treatment of, 344–345, 344f
Gastric lavage technique, 435b
   for gastric dilation and volvulus, 345
Gastritis, in ferret emergencies, 468–469
Gastrointestinal emergencies, 332–350, 334b, 339b
   abdominal radiographs in, 336–337, 337f
   anesthesia and surgery in, 340–341
   catheter care in, 339
   and circulation, assessment in, 335
   conclusion for, 348
   diagnosis of, 336–337

Gastrointestinal emergencies *(Continued)*
　enteral feeding and, 338b
　enteral nutrition in, 339
　first aid measures in, 333–334
　hypothermia and, 339
　medical treatment of, 337–340
　monitoring in, 340
　nasogastric tubes in, 339
　nonsteroidal antiinflammatory drugs in,
　　338–339
　pain in, 338, 338b
　parenteral nutrition in, 339–340
　physical examination in, 334–335
　postoperative care in, 341
　record keeping in, 340, 340b
　resuscitation of critical patient in, 335–336
　technician, role of, 333b
Gastrointestinal foreign bodies, 342–343
　clinical signs of, 342
　diagnosis of, 342–343
　history of, 342
　treatment of, 343
Gastrostomy (G) tube, 111t, 112–116
　volume for, 117
Gastrotomy, for toxicologic emergencies, 435
Gelatins, 71–72
Generalized seizures, 416
Genetic epileptics, 416–417
GI stasis, in rabbit and rodent emergencies,
　474
Glaucoma, 407
　ophthalmic drugs for, 406t–407t
Globe, ocular emergencies of, 407–409
Gloves, in infection control, 194–195
Glow jewelry, in toxicologic emergencies,
　447
Glucocorticoids (cortisol), 357, 359–360, 364
Glucose, preparations of, 118
Glycoprotein A, 439
Glycopyrrolate, 173–174, 173t–174t
Grapes, in toxicologic emergencies, 439
Graveyard shift, 510
Green slime disease, 469
Grief, 220
Guidewire technique, 47–54, 50b–52b, 54f
Guinea pig(s)
　cystic calculi in, 475
　intravenous catheterization site in, 467t
　physiologic values of, 466t
　restraint for, 470
　venipuncture for, 471

H

Hageman factor, 270t
Hairballs (trichobezoars), in rabbit and
　rodent emergencies, 474
Hamster(s)
　physiologic values of, 466t
　restraint for, 470
　venipuncture for, 471
"Hand-bagging," 135–136, 136f
Hand hygiene, 191–192, 194

Head/facial trauma, 264
　assessment of, 264
　management of, 264
　monitoring of, 264
Head trauma, 427–429
　diagnostic procedures of, 427–429
　hypotension and, 428
　hypoxia and, 428
　pathophysiology of, 427
　steroids for, 429
　treatment plans of, 427–429
Heart
　backward failure of, 304
　congestive failure of, 304
　contractility of, 302–303
　diastolic function, 303
　forward failure of, 303–304
　low-output failure of, 303–304
　rate and rhythm of, 303
　systolic function of, 302
Heart disease
　common signs in, 294b
　diagnosis of, 293–302
　echocardiography for, 299–302, 302b
　electrocardiogram for, 296, 297t
　　cardiac rhythm disorders, determination
　　　with, 298t
　emergencies associated with
　　canine, 295t
　　feline, 295t
　history in, 294
　signalment in, 294
　thoracic radiographs in, 296–298
　troponin and, 293–294
Heart failure, 303–304
　classification of, 303b
　client complaints of, 304
　common causes of, 305b
　diagnostic imaging and electrocardiogram
　　of, 304–305
　diuretic therapy for, 306
　　monitoring for, 308
　drugs used to treat, 306t
　goals in emergency treatment of, 306t
　hemodynamic measurements and clinical
　　signs of, relationship between, 304
　identification of patients with, 304–307
　monitoring for, 307–308, 307b
　oxygen therapy for, 306–307, 306b
　physical findings, 304
　positive inotropic therapy, 307
　　monitoring for, 308
　sympathomimetic drugs for, 307
　vasodilator therapy for, 307
　　monitoring for, 307–308
Heart murmurs, 294
　intensity of, 296
Heart rate, shock and, 226–227, 226t
Heart tones, anesthesia and, 167
Heartworm disease, 312–314, 314f
　Caval syndrome, 312–313
　emergencies associated with, 295t
Heinz body anemia, 283

Helicobacter mustelae, in ferret emergencies,
　468–469
Hematocrit (HCT), 16
　shock and, 232
Hematologic analysis, 17–19, 17b
　blood smear technique for, 18–19, 18f, 19b
　equipment for, 18
　indications for, 18
　interpretation for, 19
　reference ranges for, 19
　troubleshooting for, 19
Hematologic emergencies, 269–291
　bleeding time test, 278–279, 278f, 278b
　clinical assessment of, 276–280
　history of, 276–277
　laboratory tests in, 277
　physical examination in, 277, 277f
　platelet estimation in, 278
　primary hemostatic tests in, 277–278
　secondary hemostatic tests in, 279–280
Hematology, manufacturers of equipment, 41
Hemodialysis, for chronic kidney failure,
　388, 388f
Hemoglobin (Hb)
　levels, anesthesia and, 166–167
　in oxygen delivery, 224
Hemoglobin-based oxygen carriers, 71
　solutions, 102
Hemoglobinuria, 282
Hemogram, 287–288
Hemolysis, 15f, 16, 102, 281
　causes of, 284
Hemolyzed serum, 16
Hemophilias, 274
Hemorrhage, control of, in traumatic
　emergencies, 258–259, 258f
Hemorrhagic gastroenteritis, 345–346
　clinical signs of, 345
　diagnosis of, 345–346
　history of, 345
　treatment of, 346
Hemostasis, 269–276, 271b
　primary, 270
　　disorders of, 272–274
　secondary, 270
　　disorders of, 274–275
Hemothorax, 326
Hereditary bleeding disorders, 272t, 278f, 278b
Hereditary coagulopathies, 272t, 274
Hernia, diaphragmatic, 326–327
Hetastarch, 72
Histoplasmosis, 330
hIVIG. *see* Human intravenous
　immunoglobulin (hIVIG)
Holter system, 308, 309f
Horner's syndrome, 409
　clinical signs of, 421–422, 421b
Hospital preparedness, for exotic patients,
　453
Hospitalization, nutritional support during,
　107–110
Huddles, 209
　example of, 209–210

Human intravenous immunoglobulin (hIVIG), 82
Human serum albumin (HSA), 82
Hurricane Katrina
    decontamination during, 497–498
    disaster medicine and, 488–489
Hydrocortisone acetate, 360t
Hydrocortisone phosphate, 360t
Hydrocortisone sodium hemisuccinate, 360t
Hydrogen peroxide, 434
    accelerated, as disinfectants, 199t–200t
Hydromorphone, 153, 156, 172
    CRI dosage for
        in cats, 158t
        in dogs, 159t
    dose for, 156
    for spinal cord injury, 425
Hydroxyethyl starches (HES), 72
Hyperbaric oxygen therapy (HBOT), 131–132
Hyperbilirubinemia, 282, 283f
Hypercalcemia, 362–365
    causes of, 362, 362b
    clinical signs of, 363t
    definition of, 362
    monitoring of, 364–365
    nursing care of, 364–365
    presentation of, 363
    treatment of, 363–364
Hypercalciuria, 366
Hypercapnic respiratory failure, 137–138, 137t
Hypercoagulability, 275
Hyperkalemia, 21, 309
    ECG for, 375, 375f
    treatment of, 311, 312f–313f, 313t
Hyperlactatemia, 228
Hypernatremia, 21
Hypertension, anesthesia and, 184t–188t
Hyperthermia/hypothermia, in disaster medicine, 494
Hypertonic crystalloids, 229–230
    doses of, 71t
    solutions, 69, 71t
Hypertonic saline (HTS), 69b
Hypertonic solutions, 69
Hypertrophic cardiomyopathy, emergencies associated with, 295t
Hyphema, 408, 411
Hypoadrenocorticism, 356–361
    case study of, 361
    clinical signs of, 357t
    clinicopathologic findings of, 359t
    definition of, 356–357
    ECG of, 358f–359f
    medications and doses for, 360t
    monitoring of, 360–361
    nursing care of, 360–361
    presentation of, 357
    treatment of, 357–360, 359b
Hypocalcemia, 21, 365–368, 400
    calcitriol for, 367t
    calcium carbonate for, 367t
    calcium chloride for, 367t

Hypocalcemia (Continued)
    calcium gluconate for, 367t
    calcium lactate for, 367t
    causes of, 365–366, 366b
    clinical signs of, 365b
    definition of, 365–366
    dihydrotachysterol for, 367t
    drugs for, 367t
    ECG of, 367f
    ergocalciferol for, 367t
    monitoring of, 368
    nursing care of, 368
    parenteral calcium for, 367t
    presentation of, 366
    supplements for, 367t
    treatment of, 366–368
    vitamin D for, 367t
Hypochlorite, as disinfectants, 199t–200t
Hypochromic anemia, 287–288
Hypofibrinolysis, 275
Hypoglycemia, 21, 368–371
    causes of, 368–369, 368b
    clinical signs of, 369b
    definition of, 368–369
    monitoring of, 371
    nursing care of, 371
    presentation of, 369–370
    treatment for, 370–371
Hypomagnesemia, cardiac arrhythmia and, 309
Hypoparathyroidism, 365
Hypoplasminogenemia, 275
Hypotension, 35, 396
    anesthesia and, 184t–188t
    head trauma and, 428
Hypothermia
    gastrointestinal emergencies and, 339
    prevention of, anesthesia and, 183, 183f
    surgery and, 341
    trauma and, 256
Hypotonic solutions, 69
    crystalloid, 70t
Hypoventilation, anesthesia and, 166, 184t–188t
Hypovolemia, 63
Hypovolemic shock, 224
Hypoxemia, 124
Hypoxemic respiratory failure, 137, 137t
Hypoxemic shock, 281
Hypoxia, head trauma and, 428

I

I-PASS (Introduction, Patient summary, Action list, Situation awareness/contingency planning, Synthesis by receiver, 6, 6b
Iatrogenic blood loss, 28–29
Iatrogenic hypoadrenocorticism, 356
Iatrogenic secondary hypoadrenocorticism, 356
Icteric serum, 16
Icterus, 16
Icterus mucous membrane, 3f

Idexx Laboratories, 20f
    VetStat blood gas and electrolyte analyzer, 22f
Idiopathic epilepsy, 416–417
Idiopathic old dog (geriatric) vestibular syndrome, 421
Idiopathic thrombocytopenic purpura (ITP), 272
Immune-mediated hemolytic anemia (IMHA), 282, 283f
    secondary, 283
Immune-mediated thrombocytopenia (IMT), 272
Immunochromatographic cartridge test, 88f, 88b
Immunoglobulins, 82
In-hospital isolation, 204
In-hospital monitoring, fluid therapy of, 66–68
Incident command staff graph, 503f
Incident command system (ICS), in disaster medicine, 503
Incubators, for exotic patient, 453
Indirect blood pressure monitoring, 33–35, 34b
Induction, of anesthesia, 170b, 174–175, 174b
Infection
    control of. see Infection control
    prevention of, isolation for, 191
    risks of, in veterinary clinics, 192
Infection control, programs for, 192–201
    attire in, 195, 195b
    biosecurity in, 193–194
    cleaning and disinfection in, 197–201
    footwear in, 197, 197f
    gloves in, 194–195
    hand hygiene in, 194
    laundry in, 195, 196f
    personal protective equipment in, 195–197, 197f, 197b
Infectious disease screening
    for canine, 87t
    for feline, 89t
Infective endocarditis, emergencies associated with, 295t
Ingested toxins, in toxicologic emergencies, 434–435
Inhalants, 176
Injuries. see also Traumatic emergencies.
    to abdomen, 266
    to cervical soft tissue, 264–265
    chest, 265–266
    to musculoskeletal system, 266–267
    orthopedic, in disaster medicine, 494
    prevention, in disaster medicine, 494b
    soft tissue, in disaster medicine, 494
Innocent murmurs, 294
Insecticide, in toxicologic emergencies, 432
Insulin, 353
    action duration of, 355t
    maximal effect time of, 355t
    onset time of, 355t
    types of, 355t

Insulinoma, in ferret emergencies, 468
Intensive care unit (ICU), monitoring tool in, 32
Interfetal gas patterns, 394
Internal cardiac compression, 238–239, 238b
Interposed abdominal compression (IAC), 239
Interpretation, as concept, 5
Interpretation skill, 1–8
Intervertebral disc herniation (IVDH), 423, 424f
Intestinal "accidents," 345
   clinical signs of, 345
   diagnosis of, 345
   history of, 345
   treatment of, 345
Intracellular space, 62
Intraocular pressure, 408
Intraosseous, routes of administration, 63t
Intraosseous bolus volumes, in avian emergencies, 460b
Intraosseous cannulization, 58
Intraosseous (IO) catheter
   fluid administration via, 229f
   placement of
      for avian emergencies, 460, 460b
      for rabbit and rodent emergencies, 473
      for reptile emergencies, 481–482
Intraosseous catheterization, 56
Intratracheal route, of drug administration, 242, 242b
Intravenous, routes of administration, 63t
Intravenous bolus volumes, in avian emergencies, 460b
Intravenous catheter, 43–60
   antimicrobial impregnated central, 44
   cantankerous canine and, 57–58
   challenges with, 57–58
   choosing right, 45–46
   fractious feline and, 57–58
   intraosseous, 56
   length of, 46, 46f
   maintenance of, 58–59
   material for, 45–46
   multi-lumen, 44–45, 45f
   neonates challenge with, 57
   over-the-needle, 44
   placement of, 46–47, 47b
      prevention and management of complications during, 53
   size of, 46
   stabilization of, 54–56
   suggested readings for, 59
   through-the-needle for, 44, 52b–53b
   types of, 44, 44f
   vascular access points for, 46
   vascular access ports for, 45
Intravenous fluid administration, 71t
Intravenous (IV) fluid therapy, for diabetic ketoacidosis, 352–353
Intravenous fluids, for traumatic emergencies, 250

Intubation, 177–178
   airway swelling/ obstruction and, 178, 178b
   with possible airway disruption, 178
Ion trapping, for toxicologic emergencies, 436
Irreversible shock, 227–228
Isoflurane, 176
Isolation
   facilities, 202–204
      antimicrobial stewardship in, 204
      footbaths/footmats in, 203
      improvised isolation in, 204
      nursing patients in, 203–204
      room, 202–203
      waste disposal in, 204
   improvised, 204
   nursing patients in, 203–204
   protocols, 201–202, 201b
   techniques, 191–206
Isotonic crystalloid(s), 69, 229
   for diabetic ketoacidosis, 352–353
   doses, 71t
Isotonic replacement fluids, 70t
IV bicarbonate (HCO_3-) therapy, for diabetic ketoacidosis, 355
IV catheter, placement of
   in avian emergencies, 459–460, 459f, 459t, 460b
   for reptile emergencies, 482–483, 482t
Ivermectin, in toxicologic emergencies, 443

J

J tube. see Jejunostomy (J) tube
Jejunostomy (J) tube, 111t, 116
Joint space, analgesia injection in, 155
Jugular catheter, 54b, 55–56, 55f, 57f–58f
Jugular vein(s)
   evaluation of, anesthesia and, 167b
   gastrointestinal emergencies and, 335

K

Keratitis, 410
Keratoconjunctivitis sicca (KCS), 410, 411f
Ketamine, 157, 175–176, 176b
   CRI dosage for
      in cats, 158t
      in dogs, 159t
   dose for, 157
Kidney, 383
Kidney disease, 383–385
Kidney failure, 383–385. see also Acute kidney injury (AKI); Chronic kidney failure (CKF)

L

Lactate, levels of, in gastric dilation and volvulus, 344
Lactate concentration, 27–28
   equipment for, 27
   indications for, 27, 27b

Lactate concentration (Continued)
   interpretation of results, 27–28
   shock and, 228
   technique for, 27
   troubleshooting for, 27
Lactate POC analyzer, manufacturers of equipment, 41
Lactic acidosis, 228
Laryngeal paralysis, 328
Latanoprost, 408, 411–412
Laundry, in infection control, 195, 196f
Lead, in toxicologic emergencies, 449–450
Lead ingestion, in avian emergencies, 463–464
Lectins, 439
Left atrium/aortic root ratio, heart disease and, 301–302
Left ventricular chamber measured during diastole (LVIDd), 300
   increasing, 302
Left ventricular chamber measured during systole (LVIDs), 300
   increasing, 302
Lens, ocular emergencies of, 411–412
Less toxic environmental toxins, in toxicologic emergencies, 447
Less toxic/nontoxic plants, in toxicologic emergencies, 439
Leukoreduction, 96
Level of severity, 216
Lidocaine, 157, 172, 178, 309–310
   in advanced life support, 240–241
   CRI dosage for
      in cats, 158t
      in dogs, 159t
   dose for, 157
Life threatening, approach for, in emergency receiving, 214
Lilies, in toxicologic emergencies, 437–438
Lily toxicosis, 437
Lipemia, 15–16, 15f, 16b
Lipemic serum, 15–16, 16b
Lipids, for toxicologic emergencies, 436–437
Liquid plasma (LP), 81
Lizards
   catheterization site in, 482t
   IV catheter placement in, 482
   restraint for, 478–479, 478b
   venipuncture for, 479f, 480
Local anesthesia, 172
Local infiltration, 155
Local/regional anesthetics, 154
   for NE tube placement, 111–112
Low-output failure, of heart, 303–304
LP. see Liquid plasma (LP)
Luer-Lock injection cap, 24
Lymphoma, hypercalcemia and, 362

M

Macrocytic anemia, 287–288
Macrovascular thrombosis, 275
Mainstream sensors, in capnometry, 182–183
Malignancy, hypercalcemia of, 362

Malignant hyperthermia, anesthesia and, 184t–188t
Malnutrition
  indicators of, 107
  severe, 107–110
Mannitol, 408, 411–412, 428
Maropitant, for gastrointestinal emergencies, 337–338
Maropitant citrate, 422
Masimo pulse oximeter, 31f
Mask oxygen, 126–127, 127t
Mastitis, 398, 398b
Maximal sterile barrier, 53
MBD. see Metabolic bone disease (MBD)
Mean cell volume (MCV), 287–288
Measured osmolality, 68
Mechanical ventilation, 135–145
  conditions requiring, 138b
  criteria for, 138
  indications for, 137–138, 137t
  maintenance of patient on, 140–142, 141b, 142f
  monitoring in, 140, 140b
  nursing considerations for, 140–142
  placing patient on, 138–139, 139f, 139b
  references for, 143
  strategies according to disease type, 138, 138b
  summary of, 143
  troubleshooting in, 142
Medetomidine, 155, 175
  CRI dosage for
    in cats, 158t
    in dogs, 159t
Medications, administered via E tube, 112
Meibomian gland abscess, 409
Melanosis, 408
Melatonin supplements, 512
Mentation, shock and, 226, 226t
Metabolic bone disease (MBD), in reptile emergencies, 484–485, 484f–485f
Metabolic/endocrine emergencies, 351–372
Metabolic rate, associated with temperature, 14
Metal ingestion, in avian emergencies, 463–464, 464b
Metaldehyde, in toxicologic emergencies, 442–443
Metals, in toxicologic emergencies, 448–450
Methadone, 172
  CRI dosage for
    in cats, 158t
    in dogs, 159t
Methemoglobin, 285
Methemoglobinemia, 285
Methylxanthines, in toxicologic emergencies, 440
Metoclopramide, 422
  for gastrointestinal emergencies, 337–338
Mice
  physiologic values of, 466t
  restraint for, 470
  venipuncture for, 471
Microenteral nutrition, gastrointestinal emergencies and, 339

Microvascular thrombosis, 275
Micturition, 374
Midazolam, 175
MIND scheme, 418f
Mindray multiparameter monitor, 41f
Mineralocorticoids (aldosterone), 357, 360
Minute volume (MV), 137
Missouri Task Force One, during 9/11, 496f
Mixed agonist, antagonist opioids and, 153–154
"Mixed signals," 518
M-mode echocardiography, 300
  normal measurements in, 301t
Modified Glasgow coma scoring scale, 216, 217f–218f
Mold, in toxicologic emergencies, 441
Mole, unit, 68
Monitoring, record keeping and, 9–13
Monitoring equipment
  for anesthesia, 170b
  in intensive care unit, 32
  for traumatic emergencies, 249
Moraxella spp., in rabbit and rodent emergencies, 475
Morphine, 156
  CRI dosage for
    in cats, 158t
    in dogs, 159t
  dose for, 156
Morphine sulfate, 153
Mouse. see Mice
Mouth care, in ventilator patient maintenance, 141, 142f
Mucous membrane(s)
  brick red, 13f
  color of, shock and, 226, 226t
  moisture, 64
  pale, 13f
Multi-lumen catheter, 44–45, 45f
  jugular, 55
Multifocal ventricular premature contractions, anesthesia and, 184t–188t
Multifunction monitors, manufacturers of equipment, 41
Multiparameter monitoring equipment, 40–41
Musculoskeletal system, injury to, 266–267
  assessment of, 266
  management of, 266–267
  monitoring of, 267
Muzzles, for safety, in traumatic emergencies, 252–253
MV. see Minute volume (MV)
Mycoplasma haemofelis, 89
Mycoplasma haemominutum, 89
Mycotoxins, in avian emergencies, 463
Myelophthisis, 284

N

Nasal cannula, 127t, 129, 129f
Nasal "prongs." see Nasal cannula
Nasoesophageal (NE) tube, 111–112, 111t
  disadvantages of, 111–112

Nasogastric tube, 339
  in surgery, 341
  for vomiting, 333
Naso-oxygen catheter, 127t, 129–130, 130f
  placement of, 131b
Nasopharyngeal polyps, 421–422
Natural colloids, 26
NE tube. see Nasoesophageal (NE) tube
Near drowning, in disaster medicine, 495
Negative airflow system, in isolation unit, 203
Neonatal isoerythrolysis, 90
Neonates
  care of, 397
  postoperative, 396
Neonates challenge
  with intravenous catheter, 57
  restraint for, 57, 57f
Neuroanatomic diagnosis, 415
Neuroanatomy, components of, 415t
Neuroleptanalgesia, 175
Neurologic emergencies, 414–430
Neurologic examination, 415
  components of, 415t
Neurologic injuries, in disaster medicine, 494
Neuromuscular blocking agents, 176–177
  monitoring with, 177, 177b
Nicotine ingestion, in avian emergencies, 463
Night shift, art of scheduling and, 510, 513
  after shift, 513
9/11 terrorist attack, 488–489, 489f
  Missouri Task Force One during, 496f
Nociception, loss of, 422
Nociceptors, 148
Noncardiogenic (neurogenic) pulmonary edema, 418
Nondepolarizing neuromuscular blocking agents, 177, 177b
Nonpharmacologic interventions, for pain, 149–150, 150f–151f
Nonregenerative anemia, 285
Nonsteroidal antiinflammatory drugs (NSAIDs), 152
  gastrointestinal emergencies and, 338–339
  in toxicologic emergencies, 448
Nonurgent, approach for, in emergency receiving, 214
Nonverbal communication, 517–518, 518f
Norepinephrine, hypovolemic shock and, 225
Noticing, as concept, 5
NSAIDs. see Nonsteroidal antiinflammatory drugs (NSAIDS)
Nuclear sclerosis, 412
Nursing care, 3
Nutrition. see also Enteral nutrition; Parenteral nutrition (PN); Total parenteral nutrition (TPN)
  assessment of, 107, 108f–109f
  plan, 110
  requirements, calculation of, 110
  trauma and, 262–263
Nutritional support
  for acute kidney injury, 386
  for chronic kidney failure, 387

Nutritional support (Continued)
  for critically ill patient, 106–122
  duration of, 110
  enteral, 110–117
  goals of, 107–120
  parenteral, 117–118
  products listed for, 120
  suggested readings for, 120
  summary of, 120
  veterinary technician's role in, 110

O

Observation skill, 1–8
Obstructive shock, 224
Ocular disease, breed predisposition
    for, 405t
Ocular emergencies, 404–413, 404b
  of anterior chamber, 411
  of cornea, 410–411
  of eyelid, 409
  of globe, 407–409
  of lens, 411–412
  ophthalmic drugs for, 406t–407t
Ocular exposure, 495
  in toxicologic emergencies, 434
Oliguria, fluids for, 72t
Omeprazole, for gastrointestinal emergencies,
    338
Onions, in toxicologic emergencies,
    439–440
Open abdominal drainage
  complications of, 348
  for peritonitis, 347, 348f
Open-ended questions, 519
Open posture, 517–518
Ophthaine, 409
Opioids, 152–153, 171–172
  for spinal cord injury, 425
Optimal shift, for employees, 510–512
Optimmune ophthalmic ointment, 410
Oral, routes of administration, 63t
Oral exposure, 495
Orchitis, 401
Organophosphates, in toxicologic
    emergencies, 442
Orthopedic injuries, in disaster medicine,
    494
Orthopnea, 320, 320f
Oscillometric devices, 34, 181
Osmolality, fluid therapy and, 68
Osmole, unit, 68
Osmometer, manufacturers of equipment,
    41
Otitis interna, 421–422
Otitis media, 421–422
Ovarian cycle, four phases of, 391–392
Over-the-needle catheter unit
  intravenous catheter, 44
  placement technique, 54b
Overlapping shifts, 511
Overnight shift, 511, 511b
Owner, in disaster medicine, 493, 493b

Oxygen
  cage, 127–129, 127t, 128f
  content, equation for, 224, 224f
  delivery (DO_2), 126–132, 127t, 280–281, 281b
    determinants of, 224f
    flow-by, 126, 127f, 127t
    mask, 126–127, 127t
    nasal cannula, 127t, 129, 129f
    naso-oxygen catheter, 127t, 129–130,
        130f, 131b
    shock and, 224
    therapy to improve, 231b
    transtracheal catheter, 130–131, 131f–
        132f, 131b
  flow rate of, 126
  hood, 127–129, 127t, 128f
  levels, assessment of, 124–126, 124b
  need for, assessment of, 124
  saturation, shock and, 231
  therapy
    conclusion of, 132
    equipment for, 127t
    for heart failure, 306–307, 306b
    hyperbaric, 131–132
    for shock, 228–229
    for smoke inhalation, 327–328
    suggested readings for, 133
    techniques of, 123–134, 124b
  toxicity, 132, 132b
Oxygen extraction ratio (OER or O_2ER), 281
Oxygen hood, 127–129, 127t, 128f
Oxygen saturation, decreased, anesthesia and,
    184t–188t
Oxygenation, 226
  monitoring of, anesthesia and, 181–182
  in traumatic emergencies, 257
Oxyglobin®, 102
Oxyhemoglobin, 125b
Oxyhemoglobin dissociation curve, 124,
    125b, 126f
Oxymorphone, 153, 172

P

P/F ratio, 124
Pacemaker therapy, for cardiac arrhythmias,
    311–312, 313f
Packed cell volume (PCV), 16–17, 323
  fluid therapy for, 65
  total plasma protein measurements and,
      16–17, 17b
    equipment for, 16
    general guidelines for, 17, 17b
    indications for, 16
    interpretation of, 17
    technique for, 16
    troubleshooting for, 16–17
Packed red blood cells (PRBCs), 80, 80b,
    84t–85t
Pain
  analgesic drugs for, 150–152
  assessment of, 148–149
  beliefs on, 146

Pain (Continued)
  breed variations in, 147
  deleterious physiologic effects of, 149
  drug options for, 152–153
  epidural anesthesia and analgesia for, 160,
      160f
  indicators of, 148
  local and regional anesthetics for, 154
  management of, 147, 160–163
  nonpharmacologic interventions for,
      149–150, 150f–151f
  patient questions on, 150
  physiology of, 148
  reasons to withhold analgesia for, 149
  recognition of, 148–149
  relief for, 149–153
  suggested readings for, 163
  treatment of, 149, 149f
Pain management
  checklist for, 160–163
  drug effect monitoring in, 160
Pain scales, 161f–162f
Pale mucous membrane, 3f
Palpation, 14
Pancreatitis, 346–347
  clinical signs of, 346
  diagnosis of, 346–347
  history of, 346
  pathophysiology of, 346
  treatment of, 347
Pannus, 411
Panophthalmitis, 408, 408f
Pantoprazole, for gastrointestinal
    emergencies, 338
Paraphimosis, 401, 401b
Paraverbal communication, 517–518
Parenteral calcium, for hypocalcemia, 367t
Parenteral nutrition (PN), 117–118, 118f, 119b
  complications of, 119
  gastrointestinal emergencies and, 339–340
  indications for, 117
  solutions for, 118
Partial parenteral nutrition (PPN), 117
Partial pressure of carbon dioxide (PCO_2), 24–25
Partial pressure of oxygen (PaO_2), 24–25,
    124, 281
Partial seizures, 416
Partial thromboplastin time (aPTT), 323
Parturition, stages of, 392–393, 392f, 392b
Pasteurella multocida, in rabbit and rodent
    emergencies, 475
Patent ductus arteriosus (PDA), emergencies
    associated with, 295t
Patient assessment
  in emergency receiving, 212
  of fluid therapy, 63–66
  in traumatic emergencies, 253–256
    diagnostic tests for, 255–256, 255f
    history in, 254–255
    initial database in, 254
    primary and secondary survey in, 253–254
    scoring systems in, 256, 256t
    triage in, 253, 253b

Patient positioning, anesthetic plan and, 169
Peak inspiratory pressure (PIP), 137
Peel-away sheath technique, 48b–49b
PEEP. *see* Positive end-expiratory pressure (PEEP)
PEG tube. *see* Percutaneous endoscopically placed gastrostomy (PEG) tube
Penetrating trauma, 263
Penile trauma, 402
Pentastarch, 72
Perceived wait time, 519
Percussion, method and interpretation of, 254b
Percutaneous endoscopically placed gastrostomy (PEG) tube, 111t, 112–116, 116f
Perfusion parameters, shock and, 226, 226t
Pericardial disease, emergencies associated with, 295t
Pericardial effusion
    cardiac tamponade and, 314–315
    client complaints in, 314–315
    clinical signs, 315
    diagnostic imaging and electrocardiogram of, 315
    monitoring of, 315
    treatment of, 315
Pericardiocentesis, for cardiac tamponade and pericardial effusion, 315
Peripheral catheters, 54–55
Peripheral edema, 58
Peripheral nerve stimulators, 177
Peripheral nervous system emergencies, 426–427
    diagnostic procedures of, 426–427
    treatment plans of, 426–427
Peripheral vestibular disorders, and central vestibular disorders, 421t
Peripherally inserted central catheters (PICCs), 46
Peritoneal dialysis, for chronic kidney failure, 387–388
Peritoneal space, analgesia injection in, 155
Peritonitis, 337, 337b, 347–348
    clinical signs of, 347
    diagnosis of, 347
    history of, 347
    treatment of, 347–348
Perivascular injection, anesthesia and, 184t–188t
Permethrins, in toxicologic emergencies, 441–442
Peroxygen, as disinfectants, 199t–200t
Personal protective equipment (PPE), 195–197, 197f, 197b
Pesticides, in toxicologic emergencies, 441–443
Petechia, 18f
PETS Act, 488–489
Pharmaceuticals, in toxicologic emergencies, 447–448
Pharmacokinetics, 147
Pharmacology, 432

Phenobarbital, 420
Phenols, as disinfectants, 199t–200t
Phenothiazines, 174
    for gastrointestinal emergencies, 337–338
Phenylephrine, 409
Phosphate enemas (Fleet® enemas), 365–366
Phosphofructokinase deficiency, 283
Physical exam, of fluid therapy, 63–64, 64f
Physical examination
    for avian emergencies, 455–462, 455f–456f, 455b
    for exotic small mammal emergencies, 465–468, 465b, 466t
    preanesthetic, 167
    for reptile emergencies, 476–484, 476b, 477f
PICCs. *see* Peripherally inserted central catheters (PICCs)
Piezoelectric crystal, 33
PIP. *see* Peak inspiratory pressure (PIP)
Placenta, drugs cross in, 395–396
Plants, in toxicologic emergencies, 437–439
Plasma
    components of, 80–82
    fresh frozen, 81
    frozen, 81, 84t–85t
    liquid, 81
Plasma proteins, lack of, 26
Plasma thromboplastin antecedent, 270t
Platelet(s), 83
    activation of, 270
    adhesion of, 270
    concentrate solutions, 83, 84t–85t
    hyper-reactivity of, 275
Platelet count, 277
    for anemia, 288
Platelet-rich plasma (PRP), 83, 84t–85t
Platelet transfusion, 273
    indications for, 273
Pleth variability index (PVI), 182
Plethysmography, 182, 182f
Pleural space
    analgesia injection in, 155
    conditions in, 326–327
PN. *see* Parenteral nutrition (PN)
Pneumonia, 329–331
    aspiration, 330–331
    bacterial, 329–330
    fungal, 330
    viral, 330
Pneumothorax, 326
Poinsettia plants, in toxicologic emergencies, 439
Point of care (POC) testing, 18
    manufacturers of equipment, 41
    quality control for, 20–21
Point of maximum intensity (PMI), of murmurs, 296
Polyradiculoneuritis, 426
Polyuria, 22
    fluids for, 72t
Poor husbandry, 452
Positive end-expiratory pressure (PEEP), 137

Positive inotropic therapy, for heart failure, 307
    monitoring for, 308
Positive pressure ventilation, in preanesthetic stabilization, 168
Post-cardiac arrest care, 244–245, 244b
Postresuscitation care, trauma and, 262
Posttraumatic stress disorder (PTSD), 493b
Potassium supplementation recommendations, for DKA, 354, 355t
Povidone iodine, as disinfectants, 199t–200t
PPE. *see* Personal protective equipment (PPE)
PPN. *see* Partial parenteral nutrition (PPN)
PRBCs. *see* Packed red blood cells (PRBCs)
Preanesthetic agents, 171–176
Preanesthetic exam, 167b
Preanesthetic preparedness, 169–170
Preanesthetic stabilization, 168–169, 168b
Precordial thumps, 243
    in treatment of arrhythmias, 312
Prednisolone sodium succinate, 360t
Preload, 302
Pressure gradient
    for pulmonary hypertension, 300t
    for semilunar valve stenosis, 300t
Primary hemostasis, 29b, 270
    disorders of, 272–274
Primary survey, for traumatic emergencies, 253–254
Proaccelerin, 270t
Procainamide, 309–310
ProcalAmine (McGraw), 118, 119b
Proconvertin, 270t
Proestrus, 391–392
Projectile vomiting, 333
Propofol, 176
Proprioceptive ataxia, 422
Proptosis, 408, 408f
N-propyl disulfide, 283
Prostate, enlarged, 400f
Prostate cancer, 400
Prostate disorders, 400–401
Prostate-specific antigen (PSA), 400
Prostatic abscesses, 400
Prostatic cysts, 400
Prostatitis, acute bacterial, 401
Protein C, deficiency of, 275
Prothrombin, 270t
Prothrombin time (PT), 279, 279f, 323
PRP. *see* Platelet-rich plasma (PRP)
PT. *see* Prothrombin time
Pulmonary contusions, 327
Pulmonary edema, 76, 76f, 329
    cardiogenic, 329
    noncardiogenic, 329
    treatment for, 305–306
Pulmonary effusion, 76, 76f
Pulmonic stenosis, emergencies associated with, 295t
Pulse oximeter, 124, 124b
Pulse oximeter probe, 31f

Pulse oximetry, 30–32, 181–183
    equipment for, 31
    indications for, 31
    interpretation for, 32
    technique for, 31
    troubleshooting for, 31–32
Pulse quality, shock and, 226t, 227
Pulse rate, fluid therapy and, 64
Pulseless electrical activity, 243, 243f, 243b
Pulseless rhythm, electrocardiogram of, 243f
Pure (full) agonists, 153
Pyloric obstruction, fluids for, 72t
Pyometra, 398–399, 399f
    diagnosis of, 399
    signs of, 399
Pyrethrins, in toxicologic emergencies, 441
Pyrethroids, in toxicologic emergencies, 441–442
Pyruvate kinase deficiency, 283

Q

Quaternary ammonium compounds, as disinfectants, 199t–200t

R

Rabbit
    intravenous catheterization site in, 467t
    physiologic values of, 466t
Rabbit/rodent emergencies, 469–474
    abscesses and, 475
    bacterial enteritis in, 474–475
    Bordetella bronchiseptica in, 475
    catheter placement for, 471–472, 471b–472b, 472f
    common, 474–476
    cystic calculi in, 475
    cystitis in, 475
    dental disease and, 474–476, 474f
    GI stasis in, 474
    hairballs in, 474
    Moraxella spp. in, 475
    Pasteurella multocida in, 475
    respiratory tract infections in, 475
    restraint for, 469, 470f
    supplies for, 465
    uterine adenocarcinoma and, 475–476
    venipuncture for, 470–471
Rabbit V-gel device, 453–454, 453f, 454b
Rabies, 429
    diagnostic procedures of, 429
    treatment plans of, 429
Radiographs, fluid therapy and, 76f
Radiology, for traumatic emergencies, 250–251
Raisins, in toxicologic emergencies, 439
RAP status, 492–493
Rapid intubation sequence, 322–323, 323f
Rat(s)
    physiologic values of, 466t
    restraint for, 470
    venipuncture for, 471

Readiness assessment, 209–210
Record keeping, monitoring and, 9–13
Rectal thermometers, for gastrointestinal emergencies, 335
Red blood cells (RBCs), 17
    canine, red cell shelf life of, 91t
    destruction of, 282–284
    dosing formula, 99b
    loss of, 281–282
    packed, shock and, 230
    trauma to, 102
Red rubber tubes, in crash cart, 249, 249f
Reduced or ineffective erythropoiesis, 284–285
Re-energizing, in emergency receiving, 216–220, 220f
Reference ranges, for hematology analyzers, 19
Referral practices, communication with, 521
Reflection, as concept, 5, 5f
Reflective listening, 519, 521
Refractometer, 16
Refractory anemia, 285
Regional anesthesia, 172
Regurgitation
    anesthesia and, 184t–188t
    vomiting and, 333
Renal disease, 374
Renal failure, in reptile emergencies, 485
Renal transplantation, for chronic kidney failure, 388, 389f
Reproduction system, 391
Reproductive emergencies, 391–403
    in female, 392–400
    in males, 400–402
    in rodents, 476
Reproductive tract
    female, 391
    male, 391
Reptile emergencies, 476–486
    abscesses in, 485
    anesthesia for, 483–484
    dystocia in, 485
    egg binding in, 485
    fluid therapy for, 483
    foreign bodies in, 485, 486f
    injections for, 483
    IV catheter placement for, 482–483, 482t
    MBD in, 484–485, 484f–485f
    physical examination for, 476–484, 476b, 477f
    renal failure in, 485
    restraint for, 478–479
    supplies for, 476
    tube feeding for, 483
    venipuncture for, 480–481
RER. *see* Resting energy requirement (RER)
Respiration, 319
Respiratory emergencies, 319–331, 320f, 321b–322b, 325b
    airway disorders in, 328–329
    continued management in, 325
    patient presentation in, 319–321

Respiratory emergencies *(Continued)*
    pneumonia, 329–331
    preparedness in, 321–322
    primary survey and minimum database, 323
    pulmonary edema and, 329
    rapid intubation sequence in, 322–323, 323f
    secondary survey in, 323–325
    technician's role in, 330–331
    thoracentesis in, 324b
    traumatic conditions in, 325–328
    vascular access in, 322
Respiratory exposure, 495
Respiratory failure, categories of, 137t
Respiratory rate, anesthesia and, 167
Respiratory tract infections, in rabbit and rodent emergencies, 475
Responding, as concept, 5
Resting energy requirement (RER), 110, 119–120
Restraint
    for avian emergencies, 455–458, 455b, 457f
    for ferret emergencies, 466, 466f, 466b
    neonates challenge for, 57, 57f
    for rabbit and rodent emergencies, 469, 470f
    for reptile emergencies, 478–479
Restrictive cardiomyopathy, emergencies associated with, 295t
Resuscitation
    in gastrointestinal emergencies, 335–336, 345
    in traumatic emergencies, 256–259
        fluid administration and, 257–258
        goals of, 256–257
        hemorrhage control and, 258–259, 258f
        oxygenation and, 257
        with severe intraabdominal hemorrhage, 259
        surgical, 260
        ventilation and, 257
Reticulocyte count, anemia and, 287
Reticulocytosis, anemia and, 287
Retrobulbar masses, 408
Reversal agents, in advanced life support, 241
Ricin, 439
Rodenticides
    in toxicologic emergencies, 443–446
    types of, 443
Rolled gauze, 55

S

Safe housing, for hospitalized exotic patients, 453
Safety, for traumatic emergencies, 252–253
Saline agglutination test, for anemia, 288
SART. *see* State Animal Response Team (SART)
SAVE method, for triaging, 493
SBAR (S, situation; B, background; A, assessment; R, recommendation), 6, 6b

Schiff-Sherrington syndrome, 425
Scoring systems, for trauma, 256, 256t
Scrotal disorders, 401–402
Scrotal neoplasia, 401–402
Search and rescue canines, 490
  decontamination of, 497–498, 498f, 498b
  in disaster medicine, 495–498, 495b, 496f
  stray animals and, 496–497, 497b
Secondary hemostasis, 29–30, 270
  disorders of, 274–275
Secondary hypoadrenocorticism, 356
Secondary survey, for traumatic emergencies, 253–254
Sedation, in respiratory emergency, 322, 322b
  for cats, 322
Seizures, 415–420
  causes of, 415, 418f
  classification of, 415–416
  conditions easily mistaken for, 417b
  definition of, 416
  descriptors of, 416t
  diagnostic procedures of, 417–420, 419b–420b
  episodic disorders, 416
  focal, 416
  generalized, 416
  identification of, 417
  partial, 416
  treatment plans of, 417–420, 419b–420b
  types of, 416
Seldinger technique, 47–54, 50b–52b
Sepsis, distributive shock from, 225
Serotonin antagonists, for gastrointestinal emergencies, 337–338
Sertoli cell tumor, 401–402
Severe hypotension, anesthesia and, 184t–188t
Sevoflurane, 176
Shared mental model, 4
Shift work, 508
Shift work maladaptive syndrome (SMS), 508
Shifts, length of, 511–512, 512b
Shock
  arterial blood pressure and, 231
  arterial pH and, 232
  blood gases and, 232
  cardiogenic, 224
  central venous pressure and, 231–232
  colloid osmotic pressure and, 232
  definition of, 223
  in disaster medicine, 494
  distributive, 224
  electrocardiogram and, 231
  electrolytes and, 232
  hematocrit and, 232
  hypovolemic, 224
  initial assessment of, 226–228
  laboratory parameters of, 232
  lactate concentration and, 228
  management of, 223–233
  monitoring of, 231–232
  obstructive, 224
  oxygen delivery and, 224

Shock (Continued)
  oxygen saturation and, 231
  pathophysiology of, 224–225
  physical assessment of, 226–228, 226t, 228b
  physiologic monitoring parameters of, 231–232
  recognition of, 226–228
  therapy for, 228–231
  total protein and, 232
  types of, 224, 224b
  urinary output and, 232
  vasomotor tone and, 227–228, 228t
  venous access and, 229, 229f, 229t
Shock index, 228
Sick sinus syndrome, 311, 313f
Sidestream monitors, in capnometry, 182–183
Siemens RAPIDlab blood gas analyzer, 22f
Sight, heart disease and, 294–295
Signalment, heart disease and, 294
Simple blood gas analysis, 25
Sinus arrest, anesthesia and, 184t–188t
Sinus rhythm, 296
Skin tent, fluid therapy and, 64
Skin turgor, fluid therapy and, 64
Sleep deprivation, art of scheduling and, 510, 510b
Sleep-deprived people, 510
Sleeping pills, 512
Slide method, of blood crossmatch, 97, 98b
Small human blood ketone meters, 356
Small rodents, intravenous catheterization site in, 467t
Smoke, in disaster medicine, 494–495
Smoke inhalation, 327–328
Snail/slug killers, in toxicologic emergencies, 442–443
Snake emergencies, 484
Snakes
  catheterization site in, 482t
  IV catheter placement in, 482
  restraint for, 478, 478b
  venipuncture for, 480
Sodium bicarbonate, in advanced life support, 241
Sodium sulfate, as cathartic, 449–450
Soft tissue injuries, in disaster medicine, 494
Sound, heart disease and, 295
Spastic paresis, 425
Spermatic cord torsions, 401
Spinal cord injury, 422–426
  causes of, 422–423
  clinical signs of, 423b
  diagnostic procedures of, 425–426
  neurologic findings with, 423f
  treatment plans of, 425–426
Spinal shock, 425
Spinosad, 443
Splints, in traumatic emergencies, 259–260, 260f
Spun capillary tubes, 16
Stabilization, preanesthetic, 168–169

START method
  color code system for, 493t
  for triaging, 492–493
State Animal Response Team (SART), 500–501
Status epilepticus, 417
Sterile adhesive bandage, 55
Sterile gauze pad, 55
Sterile prep, complete, 47, 47f, 53
Steroids, for head trauma, 429
Stranguria, 375
Stray animals, search and rescue canines and, 496–497, 497b
Stress, trauma-induced, 218
Stroke volume, 224
Struvite, 382
Stuart factor, 270t
Subaortic stenosis, emergencies associated with, 295t
Subcutaneous, routes of administration, 63t
Succinylcholine, 177
Sucking chest wound, 327
Suction canister, in surgery set up, 170
Suction equipment, for traumatic emergencies, 249–250
Suctioning, gastrointestinal emergencies and, 339
Sulfhemoglobin, 285
Supraventricular tachycardia
  anesthesia and, 184t–188t
  treatment of, 310, 311f
    drugs used in, 311t
Surgery
  for disaster medicine, 498
  in gastrointestinal emergencies, 340–341
  for gastrointestinal foreign bodies, 343
  set up, anesthesia and, 170, 170b
  for traumatic emergencies, 251, 251b
  urologic emergencies, 374, 374b
Surgical resuscitation, 260
Symblepharon, 409
Sympathomimetics, 230–231
Synthetic colloids, 71, 73f, 229–230
  doses of, 71t
Synthetic crystalloids, doses, 71t
Syringe feeding techniques, 111
  for rabbit and rodent emergencies, 473–474, 473b–474b
Systemic inflammatory response syndrome, gastrointestinal emergencies and, 336
Systolic dysfunction, causes of, 225
Systolic function, 302

T

Tachycardia
  anesthesia and, 166, 184t–188t
  circulatory shock and, 227
Tachypnea, 307
TACO. see Transfusion-associated circulatory overload (TACO)
Tacrolimus, 410
Tanner's clinical judgment model, 5

Technician, role of
  in gastrointestinal emergencies, 333b
  in respiratory emergency, 330–331
Telephone calls, 516–517, 516f
Temperature
  anesthesia and
    conservation of, 183, 183f
    monitoring of, 180–181
  metabolic rate, associated with, 14, 14b
Terrorism, 490
Test tube crossmatch, 97, 98b
Testicular disorders, 401–402
Tetralogy of Fallot, emergencies associated
    with, 295t
Thalamocortex, four neurologic tests for, 416b
The Joint Commission (TJC) analysis, 5
Theobromine, in toxicologic emergencies, 440
Thermometers, rectal, for gastrointestinal
    emergencies, 335
Third-space losses, 22b
  fluid therapy, 66b
Thoracentesis, 324b
  for pneumothorax, 326, 326f
Thoracic expansion, lack of, anesthesia and,
    184t–188t
Thoracic pump mechanism, of blood flow, 237
Thoracic radiographs
  for heart disease, 296–298
  in preanesthetic exam, 168, 168b
Thrombin, 271
Thrombin clotting time, 280
Thrombocytopenia, 272
Thromboelastography, 280, 280f
Thrombopathia, 272–273
Thrombosis, 275
  in disseminated intravascular coagulation,
    276
Through-the-needle catheter unit
  intravenous catheter, 44, 52b–53b
  jugular, 55–56
  placement technique, 47–54
Tick paralysis, 426
  diagnostic confirmation of, 427
Tick titers, for anemia, 288
Tidal volume (TV), 136
Tier 1 patients, in biosecurity, 193
Tier 2 patients, in biosecurity, 193
Tier 3 patients, in biosecurity, 193–194
Tier 4 patients, in biosecurity, 194
Tissue dilator, 45
Tissue factor, 270t
Tissue factor pathway inhibitor (TFPI),
    deficiencies in, 275
Tongue clips, in pulse oximetry, 181–182
Topical analgesia, 154
Topical exposure, in toxicologic emergencies,
    434
Tornadoes, disaster medicine and, 492
Total parenteral nutrition (TPN), 117
Total plasma protein measurements, packed
    cell volume and, 16–17, 17b
  equipment for, 16
  general guidelines for, 17, 17b

Total plasma protein measurements, packed
    cell volume and (Continued)
  indications for, 16
  interpretation for, 17
  technique for, 16
  troubleshooting for, 16–17
Total protein, shock and, 232
Total solids (TSs), 323
Touch, heart disease and, 295
Toxicologic emergencies, 431–451
  absorption prevention in, 433–435
  acetaminophen in, 447–448
  activated charcoal for, 436
  antidotes for, 436, 436t
  antiparasitics in, 441–443
  with bromethalin, 444–445
  caffeine in, 440
  cathartic for, 436
  chocolate in, 440
  with cholecalciferol, 445
  emesis for, 434
  enhanced elimination techniques for, 436
  environmental toxins in, 446–447
  ethylene glycol in, 446–447
  foods in, 439–441
  garbage toxicity in, 441
  gastrotomy for, 435
  ingested toxins in, 434–435
  insecticide in, 432
  ion trapping for, 436
  lipids for, 436–437
  metals in, 448–450
  methylxanthines in, 440
  ocular exposure in, 434
  organophosphates in, 442
  permethrins in, 441–442
  pesticides in, 441–443
  pharmaceuticals in, 447–448
  phone advice for, 433b
  plants in, 437–439
  pyrethroids in, 441–442
  rodenticides in, 443–446
  snail or slug killers in, 442–443
  supportive care for, 437
  theobromine in, 440
  topical exposure in, 434
  toxicity types of, 437–446
  treatment for, 433
  zinc phosphide in, 445–446
Toxicology, 432
  in veterinary hospital, 450
Toxins, 431, 436t
  ingested, in avian emergencies, 463–464
  inhaled, in avian emergencies, 464, 464b
TPN. see Total parenteral nutrition (TPN)
Tracheostomy tube placement, 324b
TRALI. see Transfusion-related acute lung
    injury (TRALI)
Transcutaneous pacing, 313f
Transfusion, for anemia, 289
Transfusion-associated circulatory overload
    (TACO), 101
Transfusion complication, 101

Transfusion medicine, 78–105
Transfusion reactions, 90, 100–102, 100f, 102b
Transfusion-related acute lung injury
    (TRALI), 101
Transfusion-related immunomodulation
    (TRIM), 101
Transfusion therapy, 84t–85t
  administration rates and, 99–100
  administration routes and, 99
  administration volume and, 99, 99b
  blood filters in, 100
  methods of, 100
  references and further readings for, 103
Transtracheal oxygen catheter, 130–131,
    131f–132f, 131b
Transvenous pacing lead, 311–312, 313f
Trauma patient scoring scale, 216, 217f–218f
Trauma-induced stress, 218
Traumatic conditions, respiratory
    emergencies and, 325–328
  laryngeal, 326
  tracheal, 326
Traumatic emergencies, 247–268, 248b
  advanced monitoring for, 261–262
  analgesia, 259, 259b
  assessment of, 263–267
  autotransfusion for, 250, 250f
  basic monitoring in, 260–261
  communication with owner and, 263,
    263b
  crash cart for, 248–249, 249f
  first aid and safety for, 252–253
  fluid administration in, 257–258
  head and facial, 264
  hemorrhage control in, 258–259, 258f
  intravenous fluids for, 250
  introduction to, 248
  laboratory equipment for, 251
  management of, 263–267
  measured parameters for, 261t
  oxygenation in, 257
  patient assessment in, 253–256
    diagnostic tests for, 255–256, 255f
    history in, 254–255
    initial database in, 254
    primary and secondary survey in,
      253–254
    scoring systems in, 256, 256t
    triage in, 253, 253b
  postresuscitation care in, 262
  primary survey for, 253–254
  protocols for, 252
  radiology for, 250–251
  readiness for, 248–253
  responsibilities of veterinary technician
    in, 248b
  resuscitation in, 256–259
  secondary survey for, 253–254
  suction equipment for, 249–250
  surgery for, 251, 251b
  triad of death in, 256
  triage for, 253, 253b
  ultrasound for, 250–251

Traumatic emergencies (Continued)
  ventilation in, 257
  veterinary team in, 252
  warming devices for, 251–252
Treatment area, of emergency receiving, 210–211, 211f–212f
Treatment sheets, 3
Tremorgenic mycotoxins, 441
Triage
  in disaster medicine, 492–493, 492b
  in emergency receiving scenarios, 212, 215f
  SAVE method for, 493
  START method for, 492–493
  for traumatic emergencies, 253, 253b
Tricuspid dysplasia, emergencies associated with, 295t
TRIM. see Transfusion-related immunomodulation (TRIM)
Troponin, heart disease and, 293–294
Tube feeding
  for avian emergencies, 460–461, 460b, 461f
  for reptile emergencies, 483
Tube welders, 91
Turgid bladder, 380
TV. see Tidal volume (TV)
T waves, tall, in preanesthetic exam, 168, 168f
Two-dimensional echocardiography, 300

U

Ulcer(s)
  collagenase, 410
  corneal, 410, 410f
  prophylaxis of, gastrointestinal emergencies and, 338
  viral, 410, 411f
Ultrasound, for traumatic emergencies, 250–251
Urethral catheterization, in ferret emergencies, 468, 468b
Urethral prolapse, 402, 402b
Urgent, approach for, in emergency receiving, 214
Urinalysis, for anemia, 288
Urinary calculi, 374
Urinary obstruction, 374–383
  cats with, 374–379
  contrast medium for, 380, 380f
  in dog, 379–383
  ultrasound depiction of, 374, 374f
Urinary output, shock and, 232
Urine, volume and specific gravity of, 21–22
  equipment for, 21–22
  indications for, 21
  interpretation for, 22
  technique for, 22, 22b
Urine concentration, in diabetic ketoacidosis, 356
Urine production, fluid therapy and, 66
Urohydropropulsion, blocked dog and, 381–382
Uroliths, 380
Urologic emergencies, 373–390
  etiology of, 373
  surgery, 374, 374b

Uterine adenocarcinoma, rabbit and rodent emergencies and, 475–476
Uterine prolapse, 397–398, 397f–398f
Uterine torsions, 399–400
Uveitis, 411

V

Vaginal prolapse, 397–398, 398f
VAP. see Ventilator-associated pneumonia (VAP)
Vascular access, in respiratory emergencies, 322
Vascular access points, intravenous catheter, 45–46
Vascular access ports, intravenous catheter, 45, 45f
Vasoconstriction, 270
  pulse quality and, 227
Vasodilator therapy, for heart failure, 307
  monitoring for, 307–308
Vasodilatory shock, 228
Vasomotor tone, shock and, 227–228, 228t
Vasopressin, in advanced life support, 240
Vector-borne transmission, of disease, 193
Venipuncture
  for anemia, 289
  for avian emergencies, 457–459, 458f, 458b
  for ferret emergencies, 466–467, 467f
  for rabbit and rodent emergencies, 470–471
  for reptile emergencies, 480–481
Venous access
  emergency supplies and, 236b
  shock and, 229, 229f, 229t
Venous blood gas, in preanesthetic exam, 168
Ventilation
  anesthesia and, 171–172
  in basic life support, 239, 239b
  controlled, 179, 179f
  in patient recovery, from anesthesia, 189
  in traumatic emergencies, 257
  weaning of, 143
Ventilator-associated pneumonia (VAP), 141
Ventricular arrhythmias, drugs used to treat, 310t
Ventricular fibrillation, 243, 244f, 244b
Ventricular septal defect, emergencies associated with, 295t
Ventricular tachycardia
  anesthesia and, 184t–188t
  gastric dilation and volvulus, 344–345, 344f
  treatment of, 309–310, 310f
Vertebra, transverse section of, 424f
Vertebral canal, sagittal section of, 424f
Vertebral heart scale (VHS), 296
  landmarks for measurement of
    in cats, 299f
    in dogs, 299f
  normal range for, 299t
  ranges of severity of, 299t
Vestibular disorders, 420–422
  diagnostic procedures of, 422
  treatment plans of, 422

Vestibular syndromes, 420–421
Veterinary Emergency and Critical Care Society (VECCS), 210
Veterinary field hospital, 490f
Veterinary hospital, toxicology in, 450
Veterinary Information Network, 20
Veterinary technician(s), 414
  in J tube placement, 111
  in nutritional support, 110
Viral pneumonia, 330
Viral ulcers, 410, 411f
Vitamin D, for hypocalcemia, 367t
Vitamin K, 274
Vitamin K antagonism, 274
  protein induced by, 279
Volume overload, 74–77
Voluven, 72
Vomiting, 333
  anesthesia and, 184t–188t
  assessment of, 334b
  projectile, 333
von Willebrand's disease, 273–274
  canine, 273t
von Willebrand's factor (vWF), 270

W

Waiting room, of emergency receiving, 210
Warming devices, for traumatic emergencies, 251–252
Waste disposal, infection control and, 204
Weaning, from ventilator, 143
Weight, evaluation of, anesthesia and, 167
Wellness, 218
Wescor Inc. colloid osmometer, 26f
Whole blood, 79–80
  components of, 79–83
  processing of, 79
  shock and, 230
  stored, 79–80, 84t–85t
Whole bowel irrigation, 435
Wounds
  in disaster medicine, 494
  in traumatic emergencies, 259–260
WSAVA Nutritional Assessment Checklist, 107, 108f–109f

X

Xenotransfusion, 102–103, 103b
Xylazine, 155
Xylazine hydrochloride, 435
Xylitol, in toxicologic emergencies, 440–441

Z

Zinc, in toxicologic emergencies, 448–449
Zinc ingestion, in avian emergencies, 463–464
Zinc phosphide, in toxicologic emergencies, 445–446
Zinc toxicosis, 283–284